Competency Skills for the Dental Assistant

Charline M. Dofka, CDA, RDH, MS

 Delmar Publishers

I(T)P An International Thomson Publishing Company

Albany • Bonn • Boston • Cincinnati • Detroit • London • Madrid • Melbourne
Mexico City • New York • Pacific Grove • Paris • San Francisco • Singapore • Tokyo
Toronto • Washington

WP

NOTICE TO THE READER

Cover Credit: Vincent S. Berger

Publishing Team:

Publisher: David C. Gordon
Acquisitions Editor: Kimberly Davies
Developmental Editor: Jill Rembetski
Editorial Assistant: Donna Leto

Project Editor: Melissa Conan
Production Coordinator: Karen Leet
Art and Design Coordinator: Vincent S. Berger

Copyright © 1996
By Delmar Publishers
A division of International Thomson Publishing Inc.

The ITP logo is a trademark under license

Printed in the United States of America

For more information, contact:

Delmar Publishers
3 Columbia Circle, Box 15015
Albany, New York 12212-5015

International Thomson Publishing Europe
Berkshire House 168-173
High Holborn
London, WC1V7AA
England

Thomas Nelson Australia
102 Dodds Street
South Melbourne, 3205
Victoria, Australia

Nelson Canada
1120 Birchmount Road
Scarborough, Ontario
Canada M1K 5G4

International Thomson Publishing—Japan
Hirakawacho Kyowa Building, 3F
2-2-1 Hirakawacho
Chiyoda-ku, Tokyo 102
Japan

International Thomson Editores
Campos Eliseos 385, Piso 7
Col Polanco
11560 Mexico D F Mexico

International Thomson Publishing GmbH
Königswinterer Strasse 418
53227 Bonn
Germany

International Thomson Publishing Asia
221 Henderson Road
#05-10 Henderson Building
Singapore 0315

1 2 3 4 5 6 7 8 9 10 XXX 01 00 99 98 97 96 95

Library of Congress Cataloging-in-Publication Data
Dofka, Charline M.
    Competency skills for the dental assistant / Charline M. Dofka.
      p. cm.
    Includes index.
    ISBN 0-8273-6685-X
    1. Dental assistants. 2. Dentistry. I. Title.
    [DNLM: 1. Dental Assistants 2. Clinical Competence. WU 90
D653s   1996]
RK60.5.D64   1996
617.6'0233—dc20
DNLM/DLC
for Library of Congress

94-24642
CIP

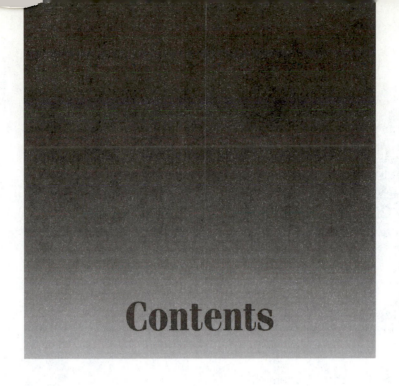

Contents

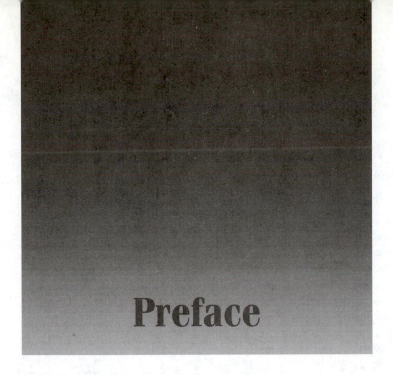

Preface

Outline

Competency Skills for the Dental Assistant is an interactive worktext designed to provide dental assistants with a working knowledge of basic chairside and office procedures. The competency-based approach allows assistants to master one skill, then build upon this knowledge as they move onto the next lesson. Both entry-level students still in training and experienced dental assistants wishing to brush up on skills will benefit from the simple, step-by-step format of this text.

This worktext contains eleven units grouped by specific topics. The units contain separate lessons and are self-contained, allowing the instructor or more advanced student to begin at any point in the text. A total of sixty-five chairside and office procedures are broken down into easy-to-follow steps and coded to specific Competency Evaluation Sheets, located in Appendix C, which provide the student with immediate feedback on proficiency. Assignment Sheets, located in Appendix B, correspond to individual lessons, providing students with additional learning activities to reinforce material. The answers to the Theory Recalls, Post Tests, and Assignment Sheets appear in Appendix A. The "Passport to Progress" may be used to record all lesson and testing dates as well as test results. The text also contains a Reference section for further reading, a detailed Glossary of common dental terms and an Index. Each unit includes:

- individual lessons containing background theory and a step-by-step, numbered breakdown of each procedure.
- measurable objectives and lists of key terms for each lesson

- Theory Recall quizzes at the end of each lesson that correspond to the objectives and emphasize the material just covered
- numerous photographs, illustrations, and tables to clarify and enhance concepts
- Tests to evaluate student's progression in specific areas and provide the opportunity to review areas of weaknesses

How to Use the Competency Evaluation Sheets

The Competency Evaluation Sheets, located in Appendix C at the back of this text, are numbered to match each of the sixty-five procedures. After reading the steps of each procedure and completing the Theory Recall readers are instructed to turn to the appropriate Competency Evaluation Sheet where they will find a detailed breakdown of the procedure. Each step of the procedure is divided into its component parts and assigned points. One scoring column allows for peer review in a practice situation. Another column provides for review by the instructor, who may grade while participating as the operator or who may evaluate two students working as an operator-assistant team. These sheets have been perforated for easy removal.

A student must achieve a score of 80% to pass the Competency Evaluation Test. If a step is performed incorrectly or forgotten, the instructor may indicate this in the review column. The student can refer back to the theory section of the text to retrain. A completed Competency Evaluation Sheet serves as a written record of the student's proficiency in a procedure.

Once the procedure has been tested and successfully completed, the instructor may enter the results in the Passport to Progress chart, which is a running record of instruction and testing dates, and the results of the evaluation. Students will have a written record of their entire progression and many use this chart during a job interview to verify training and evaluation of completed dental assisting procedures.

How to Use the Assignment Sheets

Appendix B contains twenty-four Assignment Sheets, which correspond to all lessons in the text that do not include procedures. These worksheets contain projects that give students the opportunity to demonstrate their hands-on understanding of the theory discussed in a particular lesson. For example, the activity in Assignment Sheet 1.7 "Composing a Resume and Cover Letter", corresponds to the lesson in Unit 1. The instructor is at liberty to create a grade point system for the Assignment Sheets or to assign them as extra reinforcement for the student before he or she progresses to another lesson.

Summary

The competency-based style of this worktext allows readers to pace themselves as they participate in their own hands-on training. The simple style and clearly defined procedures provide entry-level dental assisting students with a tangible outline of what is expected of them; the graded Competency Evaluation Sheets identify their weaknesses and provide proof of competence. Advanced students and practicing dental assistants will find this worktext a useful tool for reinforcement of concepts and skills. Instructors will benefit from the user-friendly style and the documented evidence, in the form of the Competency Evaluation Sheets and the Passport to Progress, that theory and procedures have been taught.

Competency Skills for the Dental Assistant may be used solely as an instructional tool or supplemented with additional references and materials, depending on the nature of a program. Completion of this worktext should result in competent, self-assured individuals ready to enter the exciting work of dental assisting.

The lightbulb icon and asterisks throughout the text indicate important information for the students to know.

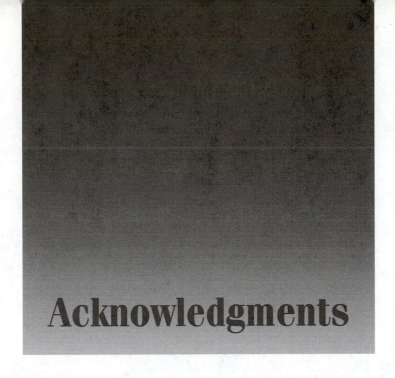

Acknowledgments

Without the help and encouragement from some wonderful people, this book could not have been completed. I am most grateful for the professional advice and assistance from the staff at Delmar Publishers. I would like to thank Adrianne Williams and Kimberly Davies, Acquisitions Editors; Jill Rembetski, Developmental Editor; Mary Siener and Vincent Berger, Art and Design Coordinators; Melissa Conan, Project Editor; Karen Leet, Production Coordinator; and Donna Leto, Editorial Assistant.

Appreciation is expressed for the insight, opinions, and general advice of the following reviewers who contributed to the development of this project: Tamara Erickson, CDA, Concorde Career Institute; Dianne McCarley, RDA, CDA, National Education Centers; Dona M. Metts, RDH, DeKalb Occupational Education Center North; Judith E Sheets, CDA, AA, Des Moines Area Community College; and Suzanne Wright, RDH, AS, North Montgomery County Vocational Technical School.

Special thanks are offered to the various manufacturers and company and association representatives who have reviewed items and submitted photos and research material used in these pages.

Equally helpful were Dr. Donald Lough and Dr. Arthur Rybeck and their excellent staff who loaned their office, equipment, materials, energy, and smiles for the photo shoot with our patient photographer, Dick Cress.

A grateful mention should be made of my brother, Tom Manion, for all his help with the computer, making the task of completing the manuscript so much easier.

Finally, appreciation and thanks go to my husband, Patrick, and my parents, children, grandchildren, family, friends, and neighbors. Your love and support have sustained and blessed me.

Delmar Publishers' Online Services

To access Delmar on the World Wide Web, point your browser to:
http://www.delmar.com/delmar.html

To access through Gopher: gopher://gopher.delmar.com

(Delmar Online is part of "thomson.com", and Internet site with information on more than 30 publishers of the International Thomson Publishing organization.)

For more information on our products and services:

email: info@delmar.com

or call 800-347-7707

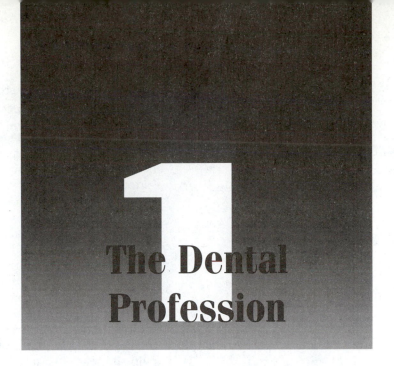

1

The Dental Profession

OBJECTIVES

Upon completion of this unit, the student will achieve a score of 80% or better on the Post Test covering the following material.

1. List the various members of the dental team. Describe the educational requirements, professional roles, responsibilities, and duties of each.
2. Discuss the educational requirements, employment, professional involvement, and certificate opportunities available for the dental assistant.
3. Demonstrate knowledge of the necessary attributes for the professional, personal, and job qualities of the dental assistant.
4. Define the meaning of ethics and give examples of ethical standards from the "Code of Ethics of the American Dental Assistants Association."
5. State the various types of legal restrictions and statutes regarding the practice of dentistry and how a dental assistant may conform to the legal boundaries of the profession.
6. Discuss the various methods and avenues of obtaining information for job placement in the dental community.
7. Demonstrate the method and style for preparing a personal resume, cover letter, and job application form for a position as a dental assistant.
8. Demonstrate good job interviewing skills by role-playing practice situations.

KEY TERMS

applicant
associate degree
attributes
chronological
classified ad
competent
confidential
consent
consultant
cover letter
DDS or DMD
dental assistant
dental
 equipment
 serviceperson
dental hygienist
detail or
 salesperson
disparaging

endodontics
ethics
functional
interview
jurisprudence
laboratory
 technician
liability
license
malpractice
negligence
networking
obligation
on-the-job
 training
 (OJT)
oral and
 maxillofacial
 surgery

oral pathology
orthodontics
para-dental
 professionals
pediatric dentistry
periodontics
placement
postsecondary
prosthodontics
public health
 dentistry
reference
resume
specialist
State Dental
 Practice Act
statutes
supervision

THE PROFESSIONAL DENTAL TEAM

To function properly in the position of a dental assistant, the person aspiring for employment must know the various members of the dental team and the procedures and duties each performs.

The professional dental team consists of the following members:

dentist
dental hygienist
dental assistant
dental laboratory technician
dental company detail or salesperson
dental equipment serviceperson
para-dental professionals

The Dentist

The dentist is the key figure in the dental team. The dentist is responsible for the treatment and care of the patients and liable for the actions committed by self and employees.

To earn the title of **DDS** (Doctor of Dental Surgery) or **DMD** (Doctor of Medical Dentistry), an individual must complete at least two to four years of college work concentrating on specific scientific courses, plus another three to four years of specialized study in the field of dentistry. Upon successful completion of the requirements, the individual is awarded the title of doctor of dentistry and then completes a written and clinical test in the state where the dentist wishes to practice.

After fulfilling the requirements of the **State Dental Practice Act** (SDPA) and passing the written and clinical boards of the state where the practice will be located, the dentist is legally permitted to perform the art and science of dentistry, performing dental procedures in all skill areas. Some dentists prefer and are more adept at one type of practice procedure than another. A dentist may choose to limit the practice to a specific type or may refer patients requiring certain procedures to a **specialist**, another dentist who has received more advanced and thorough training in a particular field.

There are presently eight recognized dental specialties. Each specialty determines its own requirements for study, training, practice, and testing before bestowing the title of specialist. Once a dentist has become a specialist in a particular field, the other areas of dental procedures are forsaken. Patients are either sent to another specialist or to the general dentist for work in areas other than the specialty.

The eight specialties are:

1. **prosthodontics**—concerned with the restoration and maintenance of normal dental functions through the application of artificial teeth and replacement appliances.
2. **periodontics**—concerned with the treatment and prevention of diseases to the oral periodontium, gum, and supporting gingival tissues.
3. **oral and maxillofacial surgery**—concerned with the diagnosis and treatment of diseases, deformities, injuries, and malfunctions of the jaws and surrounding structures.
4. **oral pathology**—concerned with the diagnosis, study, and treatment of diseases of the oral cavity and surrounding structures and the effect of dental disease upon the whole body.
5. **orthodontics**—concerned with the correction of deformities and dental anomalies through the art of adjustment, alignment, and movement of the dental tissues and structures.
6. **endodontics**—concerned with the diagnosis, cause, prevention, and treatment of diseases of the pulp and related tissues.
7. **pediatric dentistry**—concerned with the care, treatment, and maintenance of good oral health for children.
8. **public health dentistry**—concerned with the study, prevention, and treatment of dental disease through community resources, such as federal, state, and local agencies.

The Dental Hygienist

The **dental hygienist** is a member of the dental team whose primary goal is to aid in the prevention of dental disease. The hygienist must complete at least a two-year **postsecondary** program and may be awarded a diploma or an **associate degree**. Students who complete the four-year college program can receive a bachelor of science degree in dental hygiene. Some graduate schools offer a master of science in dental hygiene to the hygienist who desires further education for teaching or administrative work.

The hygienist must also have a **license** to work in the state where the practice is located. Passing the state boards enables the hygienist to perform the allotted duties under the direct or indirect supervision of a dentist. Each state mandates the duties and **supervision** of the hygienist. Some states permit a solo practice while others require direct supervision of hygienist duties, which may involve prophylaxis, exposure of radiographs, polishing of restorations, education of patients, and preventive treatments, such as sealant and fluoride application.

The American Dental Hygienist Association is the national professional association for the hygienist. There are state and local branches of this professional group.

The Dental Assistant

The **dental assistant** is another member of the dental team who usually works directly with the dentist and at times must be versatile (Figure 1–1). The assistant may be given **on-the-job training (OJT)** or receive formal school education in vocational, secondary, and postsecondary sites, or community colleges.

Dental assisting duties and skills are varied. They are grouped sometimes into areas, such as chairside, laboratory, receptionist/secretarial, expanded duty, and support. The assistant may become certified by the Dental Assisting National Board in general dental assisting (CDA) encompassing all areas or may sit for tests in specialized areas of expertise, such as radiology and dental specialties. Many states approve these national boards and accept completion of the boards as recognition of knowledge in a certain area, such as radiology. Passage may permit the assistant certification and SDPA permission to expose radiographs.

The American Dental Assistants Association is the national professional association for assistants. There are state and local branches of this professional group.

The Dental Laboratory Technician

The primary service of the dental **laboratory technician** is completing the cases in the dental laboratory. The technician constructs or repairs appliances, case models, restorations, dentures, and all other prosthodontic work for the dental practice.

The technician receives training on the job or in school. Many large companies conduct training classes for dental laboratory technicians, or a person may obtain work in a large dental laboratory and learn the various techniques by firsthand practice. All dental work completed in the dental laboratory is done to the prescription of the authorizing dentist.

The Dental Company Detail or Salesperson

Dental practices must stay current and be supplied with goods and products regularly. The company

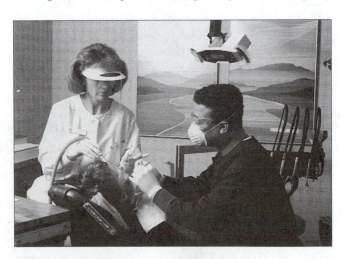

FIGURE 1–1 The dentist and assistant work as a team to provide dental care for the patient.

detail or salesperson is employed by a supply house or large manufacturer to call upon the dental practice. The salesperson may or may not have had dental training. All salespersons are trained in their particular company products and inform the dentist of all new products and materials available.

The Dental Equipment Serviceperson

The assistant and the dentist provide proper maintenance and handling of the dental equipment; however, the expertise of a **dental equipment serviceperson** sometimes is called upon to keep the machinery, which is often quite expensive, working properly. Many times servicepersons trained by the manufacturing company are employed to install new equipment or repair and maintain existing equipment.

Para-dental Professionals

Occasionally, the dentist must involve **para-dental professionals** in the treatment and care of a patient. The dentist may use the services of a pharmacist or medical laboratory when extensive disease is involved. Patients who suffer from improper eating habits may need consultations with a dietitian for good general health.

A dental **consultant** may be employed to analyze a dental practice. These professionals monitor the various methods and procedures performed throughout the work day. At the end of the two- or three-day visit, the consultant indicates to the dentist money- and effort-saving procedures that may produce a more efficiently and effectively run practice. ▲

THEORY RECALL

The Professional Dental Team

1. Who is ultimately responsible for the treatment of the patient and the care given by the office personnel?

   _____

2. What tests must a dentist complete before beginning practice in a particular state?

   _____

3. How many recognized dental specialties are there?

   _____

4. What is the primary duty of the dental hygienist?

   _____

5. Who mandates the duties and responsibilities of the hygienist?

   _____

6. Where does the dental assistant receive training?

_____

7. List three work areas in the dental practice in which the assistant may have specific duties.

a. _____

b. _____

c. _____

8. What is the name of the national professional organization for dental assistants?

_____

9. What type of work does the dental laboratory technician do?

_____

10. List three para-dental professionals a dentist may call upon to assist with providing care to the patient.

a. _____

b. _____

c. _____

For additional activities related to this lesson, turn to Assignment Sheet 1.1, The Professional Dental Team, located in Appendix B of this text.

THE ROLE OF THE DENTAL ASSISTANT

Dental assistants should be aware of the educational requirements, employment opportunities, and basic duties expected of their position. A well-informed person may participate and function easily when prepared. The history, educational opportunities, division of duties, professional organization, and certification processes of the dental assistant follow.

A Member of the Dental Team

Dr. C. Edmund Kells is credited by many to be the first to employ a woman as a dental assistant. Around 1855, partially in need and partially to satisfy social propriety of having another woman present in the room for female and children patients, Dr. Kells hired and trained a young woman to assist him in his practice. He advertised "Lady in Waiting" on a poster in his window. The venture was so successful that in a few years he had a staff of three trained and able aides. Thus began on-the-job training for the dental assistant. OJT was the only method of education as a dental assistant for many years and is still in use today.

As dentistry progressed and new materials, equipment, and procedures became more involved, it was evident that it took quite a bit of time, effort, and office expense to train a **competent** dental assistant. As a result, schools were formed to complete this task. The dental assistant candidate may now learn from OJT or seek an education and a diploma in a local vocational or proprietary school, either as a secondary student or in an adult education class.

Many cities have community college courses to educate individuals interested in becoming dental assistants. These colleges award a successful student with a diploma in dental assisting or expand the course offerings to include other classes that permit the student to obtain an associate degree in dental assisting or health studies.

There are many methods to obtain the knowledge needed to be a dental assistant; only the avenues of availability limit the choice. The potential assistant should search carefully to find the appropriate school that will provide the training necessary for gainful employment in the dental field.

Opportunities for Employment

The dental assistant has many opportunities for employment. The most numerous are positions available in the dental office, whether it be a solo (one dentist) practice or a group (two or more dentists) practice. Private and commercial medical and dental clinics hire talented, trained personnel. The dental assistant who is part of an oral hygiene or health team works side by side with other dental professionals in state, federal, or international mobile dental units. These teams travel to rural areas bringing care to persons unable to come to dental facilities.

Hospitals and nursing homes as well as dental school clinics employ dental assistants to work with the dentists who serve on their dental and oral surgery staff. Many assistants find employment in public health facilities assisting with care of homeless and needy persons. Dental specialists such as orthodontists, periodontists, oral surgeons, and endodontists need assistants with a good general knowledge of dentistry and specific knowledge and training in the specialized field.

Dental assistants with education and experience eventually may become educators and instructors who will train future assistants. Dental supply companies employ experienced dental assistants to travel from area to area visiting offices to demonstrate dental products to the dentist. The assistant may become part of a research team working to improve dental techniques, equipment, materials, or drugs. Insurance companies hire trained dental assistants to use their expertise in reviewing insurance claims. The choices and selections of employment are unlimited, and each assistant's desire may be fulfilled.

Duties and Responsibilities

The duties and responsibilities of a dental assistant are as varied as the education and places of employment. A dental facility that employs only one assistant most likely will require that person to assume all the assistant duties. Offices or facilities employing more than one assistant may divide the responsibilities of the personnel, usually into the roles of chairside assistant, expanded function assistant, business manager/receptionist, insurance clerk, dental laboratory assistant, infection control, and clinical support assistant. Each assistant should be aware of the duties of the others so when one is ill or absent, the other may fill in and perform the work (Figure 1–2).

Chairside assisting can be subdivided into regular and expanded duty. Each state regulates the training and testing required before an assistant can perform procedures determined to be "expanded" or demanding of special training. A chairside assistant may become an oral health instructor, teaching and monitoring the patient in home care. In some states, a few duties, such as exposure of x-rays or coronal polishing, require testing and certification, while other states do not grant the assistant permission to complete these tasks. Each state regulates the duties an assistant may perform. It is the responsibility of the assistant to be familiar with the state laws before seeking employment in a particular state.

Some dental assistants are employed as clinical support personnel. These persons perform office duties, maintaining organization. The support personnel may perform the sterilization and disinfection of the operatories between patients, seat the patients, and in general, keep everything organized and on time.

Dental laboratory assistants may complete general services in the laboratory setting. Dental lab assistants

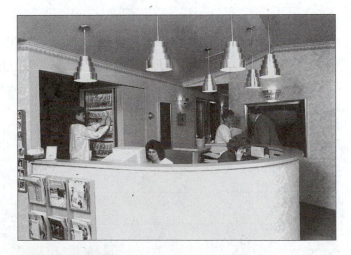

FIGURE 1–2 Dental assistants perform many and varied duties in a dental facility.

may pour the impressions, trim models, and prepare orthodontic appliances and equipment; yet they do not perform the complex duties of the dental laboratory technician.

Professional Involvement

The dental assistant may become a member of the American Dental Assistants Association (ADAA). The ADAA is a professional association that represents all persons employed as dental assistants, including certified, noncertified, chairside, laboratory, and support assistants or business and practice managers or receptionists.

Membership in this professional organization is based on a three-level involvement. The assistant attends and participates in local monthly or bimonthly meetings with other assistants in the region. They share their expertise or invite experts to speak and provide demonstrations of new or expanded dental materials and equipment. The local group may put on fund-raising events to sponsor community dental activities, such as a children's dental health poster contest or dental care clinics for the needy.

State-wide structure of the organization involves all local societies. State organizations meet periodically and work on projects and community involvement. Representatives from the state association attend national meetings and represent their local and state members.

Some of the privileges that are the result of ADAA membership are professional liability and accidental death and dismemberment coverage, home study courses, legislative representation, group insurance coverage at discounted rates, loan assistance, professional magazine subscriptions to *The Dental Assistant* and *Update*, credit card programs, commercial discounts, as well as professional growth and assistance from fellow members.

Certification

Dental assistants may become certified through the Dental Assisting National Board (DANB). In addition to the basic dental assisting certification (CDA), this organization offers examinations in infection control (ICE), dental radiation health and safety (RHS), oral and maxillofacial surgery assisting (COMSA), dental practice management assisting (CDPMA), and orthodontic assisting (COA).

The infection control exam (ICE) and the dental radiation health and safety examination (RHS) may be taken by any individual. Although DANB does not set eligibility requirements for sitting for these exams, some states may require various eligibility standards because successful completion of these exams may complete that state's requirements for certification. The contents of the ICE (100 questions) and RHS (100 questions) exams comprise two-thirds of the CDA exam. The other one-third consists of general chairside questions (120).

Only candidates who have completed eligibility requirements are permitted to take the CDA, COMSA, CDPMA, and COA exams. The requirements that must be met for CDA are either graduation from a dental assisting program accredited by the American Dental Association Commission on Dental Accreditation, two years full-time employment work experience (3,500 hours) with a high school diploma or equivalent, or previous certification with a lapsed status of 18 months or more. All candidates must have a current cardiopulmonary resuscitation (CPR) certification. The certified specialty eligibility requirements are very similar to the CDA requirements or prerequisites.

Persons who have taken and successfully completed the various certification exams may place the appropriate certification initials behind their name and wear the DANB pin (Figure 1–3). These individuals must maintain their certification by completing 12 continuing dental education units each year. CDE hours may be obtained from numerous sources, including dental and dental assisting meetings, educational programs, home study courses, readings and tapes, community participation, college courses, CPR courses, and successful examination participation.

Some state dental boards offer testing and certification in areas such as expanded duties assisting, radiation health and safety, and other specialty areas. Such certification is valid only in the issuing state. When an assistant becomes employed, he or she must seek and follow that particular state's certification and regulation policies.▲

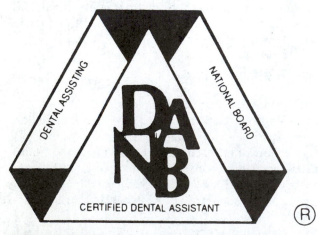

FIGURE 1–3 Only those who have successfully passed the certification tests and maintain the certification status may wear the Dental Assistant National Board certification pin. (Courtesy of the Dental Assisting National Board.)

THEORY RECALL

The Role of the Dental Assistant

1. What do the initials OJT stand for?

2. List three places where a person may be educated as a dental assistant.
   a.
   b.
   c.

3. List three areas in which a dental assistant may find employment.
   a.
   b.
   c.

4. What are the duties of the clinical support dental assistant?

5. What work may a dental laboratory assistant perform?

6. What is the name of the national organization that represents dental assistants?

7. What are the three levels of professional organization memberships?
   a.
   b.
   c.

8. Through what organization may dental assistants become certified?

9. List five specialized certification exams given by the DANB.
   a.
   b.
   c.
   d.
   e.

10. Where is state certification of a dental assistant valid?

For additional activities related to this lesson, turn to Assignment Sheet 1.2, The Role of the Dental Assistant, located in Appendix B of this text.

QUALITIES OF THE DENTAL ASSISTANT

The dental assistant is an extension of the dental practice and actually may give the patient his or her first impression of the practice. The assistant starts the patient-staff relationship and sets the tone for office behavior; therefore, it is important for the dental assistant to know what qualities are expected of the professional.

The desirable qualities of the dental assistant may be divided into three groups: professional, personal, and job qualities.

Professional Qualities

The professional dental assistant should maintain all confidences of the practice. Records and information taken during treatment, dentist-patient relationships, financial and business matters, and all data are kept private and confidential. The assistant will not discuss or release any data unless instructed by the dentist, who will insist upon written release forms for permission.

The assistant should demonstrate an interest in the patient's welfare, assuring the person that professional treatment will be rendered. By recognizing the needs of others and the emotions and feelings of the patient, the assistant may relate to the patient better. Performing the Golden Rule of "do unto others as you wish done unto you" will guide the professional into a caring and sharing individual.

Following instructions carefully and accurately is a trait of a professional dental assistant. Maintaining accurate and neat records and performing duties correctly are the standards of a quality assistant.

A professional dental assistant performs only the duties and procedures that are legally and ethically expected. Only knowledgeable skills that have been properly delegated are performed by the assistant.

Personal Qualities

The dental assistant should be dependable and honest in all dealings. When the assistant can be relied upon to do the work delegated or perform the task correctly, the individual can be considered reliable.

The dentist should be confident that the assistant will be punctual and come prepared for work. The assistant should dress in a professional manner and be well groomed. Hair should be clean and worn in a reserved style. Nails should be short and clean with snag-free edges. Shoes should be shined or cleaned. Posture should be straight and alert looking. When the assistant exhibits a positive self-image of confidence and assurance, the patient feels comfortable and properly cared for.

Good communication skills are essential for the dental assistant. After a person has made a first impression with appearance, the second impression is made with speech. The assistant should speak in a calm, clear voice, use correct language, and avoid slang words or expressions.

Job Qualities

When performing work tasks, the dental assistant should be willing to learn. No matter how many times or how many days a person works at a job or profession, there is always room for new ideas or learning situations. The assistant should maintain an open mind and seek to improve each day.

Adapting to the situation at hand is a very important trait. There may be days when things do not go as planned and situations are hurried or hectic. The assistant must be able to adapt to all situations and perform to the best of his or her ability.

Listening to criticism constructively and using it as an improvement tool is a quality of the professional assistant. Learning from mistakes and accepting suggestions help to improve the services of the assistant (Figure 1–4).

Safety rules must be followed at all times. The assistant must protect the patient and self by applying all safety regulations. Shortcuts may endanger a person. The assistant should be aware of the needed

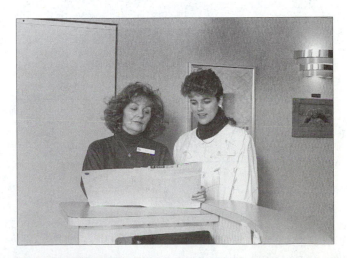

FIGURE 1–4 A dental assistant should listen to criticism and accept it as a positive learning experience.

safety precautions and should look up the hazards and controls needed for them if not sure.

At all times the assistant should be a team member, remembering that the practice of dentistry needs team efforts. As a willing worker who is concerned with the welfare of the practice and concern for the dentist and patient, the assistant will prove to be very valuable.▲

THEORY RECALL

Qualities of the Dental Assistant

1. What types of patient records are considered confidential?

_____

2. How may the dental assistant demonstrate an interest in the patient's welfare?

_____

3. In what manner should the dental assistant maintain professional records?

_____

4. What must a dental assistant do on the job to be considered reliable?

_____

5. How can the dental assistant dress in a professional manner?

_____

6. How can a dental assistant improve communication skills?

_____

7. List three ways a dental assistant can exhibit good job qualities.

   a. _____

   b. _____

   c. _____

8. For whom must the dental assistant strive to provide safety?

_____

9. How can the dental assistant observe safety rules?

_____

10. How can the dental assistant become a team member?

_____

For additional activities related to this lesson, turn to Assignment Sheet 1.3, Qualities of the Dental Assistant, located in Appendix B of this text.

ETHICS FOR THE DENTAL ASSISTANT

Each person involved in a profession is expected to act in an ethical manner. Therefore, the dental assistant should understand the meaning of **ethics** and general actions stressed in the "Code of Ethics of the American Dental Assistants Association."

Ethics is a code of discipline or a statement of moral **obligations** imposed by the members of a profession. The ethical standards of each profession are developed by its professional organization. Those practicing that art are morally required to present themselves in an ethical manner.

The dental assistant, as an agent of the dentist, must follow the ethical standards of the dental practice as well as perform actions that govern the profession of dental assisting. A formal statement of conduct has been developed called the "Code of Ethics of the American Dental Assistants Association" (Figure 1–5). This code, in essence, states the dental assistant should:

▶ Treat others as they wish to be treated. In other words, practice the Golden Rule. Treat each and every person as an important individual regardless of their age, sex, race, religion, or social status.
▶ Be honest and loyal in actions and demonstrate a desire to serve the dentist and patients. Be sincere and trustworthy in actions and relations with the patients, dentist, and other staff members.
▶ Hold in confidence all details of the professional services rendered. Do not talk about patient cases to others. Keep conversations and records private and **confidential**.

Code of Ethics of American Dental Assistants Association

The spirit of the Golden Rule should be the guiding principle of conduct for the dental assistant. In all her contacts with the dental profession and society she should maintain honesty, loyalty, and a desire to serve to the best of her ability her employer and his patients.

The dental assistant should give to her employer the cooperation he needs to serve his patients capably and efficiently. She will hold in confidence the details of professional services rendered by her employer. She should refrain from performing any service for patients which requires the professional competence of the dentist, or which may be prohibited by the dental practice act of the state in which she is employed.

She should avoid making any disparaging remarks about the conduct of the profession she serves, or of her employer's treatment of his patients.

The dental assistant has the obligation of increasing her skill and efficiency by availing herself of the educational opportunities provided by the Association and its component societies. She should take part in the efforts of these groups to improve the educational status of the dental assistant and should support this Code of Ethics.

FIGURE 1–5 "Code of Ethics of the American Dental Assistants Association."

▶ Refrain from performing any service prohibited by the State Practice Act or requiring the competence of a dentist. Do not attempt to care for a patient in any manner prohibited by law or personal ability.

▶ Avoid **disparaging** remarks about the conduct or performance of the employer or profession. Do not grumble about the practice. Be aware of body language and facial expressions. Have a positive attitude.

▶ Increase skills and efficiency by taking advantage of education opportunities. Attend workshops, meetings, and other informative classes.

▶ Take part in professional organizations. Support the profession of dental assisting. Join with others to increase skills and interests.▲

THEORY RECALL

Ethics for the Dental Assistant

1. Define the term ethics.

   _____

2. Who develops the ethical standards of a professional organization?

   _____

3. Who is morally required to present themselves in an ethical manner?

   _____

4. What is the "Code of Ethics of the American Dental Assistants Association"?

   _____

5. What action does the Golden Rule dictate?

   _____

6. In what manner should the assistant hold the details of the professional services rendered in the dental office?

   _____

7. About what should the assistant avoid negative or disparaging remarks?

   _____

8. How can the assistant increase skills and efficiency?

   _____

9. What actions should the assistant take toward the professional dental organizations?

   _____

For additional activities related to this lesson, turn to Assignment Sheet 1.4, Ethics for the Dental Assistant, located in Appendix B of this text.

DENTAL JURISPRUDENCE—LEGAL CONSIDERATIONS

Dental **jurisprudence** is the application of legal **statutes** and regulations covering the practice of dentistry. The dentist must adhere to federal, state, and civil law in all relations with the public. As an agent of the dentist, the assistant should be aware of the different forms of jurisprudence and the role the assistant may play in each case.

On the federal level dental jurisprudence involves the requirement for the dentist to file and obtain a federal narcotics stamp each year from the United States Treasury Office. This stamp number entitles the dentist to prescribe narcotic medicines used in the practice of dentistry and is present on the prescription form. The assistant must renew the stamp number each year by filing the proper renewal papers and fee.

State legal statutes govern the practice of dentistry. The State Practice Act regulates who may practice and in what manner. Dentists, dental hygienists, and, in some states, dental assistants are licensed or certified to practice certain procedures while in that state. These individuals are required to display their license and renewal card each year. Many states require not only a renewal fee but proof of continuing education credits before renewing the license.

The examination, registration, licensing, and enforcement of the State Practice Act is completed by the State Dental Board, a governing body consisting of appointed dental professionals. The board suggests regulations to the state legislature, which enacts these items into law. The board monitors the dental profession and enforces the statutes in the state. A person practicing dentistry without a license or performing a dental procedure not included in the legal delegation of duties of that individual's license may be fined and imprisoned. It is the duty of the practitioner to know which duties or procedures are permitted. Ignorance of the law is no excuse.

The dental practice is also governed by the legal code, which may be divided into civil and criminal law. The dentist may be sued for personal injury claims or for **malpractice**. If a patient or guest slips and falls on a loose rug or waxed floor, the injured party may sue the dentist or practice for injury incurred and damages resulting from the accident. The assistant must be on the lookout for possible hazards and perform all tasks with safety and patient regard in mind.

Malpractice may occur from performing an act or failure to correctly perform a service that results in an injury to the patient. This act may be committed by the dentist or a member of the staff. The dentist is responsible for all employed in the practice and may be sued for the actions of the dentist, hygienist, expanded duty assistant, or any delegated staff member. In most cases, only the dentist is sued; but a suit may be brought for the offending staff member also. The employer dentist and any personnel performing direct patient care procedures should maintain **liability** insurance.

Some reasons for malpractice suits may be that the practitioner:

1. Did not perform the "standard of treatment," or what is usually done by most dentists, dental hygienists, and assistants.
2. Performed an action that caused injury from ignorance, carelessness, lack of skill, disregard for rules or principles, **negligence**, or with intent.
3. Did not fully instruct or advise the patient in pre- or postoperative treatment.
4. Did not seek competent care by referring to a specialist.
5. Committed a lack of treatment by not performing a procedure when needed.
6. Did not use all methods available to obtain a proper diagnosis.
7. Violated the patient's privacy.
8. Did not give proper attention to symptoms or patient's complaints.
9. Did not fulfill a dental contract or promise.

Criminal charges may be filed against a dentist for malicious injury, income tax evasion, narcotics misuse, or any other criminal reason.

The assistant may help to avoid malpractice occurrences by completing assigned duties properly and always being on the lookout for potential safety or health hazards (Figure 1–6). Sterilization and preparation procedures must be thorough. The assistant should perform only duties in which he or she has been fully trained and those permitted by law. Hazards should be avoided by maintaining the equipment

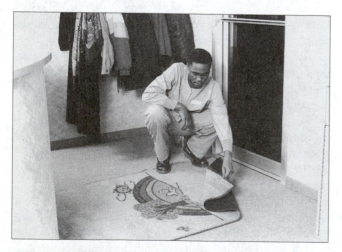

FIGURE 1–6 The alert dental assistant may prevent accidents and injuries by fixing loose rugs and looking for possible hazards.

in good working order, and safety features should be observed.

Dental and business records must be neat, legible, and accurate in all details. If an entry is mistakenly entered, the assistant should avoid using an eraser for correction. The mistake should be marked through and the correct entry made with the assistant placing initials nearby for confirmation. All records must be kept confidential. If a patient requests information to be sent elsewhere, the assistant should ask for written notification before sending the material.

When giving pre- or postoperative instructions to a patient, the assistant must make sure the patient understands them fully. When working with a minor or a premedicated person, the assistant should review the instructions with the patient's parent or companion. Printed forms are good to give to the patient to take home. **Consent** to operate must be obtained for major surgeries, complicated procedures, and minor children. The assistant will gather these slips and place them in the patient's records.

The assistant should be updated in CPR and first aid classes and prepared to assist in any emergency. In an emergency, the assistant should say nothing. Statements like "I never saw that before" could be used in a legal case. The assistant should speak highly of the employer dentist and not criticize other dental professionals and their work.▲

THEORY RECALL

Dental Jurisprudence—Legal Considerations

1. What is dental jurisprudence?

   _____

2. What legal federal regulation must the dentist complete?

   _____

3. Who regulates and monitors the practice of dentistry in a state?

   _____

4. What may happen to a person practicing dentistry without a license?

   _____

5. How may malpractice occur?

   _____

6. List three reasons for malpractice suits.

   a. _____

   b. _____

   c. _____

7. How can the assistant help avoid malpractice suits in relation to duties?

_____

8. How can the assistant help avoid malpractice suits in relation to records?

_____

9. How can the assistant help avoid malpractice suits in relation to giving instructions to a patient?

_____

10. How can the assistant help avoid malpractice suits in relation to an emergency?

_____

For additional activities related to this lesson, turn to Assignment Sheet 1.5, Dental Jurisprudence—Legal Considerations, located in Appendix B of this text.

JOB SOURCES

Seeking employment can be a very demanding task. If the **applicant** knows how to locate a job, apply, and perform a good interview, the experience may be a rewarding one.

The first step in obtaining future employment is locating a job source. By knowing where to look for openings, the applicant can find a proper situation. The most common avenues of locating jobs or careers are classified advertisements, school placement departments, networking, professional associations, employment agencies, and independent search.

Classified Advertisements

Want ads in the newspaper are the most common method of looking for employment. **Classified ads** are paid advertisements placed by businesses searching for employees to hire. The Sunday edition of most newspapers contains the largest selection of openings. Some newspapers' classified sections are so large that help-wanted advertisements are broken into divisions, such as health, domestics, clerical, and legal.

Many companies identify themselves, and state the position open, the education desired of the employee, the hours, such as full time (FT) or part time (PT), and the duties involved. Some companies merely give the position and a box number to apply. These are called blind ads, because the business that is hiring is not identified (Figure 1–7). Blind ads can be dangerous if an employee desires a change and wishes to look for another placement but does not know to whom the reply is sent. There is always a possibility that the blind ad may be related to the present placement. Some newspapers offer a confidential service in which

---

Help Wanted

FT chairside dental assistant needed for progressive office. Training or experience preferred. Send resume to Box 1511 ᶜ/o this paper.

FIGURE 1–7 **Blind advertisements tell of job openings. They do not indicate the name of the facility or employment site.**

a person replying to a blind ad may place the letter addressed to the box number and a note stating with whom not to place the reply. In this way, the newspaper can maintain the anonymity of the advertiser while protecting the job seeker.

When seeking a job, the assistant should read every ad placed in the classified section. Many advertisements are incorrectly stated or placed in a wrong section. For instance, a secretarial position may include chairside duties. Scanning the want ad section may take a long time, but the rewards may be well worth the effort.

Placement Department

Many schools maintain a **placement** department, a division of the institution that investigates the possibility of employment in area businesses and handles calls from local employers for potential new employees. A short time before graduation, the assistant should visit the placement department and register with the office. Let them know of the desire for employment and the method to contact the applicant after graduation.

Former instructors are good sources of employment. They maintain contacts with dentists and dental facilities through their work. If an instructor is aware of the assistant's desire for employment, a **reference** may be made. It is wise to give the instructor a current resume that may be photocopied and available for distribution to possible employers.

Networking

The assistant searching for a job should let everyone know that employment is desired. It is amazing how many opportunities occur because someone knew the "right" person. Many times the "right" person just happens to hear that an assistant desires a job and hires the friend, son, or daughter of a good employee, hoping to find another faithful worker. Patients in the dental chair hearing that an assistant is leaving soon may suggest to their dentist to employ you. **Networking** yourself by letting everyone help to search for a job may prove to find the very opening needed.

Professional Associations

Attending local professional organization meetings helps the assistant keep current in knowledge and establish contacts with other members of the profession. Job opportunities may be offered through other professionals who are aware of openings.

Employment agencies are businesses that find employment for their clients. The state offers a free employment service in which a person may register skills, education, and particulars. If a position in that area becomes available, the state employment officer will contact the applicant and arrange an interview. The state agency also provides bulletins of state and federal positions seeking employees. Any resident may take advantage of the free employment services of the state facility.

Employment Agencies

Commercial employment agencies offer placement services for a fee. The cost is paid by either the employer or the newly hired employee. The person seeking the job may specify they accept only jobs whose fees are prepaid or may make a contract to pay the employment service for the placement. If contracting for placement service, the assistant should be cautious about a few things. The service should be licensed and agree to keep the applicant's records confidential. The contract should be read carefully before signing. The contract should state what would happen if the new employee is laid off or does not care for the job and resigns after a few weeks. The payment time and method should be outlined.

Some temporary help agencies are good sources of employment. Although the job does not offer security or benefits, temporary assignments may lead to possibilities and contacts in the profession. Temporary help employment also looks good in a job **interview** should you be asked what you have done since school.

Each state operates an employment bureau to assist residents in the job search. Local, state, and federal job availabilities are posted regularly. Many military or federal hospitals and clinic openings are listed throughout the country. If an assistant wishes to relocate, employment in another area may be available. If there are no openings, the assistant may fill out an information card and be called if a suitable situation arises.

Independent Search

The job-seeking assistant may contact independently places of employment. The assistant may telephone a facility or dental office and inquire if any positions are open. This is a difficult procedure because no one wants rejection, but it may become easier with prac-

tice. Having a resume with personal and employment history handy during the conversation may prove to be helpful if asked questions. If an opening is available, request an interview to apply for the position.

The assistant may also go directly to a facility or dental office and inquire of the receptionist if a resume for a job may be placed in the office file. The receptionist may at that time take the resume to the dentist or offer to do so at a later time. The assistant should thank the person then call in a week to inquire if the resume was reviewed. Such tactics may lead to employment in that particular office or in another related office or facility.

Employment searching can be easy or difficult. All avenues and tactics should be attempted and the assistant must not lose heart but keep trying. Just when all seems blue, a perfect job may come along.▲

THEORY RECALL

Job Sources

1. Which edition contains the most want ads in the newspaper?

2. Why should the assistant read all employment ads in the classified section?

3. What are the duties of the school placement office?

4. How may a former instructor be a source for employment?

5. What is networking?

6. How can attending a local professional organization meeting help in job placement?

7. Who offers a free employment service for job placement?

8. When dealing with a commercial agency, what items of a contract should the assistant examine closely?

9. How may a temporary employment agency help in job placement?

10. After leaving a resume with a facility, how long should the assistant wait before calling back to determine the status of the resume?

For additional activities related to this lesson, turn to Assignment Sheet 1.6, Job Sources, located in Appendix B of this text.

COMPOSING A RESUME AND COVER LETTER

A resume is a fact sheet describing skills, experiences, and education of an applicant applying for a job position. The resume is the employer's first glance at an individual and represents the chance for further interest in filling an employment post (Figure 1–8).

Resume Preparation

The resume should be printed on quality, bonded paper. Pastel or neutral colors as well as the standard white, shaded paper are acceptable. The resume should

---

Betsy Sue Logan
102 Mirror Avenue
Anywhere, US 12345

(123)555-7890

Career Objective

To pursue a career as a Dental Assistant, specializing in chairside assisting.

Education

Healthful Arts Career School	Anywhere, US 12345
September 19xx–June 19xx	Dental Assistant Diploma
Anywhere High School	Anywhere, US 12345
September 19xx–June 19xx	Diploma
Anywhere City Hospital	Anywhere, US 12345
EMT 107-hour course	EMT Certificate

Professional Skills

Clinical—chairside assisting, patient education, laboratory procedures, infection control practices, vital signs, emergency care, radiology, and CPR and EMT training
Administrative—typing and computer training, insurance forms, health history, patient scheduling, filing and bookkeeping skills

Work Experience

Dr. James Bell	April 19xx–May 19xx
Anywhere, US 12345	Externship
Downtown Health Center	June 19xx–to present
1200 Market Street	Child-care worker
Anywhere, US 12345	

Duties include babysitting, supervising play area, assisting with educational and constructive play sessions for children of health center patrons

Anywhere City Park	Summer employment
Anywhere, US 12345	

Duties involved counter work, food preparation, sanitation, and general assistance in park's food center

Activities

Honor student	Healthful Arts Career School
National Honor Society	Anywhere High School
Sports letters for track and basketball	Anywhere High School

References

Available upon request

FIGURE 1–8 **A resume must be neat and correct because it may be the applicant's first contact with the employer.**

be typed using a good quality ribbon and in a professional script. Handwriting and italic scripts are not desirable in the business world as well as letters all typed in a capital case mode.

The applicant must review and check the material to be sure there are no misspelled words, punctuation errors, or abbreviations. A sloppy letter will reflect upon the applicant's work. Margins must be correct. The finished letter must be centered in the middle of the page for easy and balanced reading.

All data and items discussed on the resume must be brief and to the point. It is better to have a one-page resume and discuss the data at greater length during the job interview.

The resume should include personal data—the applicant's name, address, and phone number. It is wise to give two phone numbers if the applicant works or is away from home for periods of time. Personal data, such as age, race, dependents, marital status, religion, and national origin, is not required but may be voluntarily submitted by the applicant.

The resume should state job objectives of the applicant, so the employer is aware of the employee's goals. If the applicant desires a position in more than one area, the objectives are listed in the order of choice.

Positive **attributes** and experiences are stressed, while negative occurrences are avoided. The truth must be stated at all times, because the potential employer may make inquiries into the applicant's past experiences before hiring. Concentration on the strengths of the applicant may overshadow any shortcomings the potential employee may have.

Resumes may be formatted in a **chronological** (time sequence) order, a **functional** fact mode, or a combination of the two. The functional style may be more favorable for a person without much work experience. A person with training and education could stress the talents achieved that will aid in the work position. The chronological style places more emphasis on work experience, listing the most recent experiences first and moving into the past with each entry.

Whichever style is used, the contents must show action. Avoid personal pronouns. State experience or education in terms of completing a specific action. List skills, special training, externships, awards, and items that present an interested and talented potential employee.

References need not be placed on the resume, but the applicant should be prepared to offer at least three at the interview session. All persons listed as references should be contacted and permission should be granted before listing a reference.

Composing the Cover Letter

It may be possible to take a resume on a job search and leave it with an office for review, but it is not proper to send a resume to an office or facility without some letter of explanation. A **cover letter** is included with the resume when mailing the form. A cover letter's appearance should follow the same guidelines as the resume (Figure 1–9).

The cover letter should contain at least three paragraphs. The first paragraph explains why the letter and resume have been sent to the facility. The second paragraph "sings the praises" of the applicant, telling the employer why this person should be hired. The third paragraph indicates the desire for an interview and the availability of the applicant.

Photographs are not included in a cover letter and resume approach, but copies of certificates of education or awards, if pertaining directly to the desired job, may be included. All work should be checked and double-checked before sending. It may be advisable to show the material to a friend and ask for an honest critique of the work.▲

102 Mirror Avenue
Anywhere, US 12345
June 5, 19xx

Box 115
Home Daily News
1400 Main Street
Anywhere, US 12345

Dear Doctor,

I am writing in response to your advertisement in the *Home Daily News* of June 4 describing the chairside dental assisting position opening. My enclosed resume will acquaint you with my background.

As a recent graduate of dental assistant training at the Healthful Arts Career School, I am qualified to perform the chairside assisting duties. I completed a six-week externship in the office of Dr. James Bell, which has prepared me with the skills and professionalism required.

I may be reached at (123)555-7890 to schedule an interview. Thank you for your attention to my resume. I look forward to hearing from you soon.

Sincerely,

Betsy Sue Logan
Betsy Sue Logan

Enclosure

FIGURE 1–9 **Cover letters are sent with the resume. These letters introduce the applicant and state the reason for the resume.**

THEORY RECALL

Composing a Resume and Cover Letter

1. What is a resume?

2. Why are the correctness and appearance of the resume important?

3. How many pages long should a resume be?

4. How does the employer get to know the goals and objectives of the applicant from a resume?

5. What does the functional style of a resume stress?

6. How are experiences and education listed on a chronological resume?

7. Must references be placed on a resume?

8. What is a cover letter?

9. What should the three paragraphs of the cover letter state?

   a. _____

   b. _____

   c. _____

10. What may be included in the cover letter and resume?

For additional activities related to this lesson, turn to Assignment Sheet 1.7, Composing a Resume and Cover Letter, located in Appendix B of this text.

COMPLETING A JOB APPLICATION FORM

A job application form is given to a potential employee when the applicant arrives for an interview, or it may be requested from a facility or place of employment. The information required on an application form is more direct and intense than the information given on a resume. Some offices or facilities do not use job application forms but interview using the applicant's resume. Other facilities may require the applicant to fill out a particular form chosen by the firm (Figure 1–10).

Application for Employment
(Please Print Clearly)

Confidential

Personal Information

Date of Application: June 7, 19XX   Date Available: Immediate

Name: Logan (Last) Betsy (First) Sue (Middle)

Social Security Number: 123-48-1501

Present Address: 102 Mirror Ave. (Street) Lewis (City) NE (State) 12345 (Zip Code)

Phone Number: 555-1230

Permanent Address (if Different than Present Address): ____ (Street) ____ (City) ____ (State) ____ (Zip Code) Phone Number: ____

If you cannot be reached at above phone number, where may we contact you? Name of Person: N/A   Phone: ____

Employment Desired

Type of Work Desired	Shift	Salary
First Choice: Chairside	all	open
Second Choice: Front desk	all	open
Third Choice:		

Will You Accept Employment of: ☒ Full Time? ☐ Part Time? ☐ Temporary?

Are You 18 Yrs. of Age or Older? ☒ Yes ☐ No

Are You Employed Now? ☐ Yes ☒ No

May We Contact Your Present Employer? ☐ Yes ☐ No

How Did You Learn Of This Opening? Classified Ad

Education

Circle Highest Grade Completed: 8 9 10 11 (12) 13 14 15 16

Scholastic Honors Received: National Honor Society

	Name of School	Location (City, State)	Courses Taken	Completed	Type of Degree or Certificate Received
Grammar or Grade School	Madison Ave	Lewis, NE	—	☒ Yes	
High School	Lewis Central	Lewis, NE	Academic	☒ Yes	
College				☐ Yes ___	
Vocational or Business				☐ Yes ___	
Professional Education	Healthful Arts Career School	Graham, NE	Dental Assisting	☒ Yes; 6.1.XX	Certificate
Laboratory or X-Ray Training	Lewis General Hospital	Lewis, NE	X-Ray, CPR, EMT	☒ Yes; 9.15XX	EMT Certificate

Extracurricular Activities While in School: Sports, National Honor Society, Drama Club

Member of Professional Organizations: Health Career Student Association

Honors Received, Volunteer or Community Service or Other Qualifications You Have Which You Feel Are Related to the Position for Which You Are Applying: Volunteer Red Cross Blood Bank, Meals on Wheels

Were you in the U.S. Armed Forces? ☐ Yes ☒ No If yes, what branch? ____

Dates of Duty: From ___/___/___ (Month/Day/Year) To ___/___/___ (Month/Day/Year) Rank at Discharge ____

Professional Licenses and/or Certifications

Type	Organization or State Issued	Date Issued	Number	Verif.
Dental Asst.	Healthful Arts Career School, NE	6-1-XX		
EMT	National EMT Service	9.15.XX	1234-B	

Form 3294R BRIGGS, Des Moines, IA 50306 (800) 247-2343 PRINTED IN U.S.A.

Rev. 4/92

FIGURE 1-10 Job application forms can be simple or quite complicated. The applicant should read the form over before filling it in. [Reprinted with permission of Briggs Corporation, Des Moines, IA 50306, (800) 247-2343.]

16

This Page For Institution and Interviewers' Use Only

Interviewers Comments

Interviewer	Date	Comments

Reference and Prior Employment Check

Individual Contacted	Name of Firm	Results of Check

For Personnel Office Use

Hired _____ For what department _____ Position _____

Salary _____ per Year Month Hour   Starting Date _____

(Continued)

Job application forms vary. Some are relatively easy to complete while others may be quite involved. Some offices request the applicant to fill out a four- or five-page psychological form requesting the applicant's favorite color, last book read, and type of movies watched, hoping to match the personality of the applicant with the other staff members.

Most facilities require the applicant to complete a basic questionnaire about skills, work experience, and education. The applicant can be prepared for these questions by taking along the information to the interview. A small wallet-sized form listing pertinent information, dates, and data is a handy item to carry when job seeking. Being prepared can prevent leaving blanks or making erasures or scratch outs on the form and will increase accuracy of dates and addresses.

The applicant should read the application before filling in information, being careful to follow directions. Some applications ask for pencil or printing to see if the applicant is observant. If pencil is not requested, the assistant should fill the form out in ink, dark enough and firm enough to be easily read.

Questions regarding work and education experiences should be filled in as completely as possible in chronological order. The most recent work experience or school attended is listed first with the next attended listed second and so on.

All blanks and question lines should be completed. If a question does not apply to the applicant, a simple "NA" (not applicable) in the blank shows the question was read. Answers should be truthful as most employers check references and former places of employment before hiring.

The applicant should ask for an explanation if there is a question that is unclear on the application form. It is better to ask than to fill in an incorrect answer. Questions on salary desired or previous salary can be answered by writing in "open" or "negotiable" and can be discussed in the interview session.

All smudges and marks should be neatly erased before handing in the application form. A clean, correct, and accurate job application form is an example of the type of work the potential employee can contribute.▲

THEORY RECALL
Completing a Job Application Form

1. When is a job application form given to a potential employee?

2. How do job application forms differ?

3. How can the applicant be prepared for filling out a job application form?

4. How can being prepared with the information to be placed on the job application form help the applicant complete the form?

5. What should the applicant do before filling out the application form?

6. If a question does not apply to the applicant, what should that person do?

7. Why should all answers be truthful?

8. If there is a question that the applicant does not understand, what should the applicant do?

9. What does the appearance of the job application form reveal about the potential of an employee?

For additional activities related to this lesson, turn to Assignment Sheet 1.8, Completing a Job Application Form, located in Appendix B of this text.

DEMONSTRATING JOB INTERVIEW SKILLS

The interview is the most important part of the job-seeking process. During this question-and-answer period, decisions are made by the applicant as well as the employer. An interview is two-sided. The employer must expect the applicant to be able to complete the job position responsibilities and the applicant must feel comfortable in assuming them.

A pleasant interview can not only land a job for an applicant but can also set the tone for the future relationship in the position. Some helpful tips for a good interview follow.

The assistant should arrive a bit early for a job interview appointment, but not too early. Entering the office 10 to 15 minutes before the appointment will give the applicant time to acclimate to the surroundings and prepare for the meeting. This period can also permit the assistant to watch the staff-patient relationship and office atmosphere.

If unsure of the office location, try a dry run the night before the interview to locate the correct place to go. Rushing in at the last moment gives a hurried appearance. The applicant may always feel a little behind.

The assistant must come to the interview alone. If a friend or relative has driven the applicant to the interview, the friend should be asked to wait outside, away from any view, until the interview is over. A potential employer does not want to see an applicant who is afraid or too dependent upon others.

The applicant should be dressed in clean and neat business attire. Hair and nails must be well kept as the employer is aware that the assistant will wear a facility-supplied barrier uniform while working in the office but the hair and nail upkeep is the responsibility of the applicant.

Perfume or cologne and makeup are generally worn but tastefully done. The perfume or cologne should not be overwhelming, and the makeup should be daytime colors and style.

Physical movement, or body language, as some people call it, tells a lot about a person. If the applicant enters the room with a smile, shakes hands, and uses the interviewer's name, the person will be impressed. Eye contact throughout the interview shows a definite interest in the job and the interviewer.

Wait to be asked to be seated and then sit erect. Do not slump down in the chair or hang over the edges. Do not perform annoying mannerisms such as thumping fingers, shaking or bouncing a leg, or any other habit that may distract from the interview (Figure 1–11).

It is said that the first thing a person notices about a new person is their appearance. The second item is a person's speech or grammar. A dental assistant must use good grammar when speaking during the meeting. The grammar of the staff indicates the image of the office. Most employers want to place high standards on the office and must have personnel who enunciate clearly and are easily understood by others. If an applicant has something to say, it should be said in a pleasant voice using full sentences, not just yes and no.

The assistant must show a good attitude. Approach everything from a positive side; stress the good and downplay the negative or weak issues. Be enthusiastic about working. The applicant must display a desire to work. If asked about former employment that was not satisfactory, talk about what was good and never talk negatively about a former employer. Simply state "Our philosophies were different" or "I would like to experience a change of pace."

The assistant must display knowledge in the field. The applicant must show the interviewer that research has been done. The assistant must have an idea of the type of work required and discuss the ability to do the work. No one knows everything about a subject. If a procedure is brought up that the assistant feels weak in or does not know, be truthful and admit that it is a new area. Quickly add "I am willing to learn it."

There will be questions throughout the meeting. The applicant should let the interviewer take the lead and ask the questions. Sometime during the interview, the assistant may be asked if he or she has any questions. If salary and benefits have not been discussed, the assistant may inquire by stating he or she has a budget to maintain and wishes to know the pay scale, hours, or benefits.

The interviewer indicates when the meeting is over. The assistant must follow the lead and prepare to leave. A smile and "thank you" with a handshake will leave a pleasant memory. The applicant should not linger about, as there may be other applicants to be interviewed or the employer may have a schedule to maintain.

The following day, the assistant should send a thank-you letter to the employer who gave the interview. This is a polite method to remind the employer of the applicant. The letter should be done on quality paper in white or a pastel shade. It should be typed in a business script and contain at least three paragraphs. The first paragraph should thank the person for the interview. A mention of the tour of the office or friendliness of the staff may merit a comment. The second paragraph should restate the applicant's interest and ability to do the job, while the third paragraph should state that the applicant is available for more interviewing, if needed. Sometimes the letter is the final deciding point in the favor of the applicant and the job becomes a reality.

It is acceptable to call an office a week after the interview to ask about the status of the position. Some offices take a long time to interview or to make decisions, and a current expression of interest may work in the applicant's favor. If the job has been filled, the assistant should thank the receptionist. If a conversation is pleasant, the applicant may inquire as to what areas can be improved for future job seeking. Always leave the conversation on a pleasant note, as more openings may occur in the future and the applicant may be remembered.▲

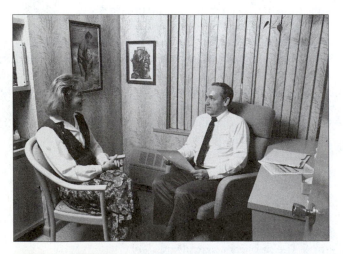

FIGURE 1–11 The interview is the most important part of the job-seeking procedure.

THEORY RECALL

Demonstrating Job Interview Skills

1. What can the assistant do during the time between the arrival at the facility and the interview?

2. If not sure of the office location for the interview, what should the assistant do before the interview appointment?

3. Why should the assistant come to an interview alone?

4. How should the assistant be dressed for the interview?

5. Should the assistant wear perfume, cologne, or makeup to an interview?

6. When seated during the interview, what should the applicant be careful not to do?

7. What does the grammar of the staff indicate to the patients?

8. How can the assistant show a positive attitude during the interview?

9. If an assistant is not aware of or does not know how to do a certain procedure, what should the assistant say to the interviewer?

10. What should the thank-you letter for an interview state?

For additional activities related to this lesson, turn to Assignment Sheet 1.9, Demonstrating Job Interview Skills, located in Appendix B of this text.

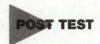

POST TEST

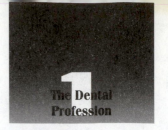
The Dental Profession

Total possible points = 100 points
80% needed for passing = 80 points

Total points this test _____ pass _____ fail _____

MATCHING: Place the letter from column B in the correct blank in column A. Each question is worth 1 point for a total of 10 points.

Column A

_____ 1. code of ethics
_____ 2. interviewer
_____ 3. outline giving applicant's attributes and positive points
_____ 4. gingival tissue specialist
_____ 5. letter introducing applicant
_____ 6. dental specialist for children
_____ 7. blind ad
_____ 8. most common method of job hunting
_____ 9. applicant
_____10. networking

Column B

a. periodontist
b. cover letter
c. discipline or manners of a profession
d. classified ads
e. person requesting employment
f. telling friends and relatives of a job need
g. pediatric dentist
h. gives little information regarding the job
i. resume
j. one attempting to hire someone

TRUE OR FALSE: Write true or false in the blank before the statement. Each question is worth 2 points for a total of 10 points.

_____ 1. Performing all dental procedures requested of the dental assistant is an indication of a trained, knowledgeable employee.

_____ 2. The title CDA is awarded to qualified dental assistants through the American Dental Assistants Association.

_____ 3. A business letter should be typed on neutral, bonded, stock paper.

_____ 4. If a question on a job application form does not relate to the applicant, the area should be left blank.

_____ 5. A short resume typed on bonded paper is considered more effective than a long resume typed on bright, contemporary, sheet paper.

MULTIPLE CHOICE: Circle the correct answer. Each question is worth 4 points for a total of 80 points.

1. Who should accompany the applicant to the job interview?
   a. no one   b. the applicant's mother   c. a friend   d. an instructor

2. What is required for the transfer or release of patient information?
   a. a call from the consulting specialist   c. a completed form request from the insurance company
   b. a call from the patient   d. a written request from the patient

3. Which of the following is *not* considered a correct title for a dentist?
   a. DDS   b. DMD   c. DMA   d. DENTIST

4. Who pays for the job placement fee when employment is accomplished by the State Employment Bureau?
   a. employer   c. neither the employer nor the applicant
   b. applicant   d. either the employer or the applicant

5. Of the following job-seeking procedures, which reveals the most information regarding the applicant?
   a. the interview   b. the application form   c. the resume   d. the report card

6. What is the intention of a disparaging remark?
   a. to offer negative criticism   c. to act insincerely
   b. to praise   d. to act indifferently

20

7. How is a code of ethics for a specific organization developed?
   a. by the National Governing Board
   b. by the organization in general
   c. by state and federal statutes
   d. through legal precedents

8. Criminal charges may be filed against the DDS for all of the following causes except
   a. improper diagnosis.
   b. income tax evasion.
   c. malicious injury.
   d. narcotic misuse.

9. Who should ask questions at a job interview?
   a. the employer
   b. the applicant
   c. both the employer and the applicant
   d. neither the employer nor the applicant

10. Which is *not* an example of information requested on a job application?
    a. physical qualities   b. work experience   c. education   d. address

11. The application of legal statutes and regulations covering the practice of dentistry is called dental
    a. laws.
    b. jurisprudence.
    c. statutes.
    d. board regulations.

12. When correcting a mistake on a patient's records, the assistant should
    a. erase the error and correct it.
    b. redo the entire record.
    c. scratch over and initial the error.
    d. pencil in the correction.

13. Who mandates the duties and responsibilities of the dental assistant?
    a. the dentist
    b. the dental hygienist
    c. the ADAA
    d. the State Dental Board

14. Which of the following situations is likely to be considered in a personal injury legal suit?
    a. removal of the wrong tooth
    b. falling on a wet floor
    c. violation of a patient's privacy
    d. neglect to treat the symptoms

15. Which type of government control is a narcotics stamp purchase?
    a. local   b. state   c. regional   d. federal

16. How long should the assistant wait to call a potential employer regarding the status of a resume or job interview?
    a. two hours   b. two days   c. one week   d. two weeks

17. During office emergencies, which is *not* the duty or responsibility of the dental assistant?
    a. to use emergency skills
    b. to assist with care
    c. to make comments
    d. to update skills

18. Which dental assistants may place the CDA initials after their names?
    a. all successful candidates
    b. assistants with 10 years of experience
    c. currently certified assistants
    d. any full-time, employed assistant

19. Job application forms should be filled in using
    a. pen.   b. pencil.   c. marker.   d. whatever is requested.

20. Which of the following dental personnel must be licensed before performing professional duties?
    a. a dental detail person
    b. a dental technician
    c. a dental hygienist
    d. a dental salesperson

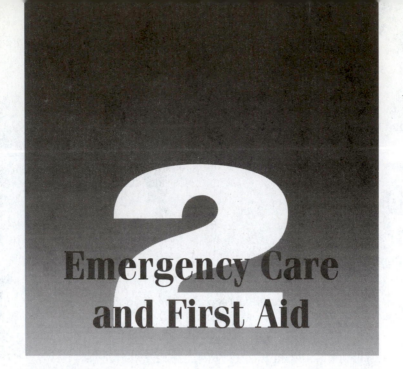

Emergency Care and First Aid

2

OBJECTIVES

Upon completion of this unit, the student will achieve a score of 80% or better on the Post Test covering the following material.

1. Briefly explain the basic emergency procedures and rules for dental office personnel.
2. Describe procedures for measuring and recording vital signs of pulse, respirations, blood pressure, and oral- and ear-style temperatures.
3. Describe methods to assist with a choking victim by identifying symptoms of inability to breathe and giving general emergency assistance techniques.
4. Discuss the Heimlich abdominal thrust maneuver for the conscious, unconscious, pregnant, or obese victim.
5. Outline steps in assisting with the one- and two-person CPR rescue methods.
6. Explain how to assist in a shock emergency, including recognizing signs and symptoms of shock, listing types of shock, and explaining procedures for care of a shock victim.

KEY TERMS

aggravate	diastolic	resuscitation
ambu bag	expiration	rhythm
anaphylactic	hemorrhagic	septic
axillary	Hg (mercury)	sphygmomanometer
brachial	inflate	sternum
cardiogenic	inspiration	stethoscope
cardiopulmonary	metabolic	supine
carotid	modification	syncope
compress	monitor	systolic
counteract	neurogenic	traumatic
dilated	psychogenic	tympanic
diaphragm	radial	xiphoid

EMERGENCY CARE PREPARATION

The most effective and efficient way of dealing with an emergency is to be prepared. Many emergencies may be prevented or minimized by following some basic health care rules. The assistant must always be alert to emergency needs. Any patient may exhibit unexpected, extreme medical problems. Stress, anxiety, or allergic reactions can happen to even the healthiest patient. Medical problems may occur during treatment of persons with diagnosed diseases and conditions. Reviewing a patient's medical history is an important step in preparation.

Remain calm and know how to seek help and offer assistance in an emergency. Knowledge of emergency tray contents and use, emergency assistance numbers, and basic emergency treatment plans helps prepare the assistant for unexpected care.

Practiced "emergencies" may provide the staff with an understanding and "know how" of operation of emergency care during stressful situations. A general review of tactics and procedures expected of staff members lessens confusion and prepares a functional team. The following steps will help the dental assistant prepare for emergency care.

Monitor Health History

Maintaining a current and correct medical history of each patient may help to avoid many emergency problems. If the office staff is aware of impending medical conditions, care may be taken to perform or administer proper treatment.

When a patient is treated for the first time in a dental office, the assistant must record medical data. The patient may be given a questionnaire to fill out or the assistant may personally interview the person regarding personal health status. The questionnaire may be lengthy or quite short, depending on the office's protocol; but particular attention should be given to present medications, allergies, drug reactions, bleeding episodes, anxiety level, and diagnosed conditions such as diabetes, epilepsy, or cardiac disorders. The history should include also the name and phone number of the patient's personal physician. All important data should be highlighted with a marking pen or indicated by bright stickers so attention is given to the condition (Figure 2–1).

Each time the patient revisits the office, the medical history should be monitored. If the interval has been a few months, the questionnaire should be reviewed. If the visit has been only a few weeks or days, the assistant should ask about the patient's health during the absence. Any replies regarding health or medical problems should be followed by questions regarding medication or treatment received during the illness.

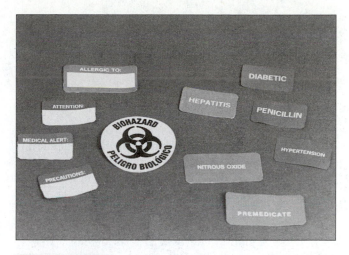

FIGURE 2–1 The dental staff is alerted by medical and health caution stickers, which are placed on patients' records in a conspicuous area. (Courtesy of Medical Arts Press, 1-800-328-2179.)

Be Alert

The dental assistant may be the first to notice an emergency is occurring. The assistant remains with the patient after a local anesthetic injection and monitors the patient following surgery, so the assistant may be first to notice a patient showing distress or experiencing some questionable problem and promptly investigate the patient's condition.

Remain Calm

The first rule the assistant must follow in an emergency is to remain calm. Panic in front of a patient can only lead to more confusion and **aggravate** the condition, causing more stress. When witnessing a malfunction, the assistant should be helpful and reassuring. A confident attitude helps assure the patient that aid will be provided.

Seek Assistance

The assistant should summon the dentist or other office help as soon as possible. Ask for help quickly and quietly, avoiding any unnecessary excitement among other patients in the office. Many dental facilities use code names for emergencies. A strong "Code Blue," "Stat" or any words can be designated as "Help, right now!"

Review Medical Records

While the assistant is awaiting help, a quick search for any medical identification tag may help with the diagnosis of the medical emergency. Many patients wear such a tag on the wrist or around the neck (Figure 2–2). The assistant should search the patient's arm and neck for a tag. A quick review of the patient's health history, looking for any alert marks, may also help diagnose the condition.

Know Emergency Numbers

To be prepared for an emergency, the assistant should have the local emergency care numbers by the telephone. Many areas have the 911 emergency number, but the assistant may have to seek help in other localities without this convenience. Local emergency numbers, including the poison control center number, should be at hand. The assistant should also search the patient's records for the personal physician's name and phone number and be prepared to call for help.

Be Familiar with the Emergency Tray

Each dental facility should have an emergency tray. The assistant should know the whereabouts of this tray and how to use the items present. Practice with the dentist and other members of the office staff to prepare all concerned for a real emergency.

Some of the items on the emergency tray are drugs used to **counteract** emergency symptoms. All drugs have a shelf life or effective period. The expiration date for the drugs on the emergency tray should be checked every few months and any drug or supply nearing the expired time limit should be reordered and replaced.

Know How to Administer Oxygen

The administration of oxygen (O_2) is indicated in most emergencies. The assistant should know the whereabouts of the oxygen supply. Oxygen is administered by the dentist, but the assistant must be prepared to assist in an emergency. In offices that use the nitrous oxide (NO_2) and oxygen central supply, the assistant should know how to place a mask and operate the gas flow (Figure 2–3). In offices that maintain a portable oxygen tank for emergency care, the assistant should know its location and how to activate and regulate the oxygen flow.

Many offices maintain an **ambu bag** on the emergency tray. This is basically a face mask with an attached balloon bulb that forces air into the patient's lungs when the bulb is squeezed. Although the air flow is not oxygen enriched, there is a higher percentage of oxygen given to the patient in this method than with mouth-to-mouth resuscitation.

Assist with Care

During an emergency, the assistant aids the dentist with care of the patient by following orders and performing duties. Being prepared and able to help with emergency drug administration, oxygen inhalation, and supportive care can be very valuable in stressful times.

Record Data

After an emergency has passed, the assistant should record the essential data on the patient's record. The date and time of the occurrence, the symptoms evidenced, and the treatment supplied are all noted and recorded. Any time periods of unconsciousness or documentation of medications used are included also. The assistant reviews the notes with the dentist to be sure everything is recorded fully and accurately (Figure 2–4).▲

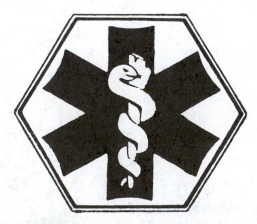

FIGURE 2–2 Persons with health problems wear necklaces, bracelets, or lapel pins with this insignia to alert care givers.

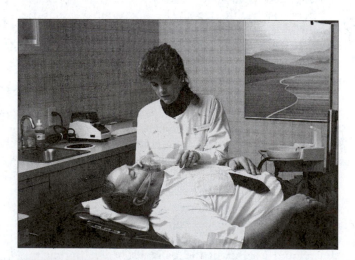

FIGURE 2–3 The dental assistant may assist with administering oxygen to an ill or distressed person.

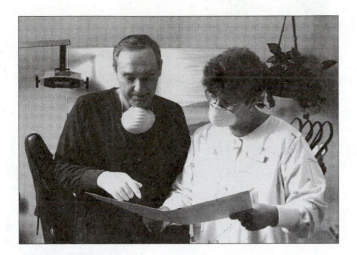

FIGURE 2-4 After an emergency, medical records are reviewed and all important information is recorded correctly.

THEORY RECALL

Emergency Care Preparation

1. What is the most effective and efficient way of dealing with an emergency?

2. How does practicing emergencies help to prepare the dental team?

3. Why is the dental assistant most often the first to notice an emergency occurring?

4. What is the first rule the assistant must follow in an emergency?

5. How may the assistant's reaction of panic affect the patient in distress?

6. What is one method to summon quick assistance in a dental office without causing unnecessary excitement?

7. What may the assistant do while waiting for aid?

8. Where should the emergency numbers be placed in the dental office?

9. What should the assistant check for on the emergency tray?

10. How may the assistant aid in the administration of oxygen in an emergency?

11. What is an ambu bag and how is it used?

12. What does the assistant record on the patient's chart after an emergency has occurred?

For additional activities related to this lesson, turn to Assignment Sheet 2.1, Emergency Care Preparation, located in Appendix B of this text.

MEASURING AND RECORDING VITAL SIGNS

Vital signs are a combination of measurements that indicate the condition of the human body. The vital signs are composed of pulse, respirations, blood pressure, and body temperature.

Pulse

Pulse is an indication of blood flow within an artery. As the heart contracts, it forces out a wave of blood causing a "beat" against the walls of the artery. In pulse point areas where the artery is situated close to the surface of the skin, the beat may be felt by applying finger pressure upon the artery and pressing toward the neighboring bone. The dental assistant counts the amount of the wave "beats" felt during a 30-second period and doubles the total for a count per minute, or the assistant might count each beat for a 1-minute period. The total count during the time period is written down as the pulse rate.

Not only the amount of beats is counted, but the **rhythm** is noticed and recorded as regular or irregular. The strength of the pulse wave is a good indication of the cardiac output. Any rippling, thready, or weak wave should be noted and recorded. Adults should have a regular, strong beat, at 65 to 90 beats per minute. Children's rates are faster at 80 to 120. Infants' pulse rates are even more rapid and may beat as much as 160 times per minute.

Respirations

Respirations, amount and type, are vital signs that may indicate the presence of anxiety or an underlying adverse health condition, such as asthma or emphysema. Any unusual breathing patterns or sounds are noted, recorded, and brought to the dentist's attention.

Blood Pressure

Blood pressure indicates the force of the flow of blood in the body during the heartbeat and in the rest period. The readings may be affected by age, personal body condition, and other external factors, such as stress, time of day, consumption of caffeine, alcohol, or nicotine.

A **stethoscope** and **sphygmomanometer** are required to take a blood pressure reading (Figure 2–5). There are three types of stethoscopes: bell, **diaphragm**, and a combination of the two. The bell-shaped stethoscope defines the low-pitched sounds while the diaphragm-type is better with high-pitched sounds and quiet murmurs. The combination stethoscope may be used in cardiac care and readings.

Sphygmomanometers are composed of three parts: the machine, the inflatable bladder cuff, and the inflation bulb with a pressure release valve. There are two types of sphygmomanometers: mercury column and aneroid dial. The mercury column types are more accurate but not as compactable and movable as the aneroid.

Body Temperature

Temperature is not taken as frequently as the other vital signs. When a patient exhibits an infected tooth or appears to be flushed, hot, or extremely tired and unresponsive, the dentist may request a temperature reading to assist with diagnosis of a probable condition.

All vital signs may be taken on a person to determine the base line readings for use in an emergency and to establish the patient's health record. Vital signs may be requested to be taken at any time in the dental office.

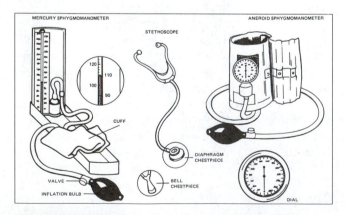

FIGURE 2-5 Blood pressure equipment used for readings. (Courtesy of Keir, Wise, and Krebs, *Medical Assisting: Administrative and Clinical Competencies*, 3rd edition, copyright 1986 by Delmar Publishers Inc.)

P R O C E D U R E   1

Measuring and Recording Vital Signs

1 Complete the Preparations

2 Measure and Record Pulse

3 Measure and Record Respirations

4 Measure and Record Blood Pressure

5 Measure and Record Temperature

6 Replace the Equipment

1 Complete the Preparations

When preparing to take and record vital signs, the assistant assembles the following equipment: watch or clock with a second hand; paper and pen for recording; sphygmomanometer and stethoscope; alcohol wipes for disinfection of earpieces, oral mercury, electric oral, or ear infrared scanner.

The assistant informs the patient that the dentist has requested a reading of the vital signs as a routine precaution. The procedure is explained.

2 Measure and Record Pulse

There are several acceptable pulse sites in the body (Figure 2–6). The **radial** pulse in the wrist is most

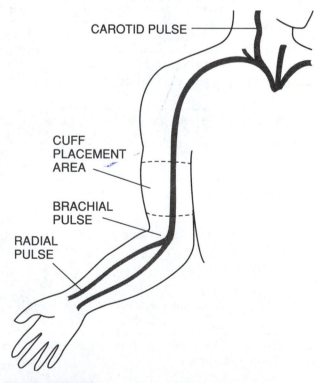

FIGURE 2-6 Correct position for taking a patient's pulse count. Pulse points may be found at the wrist (radial), elbow (brachial), or neck (carotid).

commonly used for taking the pulse count. When preparing to record the patient's pulse, the assistant bares the wrist and places the palm downward. Using the index and third fingers, press the radial artery, which is located at the wrist on the thumb side, inward. The radial artery is pressed in toward the bone until a "beat" is found. The assistant notes the time on the second hand of the clock and counts the beats of the pulse for 30 seconds or 1 minute. All 30-second readings are doubled, but the actual count is used for 1-minute readings. The total amount of beats at the end of the time period is written on the patient's chart as the pulse rate. If there is any irregularity in the rhythm or force of the beat, this is noted on the chart and brought to the dentist's attention.

3 Measure and Record Respirations

While taking the pulse, the assistant can notice the **inspirations** and **expirations** of the patient's respirations. One full inhale and exhale is counted as one full respiration. It is better not to caution the patient about taking the respirations, as the patient may control the amount and force an unnatural reading.

The assistant notices and counts the amount of respirations while taking the pulse reading. The amount of respirations at the end of the 30-second time period is doubled and written down for a count. Any shallow, labored, rasping, or noisy breathing condition is also written down and brought to the attention of the dentist. The normal respiration rate for an adult is 15 to 20 per minute. For children, 18 to 24 is considered normal.

4 Measure and Record Blood Pressure

Blood pressure (BP) measures the flow of the blood within the blood vessels at rest (**diastolic**) and under pressure (**systolic**). The assistant makes sure the patient is seated and comfortable. The arm clothing is removed or rolled up, and the deflated sphygmomanometer cuff is placed on the upper arm, around the **brachial** artery at the curve of the elbow (antecubital space). The deflated air bladder inside the cuff is centered over the artery firmly and smoothly, about two fingers above the bend of the elbow (Figure 2–7).

The assistant locates the radial pulse and **inflates** the cuff beyond a point where the pulse disappears. The release valve on the bulb is turned to permit the cuff to deflate slowly (about 2 mm **Hg** per second) until the pulse returns. The pressure reading occurring at this time is noted, and the cuff is quickly and totally deflated.

Once the systolic blood pressure point is determined, the assistant locates the brachial pulse site at the elbow crease and positions the stethoscope's diaphragm over this area. The cuff is inflated approxi-

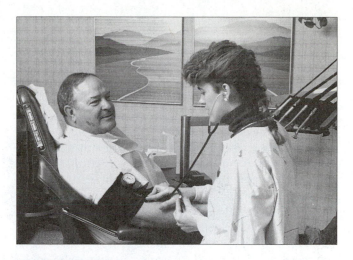

FIGURE 2–7 Position for BP reading. *Caution*: Do not maintain cuff pressure in constant position. Decrease pressure evenly and immediately.

mately 20 mm Hg beyond the determined systolic pressure point.

The cuff is deflated slowly (2 mm Hg/sec). The assistant notes the area where sounds are first heard as systolic pressure reading. When no more sounds are evident, the assistant notes this as the diastolic pressure reading.

The cuff is quickly deflated and the two noted readings are recorded. The first reading is systolic pressure and the second reading is diastolic. For example, in the reading 120/80, 120 is the systolic reading and 80 is the diastolic reading. All readings are recorded in even numbers. Systolic readings over 140 and diastolic readings over 90 are considered high and should be brought to the attention of the dentist.

The blood pressure cuff acts as a tourniquet and stops the flow of blood. Caution must be taken to avoid permitting the cuff to be inflated on the arm for a period of time. If a reading is not successfully completed on the first effort of inflation, deflate the cuff and permit recirculation of blood before another attempt is made (approximately 30 seconds).

5 Measure and Record Temperature

Temperature is a vital sign that may be taken in four areas: oral, rectal, **axillary** (armpit), and the ear. Only two methods are used in the dental office, the oral and the ear canal.

Before taking an oral temperature, the assistant should ask the patient if there has been any eating, drinking, or smoking in the last 15 minutes. Intake of cold or hot foods may alter the temperature readings if the tissues of the mouth are still warm or cold from the food or smoke.

A clean, sterile, oral thermometer that has been shaken down until the mercury is in the tip is inserted into the mouth and placed under the tongue, toward the side of the mouth. The patient is instructed to *gently* close the mouth and let the tongue cover the thermometer, which is left in the area for three minutes. At the end of the waiting period, the assistant removes the thermometer, wipes off the glass rod with a cotton ball, and reads the numbers in the column where the mercury has risen. The number is recorded as the patient's temperature. The normal temperature for an adult patient is 98.6°F.

Some offices have an electric thermometer that uses a probe cover and lessens the sterilizing duties. The assistant removes the probe from the case holder and inserts the metal probe into a clean, sterile, plastic probe cover. The probe and probe cover are inserted into the patient's mouth in the same position as the glass oral thermometer. Since the electric probe is heavier than the oral glass thermometer, the assistant may have to hold it in place for the required time. The electric thermometer does not take as long as the glass mercury column rod. The machine indicates when the temperature is reached by making a buzzing sound. The assistant removes the probe, reads the light-emitting diode (LED) printout on the bottom of the machine and records this number as the patient's temperature. The contaminated probe cover is disposed of in the contaminated trash bag by pressing on the release button on the end of the probe holder. The unsoiled machine probe is then reinserted into the probe hole of the machine.

Temperature may be taken in the ear by using the infrared **tympanic** scanner machine, which registers the heat of the tympanic membrane inside the ear (Figure 2–8). The infrared machine does not need to

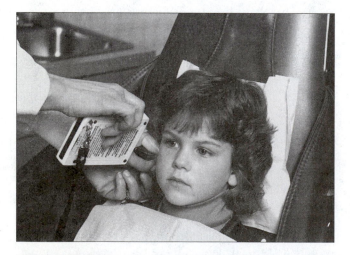

FIGURE 2–8 **The infrared scanner registers the warmth of the tympanic membrane inside the ear. It is rapid and eating or drinking does not affect the results.**

wait until the patient's mouth has cooled from eating and does not take as long to record the temperature. The machine probe end is covered with a barrier film strip, which is placed over the probe. The end of the probe is inserted in the ear canal, gently but firmly. The machine is activated by pressing the button, and the machine clicks until it finds the warmest surface. A buzz sounds to indicate when the temperature has been taken. This occurs within five seconds. The machine LED printout is read, and the temperature is recorded on the patient's chart. The barrier is removed and placed in the trash. The machine is put away.

Since this machine may be new to many patients, the assistant may demonstrate the process first by measuring the temperature of the table top or the patient's hand. When the patient can see that the process is painless, less anxiety occurs and the patient is more relaxed.

6 Replace the Equipment

After the pulse, respirations, blood pressure, and temperature have been taken and recorded, the assistant may sterilize the thermometer and the stethoscope earpieces, replace the equipment, and proceed with the patient's appointment.

The oral thermometer is cleaned with an alcohol wipe to remove film and then with a disinfectant-saturated cotton ball. The assistant grasps the barrel with the cotton ball directly below the fingers holding the thermometer. The cotton ball is rotated around the thermometer in a downward slant, running off at the tip. The assistant does not ascend the column again and in this way does not bring the microbes back up the glass rod.

The thermometer is washed with a liquid detergent-saturated cotton ball using the same motion. It is then rinsed in cool water and submerged into a chemical disinfectant bath. *The water must "feel" cool. Warm water may be too hot (over 106°F and may break the mercury column). The chemical bath may be in an emesis tray that has been lined with gauze.

When placing the thermometer into the chemical, it is recommended to record the time of insertion and removal to be sure the full sterilizing cycle is completed (8 to 10 hours for total sterilization). The thermometer is again washed off in cool water to remove the aftertaste of the chemical from the glass barrel, dried, and placed in a sterile holder until the next use.

The air is removed from the sphygmomanometer bladder by opening the pressure release valve and rolling the cuff like a jelly roll, forcing all captured air out of the bladder.

The earpieces of the stethoscope are wiped off with disinfectant-saturated gauze, and all pieces of equipment are neatly returned to the proper holding place.

Vital signs are necessary to know the patient's base readings and help if ever there is an underlying disease, problem, or emergency. ▲

Measuring and Recording Vital Signs

1. What four items compose the vital signs?

2. When discussing vital signs, what does pulse indicate?

3. How is the pulse felt?

4. Besides the count of pulse beats, what other factor is important to notice when taking the pulse?

5. What two fingers are used to place pressure when counting the radial pulse?

6. What is the normal pulse range for an adult? for a child?

7. When counting respirations on a patient, what must the assistant count to determine one respiration?

8. Why does the assistant not caution the patient when counting respirations?

9. What is the normal range of respirations per minute for an adult? for a child?

10. Is diastolic pressure the force of the blood flow when the vessel is under pressure or when it is at rest?

11. Around which artery does the assistant place the sphygmomanometer cuff to obtain a patient's blood pressure reading in the dental office?

12. Where is the diaphragm of the stethoscope placed when taking a blood pressure reading?

13. Is the systolic pressure reading taken when the sound of the heartbeat is first heard or last heard?

14. What is considered a high diastolic reading? a high systolic reading?

15. What two body areas may be used in the dental office to measure and record body temperature?

16. How long is the glass mercury thermometer kept in the mouth for a body temperature reading?

17. What is placed on the metal electric thermometer probe before inserting it into the patient's mouth?

18. Where does the infrared scanner measure body heat?

19. What is placed over the probe end of the infrared scanner?

20. How long does the infrared tympanic scanner take to record body heat?

Now turn to the Competency Evaluation Sheet for Procedure 1, Measuring and Recording Vital Signs, located in Appendix C of this text.

ASSISTING THE CHOKING VICTIM

S ometimes, without a warning, a patient may aspirate or partially swallow a large object. The foreign body may become lodged in the throat and cut off the air supply, which may cause the person's reflex action of coughing to begin.

If a person can speak, wheeze, or cough, there is some air supply entering into the lungs. The victim shows signs of great anxiety and struggles to remove the object. In the past, back blows have been recommended to assist the victim to expel the item; but it is now believed that this pressure upon the back may cause forceful inspirations that may hamper the expulsion of the foreign body. As long as the victim is suffering a partial blockage, physical assistance is not necessary. If the object becomes totally lodged and there is no air supply, the patient is not able to make any noise or cough at all. The rescuer must be ready to offer immediate assistance because the brain cannot live long without oxygen, which is supplied from the blood.

The Heimlich maneuver is a rescue method used to forcefully displace retained air in the diaphragm up and out the windpipe to dislodge a foreign object. The rescuer uses a fist-enclosed hand placed below the rib cage and under the diaphragm to administer sharp blows in an inward and upward direction. This motion is repeated 6–10 times or until the item is moved.

PROCEDURE 2

Assisting the Choking Victim

1 Be Alert

2 Seek Assistance

3 Prepare for the Heimlich Maneuver

4 Administer the Heimlich Maneuver (Standing Victim)

5 Administer the Heimlich Maneuver (Patient on the Floor)

6 Administer the Heimlich Maneuver (Seated Patient)

7 Administer the Heimlich Maneuver (Pregnant or Obese Person)

8 Search the Oral Cavity

9 Monitor the Recovered Patient

10 Record Emergency Treatment on the Patient's Chart

1 Be Alert

Sometime during the course of treatment, the assistant may notice a patient suffering distress. The person may be grasping the neck, eyes open and terror-filled, coughing, or unable to speak or breathe (Figure 2–9). A quick question "Are you choking?" should bring about a head nod meaning "yes." If the patient cannot speak or cough, there is a great possibility that the airway is totally blocked. If the patient is coughing or wheezing, but in distress, there is a possibility that there is only a partial block of the airway. In either case, the patient needs assistance.

2 Seek Assistance

The assistant must stay calm and seek help. A quick code call should bring other members of the dental team. If the dentist feels the emergency is severe enough, an order to call the emergency assistance squad may be given. The assistant should have the phone number handy and perform the call, giving the name of the caller, the nature of the emergency, and the location. The assistant should remain on the phone until the operator is finished gathering information.

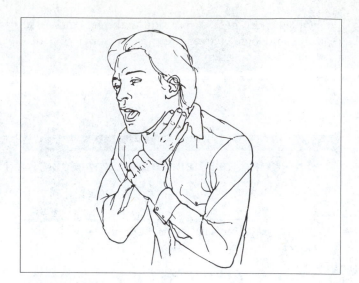

FIGURE 2–9 Choking victims cannot speak or make a noise to alert rescuers. (Courtesy of the American Red Cross. All rights reserved in all countries.)

3 Prepare for the Heimlich Maneuver

If the choking condition continues, the assistant may position the patient for a Heimlich subdiaphragmatic abdominal thrust maneuver. The patient is assisted to stand with the assistant supporting the victim.

4 Administer the Heimlich Maneuver (Standing Victim)

While the patient is standing, the assistant moves to the rear of the victim, explaining what procedure is going to take place. Both arms of the assistant encircle the patient, while supporting the patient under the armpits. The assistant closes one hand into a fist and places the fist, with the thumb side towards the victim, above the belt line and below the rib cage (Figure 2–10). The patient is instructed to lean over slightly; the assistant grabs the closed fist with the other hand and gives a quick thrust, inward and upward. The thrust is repeated six to ten times. The entire sequence is repeated again, if needed, until the object is expelled and the patient may breathe again.

5 Administer the Heimlich Maneuver (Patient on the Floor)

If the patient has fallen to the floor or is too heavy to support, the assistant places the victim in a **supine** position (on the back with the face up) and then straddles the patient. The assistant interlaces the hands with the heel of the palm of one hand against the patient and the other hand supporting the palm's heel. With the palm placed above the belt line and below

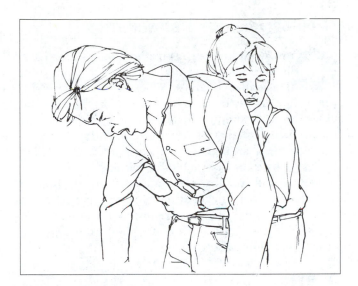

FIGURE 2–10 The Heimlich maneuver being administered to a conscious victim. (Courtesy of the American Red Cross. All rights reserved in all countries.)

the rib cage, a quick thrust is given five to ten times or as needed to remove the trapped object (Figure 2–11). If the patient begins choking, the assistant ceases the thrust and permits the patient to cough up the object.

6 Administer the Heimlich Maneuver (Seated Patient)

If the patient is seated in the dental chair or the waiting room chair, the assistant or rescue person approaches the victim from the rear and positions the patient and rescuer in the same manner as a standing maneuver. The fist is placed with the thumb side above the belt line and under the rib cage, and the thrusts are inward and upward until the object is dislodged.

7 Administer the Heimlich Maneuver (Pregnant or Obese Person)

A pregnant woman or an obese person needs some **modification** to the thrust motion. The rescuer stands behind the pregnant woman or obese person and encircles the victim, supporting from under the armpits. The fist is placed on the midsection of the person's **sternum**. The chest thrusts are performed in a backward and inward motion until the item is removed or the patient chokes and expels the object.

8 Search the Oral Cavity

The dentist or dental assistant may perform a search of the oral cavity only on an unconscious adult victim or on a child when the foreign object is in view. This type of assistance may be performed by a C-swerve

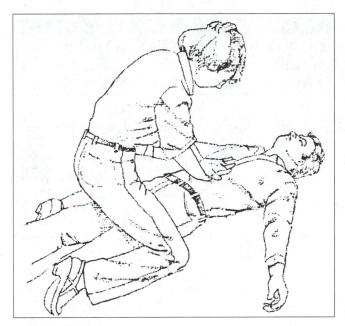

FIGURE 2–11 The Heimlich maneuver being administered to an unconscious victim. (Courtesy of the American Red Cross. All rights reserved in all countries.)

finger search, vacuum evacuator, or suction tip sweep of the mouth. In either maneuver, the rescuer must be careful not to enter directly into the mouth and push the object deeper into the throat. The sweep action must be from side to side, with a hooking action toward the front. Alternating patterns of abdominal thrusts and finger sweeps may be made on an unconscious person or child until the object is removed or coughed up.

If the victim is coughing, wheezing, or making any noise, the patient is permitted to expel the object by reflex action.

9 Monitor the Recovered Patient

When the object has been removed or expelled, the assistant **monitors** the patient reassuringly. A mask containing oxygen may be placed over the patient's nose and mouth to relieve any stress and to quiet the victim. The assistant remains with the patient until the patient is fully recovered.

10 Record Emergency Treatment on the Patient's Chart

When the patient has been dismissed, the assistant records the emergency on the patient's chart, noting the date, time, treatment, and outcome of the situation. All notes and data are reviewed with the dentist for completeness and accuracy.▲

Assisting the Choking Victim

1. List three symptoms of a choking victim.

   a. _____

   b. _____

   c. _____

2. What should the assistant say to a patient who looks as if he or she cannot breathe?

   _____

3. What is the first thing an assistant must do in a choking emergency?

   _____

4. If an assistant must make a call for the emergency squad, what should the assistant say to the operator?

   _____

5. Where is the patient positioned during a standing Heimlich maneuver?

   _____

6. Where does the assistant place the fist for the standing Heimlich maneuver?

   _____

7. If the victim is on the floor, where does the assistant position self?

   _____

8. What modification does the pregnant woman require in the Heimlich maneuver?

   _____

9. How many thrusts are given to the victim in the Heimlich maneuver?

   _____

10. What type of action should be employed in a C-swerve finger search of a choking person?

    _____

11. What should the rescuer do if the victim begins to cough?

    _____

12. What should the assistant do with the patient after the item has been dislodged or removed?

    _____

13. What is recorded on the patient's chart after the emergency has passed?

    _____

Now turn to the Competency Evaluation Sheet for Procedure 2, Assisting the Choking Victim, located in Appendix C of this text.

CARDIOPULMONARY RESUSCITATION

Cardiopulmonary resuscitation (CPR), a basic life support procedure, restores the function of the heart and lungs. When a patient has suffered an emergency and becomes unconscious, the assistant must attempt to breathe for the victim by inflating the lungs and provide circulation by compressing the heart between the chest and spine, thereby taking over the body's life-functioning tasks.

Dental and medical personnel should be trained and certified in an accepted course given by the American Heart Association or the American Red Cross. The basic principles of the CPR procedure are airway, breathing, and circulation.

Airway

Open the airway. Determine the status of the victim's breathing. Many times, the victim's tongue may drop back and block the airway. Tilting the head back and moving the chin and jaw forward lifts the tongue and opens the airway.

Breathing

Restore breathing through artificial respiration. The breath of the rescuer contains more than enough oxygen to supply a victim's immediate need for air. Mouth-to-mouth breathing should be supplied until the victim is able to breathe unassisted or professional aid is present.

Circulation

Determine the status of the victim's pulse. If there is none, restore circulation by applying chest compressions. Pressure upon the victim's chest can **compress** the lungs and force the rescuer's breath throughout the bloodstream, feeding oxygen to the brain and tissues.

Once starting the basic life-support procedures, the rescuer must continue with the care until:

▶ the patient recovers,
▶ emergency medical technicians (EMTs) take over,
▶ the patient is declared dead by a physician,
▶ the rescuer becomes totally and completely exhausted, or
▶ the scene becomes unsafe.

P R O C E D U R E   3
Cardiopulmonary Resuscitation

1 Examine the Patient

2 Position the Patient

3 Attempt to Relieve Blockage

4 Perform CPR (One Person)

5 Continue CPR

6 Perform CPR (Two Persons)

7 Exchange Rescuers

8 Record the Emergency on the Patient's Chart

1 Examine the Patient

If a patient loses consciousness, the assistant should shake the victim and try to determine if the person is breathing. If the individual does not respond and breathing is not present, the assistant calls for assistance, tilts the head back and extends the chin to open the airway. In some cases, this maneuver removes the tongue or offending object and the patient can breathe again (Figure 2–12).

The assistant must check for breathing by listening for breaths, searching the chest for rising and falling, and feeling for expelled air from the nose. If no breathing is found, the rescuer should pinch the victim's nostrils, make a tight seal around the victim's mouth and give two slow breaths ($1\frac{1}{2}$ to 2 seconds per breath) watching for a rise and fall of the chest. If the breathing technique is successful, a check of the **carotid** artery for a pulse should be made to determine if the heart has ceased beating.

To check the carotid artery, the rescuer places the index and third fingers on the patient's neck near the larynx (Adam's apple) sliding sideways into the groove on the neck. Pressure is gently applied inward and upward to feel for a pulse action (Figure 2–13).

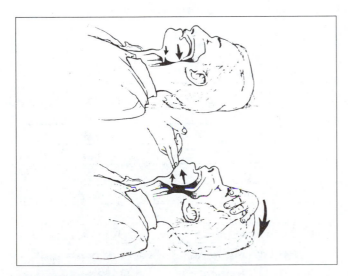

FIGURE 2–12 The airway must be open and clear before any CPR may be given. (Courtesy of the American Red Cross. All rights reserved in all countries.)

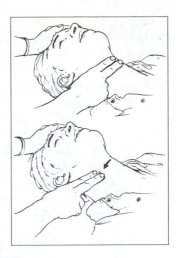

FIGURE 2–13 The assistant should practice locating the carotid artery to be familiar with the position in a time of emergency. (Courtesy of the American Red Cross. All rights reserved in all countries.)

2 Position the Patient

If no breathing or pulsation is occurring, the assistant must prepare for CPR. The patient must be placed on a hard surface. The dental chair is not hard enough to resist compression pressure. Without a backboard, this motion would be useless or ineffective. Once the patient is on the floor in a supine position, the assistant retilts the head to open the airway and prepares to inflate the lungs by pinching the nostrils with one hand and extending the mandible upward and forward with the other hand to open the airway. The mouth-to-mouth seal is reapplied and the rescuer again gives two slow, deep breaths into the victim's mouth to inflate the lungs. The assistant watches to see if the breathing causes the chest to rise and fall, which determines if the airway is open. *An alternate method to give breaths and inflate the lungs is to use an S-curve disposable airway or mask device, which is found on most dental emergency trays. The airway is carefully placed, and the rescuer breathes into the plastic airway to inflate the lungs.

3 Attempt to Relieve Blockage

If the chest does not rise and fall, the air is not getting into the lungs. Any further CPR attempts are fruitless until air inflates the lungs. An effort to reposition the chin to open the airway and reinflate the lungs can be tried. If no air is moving the chest, an attempt must be made to dislodge the blocking object by carefully inserting the finger into the mouth and sweeping from side to side to locate any object. C-swerve finger searches may be performed only on unconscious adults or on children when the foreign object is visible.

If nothing is found in the mouth, the assistant may straddle the patient and place the heel of the palm above the belt line and below the rib cage and use the other hand behind the palm heel to give a few upward thrusts to expel the obstruction (Heimlich maneuver).

If the airway opens, the assistant may proceed with CPR. Nothing can progress until the lungs are able to be inflated. If the lungs are not open, the sequence is repeated.

4 Perform CPR (One Person)

Once the airway is open, the assistant may proceed with CPR. The carotid artery is checked for pulsations. If the pulse is found, only lung inflation is attempted at the rate of one breath every 5 seconds (12 times per minute) for an adult and one breath every 4 seconds (15 times per minute) for a child. (Table 2–1 shows variations in CPR techniques for the infant, child, and adult.) If no pulse is found, the assistant must aid the body functions by compressing the heart to move the air-enriched blood through the body.

The assistant gives two breaths to the victim to inflate the lungs and then moves to the side of the patient to begin chest compressions. The rescuer locates the patient's sternum (breastbone) by tracing the rib cage margin to the chest and moves two fingers up from the **xiphoid** tip (bottom edge of the rib cage) to place the heel of the intertwined palms on

the sternum (Figure 2–14).

Kneeling above the victim with shoulders over the chest, the assistant compresses the victim's sternum approximately 1½ to 2 inches. The compression is repeated 15 times (Figure 2–15). A rhythm of 80 to 100 compressions per minute (slightly faster than one per second) is maintained. After each 15 compressions, the assistant moves to the head and gives two inflating breaths, watching the rise and fall of the chest. When

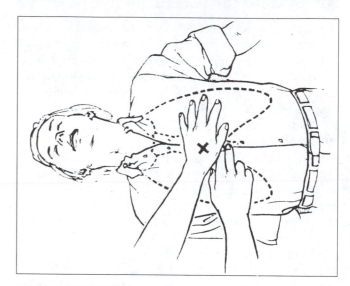

FIGURE 2–14 Correct method to observe and use for hand placement in chest compression. (Courtesy of the American Red Cross. All rights reserved in all countries.)

TABLE 2–1

Variations in CPR Techniques for the Infant, Child, and Adult (Courtesy of the American Red Cross. All rights reserved in all countries.)

AGE	INFANT 0–1 YR.	CHILD 1–8 YR.	ADULT < 8 YR.
Shake and shout	**Shake only**	Yes	Yes
Call for help	Yes	Yes	Yes
Position victim	Yes	Yes	Yes
Open airway	Yes	Yes	Yes
Look, listen, feel for breath	Yes	Yes	Yes
Two breaths	Yes	Yes	Yes
Check pulse	**Brachial**	Carotid	Carotid
Activate EMS	Yes	Yes	Yes
Locate hand position	Lower sternum	Lower sternum	Lower sternum
Compress with	**2–3 fingers**	**Heel of one hand**	**Heel of two hands**
Compression depth	**½–1 inch**	**1–1½ inches**	**1½–2 inches**
Compressions per minute	**At least 100**	80–100	80–100
Compression:Ventilation ratio	5:1	5:1	**15:2 or 5:1***

*Rates for one-rescuer (15:2) and two-rescuer (5:1) adult CPR.

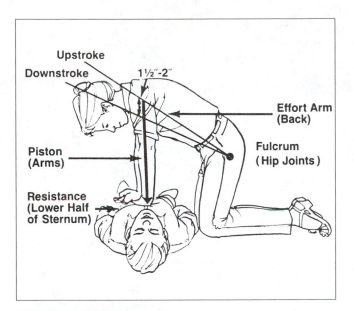

FIGURE 2-15 The shoulders must be centered over the victim's chest to provide the correct compression. (Courtesy of the American Red Cross. All rights reserved in all countries.)

inflations are completed, compressions are regiven. The cycle, 15:2, is repeated until aid arrives or a doctor confirms death.

5 Continue CPR

The assistant should recheck the carotid artery following every four cycles of compressions and breaths. If a pulse starts, the compressions are stopped and only inflations are continued until the patient breathes again.

6 Perform CPR (Two Persons)

Two-person CPR may be given if assistance arrives. The second rescuer determines if emergency aid has been summoned and does so if needed. The helper checks the victim's pulse. If one is present, only breathing aid is given. If a pulse is absent, ventilation and compression must continue.

The two rescuers have the option to continue as a team (compressor and ventilator) or alternate the role of one-person CPR assistance to the limits of each other's ability.

If working as a team, one rescuer gives breaths (ventilator) while the second rescuer gives compressions (compressor). The new rescuer positions self prepared to start compressions as the first rescuer completes the full cycle of 15 compressions and 2 breaths. After the forced breathing, the first rescuer says "Pulse check" and feels the carotid artery for approximately 5 seconds. If no pulse is determined, the second rescuer begins compressions. The first res-

cuer remains as the ventilator and gives one breath to inflate the lungs after each set of five compressions that the second rescuer gives. This cycle of 1 breath for every 5 compressions is maintained until help arrives or the rescuers tire and need to change. The breaths are never given when a compression is occurring because no air could enter the lungs during this pressure. Count one, two, three, four, five, breathe, repeat. Rescuer one may check the carotid artery more often to determine if the heart is pulsating or if the compressions are working. Whenever the heart beats independently, the compressions are stopped.

7 Exchange Rescuers

If CPR must be maintained for a long period of time, the rescuers may become tired and wish to exchange positions. The compressor rescuer orders the exchange and compresses while saying "Change-and, two-and, three-and, four-and, five." The ventilator rescuer gives the breath after count five and moves to the victim's side. Both rescuers assume the duties they have exchanged. The sternum and xiphoid are located, the palm heels are situated properly, and the new compressor waits for the signal to begin compressions. The carotid artery is checked to determine if the heart has begun beating. The new ventilator rescuer tilts the head, opens the airway, and inflates the lungs. The new compressor rescuer begins, and the CPR cycle continues until aid arrives (Figure 2–16).

8 Record the Emergency on the Patient's Chart

When the emergency is over, the assistant records the event on the patient's chart. The date, day, and time are noted. The symptoms observed and the treatment given are written down. Any times noted for unconsciousness or CPR assistance are recorded. The assistant reviews the summary with the dentist for completeness and accuracy.▲

T H E O R Y   R E C A L L

Cardiopulmonary Resuscitation

1. What do the initials CPR designate?

   _____

2. What two body functions do the rescuers take over for the victim in CPR?

   _____

3. When a patient loses consciousness, what does the assistant do?

   _____

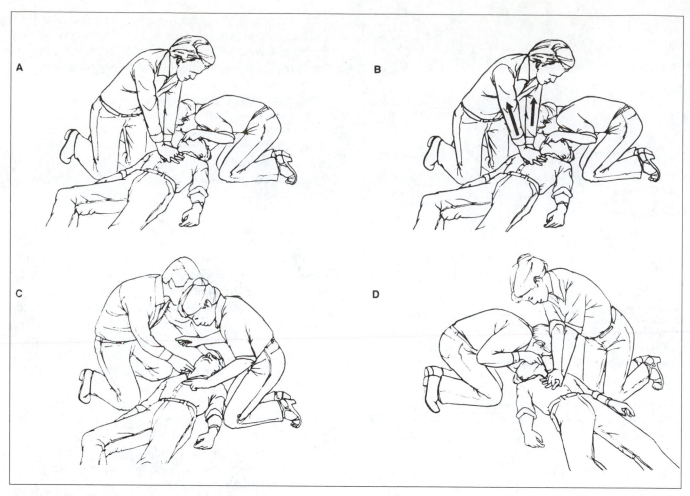

FIGURE 2-16 Exchange of rescuers is a team action. Chest compression and breath rhythm is maintained. (A) Compressor calls for exchange and counts. (B) Ventilator gives the breath at the end of the fifth compression count. (C) Ventilator moves to victim's chest and locates compression site. Compressor moves to victim's head and checks pulse. (D) New ventilator gives breath and starts cycle. (Courtesy of the American Red Cross. All rights reserved in all countries.)

4. How does the assistant check for breathing?

_____

5. How does the assistant determine if the patient's heart is beating?

_____

6. If the assistant attempts to inflate the lungs and the effort is unsuccessful, what does the assistant do next?

_____

7. If the airway is open, what must the assistant check before beginning chest compressions?

_____

8. Where does the assistant place the palm heels for chest compressions?

_____

9. How deeply does the assistant compress the chest in CPR?

_____

10. What is the rate of breaths and compressions in one-person CPR?

_____

11. How often does the assistant check the carotid artery when giving CPR?

_____

12. When two persons are available for CPR, what is the rate of the breaths and chest compressions?

_____

13. When rescuers wish to exchange positions in CPR, who issues the command?

_____

14. How long is CPR continued?

_____

15. When the emergency is over, what does the assistant do with the patient's chart?

_____

Now turn to the Competency Evaluation Sheet for Procedure 3, Cardiopulmonary Resuscitation, located in Appendix C of this text.

ASSISTING WITH A SHOCK EMERGENCY

Shock is a sign of the body functions undergoing undue stress and damage. There are early symptoms of shock that may progress to stronger signs. If left unattended and untreated, shock may result in death.

Shock may occur as a result of many different factors. The most common type in the dental office is **psychogenic** or **neurogenic** shock, which is indicated in patients who are extremely anxious and undergoing stress. Blood circulation to the brain is decreased due to tension tightening, and fainting (**syncope**) may result.

Diabetic patients who have missed breakfast or forgotten their medication may undergo a **metabolic** disturbance resulting in shock. Trembling, sweating, dizziness, paleness, and convulsions may indicate a sugar imbalance. Left untreated, the patient may suffer insulin or metabolic shock and collapse.

Patients may exhibit a severe reaction to a dental injection or materials in use. Congestion, itching, rash, and tissue swelling may cause labored breathing and an eventual body function reaction called **anaphylactic** shock. This may be very serious and needs immediate treatment.

A heart patient may undergo a malfunction of the heart, which, in turn, may cease blood circulation and cause **cardiogenic** shock. CPR and medical help must be given to this patient.

Other possible problems that are rarely seen in the dental office are **hemorrhagic** shock (excessive bleeding), **septic** shock, (infection throughout the bloodstream), and aspirated foreign objects causing cessation of breathing and respiratory shock.

The dental assistant must be prepared to deal with shock and the breakdown of body functions.

▶ P R O C E D U R E   4
Assisting with a Shock Emergency

1 Discuss Various Types of Shock and Causes

2 State General Symptoms of Shock

3 Give General Rules for Care of a Shock Patient

4 Demonstrate Care of a Fainting Victim (Syncope)

5 Demonstrate Care of an Anaphylactic Shock Victim

6 Demonstrate Care of a Heart Attack Shock Victim

7 Record the Emergency on the Patient's Chart

1 Discuss Various Types of Shock and Causes

There are various types and causes of shock. The most common type of shock in the dental office is fainting (syncope), which is brought on by anxiety and stress. This type of shock is psychogenic. Another type of shock found in the dental office is anaphylactic or allergic reaction shock. Occasionally, a person reacts to an injection or medication and the body functions undergo stress.

A patient may aspirate an object and choke. This may force the body to go into a respiratory shock. The object must be removed before the shock can be treated. Patients on insulin may undergo a metabolic shock caused from too much or too little insulin.

Any patient may suffer a heart attack, which causes the body functions to undergo stress and shock. Cardiogenic shock may be fatal without immediate assistance. Persons who have been poisoned, have blood poisoning, or have viral infections may suffer septic shock. Hemorrhage also may cause the body to go into shock. Loss of blood and body fluids force a body shutdown. Anyone who has undergone a **traumatic** accident and received massive body damage may go into traumatic shock.

2 State General Symptoms of Shock

Shock symptoms are similar in the early stages, but as shock progresses, so also do the symptoms and complications. Early visible signs of shock may be pale skin that is cool or clammy to the touch. The patient may suffer excessive perspiration and show signs of anxiety, restlessness, and panic. Vital sign readings may record a rapid, weak pulse with shallow and rapid respirations. Blood pressure also may be low.

As the shock progresses, the patient's eyes may look vacant and the pupils may become **dilated**. The victim may complain of thirst, blurred vision, and weakness, and may lose consciousness, which eventually may be fatal.

3 Give General Rules for Care of a Shock Patient

The general rules for shock are to eliminate the cause for the body stress and restore the body functions (Table 2–2). The assistant should stay calm, seek assistance, try to help restore oxygen to the system, keep the patient warm, and maintain body functioning.

4 Demonstrate Care of a Fainting Victim (Syncope)

When a person faints or suffers syncope, the assistant should remain calm, seek assistance, and lower the patient's head to increase the flow of oxygen to the patient's brain (Figure 2–17). Spirits of ammonia

TABLE 2-2

Emergency Conditions—Causes, Symptoms, and Treatment

Emergency	Causes	Symptoms	Treatment
Syncope	partial or complete loss of blood supply to the brain	tingling of hands and feet, numbness, sweating, pallor, low skin temperature, dizziness, vision disturbances, loss of consciousness	place patient in supine position, raise legs and hips to elevate height, loosen tight clothing, give spirits of ammonia, maintain airway
Hyperventilation	imbalance of respiratory gases due to fear, stress, activity	anxiety, chest pain, lightheadedness, numbness and tingling of fingers and toes, increased pulse, increased BP, increased respirations, shallower exhale of air	end treatment, remove anxiety reason, position patient upright for breathing, remove materials from mouth, calm and reassure the patient, let the patient breathe into a paper bag (6–8 times per minute)
Shock	depressed state of vital functions caused by different factors—stress, injury, allergic reaction, loss of blood, etc.	weak, fast, irregular pulse; low BP rate; increased breathing, weakness, nausea, or vomiting; pale, clammy skin	place patient in supine position, elevate legs, keep warm, give fluids if not unconscious, consult MD
Asthmatic attack	allergic reaction or extreme stress	patient usually aware of onset; labored, wheezy breathing; high BP; flushed; sweating	use patient's own medicine, calm patient, make comfortable
Allergic reaction	response to specific irritant	congestion, rash, restlessness, pale or bluish skin, itch, mucous membrane swelling, labored breathing, headache	if severe call MD, place in supine position, administer O_2, monitor vital signs
Heart attack	coronary artery occlusion	extreme chest pain, sweating, pallor, radiating pain in left arm and shoulder, labored breathing, weakness, loss of consciousness	summon medical aid at once, put in position of comfort, maintain airway and circulation
Insulin shock	excessive amount of insulin in blood supply	trembling, sweating, dizziness, rapid pulse, paleness, convulsions, collapse	consult patient's MD, supine position, keep warm, give sugar
Diabetic coma	insufficient supply of insulin in blood supply	flushed, hot, red complexion, irregular breathing, acetone-odor breath, drowsiness	consult MD, supine position, keep warm, give insulin, monitor vital signs

Emergency	Causes	Symptoms	Treatment
Hemorrhage	excessive bleeding from wound or lack of ability to clot	bright red flow from arteries, dark red flow from veins	direct pressure, elevate pressure point, get medical aid
Epileptic seizure	unknown origin, may be stimulated by bright light flashes	Grand Mal—possible mention of aura before attack, chewing and biting on tongue, involuntary urination and defecation, muscles twitch and rigid, loss of consciousness Petit Mal—interrupted speech; staring; lip smacking; arm, leg, or eyelid twitch	protect patient from self-injury, support vital signs, administer O_2, seek EMT help to transport to MD

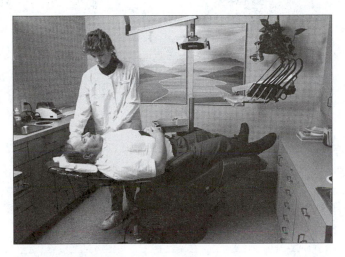

FIGURE 2-17 The fainting patient's head is lowered and oxygen is administered.

should be administered by smashing the vial away from the victim's face, then waving the contents below the nose of the individual. Care must be taken not to hold the vial too close to the patient or for too long a period. Gentle wiffing motions place enough restorative fumes. A mask with oxygen may be applied for the patient's comfort, and the assistant should reassure the victim and remain with the person until the crisis passes. Vital signs are taken frequently during the emergency to determine the body functions.

5 Demonstrate Care of an Anaphylactic Shock Victim

If a patient has an allergic reaction to an injection or medication, the shock symptoms are more severe and skin signs may appear. The patient may wheeze, show a rash, and complain of the "funny, thickening feel of the tongue." A person in anaphylactic shock requires the same treatment as the fainting person, but the dentist may request the assistant to call the emergency squad assistance and prepare for an injection of an antihistamine, usually epinephrine. The assistant may obtain the emergency carpule of epinephrine from the emergency tray, remove the anesthetic carpule from the syringe and replace it with the epinephrine. The prepared syringe is passed to the dentist, who injects the patient.

Oxygen is given to the anaphylactic shock patient. Vital signs are monitored and the patient is kept warm until the medication takes effect and the emergency passes or the EMT arrives and takes over.

6 Demonstrate Care of a Heart Attack Shock Victim

Patients who suffer heart attacks are most in danger of severe shock in the dental office. The patient may complain of a pain in the chest or left arm or heat in the room, or he or she may become unconscious. The assistant remains calm, seeks assistance, and helps to administer oxygen. The heart patient may be more comfortable in a seated position, rather than one with the head lowered. The assistant may help to apply the oxygen mask and regulate the flow to ease the patient's pain and stress. Patients with heart problems often carry their own medication for emergency use, which may be given to the distressed victim.

An emergency squad should be summoned. A phone call to the patient's physician may be made. The dentist may offer the victim a nitroglycerin tablet to place under the tongue for pain relief. The patient's vital signs are monitored, the oxygen flow maintained, and the patient is kept warm until the emergency squad arrives.

If the patient lapses into unconsciousness and there is no breathing or pulse, CPR must be started and maintained until help arrives.

7 Record the Emergency on the Patient's Chart

When the emergency has passed, the assistant records the events on the patient's chart, and notes the date, day, and time. The symptoms observed and the treatment given are recorded. If the patient reacted negatively to a medication, it should be noted in large red letters to avoid a similar occurrence. All data is reviewed with the dentist for completeness and accuracy.▲

THEORY RECALL

Assisting with a Shock Emergency

1. What is shock?

   _____

2. What is the most common type of shock in the dental office?

   _____

3. What is anaphylactic shock?

   _____

4. A patient who chokes on an object can go into what kind of shock?

   _____

5. Patients who are taking insulin may go into what kind of shock?

   _____

6. List three visible signs of shock.

   a. _____

   b. _____

   c. _____

7. List three rules for the treatment of shock.

   a. _____

   b. _____

   c. _____

8. What is syncope?

   _____

9. What medication should be used on a syncope victim?

   _____

10. What body signs may be evident in an anaphylactic shock patient?

    _____

11. What type of medication does the dentist give to an anaphylactic victim?

    _____

12. Which type of patient is most in danger of severe shock in the dental office?

    _____

13. If the heart patient lapses into unconsciousness, what should the dental assistant do?

    _____

14. What medication may the dentist give the heart patient to ease pain?

    _____

15. How should the medication that caused the anaphylactic reaction be noted on the patient's chart?

    _____

Now turn to the Competency Evaluation Sheet for Procedure 4, Assisting with a Shock Emergency, located in Appendix C of this text.

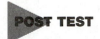
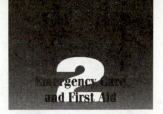

Total possible points = 100 points
80% needed for passing = 80 points

Total points this test_____ pass _____ fail_____

FILL IN: Fill in the blank with the correct answer. Each question is worth 1 point for a total of 4 points.

1. The rescuer who inflates the lungs during two-person CPR is called the _____.

2. The artery located in the neck is the _____.

3. Respiration, temperature, pulse, and blood pressure are collectively called _____ _____.

4. The ear thermometer measures the heat of the _____ membrane.

MATCHING: Write the letter from column B that best describes or matches the word in column A.
Each question is worth 2 points for a total of 16 points.

Column A (Shock)	Column B (Cause)
_____ 1. psychogenic	a. massive body damage
_____ 2. metabolic	b. allergic reaction
_____ 3. anaphylactic	c. excessive blood loss
_____ 4. cardiogenic	d. blocked airway
_____ 5. hemorrhagic	e. syncope
_____ 6. septic	f. blood infection
_____ 7. respiratory	g. insulin imbalance
_____ 8. traumatic	h. heart problem

MULTIPLE CHOICE: Circle the correct answer. Each question is worth 4 points for a total of 80 points.

1. Which artery is used when taking a blood pressure reading?
   a. radial   b. brachial   c. arterial   d. femoral

2. What is the most common emergency in the dental office?
   a. heart attack   b. diabetic shock   c. seizures   d. syncope

3. When administering the Heimlich maneuver on a pregnant woman, where is the fist placed?
   a. at the midsection of the sternum   c. between the ribs and the waist
   b. 2 inches above the belt line   d. under the sternum and between the ribs

4. Which of the following blood pressure readings should be reported to the dentist?
   a. 106/78   b. 120/80   c. 128/88   d. 150/98

5. What does the ambu bag force into the patient's lungs?
   a. medicated air   b. the rescuer's breath   c. atmosphere air   d. NO_2 and O_2

6. The systolic pressure of a blood pressure reading is a record of the heart
   a. while at rest.   b. under medication.   c. while beating.   d. at death.

7. The most efficient way to handle an emergency is to
   a. be prepared.   b. remain calm.   c. update skills.   d. do a, b, and c.

8. A wheezing patient developing a rash and a thick tongue could be suffering from which type of shock?
   a. anaphylactic   b. diabetic   c. heart attack   d. psychogenic

9. What is the depth of chest compressions for an adult CPR patient?
   a. 1 inch   b. 1½ inches   c. 2½ inches   d. 4 inches

10. A C-swerve finger search to remove mouth objects is performed on
    a. all choking patients.   c. adult patients only.
    b. unconscious adults and children.   d. pregnant women only.

11. Which is the best medication for a victim of syncope?
    a. insulin   b. epinephrine   c. nitroglycerin   d. spirits of ammonia

12. Which of the following is *not* considered a vital sign?
    a. weight   b. blood pressure   c. pulse   d. temperature

13. When performing CPR, the rescuer takes over which body functions?
    a. circulation and respiration   c. respiration and breathing
    b. circulation and excretions   d. circulation and pulse

14. What is the first thing a dental assistant does for a choking victim?
    a. beats on the back   c. gives O_2
    b. the Heimlich maneuver   d. remains calm and gets help

15. A victim grasping the neck, with terror-filled eyes, and unable to speak could be a victim of
    a. choking.   b. a heart attack.   c. an insulin attack.   d. syncope.

16. During a standing Heimlich maneuver, the patient is situated in which position to the rescuer?
    a. in front of   b. in back of   c. to the side of   d. under

17. The normal pulse rate for an adult is
    a. 60 beats per minute.   c. 100 beats per minute.
    b. 80 beats per minute.   d. 120 beats per minute.

18. During one-person CPR, how frequently should the carotid artery be checked?
    a. with every compression   c. with every four cycles of compressions and breaths
    b. with every other compression and breath cycle   d. approximately every 30 seconds

19. What medication may a dentist administer to a heart attack victim?
    a. salt tablets   b. nitroglycerin tablets   c. sugar   d. insulin

20. A victim with a bluish, cool, clammy skin; excessive perspiration; anxiety and nervousness; rapid weak pulse; and rapid respirations could be suffering from a
    a. heart attack.   b. diabetic coma.   c. heat stroke.   d. seizure.

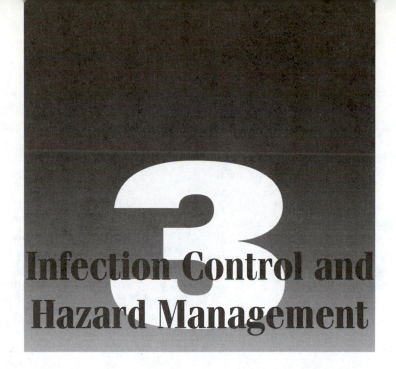

3

Infection Control and Hazard Management

▶ OBJECTIVES

Upon completion of this unit, the student will achieve a score of 80% or better on the Post Test covering the following material.

1. Identify the regulatory agencies concerned with the dental office, citing job classification, hepatitis vaccination, employee training, recording and exposure plans, and protection practices.
2. Discuss the term "chain of asepsis" and the importance of using universal precautions beginning with the steps and performance of a proper handwashing technique.
3. Describe and demonstrate the method for donning and removing barrier attire.
4. Explain the importance and demonstrate the use of the ultrasonic cleaner.
5. Demonstrate the procedure for preparing for and using the autoclave.
6. Discuss sterilization procedures using dry heat, vapor chemicals, and sterilizing indicators.
7. Discuss methods for cleanup and disposal of wastes, including the handling of sharps and disposal of hazardous materials.
8. Describe hazard and safety controls and general precautions in the dental office for model trimmers, dental lathes, chemicals, and vapors.
9. State precautions and measures to be used for fire control, and demonstrate the use of a fire extinguisher.

▶ KEY TERMS

activator	clinical attire	pressurized
ambidextrous	compliance	regulates
antimicrobial	contaminated	sanitation
asepsis	deodorize	sequence
beaker	disinfection	sterilization
biohazard	hazardous	techniques
bloodborne	immunization	ultrasonic cleaner
cassette	infectious	universal
caustic	pathogens	precautions
cavitate	penetrate	verification

COMPLYING WITH STATE AND FEDERAL REGULATIONS

In every occupation, from astronaut to zookeeper, there are perils and problems that require prevention and control practices. Dental assisting, as a profession, is a member of the health occupations cluster, the second largest employer in the United States. With so many people employed in the 2,000 or more different medical and dental occupations, there are a multitude of government controls and regulations to provide for the well-being of the employees as well as for the patients and environment.

State and Federal Agencies

Three of the major agencies concerned with safety, infection control, and hazard prevention in the dental setting are the State Dental Practice Act (SDPA), the Environmental Protection Agency (EPA), and the Occupational Safety and Health Administration (OSHA).

THE STATE DENTAL PRACTICE ACT (SDPA). Each person employed in a dental setting is governed by a state regulatory board, called the State Dental Board, or some other similar title. The State Dental Board **regulates** the level of dental care given to the public. By establishing standards for the State Dental Practice Act, this policy-making board determines who is competent to be licensed and sets forth the limitations of practice a person may be able to deliver. Each state has its own board and the standards and rules are different from state to state. Only federal employees who work in federal installations are exempt from state regulation.

State dental boards also set rules and regulations for the proper method of infection control or dental practice **sanitation** procedures. Again, these standards also differ from state to state and must be followed by those practicing dentistry in that state. In most instances, these safety and protection rules are similar to the federal OSHA guidelines; adhering to OSHA regulations will cover **compliances** with most state dental boards. It is the duty of anyone employed in a dental setting to investigate the particular dental practice regulations of the state in which they are employed. Ignorance of the law is considered no excuse.

THE ENVIRONMENTAL PROTECTION AGENCY (EPA). The EPA is a federal agency with environmental protection regulations. The EPA administers the Clean Air Act, the Clean Water Act, the Resource Conservation and Recovery Act, and other federal environmental laws.

At the state level, the EPA concentrates on the use and disposal of chemicals, materials, and wastes that are **hazardous** to the worker and the environment. The EPA has established various rules and controls for the proper utilization and care of many products related to dental practice in many states. How these concerns are written, monitored, and enforced differs from state to state. Many of the health and safety regulations of these various EPA enforcing agencies overlap with state dental practice laws and federal OSHA standards, showing us there is a need for care in infection control and hazards management at the work site.

THE OCCUPATIONAL SAFETY AND HEALTH ADMINISTRATION (OSHA). In 1970, Congress established OSHA, a federal agency with the purpose of protecting employees in the work place. In dentistry, one of the main concerns for employee safety is protection from infection related to the human immunodeficiency virus (HIV) and the hepatitis B virus (HBV). Since both are caused from **bloodborne pathogens**, OSHA has developed standards on exposure to these pathogens to cover health settings such as hospitals, nursing homes, physicians' offices, health care facilities, EMT programs, funeral parlors, and dental offices (Figure 3–1).

Many of the OSHA standards address concerns and laws of other regulatory agencies. When a conflict of procedure occurs among the agencies, the most stringent is observed, thereby satisfying most regulations.

Infection Protection Control

JOB CLASSIFICATION. Each employee in the dental office is covered by OSHA standards regulations. The extent of practice controls varies according to the classification of their position. OSHA has established three categories of office employees based on the expected amount of exposure related to the job duties. The first category is the occupational worker who is exposed to blood, saliva, and potentially **infectious** materials. This category includes the dentist, hygienist, and chairside assistant.

The second category covers the person who does not have occupational exposure to blood, saliva, and infectious materials during their normal job performance but may assist with chairside cleanup or laboratory work. This division may cover the receptionist and the laboratory technician.

The final category covers those who are not exposed throughout their work performance and do not handle or work with blood, saliva, or infectious materials. A secretarial or financial manager may be included in this category. It is interesting to note that OSHA treats all exposures to saliva as blood potentials, in that blood may be present; therefore, saliva must be considered infectious.

HEPATITIS VACCINATION. Once employee duties have been determined and classification is made, a plan for exposure control must be formally written, practiced,

JOB SAFETY & HEALTH PROTECTION

The Occupational Safety and Health Act of 1970 provides job safety and health protection for workers by promoting safe and healthful working conditions throughout the Nation. Provisions of the Act include the following:

Employers

All employers must furnish to employees employment and a place of employment free from recognized hazards that are causing or are likely to cause death or serious harm to employees. Employers must comply with occupational safety and health standards issued under the Act.

Employees

Employees must comply with all occupational safety and health standards, rules, regulations and orders issued under the Act that apply to their own actions and conduct on the job.

The Occupational Safety and Health Administration (OSHA) of the U.S. Department of Labor has the primary responsibility for administering the Act. OSHA issues occupational safety and health standards, and its Compliance Safety and Health Officers conduct jobsite inspections to help ensure compliance with the Act.

Inspection

The Act requires that a representative of the employer and a representative authorized by the employees be given an opportunity to accompany the OSHA inspector for the purpose of aiding the inspection.

Where there is no authorized employee representative, the OSHA Compliance Officer must consult with a reasonable number of employees concerning safety and health conditions in the workplace.

Complaint

Employees or their representatives have the right to file a complaint with the nearest OSHA office requesting an inspection if they believe unsafe or unhealthful conditions exist in their workplace. OSHA will withhold, on request, names of employees complaining.

The Act provides that employees may not be discharged or discriminated against in any way for filing safety and health complaints or for otherwise exercising their rights under the Act.

Employees who believe they have been discriminated against may file a complaint with their nearest OSHA office within 30 days of the alleged discriminatory action.

Citation

If upon inspection OSHA believes an employer has violated the Act, a citation alleging such violations will be issued to the employer. Each citation will specify a time period within which the alleged violation must be corrected.

The OSHA citation must be prominently displayed at or near the place of alleged violation for three days, or until it is corrected, whichever is later, to warn employees of dangers that may exist there.

Proposed Penalty

The Act provides for mandatory civil penalties against employers of up to $7,000 for each serious violation and for optional penalties of up to $7,000 for each nonserious violation. Penalties of up to $7,000 per day may be proposed for failure to correct violations within the proposed time period and for each day the violation continues beyond the prescribed abatement date. Also, any employer who willfully or repeatedly violates the Act may be assessed penalties of up to $70,000 for each such violation. A minimum penalty of $5,000 may be imposed for each willful violation. A violation of posting requirements can bring a penalty of up to $7,000.

There are also provisions for criminal penalties. Any willful violation resulting in the death of any employee, upon conviction, is punishable by a fine of up to $250,000 (or $500,000 if the employer is a corporation), or by imprisonment for up to six months, or both. A second conviction of an employer doubles the possible term of imprisonment. Falsifying records, reports, or applications is punishable by a fine of $10,000 or up to six months in jail or both.

Voluntary Activity

While providing penalties for violations, the Act also encourages efforts by labor and management, before an OSHA inspection, to reduce workplace hazards voluntarily and to develop and improve safety and health programs in all workplaces and industries. OSHA's Voluntary Protection Programs recognize outstanding efforts of this nature.

OSHA has published Safety and Health Program Management Guidelines to assist employers in establishing or perfecting programs to prevent or control employee exposure to workplace hazards. There are many public and private organizations that can provide information and assistance in this effort, if requested. Also, your local OSHA office can provide considerable help and advice on solving safety and health problems or can refer you to other sources for help such as training.

Consultation

Free assistance in identifying and correcting hazards and in improving safety and health management is available to employers, without citation or penalty, through OSHA-supported programs in each State. These programs are usually administered by the State Labor or Health department or a State university.

Posting Instructions

Employers in States operating OSHA approved State Plans should obtain and post the State's equivalent poster.

Under provisions of Title 29, Code of Federal Regulations, Part 1903.2(a)(1) employers must post this notice (or facsimile) in a conspicuous place where notices to employees are customarily posted.

More Information

Additional information and copies of the Act, specific OSHA safety and health standards, and other applicable regulations may be obtained from your employer or from the nearest OSHA Regional Office in the following locations:

Atlanta, GA	(404) 347-3573
Boston, MA	(617) 565-7164
Chicago, IL	(312) 353-2220
Dallas, TX	(214) 767-4731
Denver, CO	(303) 844-3061
Kansas City, MO	(816) 426-5861
New York, NY	(212) 337-2378
Philadelphia, PA	(215) 596-1201
San Francisco, CA	(415) 744-6670
Seattle, WA	(206) 442-5930

Lynn Martin

Lynn Martin, Secretary of Labor

U.S. Department of Labor

Occupational Safety and Health Administration

Washington, DC
1991 (Reprinted)
OSHA 2203

FIGURE 3-1 OSHA provisions of the Occupational and Health Act of 1970. Health care workers must be particularly careful to protect against bloodborne pathogens.

46

and recorded. All part-time, temporary, and probationary employees must be offered free vaccination against hepatitis B within ten days of the start of active employment. Hepatitis vaccine is delivered in a series of three injections within a six-month period. An employee may decline **immunization** but must sign a release form showing vaccination was offered. If the employee changes his or her mind at a later date, the offer is still available. All employees who have received the hepatitis B series are later tested for vaccine effectiveness. It has not been determined yet if a booster injection is needed.

REPORTING EXPOSURE INCIDENTS. OSHA standards must be followed if an unfortunate accident occurs, such as a needle stab during cleanup, or if some other method of exposure happens in the dental office. When an incident takes place, immediate action must be started. The incident must be reported to the facility's safety officer to permit a medical follow-up. Employers are required to provide free medical examinations and treatment to employees who have experienced an exposure incident.

The employee is referred to a licensed health care provider to determine the serious nature of the occurrence. The provider examines any symptoms to see if they are related to HIV or HBV development. The employee is requested to give permission for blood to be drawn for testing. The employee has the right to determine if the blood is to be tested at that time or at a future date. The blood sample is maintained for 90 days to see if any HIV or HBV symptoms develop.

The health care provider counsels the employee and makes out a written report of the incident, which is filed and remains confidential. Medical records are not made available to the employer but are private records of the employee. All records of the incident are maintained for 30 years in accordance with OSHA standards.

EMPLOYEE TRAINING. Each employee must be trained in the exposure and control plan immediately upon assuming duties. All staff members must have periodic review training. The training should include an explanation of OSHA's standards, disease transmission, exposure control, office procedure protocol for use and practice of barrier **techniques**, methods to lessen exposure, emergency practices, incidence reports, and **biohazard** label systems.

Records of each training session must be noted and recorded along with all papers and outlines for each training item. Each office maintains a safety manual outlining the office's standard operating procedures and kept on hand for OSHA on-site visitations (Figure 3–2). Normally, one member of the office staff is designated safety monitor and maintains all records; but it

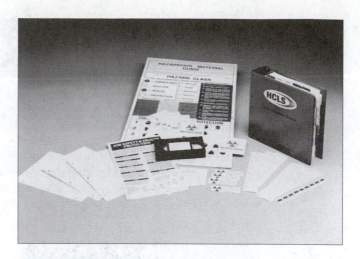

FIGURE 3–2 Each facility must maintain an office manual with exposure control plans, training material, hazard compliances, and OSHA employee records. Employees should know how to use the biohazard labels and practice safe techniques. (Courtesy of Medical Arts Press, 1-800-328-2179.)

is still mandatory that each employee is knowledgeable of the location of the manual and can produce it at any time.

DISEASE TRANSMISSION. Dental personnel must be aware of the methods or avenues of disease transmission and the procedures to use for infection control.

Infection is caused by disease-producing microbes called pathogens. These microorganisms can be transmitted through direct contact in the form of a sneeze, cough, or breathing droplets, or in dental procedures using aerospray equipment. Pathogens may be blood or airborne microorganisms that travel from person to person or are directly transmitted through contact and exchange.

Infectious diseases may also result from indirect transmission through soiled towels, hands, instruments, and articles. Improper sterilization or handling techniques may provide the opening for a pathogen to infect another person.

Some individuals may be carriers of diseases, such as tuberculosis (TB), acquired immune deficiency syndrome (AIDS), hepatitis, and other maladies, and pass these infections to people through direct or indirect transmission. Any individual, including dental personnel, may be undergoing incubation periods for diseases and may also pass these pathogens to others; therefore, infection control procedures must be carefully and fully practiced by all members of the dental team.

Asepsis is the condition of being without pathogens. To maintain a state of asepsis is the aim of the dental assistant. Using proper techniques, materials, and handling of articles from time of **sterilization** to time of use is "chain of asepsis" time. Contamination should not occur in this period. When pathogens enter the sterile field, a break in the chain is said to have occurred, and infection may result.

All articles of a dental procedure must be sanitized and sterilized or disinfected because even unused items may have become contaminated through spraying or splattering during the appointment.

SANITATION.   Sanitation involves the precleaning of instruments and equipment. All articles to be sterilized or disinfected must be clean and free of trapped debris or matter. Instruments may be placed in a holding solution to prevent blood, saliva, and debris from becoming dried on the surfaces or may be immediately cleaned after use. Cleaning of instruments may be accomplished manually or done in an **ultrasonic cleaner.** Equipment and large areas are sanitized by wiping the surfaces with a detergent type of disinfectant solution in a spray-wipe-spray method.

STERILIZATION.   Sterilization is the procedure employed to destroy all living forms of life. Items on which no pathogenic or nonpathogenic microbes are present is said to be sterile. Sterilization may be accomplished by the application of heat. The most common methods of office heat sterilization are autoclaving, chemical vapor sterilizing, and dry heat sterilizing. Some chemicals have the ability to sterilize instruments when properly mixed and used over a long time span (10 hours).

DISINFECTION.   **Disinfection** is an action that may be taken to destroy and inhibit the growth of pathogenic microbes. Disinfectant chemicals should be marked "Hospital Grade" and registered with the EPA. These solutions are generally used on surfaces, equipment, and items unable or too large to be sterilized, or in a chemical bath container, sometimes referred to as a "cold sterilizer." When prepared and used following the manufacturer's recommendations, disinfectants are helpful in maintaining and providing infection control.

Many chemical disinfectants may have detergent qualities and may be used for cleaning and disinfecting. Some solutions may leave protective **antimicrobial** surfaces, while others may stain or etch the item after prolonged use. The assistant must carefully follow the manufacturer's directions when preparing, storing, using, and disposing of the disinfectant. Personal protective equipment, especially utility gloves and eyeglasses or a face shield, should be worn when using chemical disinfectants (Table 3–1).

EXPOSURE AND INFECTION CONTROL PLAN.   The best method to prevent the spread of pathogens is through **universal precautions**. OSHA has stressed the policy of universal precautions, which is basically treating blood and infectious material as infectious regardless of the perceived status of the source or individual.

By assuming *each patient is an infectious source* and employing proper hand-washing, barrier, sterilization, and disinfection techniques, we lessen the chances of spreading hepatitis B (HBV), AIDS, and other infectious diseases from patient to patient or from patient to staff or the staff's family.

ADDITIONAL PROTECTION PRACTICES.   Other office protection procedures taken for the safety of the employees are to refrain from eating, drinking, smoking, applying cosmetics or lip balm, or handling contact lenses in areas where infectious contaminants may be present.

If the office refrigerator contains any infectious or blood-bearing specimens or potential hazardous materials, there should be no storage of food or drink that may become **contaminated**. Another refrigerator or another method to store food products must be provided.

Each office or facility should have a cleaning schedule, noting time, area, and method of compliance. Each area and incidence is treated in a custom, individualized manner. Operatory room treatment is more stringent than a patient waiting room and likewise for an obvious blood spill compared to a splattering. Particular office procedures and schedules are recorded in an office manual that may be viewed by any staff member or OSHA review team, but generally it is advised to sterilize as well as possible.

Surfaces should be disinfected after each patient and at the end of the work day using a spray-wipe-spray method. The counter tops or surfaces should be sprayed with a hospital-grade tuberculocidal disinfectant or detergent and then wiped to remove blood and debris. A second spray should be completed and the disinfectant or detergent is allowed to remain for the appropriate disinfection time. The excess is removed with a towel.

In some offices, surfaces and equipment are draped with protective coverings such as plastic barrier material or aluminum foil. These coverings should be removed and replaced between patients and at the end of the work day.

Floor care should be included in the general cleaning plan. A routine wash and disinfection should be completed along with a cleaning of the waste receptacles or containers. Carpets are discouraged for use in an operatory or sterilizing/cleanup area as they are more difficult to disinfect.

Spills usually occur more frequently than we desire, but immediate attention must be given to all spills and drips. If there is a liquid mass to be cleaned up, it may be wiped with absorbent towels; or a commercial liquid treatment system material may be placed on the

TABLE 3–1

Sterilization and Disinfection Chart

Note: All items must be precleaned before processing.

Sterilization

Method	Positive Features	Negative Features	Cautions
Autoclave Steam under pressure, most widely used, economical, effective	Short cycle, penetration is good, items may be pre-wrapped, newer models have shortened time for unwrapped items, processing is automatic in some new units	May corrode some metal instruments, may dull cutting edges, may destroy heat-sensitive items	Use distilled water, sterilizing timing does not begin until proper conditions are met, do not overload chamber
Chemical Vapor Sterilizer Heats chemical that penetrates items to be sterilized	Short cycle time, does not dull cutting edges or corrode	Vapors can destroy some plastics, vapor fumes must be monitored, no sealed containers may be used, must use specific wrap	Allow proper spacing in packing, assure proper ventilation, all items must be dry before sterilization
Dry Heat Sterilizer Dry heat is forced through-out the chamber	Does not rust or dull cutting edges, safe and useful for metal instruments and mirrors, newer models (Rapid Heat Transfer) have shortened time cycles, may sterilize wrapped or cassette-boxed items, has cool down time built in	May char or discolor items, unwrapped items must be re-done after cycle, small loads are usual, may harm heat-sensitive items	Check which type of dry heat sterilizer is to be used, look over manufacturer's directions, follow scheduled times and wrapping orders, be careful in transfer to avoid operator burns from hot trays
Chemical Sterilizing Solutions Chemical action from im-mersion in solution	Can be used on items too large or too heat sensitive to be sterilized in heat sterilizers	Cannot check effectiveness of solution, only can monitor chemical level of activity, requires 10 hours of immer-sion, instruments must be rinsed with sterile water and wrapped for storage	Avoid skin and eye tissue contact, completely cover items with solution, check effective dates of solutions and preparation procedures

Disinfection

Method	Positive Features	Negative Features	Cautions
Alcohol Immerse or wipe	May remove films left from other disinfectants, can cut oil-based residues	Not EPA registered, not considered effective disinfectant	Material evaporates in too short a time to be effective, 70% alcohol has more retention time than 90% alcohol, leaves after-taste, can irritate eyes

Note: All items must be precleaned before processing.

	Method	Positive Features	Negative Features	Cautions
Chlorine	Spray, immersion, wipe	Many are EPA registered (bleach is not), economical, easy to use, have broad range of effectiveness	May be corrosive to some items, may irritate skin or mucous membranes	Bleach must be mixed daily and used only on precleaned items and surfaces; read manufacturer's directions for stronger chlorine solutions
Gluteraldehyde	Immerse	Broad range of effectiveness including TB, noncorrosive to metals, may have long shelf or storage life	Unable to check sterilizing effectiveness of solution, may be irritating to skin and respiration, may discolor some items	Some people may be allergic or sensitive, items must be washed off after immersion, check manufacturer's recommended time (10 hours) and proper temperature
Iodophors	Spray, clean, immerse	Economical for use, have a broad range of effectiveness, may leave some residual barrier action	One-day action life (undiluted solution unaffected until prepared), may need rust inhibitor if not built in, may stain areas	Follow manufacturer's recommendation for dilution of product
Phenols	Disinfectant or disinfectant and cleaner, immerse or spray	Versatile, have a broad range of effectiveness	May be **caustic** and harmful to eyes and mucous membranes, can harm or etch glass and plastics, may leave residue film on surface	Must read manufacturer's directions and look for EPA registration, read for type of phenol and use intended
Quaternary Ammonia (Superquats)	Spray, wipe, or immerse	Economical, easy to use, nonirritating, can be used as disinfectant or cleaner if EPA registered, broad range of effectiveness	Are not tubercucidal if older types of quats, must have TB-killing mixture included in solution	Read manufacturer's directions and look for EPA registration

liquid and absorbed to make a deodorized and disinfected solid. The mass may be placed in a disposable container. There are also commercial sponges impregnated with decontaminant and vapor suppressants manufactured for the sole purpose of containing mercury spills.

Any glassware broken in a spill may be a potential contaminated break and should never be picked up with bare or gloved hands. A mechanical means, such as a dustpan and brush or forceps, should be used.

SHARPS HANDLING. Broken pieces of glass may be placed into a sharps container. Each room or area where sharp instruments are used or sterilized should contain a rigid, puncture-resistant container that is colored red and labeled "Hazardous." The container must be leakproof, have a lid, and remain upright to prevent any articles from coming out. The size of the container is dictated by the amount of use it may receive. Some rooms may contain larger containers than other rooms. The form of the container varies from manufacturer to manufacturer, and each container must be routinely replaced to avoid overfilling.

The disposal of a sharps container is regulated mainly by local or state EPA laws. The lid is closed and sealed to avoid leakage. If there may be an occasion for leakage, the container is placed in a secondary container that is closed, labeled or color-coded, and leak resistant. Some sharps containers are purchased with a mail-back system in which a company disposes of the container and returns a report stating date, location, and method of disposal. The sharps container is closed, sealed, dropped into a color-coded bag and placed into a rigid box that is sealed and mailed to the manufacturer for disposal. If the dental office is required to maintain a tracking of its infectious materials, as required in some states, it can take advantage of this service, which destroys the sharps container and returns **verification** of the process to the dental office for its records.

Care must be taken when working with sharps. Contaminated sharps must never be sheared or broken, as the person performing this task may be injured in the effort. Needles should never be recapped; but if the procedure may require recapping, it must be performed with a mechanical device or in a one-handed method, such as scooping the cap with the needle and uniting the two by pushing on the table top.

Needles and sharps should not be removed from their holders without some mechanical equipment. If a needle sheath is not available, there are some sharps containers that have an unlocking device or slot on top of the container. The device may engage a needle and hold it while the assistant turns to release it from a syringe. If no such accommodation is present, there are commercial devices designed to accomplish needle

removal, or an assistant may use a hemostat or needle holder to remove the sharp needle or scalpel blade. When removing sharps from their holders or handles, care must be taken to remove the sharp in a direction away from the body to avoid injury.

HAND WASHING. Frequent hand washing lessens contamination. The employers are required to have hand-washing facilities near exposure areas or supply disinfecting towelettes for use after exposures. It is advisable to scrub hands at least four times a day with an antimicrobial disinfectant, which may leave some microorganism protection under gloves.

Hand washing begins the chain of asepsis. One of the simplest but most important actions an assistant can perform to assure a clean operative field is to wash hands. Touching, passing, and transferring of clean and sterile instruments and items with dirty hands breaks the "chain of asepsis," ruining the aseptic field, and contamination begins.

A vigorous washing of hands in a warm lather and good rinse in cool water removes many pathogens. Some fine antimicrobial soaps that not only remove pathogens but leave an antibacterial surface coating to hamper pathogenic regrowth have been developed. The assistant is encouraged to use these. Some antimicrobial lotions also are available for hand care after washing.

The hands should be washed with extreme care at the beginning and end of the work day to prevent carrying pathogens home or to the office. The hands must be washed between each procedure and each time before and after donning gloves.

Nails should be kept short and snag free not only for comfort but also to prevent accumulation of dirt and pathogens under the nails. The blunt end of a cuticle or orange stick may be used to remove matter from under the nails. Hand washing brushes can also be used to clean this area as well as the knuckles.

The hands should not touch the faucets when hand washing. If the office is not equipped with an automatic or knee control, the assistant should use towels to touch the faucet to turn it on and off and to control the temperature. The assistant disposes of the used towels in the marked container, being careful not to touch the container's sides or top.

After assembling disposable toweling, antimicrobial lotion soap, a cuticle or orange stick and a hand brush, the assistant removes all hand jewelry, including watch. Rings may harbor pathogens and interfere with glove wear.

If knee faucet controls are not available, a piece of toweling is wrapped around the faucet to obtain and regulate water temperature. The hands and wrists are held under the flow of water, and lotion antimicrobial soap is dispensed. A good lather is worked up by rubbing the palms together. The palm of one hand is used to lather and rub the back of the other hand (Figure 3–3A). Fingers are interlaced to work the lather between the fingers (Figure 3–3B). All actions are done with vigorous friction.

A hand brush may be used in a circular motion on the skin surfaces, with particular attention given to the knuckle areas. The blunt end of the cuticle or orange stick is inserted under the nails to remove any accumulated dirt or matter.

The hands are held in a downward position and rinsed under cool water until completely free of lather (Figure 3–3C). The cuticle stick and brush are also rinsed of lather and set aside. Disposable toweling is used to thoroughly dry the hands. The towels are placed in the disposal container, being careful not to touch the sides of the sink or container. Another piece of towel is used to turn the water off (Figure 3–3D). The toweling is placed between the faucet and the clean hand and is disposed of carefully when the water is off.

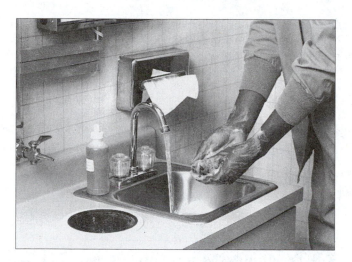

FIGURE 3–3A A good lather is necessary to perform a proper hand wash. Sudsing must extend to the wrists.

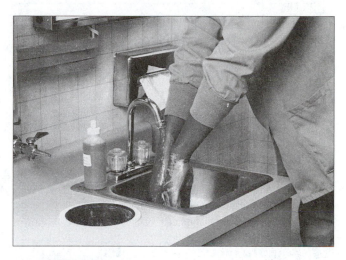

FIGURE 3–3C The hands are held in a downward position and rinsed from the wrists to the fingertips so the germs are not spread upward onto clean areas.

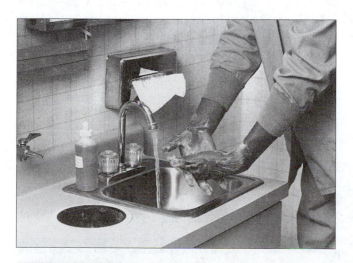

FIGURE 3–3B The fingers are interlaced to remove dirt and pathogens from between the fingers. Both sides of the hands are rubbed and cleansed.

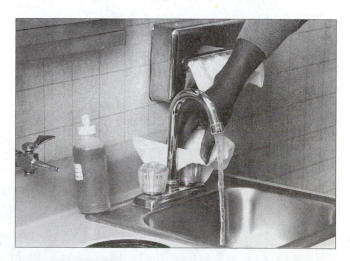

FIGURE 3–3D If automatic controls are not available, disposable towels are used to cover the handles when turning on or off and adjusting temperature.

P R O C E D U R E 5

Hand-washing Technique

1	Assemble Equipment and Materials
2	Remove Jewelry and Watch
3	Hold Paper Towel to Turn On Faucet
4	Apply Antimicrobial Soap Solution
5	Work Up a Lather
6	Work Lather Around Hands
7	Use Cuticle Stick and Brush
8	Rinse Hands
9	Dry Hands With a Paper Towel
10	Turn Off the Faucet With a Paper Towel

1 Assemble Equipment and Materials

The equipment the assistant needs for hand washing are disposable towels, lotion antimicrobial soap, cuticle or orange stick, nail brush, and a sink with running water.

2 Remove Jewelry and Watch

After assembling equipment, all hand jewelry and the watch are removed before hand washing. Rings may harbor pathogens and interfere with glove wear. A watch may be a source of germ transfer from office to home. If it is necessary to wear a watch, the assistant may have one to keep solely for office wear.

3 Hold Paper Towel to Turn On Faucet

The assistant should use the automatic or knee control to turn on warm water, or use a disposable towel to touch and use faucet to wet the hands and wrists. Germs may be transferred from patient to patient from operator contact with a contaminated faucet.

4 Apply Antimicrobial Soap Solution

A liquid soap dispenser or an electric eye container is activated to dispense liquid soap, which is used to work up a good lather. Antimicrobial lotion soap not only eliminates present pathogens but may also leave a fine skin surface coating which can defer future germ growth for a short period of time.

5 Work Up a Lather

All surfaces of the hands up to and including the wrists (where the gloves go) are washed. The palms are rubbed together, and the palm of one hand is used to lather and rub the back of the other hand, including the wrist. The fingertips on one hand are rubbed into the palm of the other and the action is then reversed.

6 Work Lather Around Hands

The fingers are interlaced to work lather between the fingers and to cleanse the inner surfaces. All actions are done with vigorous friction.

7 Use Cuticle Stick and Brush

A hand brush may be used in a circular motion on the skin surfaces, with particular attention to the nail and knuckle area. The blunt end of a cuticle or orange stick is used under the nails to remove matter.

8 Rinse Hands

The hands are held in a downward position and rinsed with cool running water until completely free of lather. Cool water is recommended to help eliminate irritation beneath the gloves. Warm water may sensitize the skin surface before the application of latex gloves. The brush and cuticle or orange stick are rinsed and set aside.

9 Dry Hands With a Paper Towel

Disposable toweling is used to thoroughly dry the hands. The hands must be dry before glove application to avoid underglove irritation and for easier insertion of the fingers. The assistant disposes of the towels in the proper container, being careful not to touch the container or container edges.

All containers holding marked contaminated or infectious matter disposal bags should have a lid, which should be operated by means of a foot lever control.

10 Turn Off the Faucet With a Paper Towel

A new disposable towel is used to grasp the faucet to turn off the water if no knee control is available. The towel may be used to wipe up the sink area, but care must be taken not to touch the sink or disposal container with the hands. The sink area should be clean and spotless when the procedure is finished.

A good hand-washing technique benefits not only the patient but the assistant as well.▲

T H E O R Y R E C A L L

Hand-washing Technique

1. What process does hand washing begin?

_____

2. Besides removing pathogens, what other service does an antimicrobial soap perform?

_____

3. When should hands be washed?

_____

4. What may be used to remove matter from beneath nails?

_____

5. If knee controls are not available for water control, what does the assistant use to work the faucets?

_____

6. What equipment should the assistant have for a proper hand-wash procedure?

_____

7. Why are rings not worn in the dental office?

_____

8. In what motion is the nail brush used? Where?

_____

9. In what position does the assistant hold the hands during the rinsing?

_____

10. What does the assistant take care *not* to do when disposing of towels?

_____

Now turn to the Competency Evaluation Sheet for Procedure 5, Hand-washing Technique, located in Appendix C of this text.

BARRIER ATTIRE

Today's dental professional arrives at the office in street clothes then dons the **clinical attire**. Uniforms to be worn in the dental office are supplied by the dentist or dental clinic and are not worn back and forth from home to office to home. The protective dress and equipment the professional dons at the office is called personal protective equipment (PPE) (Figure 3–4). Employers must provide PPE and ensure that workers wear it. The professional attire is either cleaned by a commercial laundry or is washed in an office washer and dryer located in some area away from operatory sites. Employees are not permitted to take the laundry home to be washed. Disposable attire is available from many supply houses, and some offices elect to use this type of barrier protection.

The dental assistant begins the day by removing jewelry and washing hands. The first and last hand scrub of the day are the most important, and particular care must be given to use of the hand brush and cuticle stick.

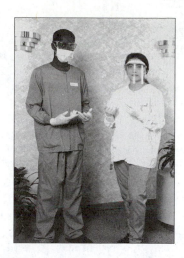

FIGURE 3–4 Personal protection equipment (PPE) provides protection for the dental personnel and helps prevent cross contamination.

Clothes worn to the office are removed or covered over by donning clinical attire. Clean stockings or hose and shoes are put on. Clinical shoes remain in the office to avoid carrying pathogens from the office site to home. When changing into the clinical shoes, the dental assistant checks to see if the shoes are clean and in good repair. Footwear to be worn all day should give good support and fit properly. There should be no blood, dirt, scuff marks, or other unappealing marks on the shoes.

Next, the assistant dons a clinical gown, pants and top, dress, or lab coat covering. Street clothes are removed or covered up. Office clothing may be of various colors, styles, and types of materials. Since much of the dental practice involves saliva and blood sprays and splattering, it is recommended to choose fluid-proof or fluid-resistant material. Because there is no universal or OSHA definition of these terms, it is wise to purchase clothing that is moisture-resistance treated.

Choice of clothing style or selection of coverage has not been dictated by OSHA. A professional may select long- or short-sleeve attire, but one should avoid skin contamination by covering body surfaces as much as possible with sleeves and high, close-fitting collars. If one desires to wear street clothes through the day, protective attire must cover all parts of the clothing in the treatment areas. Lab coats may be put on and taken off as needed.

Protective Face Cover

The dental assistant requires other protective attire while working in operative areas. The eyes, nose, and mouth of the dental staff members must be covered to prevent contamination in the practice of dentistry. These barriers are put on after the assistant prepares the operatory and seats the patient.

Masks are worn by dental professionals to protect the mucous membranes from blood and saliva splatters. Masks must be changed often. Bacteria are able to **penetrate** moist and damp areas so the assistant should choose a moisture-resistant mask and change frequently as it becomes damp in use.

There are different types of face masks. There is a flat material one with string ties or loops and a stiffer dome type with an elastic headband. The elastic band slips over the top of the head and rests around the head or loops the ears. Some professionals choose the dome type because of the looser fit. It does not get damp as fast and requires less changing. If the assistant is wearing a clear face shield, it may still be recommended to wear a face mask to avoid inhalation and splattering infection. Some masks offer face shield visor protection too.

Eyeglasses are used for two safety purposes, to protect the eyes from penetration by flying blood, debris, or objects, and to prevent contamination from sprays and splatters. High-speed rotors and concentrated air sprays splatter moisture and debris in all directions. By wearing regular or prescription impact-resistant lens glasses with side shields or over-the-glasses goggles, the professional can protect the eyes from these dangers. Some offices provide clear plastic face shield visors, which may be used instead of or with eyeglasses. These shields should extend below the chin line and wrap around the face enough to protect from splatters entering the mucous membrane of the nose, eyes, and mouth. Face shields must be disinfected, sanitized, or autoclaved between patients. Some supply houses now have disposable face shield visors, which may be used in the dental operatory.

When working with visible light curing units and not using a protective shield, the staff may wear special eyewear to protect the eyes from the harmful rays.

Barrier Gloves

Gloves are part of the universally accepted method of infection control. No longer is the patient alarmed when approached by a dental professional wearing gloves. Patients now feel more comfortable when they see their operator wearing gloves and, in fact, many demand this protection if they see it missing.

There are four types of gloves worn in the dental office: surgeon, exam, overgloves, and utility gloves. All gloves should meet Food and Drug Administration (FDA) quality standards. Sterile, rubber surgeon gloves are packed with one pair in a wrapper and are the most expensive type. These are used in surgical procedures and are manufactured for that specific purpose. They come sized and are ordered specifically for the individual operator and assistant.

Latex examination gloves are the most commonly and widely used. They are disposable and come either sized or in generalized ranges of small, medium, large, and extra large. They may be **ambidextrous**, meaning no left or right, or they can come in right and left sets or packed in mass in a box, usually 100 to a box. They vary in thickness. Some have a fine powder or talc inside for ease of donning and comfort, while others do not. Some may be flavored or one can purchase a flavoring to rub or spray on the gloves, as some people dislike the taste of latex in their mouths. Wearing gloves is one of the most efficient methods to lessen pathogen transfer.

Occasionally, an operator or assistant must leave the operatory to retrieve a forgotten piece of equipment or obtain additional supplies. Rather than removing the gloves then donning a new pair to continue, the operator or assistant can cover the contaminated gloves with a thinner, vinyl glove, such as the kind we see food handlers use. By placing these gloves over the exam gloves, a process called overgloving, a professional cuts down on expense, time, and hand irritation, while maintaining a clean environment. One word of caution: if the overgloves are in a massed box and do not dispense one at a time, the professional is encouraged to set aside a pair of overgloves for possible future use. Reaching into the box of gloves using a contaminated gloved hand will destroy the entire control process. Overgloves are discarded with the latex examination gloves in the disposal bag. Even if the overgloves were not used in the patient's mouth, they are discarded because the insides have been contaminated by covering the first gloves.

The last type of glove necessary for the dental office is the thick rubber or nitrile, all-purpose utility glove. This type of glove is used for scrubbing instruments and equipment used in sterilizing areas. Glove penetration is discouraged by the thicker density of rubber material. Safety from sharp edge cuts and needlepoint stabs is increased by using this type of glove but is not guaranteed. Care in handling must be stressed when cleaning all instruments and sharp equipment. Utility gloves are more expensive, not discarded frequently, and not considered disposable; therefore, they must be cleaned and disinfected with each use. Utility gloves can be washed with soap and water and then sprayed with a disinfecting solution and autoclaved if necessary.

Hair Care

In some elective cases, such as surgery, the professional dons a hair covering. The dental office may purchase a paper cap similar to a shower cap. This is placed over the hair and is done for the patient's and the operator's safety. Hair caps are placed on the head before the mask, as the mask may need replacing during surgery. Even if caps are worn, the professional should pay attention to the hair. It should be clean and back from the face, not loosely draping over the shoulders. There are many attractive accessories to hold hair back and many hair styles that pull the hair off the face. Clean, healthy hair worn in a professional manner enhances the assistant's clinical appearance and provides protection from infection.

Removal and Disposal of Barrier Attire

Removal of clinical attire is a very important procedure. Items that have been used in the dental operatory carry disease and sometimes bloodborne pathogens. These items must be disposed of in a manner that does not spread infection. After dismissing the patient, the assistant should gather all instruments and materials set out for the procedure. Even if an instrument was not used, it may be considered contaminated from spray or splattering.

After the instruments and equipment are placed on a tray and removed to the sterilizing area and the operatory has been disinfected, the professional may remove the latex examination gloves. The proper method to remove these gloves is to place one gloved hand, fingertips up under the cuff, on the outside surface of the other gloved hand and lift and pull out and down on that glove. This step is completed by touching only the outside surface of the contaminated gloves (Figure 3–5A).

The fingertips of the freed hand are inserted inside the cuff of the gloved hand, which is still holding the removed first glove. The freed, bare hand runs down the inside of the gloved hand turning the glove inside out and down over the first glove being held in the gloved hand, ending up with the second glove inside out and the first glove trapped inside (Figure 3–5B).

The pair of used gloves is then dropped into a marked disposal container or bag (Figure 3-5C).

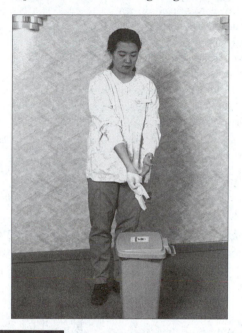

FIGURE 3–5B The assistant inserts the fingers of the freed hand inside the cuff of the second glove. She pulls the second glove down and off the hand, capturing the first glove inside.

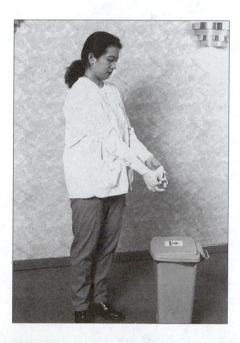

FIGURE 3–5A The assistant grasps the outside cuff of the first glove and lifts the glove off the hand. She holds the removed glove in the gloved hand.

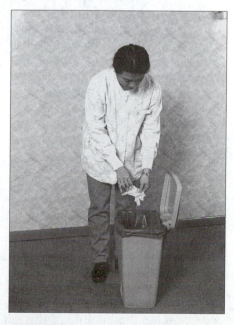

FIGURE 3–5C The assistant drops both gloves into the marked disposal bag.

Now, the assistant reaches up and unties or lifts the mask elastic off the head also dropping it into the disposal bag or container. If a face shield was worn, it is placed with the instruments to be disinfected before reuse. Eyeglasses or goggles are also placed with the instruments for disinfection before using again.

Clinical attire may or may not be discarded. If there is obvious splattering or staining, the assistant should redon a new top or lab coat. If the attire is still in good condition, it may remain until the end of the work day. An educated judgment call regulates clinical dress change. Some supply houses sell disposable aprons or operator shields to wear on top of the clinical attire. This attire is disposed of with each patient.

When the clinical attire is removed, the assistant discards it in a proper manner. Lab coats, dresses, and tops are unbuttoned or untied and one arm is removed (Figure 3–6A). The article is unwrapped around the body folding the contaminated surface to the inside. When the second arm is removed, it is folded to the inside also and the dress or coat is then folded in half (Figure 3–6B). Paper or disposable attire is dropped into the disposal bag or container, while reusable clothing to be laundered is placed in a marked laundry bag (Figure 3–6C). If the clothing has visible blood splatter or stains, the article is placed in a specially marked contaminated material laundry bag, for special care from the laundry service.

Pants and tops are removed by pulling off inside out so contaminated surfaces remain enclosed. These

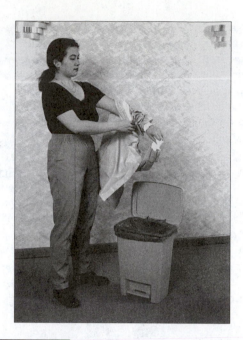

FIGURE 3–6B The assistant removes the coat with a slow, deliberate movement to avoid spreading germs.

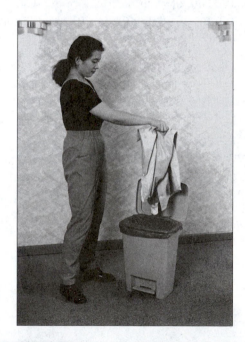

FIGURE 3–6C The contaminated coat is placed into the contaminated materials container, if disposable. If the coat is to be washed and reused, it is placed in the laundry bag and washed in a separate area or sent to a commercial laundry service.

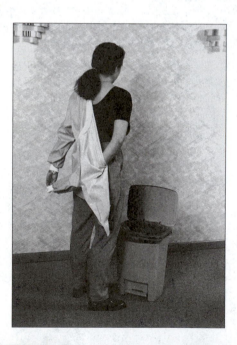

FIGURE 3–6A The assistant removes the first arm and laps or folds the outside of the lab coat inward to capture the pathogens inside the garment.

articles are also placed into the laundry bag. All removal of clothing should be done slowly to avoid thrashing around and spreading pathogens about.

Shoes should be stepped out of and hose or stockings slipped off, again inside out. The hosiery should be placed with the other laundry and the shoes should be wiped off with a disposable paper towel saturated with disinfecting solution. The towel should be held in such a manner that will keep a barrier between the hands and shoes. The used towel should be placed in the disposable contaminated bag or container. Periodically, the shoes should be polished and the shoelaces, if present, removed and laundered with the clothing in the laundry bag or disposed of in the contaminated disposable bag.

When the clothing has been removed and disposed of properly, the assistant washes hands with antimicrobial soap and redons the jewelry and street clothes to be worn home.

The laundry bag is placed in a designated area for pickup or the clothing is taken to a laundry room, which is not situated near an operatory area.

PROCEDURE 6
Donning and Disposing Clinical Attire
Donning
1 **Gather Personal Protection Equipment (PPE)**
2 **Remove Jewelry and Wash Hands**
3 **Don Clinical Attire**
4 **Don Clinical Footwear**
5 **Prepare for Procedure**
6 **Apply Mask**
7 **Don Eyeglass Protection**
8 **Don Face Shield, If Desired**
9 **Don Gloves**

Disposing
10 **Remove Instruments to Sterilizing Room**
11 **Remove Gloves**
12 **Remove Face Coverings**
13 **Remove Clinical Attire**
14 **Remove Clinical Footwear**
15 **Wash Hands and Remove Laundry Bag**

Donning
1 **Gather Personal Protection Equipment (PPE)**

The assistant needs disposable or moisture-resistant cloth dresses, pant suits, lab coats, or other dress attire for personal protection. Gloves, mask, eyewear, and shoes with clean hose or socks complete the outfit. It is the responsibility of the dental facility to supply the

needed attire for professional use. The clothing may be disposable or able to be laundered. If the clothes are to be washed, a laundry service is contracted or the facility laundry area is located away from the operatory section.

2 **Remove Jewelry and Wash Hands**

Jewelry is removed. If a watch is desired, one used only in the clinical site may be donned. Personal clothing and accessories carry pathogens home. The hands receive a thorough hand wash and drying.

3 **Don Clinical Attire**

After gathering the clinical attire, the assistant checks the cleanliness and condition of the items. Pieces with spots, tears, or unsightly areas are not worn. Personal clothing is removed or covered by properly fitting clinical attire. All ties and closures are completed.

4 **Don Clinical Footwear**

Clinical footwear, including shoelaces, is checked for cleanliness and condition. Personal shoes are not worn in the operatory and laboratory areas of the dental office. Wearing clinical shoes from office to home increases the chance of carrying infection for the staff and the staff's family. Properly fitting shoes that give support are donned over clean hose or socks.

5 **Prepare for Procedure**

The operatory is prepared for the upcoming procedure. All areas are disinfected and sterile materials are prepared and placed before the patient arrives. After greeting, seating, and positioning the patient, the assistant reviews the patient's health history and sets up the equipment and materials needed. The assistant unwraps and sets up many sterilized articles, such as a drinking cup, handpiece, and suction tips, in the presence of the patient to assure the patient that new items are being used.

6 **Apply Mask**

A fresh, dry mask is used each time a patient is scheduled for a procedure. Masks may or may not be worn if a face shield is used. If the planned procedure produces much splattering, the assistant may plan to wear both the mask and face cover. The mask must cover the nose and the mouth with either ties or loops holding it on. *If the assistant plans to wear a hair covering, the mask is placed after the cap so it may be removed if it gets wet. All masks are exchanged for fresh ones when the mask gets damp or wet.

7 Don Eyeglass Protection

Eyeglass protection may be in the form of a pair of safety glasses or goggles to wear over prescription lenses. Protection of the eyes requires side shields coverage to protect from splattering and objects. The glasses or goggles must be comfortable and fit properly. The eyewear must be clean and disinfected between each patient. The operators and assistants should have more than one pair of glasses or wear an eyeshield over the face protecting the glasses from contamination.

8 Don Face Shield, If Desired

The assistant may choose to wear a face shield with or instead of eyeglasses or goggles. The face shield must extend below the chin and have full wraparound coverage for protection. Face shields must be clean to provide proper vision, and they must be disinfected between patients. There are also disposable face shields, which are worn for one patient and then discarded.

9 Don Gloves

A new pair of gloves is worn for each patient. The assistant chooses the correct type of glove for the procedure. The gloves must fit properly and have no rips, holes, or tears in them. The assistant places a fresh pair of overgloves nearby for emergency use. If at any time a hole or tear is made or discovered, the gloves are removed and a new pair is applied after another hand wash.

Disposing

10 Remove Instruments to Sterilizing Room

When the procedure is finished and the patient is dismissed, the assistant removes all instruments and items to the sterilizing room. The face shield is removed and placed with the items to be disinfected. Suction lines are flushed, handpiece lines are cleared by running the equipment for 30 seconds, and the operatory area is picked up in preparation for the disinfection. All removable equipment is taken for sterilization regardless if it was used or not. Instruments present during the procedure may have become contaminated through splattering even if they were not used. All equipment and instruments are removed and sterilized.

11 Remove Gloves

The assistant removes the contaminated gloves by placing the fingers of one glove (1) on the outside of the other glove (2). The fingers are inserted up and under the outside surface of the cuff of glove 2, and the cuff is pulled down and out until glove 2 inverts off the hand. The removed glove 2 is held by the fingers of the hand with the glove still in place.

The bare hand is now inserted inside the gloved hand and pulls out and down on the inside of the glove until the glove inverts down and over the gloved fingers holding the first discarded glove.

Both gloves are deposited into the contaminated container and not used again.

12 Remove Face Coverings

Eyeglasses are removed and disinfected before wearing again. The mask is untied or the loops are lifted up and off the back of the head or ears. The mask is touched and carried only by the ties or loops and dropped into the contaminated container.

13 Remove Clinical Attire

If the procedures are over for the day, or if the attire needs changing, the assistant slowly unbuttons, unties, or opens the velcro closures and removes the first arm, holding onto the cuff so that the clothing arm sleeve is inverted.

The attire is unwrapped around the body and the other arm is pulled out, inverting the second sleeve in the process. The clothing, which has all contaminated surfaces folded and trapped in the inside, is folded in half; and the article is dropped into the laundry bag or the waste container, if disposable. If the clothing has obvious blood spots, the attire is placed in a specially marked biohazard laundry bag. This type of marked laundry receives special attention in processing.

Pants are removed by drawing down from the waist, inverting as removing. The pants are folded in half and placed in the laundry bag. All removal is done slowly to avoid spreading pathogens. Personal clothing is redonned if previously removed for dressing.

14 Remove Clinical Footwear

Shoes are removed and socks or hose are slowly removed inside out and placed in the laundry bag. The shoes are wiped off with a detergent-saturated paper towel to clean and remove germs. The assistant is careful not to touch the shoes with the hands, but use towels to touch the shoes. The towels are disposed of in the disposal bag. If the laces are dirty or worn, they are removed and dropped into the laundry bag or into the disposal bag. Personal footwear is redonned.

15 Wash Hands and Remove Laundry Bag

The hands are very carefully scrubbed, and jewelry may be redonned. An antimicrobial hand lotion, which leaves a fine antiseptic layer on the skin surface, may be applied to condition the hands.

The laundry bag is closed by securing from the outside edges only, tied, and taken to the laundry room or the designated pick-up area.▲

THEORY RECALL

Barrier Attire

1. Cleaning and laundering of the professional attire worn in the dental office is the responsibility of

   _____.

2. Clothing worn in the dental operatory should be made of material that is _____.

3. List two reasons why eyeglasses are worn in the dental office.

   a. _____

   b. _____

4. When should a face shield be cleaned?

   _____

5. When should a face mask be changed?

   _____

6. List four types of barrier gloves found in the dental office.

   a. _____

   b. _____

   c. _____

   d. _____

7. Where are the exam gloves and overgloves placed after use and removal?

   _____

8. What type of gloves are worn for cleaning and sterilizing?

   _____

9. Where is contaminated clinical attire that is to be washed placed after removal?

   _____

10. In what manner is the laundry bag prepared for the laundry room?

    _____

Now turn to the Competency Evaluation Sheet for Procedure 6, Donning and Disposing Clinical Attire, located in Appendix C of this text.

STERILIZING TECHNIQUES

Ultrasonic Cleaning

When the dental appointment is finished and the patient has been dismissed, the disinfection and sterilization process begins. The assistant washes hands and dons the heavy utility gloves to begin the process. There can be no sterilization or disinfection of a dirty article. Everything must be cleaned before processing. One of the most effective methods to clean an instrument is with the ultrasonic cleaner, a unit containing a water-chemical solution bath that is charged with high-pitched sonic waves. These waves, which the human ear cannot hear, cause the solution to **cavitate** (bubble). The minute bubbles rise and inwardly burst, breaking down microscopic dirt, matter, and debris, cleaning away what the brush cannot find.

The ultrasonic equipment is composed of a main solution tank with a lid, a wire tank basket, a **beaker** holder lid, auxiliary beakers with lids, a bur tray, and an assortment of cleaning solutions that add a chemical cleaning force to the physical cavitating movement (Figure 3–7). Each chemical solution is designed to work specifically with a certain debris problem, such as cement, tartar and stain, wax, gypsum, and buffing compounds. The manufacturer has a printed chart that recommends the proper solution and the proper timing to be used on each type of dirt problem.

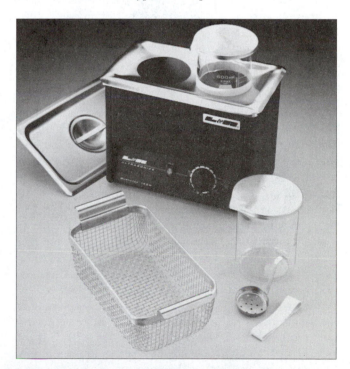

FIGURE 3–7 The ultrasonic unit uses a bubbling action to clean the gross and microscopic debris and matter from the items. (Courtesy of L & R Manufacturing Company.)

60

The main tank of the ultrasonic cleaner is filled one-half to three-quarters full with a general purpose cleaning solution that has been made up from a concentrate following the manufacturer's advice. Inside the tank is a wire basket used to hold articles through the cleaning, rinsing, and then draining. Articles placed in the wire basket may have been scrubbed or not but they all have been patted dry. Wet instruments and articles placed in the ultrasonic bath tend to dilute the solution, thereby ruining its effectiveness.

When the assistant wishes to use a different chemical solution for a specific problem, an auxiliary beaker is chosen from those supplied with the unit. An office may have a stain and tartar solution beaker, a cement solution beaker, a plaster and stone solution beaker, or any combination of solutions in different beakers.

The beaker chosen for a specific task is placed into the beaker holder lid, which suspends the glass container in the general all-purpose solution of the unit. There are beaker bands (elastics) around the beaker to permit the raising or lowering of the beaker into the unit bath to suspend the container in the solution. The beaker bottom must be partially submerged in the general all-purpose solution to cause the cavitation of the chemical solution in the beaker. Any tilting or placing the beaker on the floor of the unit may hinder the bubbling effect and ruin the cleansing purpose.

There is also a small bur basket supplied with the unit. This small, hooked basket is used to hold small items in the solution. Burs are easily obtainable by lifting the basket and removing with transfer forceps. Fingers are never used to remove items from the contaminated solutions. The trays are emptied by using transfer forceps or by dumping the contents onto disposable toweling.

All items cleaned in the ultrasonic cleaner need to be rinsed and patted dry before preparing for sterilization. Those in the wire basket may be taken to the sink and rinsed while in the basket. The basket is placed on a drain towel, and the instruments are removed by dumping the basket contents onto disposable toweling. The instruments and basket are then patted dry. Return the basket to the main unit for future use.

Periodically, the solutions need changing and the unit needs cleaning. How often this is required depends on the amount of use the unit receives. When the solution has a cloudy or dirty appearance, it is removed by draining the unit. The inside of the empty unit is scrubbed, rinsed, disinfected, and dried before the new solution is added. Beakers are treated in the same manner. Etched or highly scratched beakers are discarded, as these scratches hinder the sonic waves in their performance. The tank is never filled to the top but merely halfway. This permits room in the solution for the insertion of the beakers.

The electrical cord is plugged into the outlet at the start of the day and unplugged in the evening before going home. For safety practices, the assistant must make sure the ground prong is engaged into the receptacle in the correct manner.

To check the efficiency of the machine and to determine if the solution is cavitating properly, the assistant may hold a piece of aluminum foil in the solution for three minutes. At the end of the timing period, the foil is lifted up to the light to see if any holes have been vibrated into the material. A properly functioning machine will have produced some holes and cut areas in the foil. All instruments and items to be cleaned are immersed in the proper container. If placed in a beaker, the main tank, or a bur basket, the assistant must make sure the solution covers and is able to get to the surfaces of all submerged items. Two loads with circulation are better than one overcrowded one.

The amount of time needed to be set on the timer is best determined by following the manufacturer's recommendation, but a minimum of five minutes is set for many articles. When the unit is operating, the lids are always in place. This hampers the spread of pathogens through splattering and spraying. Lids are left on in nonoperating times to avoid evaporation and to keep the solutions cleaner. At the end of the timing cycle, the assistant removes the items or carries the wire basket to the sink and rinses away the ultrasonic solution. They are then drained, dump-removed, and patted dry with disposable towels. Fingers are never inserted into the solution. All placing and retrieving of articles is done with transfer forceps. These transfer forceps are kept near the ultrasonic unit and are used solely for this purpose. These are considered contaminated transfer forceps and are not used to transfer any sterilized articles.

Some dental facilities use an ultrasonic processing system. This utilizes a **cassette** instrument carrier that requires little manual handling and decreases the possibility of punctures (Figure 3–8). Cassettes may be made of stainless steel or a hard resin material and have slotted openings on all sides.

At the conclusion of the dental procedure, all instruments are returned to the cassette in their proper position (sequential use). Small bur blocks, instrument boxes, and clips fit inside the tray and accommodate the little items. The cassette is removed to the sterilizing area where the entire unit with instruments is submerged into the ultrasonic unit solution. There are some smaller trays that may fit into the smaller ultrasonic units but the use of the entire system requires the purchase of a large ultrasonic cleaner.

After the ultrasonic cleansing, the trays are removed to the sink, rinsed and placed on disposable toweling to drip dry. The assistant opens the tray to insert any disposables or replace any missing items and places an indicator strip inside the cassette. Lubrication of hinged instruments may be done at this time.

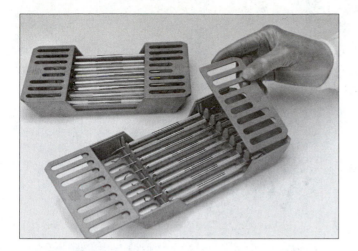

FIGURE 3-8 A cassette system helps to protect the assistant from accidental stab or puncture wounds and provides for more control of items. (Photograph courtesy of Hu-Friedy.)

Instruments cleaned by the ultrasonic cleaner are now ready for wrapping and sterilizing. Items to be autoclaved or chemical vapor sterilized may be placed in autoclave bags or wrapped with autoclave wrap coverings. Articles and instruments headed for the dry heat sterilizer may be covered with aluminum foil. Wrapping the items or cassette of items before sterilization permits the assistant to recover the objects, transfer them to their holding area and keep the items sterile until their use. Articles that are not covered or sleeved quickly lose their sterility when removed from the sterilizer.

If instruments are wrapped or bagged, it is advisable to insert a sterilization indicator strip to determine if proper conditions have been met (Figure 3–9). In-

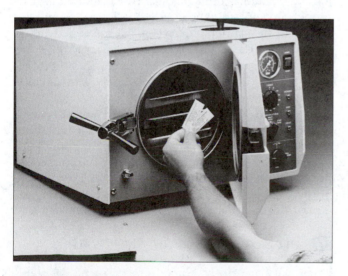

FIGURE 3-9 Indicator strips provide not only assurance of total sterilization but also legal documentation. (Courtesy of Medical Arts Press, 1-800-328-2179.)

dicator strips turn black when time and temperature requirements are met and signal to the operator that these wrapped instruments have been processed. Autoclave tape used to fasten the wrap on instruments may be marked with date and contents to identify the contents. Spore testing must still be practiced once a week to assure that the sterilizing procedure is functional.

PROCEDURE 7

Ultrasonic Cleaning

1	Prepare for the Procedure
2	Preclean the Items
3	Prepare the Ultrasonic Machine
4	Immerse the Instruments into the Solution
5	Immerse Small or Special Items into the Beakers
6	Drain the Articles
7	Use the Ultrasonic Cassette
8	Prepare Articles for Sterilization
9	Clean Up the Area and Equipment
10	Remove PPE

1 Prepare for the Procedure

The assistant washes and dries hands before donning utility gloves. The following items are needed to complete the ultrasonic cleansing of articles: main tank unit with all-purpose solution, wire basket to hold items, bur basket for small items, glass beakers filled with chemical solutions, manufacturer's chart for directions, beaker bands, beaker holder and lids for all beakers, and main tank. Cassette trays may be used in either large or regular ultrasonic units.

2 Preclean the Items

If not using a cassette system, items may be precleaned by placing them in a holding solution for a short time and then manually brushing them to remove gross debris. The items are patted dry on disposable toweling, which is placed into the marked contaminated container. Cassette-filled trays may be placed into the holding or soaking solution prior to draining and placing into the ultrasonic cleaner.

3 Prepare the Ultrasonic Machine

The assistant checks the solution in the main tank for liquid level and condition of the solution. The tank should be one-half to three-quarters full of general all-purpose solution, and the liquid must be changed if it is cloudy or dirty. All solutions are regularly cleaned according to the office manual cycle, which is determined by the amount of use and condition of instruments placed into the cleaner. A three-pronged, grounded electrical cord is engaged.

4 Immerse the Instruments into the Solution

The manufacturer's chart is consulted for the selection of the correct solution and time. General cleaning of items is completed in the main tank, which contains all-purpose solution. Specific cleaning problems, such as stain, cement, or wax, are placed into another solution chemically formulated specifically for that particular stain problem. All items are completely covered by the solution and overcrowding is avoided so there is room for the solution bubbles to cavitate around the items. The lid is put into place to avoid germ spread.

5 Immerse Small or Special Items into the Beakers

Small articles, such as burs, are placed in the small bur basket. Specific cleaning problem items are placed in a special solution geared toward the problem. These solutions are kept in 500-ml beakers, which may be placed into a beaker holder and suspended into the main tank solution. The bur tray and beaker container must be situated in the main tank's all-purpose solution to bubble. If the beaker is placed in too deeply and sits on the floor of the main tank or if not in deep enough to have the solution cover the bottom of the beaker, cavitation or bubbling will not occur (Figure 3–10).

The elastic bands around the beakers may be moved up or down the walls of the glass container to adjust the depth of the beaker's immersion. Overcrowding of the beaker, bur tray, or main tank is also avoided so the solution is able to cavitate around all the surfaces of the articles. Any surface not covered by the solution will miss the cleaning process. Lids are placed on the beaker and main tank to avoid spreading or scattering of germs.

The timer is set according to the manufacturer's direction for the solution and specific problem article. All cycles should last five minutes or more.

6 Drain the Articles

When the timer goes off, the basket is raised, drained, and taken to the sink for rinsing. The articles in the basket are placed under running water, then removed or dumped into toweling for a pat dry and preparation for sterilization. The basket is returned to the unit.

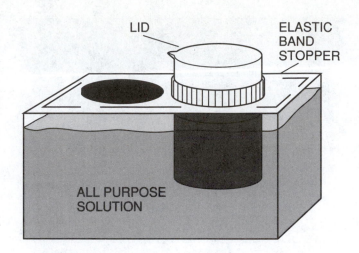

LID   ELASTIC BAND STOPPER

ALL PURPOSE SOLUTION

FIGURE 3–10 **The beaker containing a special solution must be inserted correctly to work efficiently. The bottom of the beaker must suspend into the all-purpose solution but not touch the floor of the tank.**

Never reach into the contaminated solution for items. Transfer forceps may be used to remove articles. These transfer forceps are never used to carry or move sterile items. A separate forceps that is kept in a sterile holder is used for cleaned and sterilized items. All toweling used in the processing is placed in the contaminated container.

7 Use the Ultrasonic Cassette

When using cassettes, the assistant replaces all instruments exposed throughout the procedure. Before leaving the operatory, the items will be positioned in their proper slot, in sequential order. All small items are placed in the carrier box, which is positioned inside the cassette. The entire boxed cassette is removed to the sterilizing area where it is immersed into the ultrasonic unit's solution and cavitated for the prescribed time period, usually 13 minutes.

At the end of the cycle, the cassette tray with items is removed from the unit and rinsed in the sink. The cassette is placed on disposable toweling and permitted to air dry so that the assistant may replace disposables, broken items, check the condition of the instruments, lubricate hinges, and place sterilizing indicator strips inside before wrapping for sterilization.

8 Prepare Articles for Sterilization

Items that have been cleaned are prepared for sterilization. Most articles are wrapped or placed into bags or sterilizing sleeves and taped close (Figure 3–11). The date of sterilization and type of article enclosed should be written on the bag.

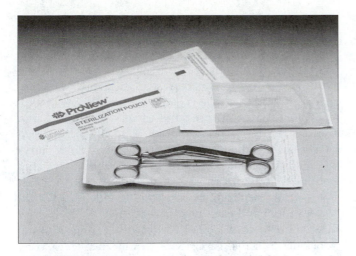

FIGURE 3–11 The marking on an autoclave bag or sleeve tape changes color when exposed to the proper sterilizing conditions. The wrapping or sleeving of the articles provides protection from contamination in handling after sterilization. (Courtesy of Medical Arts Press, 1-800-328-2179.)

Those items to be placed into dry heat may be wrapped with aluminum foil or special wrapping paper. Instruments may be set into the sterilizer without coverings, but must be carefully handled when sterilizing is over.

Cassette trays with items wrapped, sterilized, and stored may then be taken to the operatory for the indicated procedure. At this time, the wrap seal is broken, the indicator strip is checked, and the patient is aware that the items are clean and sterile.

9 Clean Up the Area and Equipment

When the ultrasonic work has been finished for the day, the unit is unplugged. Lids are kept on the main tank and the waiting beakers. If the unit has been frequently used during the day, the solution may be drained so the main tank may be washed and dried. New all-purpose solution is used to replace the liquid.

Glass beakers may be emptied, washed, dried, and refilled with new solution. Deeply scratched beakers should be discarded because the etching hampers the cavitation process. The lids and exterior of the unit are polished and cleaned up.

10 Remove PPE

When the procedure is over and the area is neat and clean, the assistant washes and dries the utility gloves, disinfects and removes them, and places them on the drying rack or hooks. The assistant's hands are washed and dried thoroughly.▲

Ultrasonic Cleaning

1. One of the most effective methods of cleaning instruments is by using_____.
2. By what method does the ultrasonic cleaner work on instruments?

   _____
3. Along with the physical means of cleaning in an ultrasonic cleaner, what other method of cleaning may be added?

   _____
4. What has the manufacturer prepared to aid the assistant with the use of the ultrasonic cleaner?

   _____
5. What is the function of the beaker band?

   _____
6. Where are burs placed in the ultrasonic cleaner?

   _____
7. How are instruments placed when cleaned and sterilized in a cassette?

   _____
8. What determines how often the solution is changed in the ultrasonic cleaner?

   _____
9. Why are etched or highly scratched beakers discarded after use in the ultrasonic cleaner?

   _____
10. Why are the lids always placed on the beakers and main tank of the ultrasonic solution?

    _____

Now turn to the Competency Evaluation Sheet for Procedure 7, Ultrasonic Cleaning, located in Appendix C of this text.

STERILIZATION BY THE AUTOCLAVE METHOD

There is a great difference between disinfection and sterilization. All forms of life, pathogenic or not, must be destroyed before the article can be considered sterilized. The sterilizing process can be accomplished in various ways. The most complete and assured manner is through autoclaving. An autoclave is basically a piece of equipment that generates pressurized steam. There are different brands of autoclaves, but they all work the same way (Figure 3–12). In each autoclave there is a chamber, an area where the objects to be sterilized are placed. Anything put in the autoclave is arranged so the steam generated later in the process can touch the objects. Overcrowding

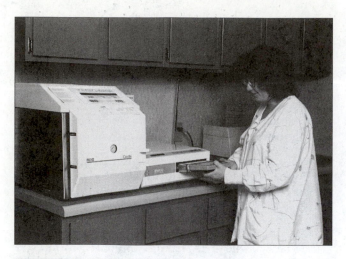

FIGURE 3-12 The autoclave is the most efficient method of sterilization. The assistant places the handpieces into the super fast autoclave, while larger items and loads are processed in the regular autoclave to her left.

hinders the process. Hinges are left open and lids are left off tilted jars in autoclaving. To reach and kill all forms of life, the steam must be permitted to circulate around the objects.

In each autoclave there is a water reservoir that is filled with distilled water. This reservoir periodically needs to be drained, washed out, and wiped clean. The assistant checks the water level line to make sure the reservoir is full and inserts the electric plug into the wall outlet, properly engaging the ground plug in the process. The prepared articles are placed carefully into the chamber, making sure not to overload. Jars and open hinges are tilted to permit steam circulation.

When the load has been arranged in the chamber, the control dial is activated by turning counterclockwise to "fill." Distilled water is released from the reservoir into the chamber. When enough water has been dispensed to cover the floor plate, the dial is again turned counterclockwise to "sterilize." The condition of the rubber door gasket inside the door is checked; the door is closed and locked according to the manufacturer's directions.

A thermostat dial is located above the control dial on the front of the machine. This dial may be adjusted to acquire the proper sterilizing temperature by rotating. Turning clockwise increases the heat and counterclockwise decreases the heat. If more heat is needed to acquire and maintain a proper sterilizing temperature, an amber light turns on. Occasionally, the assistant needs to turn the thermostat dial to adjust the unit and acquire the proper temperature. The assistant monitors the unit to see if the amber light goes out; if it does not, the assistant activates the thermostat to increase the temperature to the correct setting. Throughout the process, the assistant makes sure the amber light remains out and the cycle is completed.

When the desired pressure, usually 15 pounds, and the desired temperature of 250°F (121°C) has been reached, the timer is set for 20 minutes. Some units have an automatic timer that starts when sterilizing conditions have been met. The manufacturer's chart for specific sterilizing processing should be followed for each unit and each type of load.

At the end of the time session, a bell rings and the vent button or dial is turned to permit the steam to be driven out of the chamber. The temperature and pressure gauges return to zero. At that time, the assistant dons safety glasses and "cracks" open the door slightly to permit residue moisture to escape. There might be some moisture present, but this vaporizes in four to five minutes. *Caution:* Open the door only when the temperature and pressure gauges register zero, and then only open the door slightly. Always read manufacturer's directions before using any machine or piece of equipment.

The contents from the autoclave chamber are returned to their proper place. Wrapped packages may be transferred by hand, but bare instruments or items must be transferred with sterile forceps that are kept nearby in a dry, sterilized forceps holder. The transfer forceps and holder must be sterilized daily or more often if contaminated. As the assistant returns the articles, care is taken to rotate the stock, such as placing newer towels behind the older sterile towels. The assistant scans the cabinet drawers for cleanliness before placing the sterile items away.

When all items are returned, the assistant cleans up the area, paying particular attention to the condition of the autoclave. The door is closed and fingerprints and smudges are wiped off. The plug is removed from the socket at the end of the day.

There are some newer speed-clave machines that can perform the sterilizing process in approximately 12 minutes. These machines take only a few items (up to 13 handpieces or instruments) and work faster with no wrapping on the items (approximately 6). A cassette tray is packed with the items and an indicator strip, placed into the speed-clave, and processed. When finished, the cassette is either wrapped and stored or taken directly to the operatory for procedure use. Some autoclaves may use a higher temperature and a larger amount of pressure to complete the sterilizing process in a shorter time period. Hospitals and large facilities may prefer a more rapid autoclave procedure, but the principle is the same. The steam generated is pressurized and kills all forms of organisms.

1 Prepare for the Procedure

To prepare for the procedure, the assistant washes and dries hands to don utility gloves. All precleaned items and articles to be autoclaved are gathered to the autoclave area. Items may be wrapped or left bare. Wrapped articles require a longer exposure time in the autoclave but are easier to handle and store after processing.

2 Prepare the Autoclave

The autoclave is prepared by checking the water reservoir for water level and condition. If the water is oily or dirty, it is drained, cleaned, and replaced with fresh, distilled water. If the level is low, it is replenished with distilled water. The electrical plug is inspected for condition and properly inserted. The power is turned on, and the door is opened.

3 Load the Autoclave Chamber

The autoclave chamber is loaded. Packs are placed inside the chamber, being careful not to overcrowd or wrap the pack too full or too tight. There must be room for steam to touch all items. Lids are removed from the jars, and the jars are tilted to permit steam to enter. A 4 x 4 gauze sponge may be placed over the mouth of the jar and secured around the jar with a rubber band. This gauze material permits the **pressurized** steam to enter the jar, but still holds small objects to be sterilized. Hinges are left open on pliers and forceps so the steam can touch the inner surfaces of the instruments.

Instruments are wrapped in autoclave wrap or placed in autoclave bags and sleeves. Indicator strips may be placed within the load, while once a week a spore check indicator is placed within the center of the load and tested for effectiveness. The wraps and bags are sealed with heat indicator tape with the contents and date marked on them.

4 Fill the Chamber with Water

The control dial is turned counterclockwise to "fill," which permits water to enter the chamber floor. When the level covers the water plate in the chamber, the dial again is turned counterclockwise to "sterilize." The assistant checks the condition of the gasket on the door, closes the door securely, and locks the door.

5 Adjust the Thermostat

If the thermostat dial needs adjusting to raise or lower the temperature, maintaining the machine at 250°F, the assistant adjusts the dial. The assistant periodically checks that the machine is maintaining the proper temperature and pressure. Older machines may need adjustment of the thermostat at times.

6 Set the Timer

If the autoclave machine does not control the time through automatic processing, the timer is set for 20 minutes when the proper conditions are met. Pressure should be at 15 pounds and temperature at 250°F. If the autoclave contains a full load or many wrapped packs, the assistant may choose to permit the time for the load to exceed 20 minutes.

7 Vent the Autoclave

When the timer goes off, the assistant vents the autoclave by turning the control dial counterclockwise to "vent." Steam leaves the chamber and the gauge's dials start to drop.

After the steam has been vented out of the chamber and the gauges indicate zero, the assistant may turn the dial to "off."

8 Open the Autoclave Door

When the pressure and temperature indicate zero, the assistant may don eyeglasses and "crack" the door, opening it a little to let out the evaporation residue. After four to five minutes, this evaporation is finished and the process is completed. If the door is not "cracked" to permit this escape of evaporation, condensation occurs and the articles and items inside the chamber get wet and must be resterilized.

9 Remove the Contents

After evaporation has occurred, the articles may be removed from the chamber. Packs and wrapped items may be removed by hand and placed into storage, rotating older packs to the front and fresher ones to the rear.

Bare items must be picked up and moved to clean storage areas by dry, sterile transfer forceps, which are kept close to the autoclave in a sterile holder. These forceps and holder should be sterilized each day.

10 Clean Up the Area

The area is cleaned up. The interior and exterior of the autoclave may be wiped out and polished when the machine is cool. All items are put away. Gloves are washed, dried, and disinfected. The gloves are removed and the assistant's hands are washed and thoroughly dried.▲

THEORY RECALL
Sterilization by the Autoclave Method

1. What must be destroyed before an article can be considered sterilized?

   _____

2. What is the most complete and assured manner of sterilization?

   _____

3. List three precautions that should be observed when loading an autoclave.

   a. _____

   b. _____

   c. _____

4. With what substance is the reservoir filled before sterilizing?

   _____

5. What dial is activated to increase the heat in an autoclave?

   _____

6. What are the desired pressure, temperature, and time for autoclaving?

   _____

7. What procedure does the assistant perform when the timer bell goes off?

   _____

8. What precaution must be observed before opening the door of the warm autoclave?

   _____

9. Why does the assistant wait a few minutes before emptying the autoclave?

   _____

10. Some hospitals and facilities use an autoclave that reaches a high temperature and high amount of pressure. What happens to the amount of time needed to sterilize in these units?

_____

Now turn to the Competency Evaluation Sheet for Procedure 8, Operation of an Autoclave, located in Appendix C of this text.

DRY HEAT STERILIZATION

Another popular method of sterilizing in the dental office is through dry heat. This process is basically sterilizing using an oven. It is good to use for instruments that tend to rust in a moist autoclave, but it is slower than autoclave processing. The amount of time necessary to sterilize depends on the temperature of the oven. The assistant should read the manufacturer's directions to determine the temperature setting for processing. Usually dry heat sterilization takes one hour at 340°F or two hours at 320°F. A new, rapid-acting, dry heat sterilizer with forced circulation at the temperature of 375°F has been developed to sterilize unwrapped items in 6 to 10 minutes for small loads (Figure 3–13). If articles are wrapped or in a cassette, a longer period is required for sterilization. Manufacturer's recommendations must be followed for all types of sterilizers. Although there are different types of dry heat sterilizers, they work on the same principle.

After washing and drying hands and donning thick, utility gloves, the instruments to be sterilized are precleaned and patted dry. They may be inserted directly

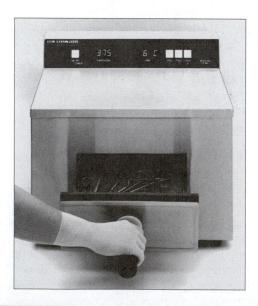

FIGURE 3–13 The assistant should use care when placing or removing the hot tray from the unit. (Courtesy of Cox Sterile Products, Inc.)

into the dry heat oven, or they may be wrapped in foil. Paper or heavy cloth may be used but these materials may char and discolor from the heat.

The three-prong electrical cord is properly inserted into the wall outlet and removed after the last load in the evening. Temperature gauges are checked and a quick review of the manufacturer's directions for the present type of load is made. The sterilizer is turned on and the temperature is permitted to rise to the proper level, either 340°F or 320°F. Occasionally, the assistant must adjust the temperature dial to activate and regulate the heating system to obtain the desired level.

Once the temperature is reached, the prepared instruments and objects are placed into the oven chamber. Much care is to be given to the proper handling in this hot area. To avoid burns, the new assistant should practice operating the loading and unloading of the oven when it is cool until the art is mastered. Articles may be placed in a cool chamber before the heating is activated but no timing of the load is begun until the sterilizing temperature is fully reached.

The articles to be sterilized are placed into the dry heat sterilizer, either wrapped or not. If the wrapping is too tight or the load is very large, extra time should be allotted. Circulation of the heat around the oven chamber must be permitted, so the chamber should not be overloaded.

When the items are loaded, the temperature is again allowed to rise to the prescribed level. At this time the sterilizing time **sequence** is begun and noted. Nothing should be added to the chamber once the timing has started. Opening the door and placing new objects into the oven chamber lowers the temperature and the cycle is ruined. Once sterilizing time is started, it should not be interrupted. At the end of the cycle the chamber is emptied, the instruments and materials are removed, and a new cycle started for another load.

The sterilized items are put away into their proper place. The wrapped items may be transferred by hand but those that are not wrapped must be moved using sterile transfer forceps.

The dry heat sterilizer should be checked periodically. The inside surfaces and trays should be cleaned only when the oven is cool. The outside of the unit should be kept smudge and fingerprint free by polishing with a dry cloth.

Chemical Vapor Sterilization

Chemicals may or may not be used for heat sterilization. In some manner they may sterilize and in other conditions they may be used to disinfect. The type of chemical and the proportion and method used helps to determine what state of asepsis is reached. (Chemical disinfection and sterilization are discussed in deeper detail later in this unit.).

Some dental offices may have a chemical vapor sterilizer. This is a piece of equipment that uses chemical steam (usually a formaldehyde mixture) instead of water steam so that instruments have less rust or corrosion in the vapor sterilizer than in the autoclave. Although it is an effective sterilizer and works in about the same time (20 minutes for 40 pounds of pressure at 270°C), it does have some setbacks that may make it an unpopular sterilizing method in the office. The major disadvantage to the chemical vapor sterilizer is that the chemical vapors are strong and have an offensive odor. The sterilizing area must have proper ventilation to use this method. Instruments must be entirely dry before placement in the chamber, or some rusting may occur. No sealed containers may be used. Items to be processed must be placed in a specific type of chemical-penetrating wrap material, and the chemical vapors may destroy some plastics. Wrapped packs must not be too large to hinder chemical vapor circulation in the chamber.

Sterilization Indicators

No matter what type or method of sterilizing is employed, the process should be periodically checked. Autoclave tapes placed on packages indicate if the prescribed pressure and temperature have been met but do not guarantee the procedure was fulfilled. To determine if the equipment is working properly and the system employed by the office personnel is exact, the assistant can include a commercial indicator in the load to be sterilized. It should be placed in the middle of the load to test effectiveness.

This indicator may be a strip, vial, or bulb that undergoes the entire sterilizing process. The indicator is either sent to a lab to be cultured and read or is placed in an office incubator for a later readout of effectiveness. In either case, the results of the sterilizing test should be recorded. The test should be performed on a regular basis, usually once a week, to assure proper sterilizing processing.

PROCEDURE 9
Operating a Dry Heat Sterilizer

1 **Prepare for the Procedure**
2 **Assemble the Equipment and Materials**
3 **Prepare the Dry Heat Sterilizer**
4 **Heat the Sterilizer**
5 **Load the Dry Heat Sterilizer**
6 **Complete the Sterilization Cycle**
7 **Remove the Articles**
8 **Store the Sterilized Items**
9 **Clean Up the Area**
10 **Remove the PPE**

1 Prepare for the Procedure

To prepare for the dry heat sterilizing procedure, the assistant washes and thoroughly dries hands before donning utility gloves. Incomplete drying of the hands may lead to under-glove irritation and bacterial growth during glove wear.

2 Assemble the Equipment and Materials

The assistant gathers the contaminated items and pre-cleans them. Instruments that are to be wrapped receive coverage. Aluminum foil is a good material to use to wrap items for the dry heat unit. Instruments may be placed into the dry heat sterilizer without coverage, but care in handling must be taken when removing the sterile objects.

3 Prepare the Dry Heat Sterilizer

The electrical plug to the unit must be carefully engaged and the temperature of the gauges checked. The manufacturer's chart should be consulted to determine desired temperature and time exposure. The amount of time involvement depends on the degree of heat in the unit. If the internal heat measures 340°F, the exposure time takes one hour. If the internal heat is 320°F, the time required is two hours. It is advisable to increase the exposure time if the load is large or there are full packs.

4 Heat the Sterilizer

The unit is turned on and the assistant monitors the equipment until the proper temperature is reached. A thermometer on the front of the unit displays the internal heat.

5 Load the Dry Heat Sterilizer

When the unit is ready, the assistant uses the supplied handle to open the door carefully and remove the sterilizer tray. The hot tray may be set on top of the unit to fill. Care must be taken to avoid overcrowding.

The loaded tray is inserted into the sterilizer, and the door is carefully closed. The unit may be filled when cold, but sterilization does not begin until the ideal temperatures have been met. Since the unit is loaded and used frequently while it is hot, the assistant should practice placing the tray in and out a few times when it is cool.

6 Complete the Sterilization Cycle

The sterilization process does not begin until the proper temperature is obtained. The assistant monitors the thermometer. When it reaches the correct temperature, the timer is set.

Once the sterilizing cycle has begun, no new articles may be placed into the unit. If something is added, the temperature drops and the cycle must be restarted to include the new item.

7 Remove the Articles

When the timer signals the end of the cycle, the assistant uses the handle to carefully open the door. The handle is engaged onto the loaded tray to remove it and place it on top of the unit. The items may be permitted to cool for awhile.

8 Store the Sterilized Items

The wrapped articles are placed into storage. All sterilized articles are rotated so newer packs are in the rear and older ones are used first.

Items that were not wrapped or covered are transferred by using sterile transfer forceps, which are kept close to the sterilizer. The items are placed in their proper area and covered to avoid contamination from dust. Sterilized articles may be placed into barrier or plastic sleeves for storage and handling. The transfer forceps and dry container are sterilized daily or more often if contamination occurs.

9 Clean Up the Area

The handle is used to pick up the tray, open the door, and return the tray to the hot oven. New articles may be sterilized at this time, or the unit may be turned off.

When the unit is cold, the assistant wipes out the interior and polishes the exterior. The plug may be removed at the end of the day.

10 Remove the PPE

When the sterilizing procedure is completed, the assistant washes, dries, and disinfects the utility gloves. The gloves are removed, and the hands are thoroughly washed and dried.▲

THEORY RECALL
Dry Heat Sterilization

1. What is one advantage a dry heat oven has over an autoclave?

2. What is one disadvantage a dry heat oven has to an autoclave?

3. What determines the amount of time necessary for dry heat sterilization?

_____

4. How much time would be required for dry heat sterilization in a 340°F oven? in a 320°F oven?

_____

5. With what material can the assistant wrap instruments for the dry oven?

_____

6. What is one precaution the assistant must observe when loading the dry oven?

_____

7. Why must the assistant wait to start timing the dry oven cycle after the instruments have been placed?

_____

8. What happens when new articles are placed into a dry oven sterilizer during a sterilizing process?

_____

9. Where are the instruments placed at the end of a dry oven sterilizing cycle?

_____

10. How soon may a new load for sterilizing be started after the first one is finished?

_____

Now turn to the Competency Evaluation Sheet for Procedure 9, Operating a Dry Heat Sterilizer, located in Appendix C of this text.

CHEMICALS AS DISINFECTANTS AND STERILIZERS

To be effective sterilizers, chemicals must be handled in a precise and exacting manner. The chemical preparation, storage, and use must be carefully monitored to be sure sterilization can occur. Many chemicals can kill pathogenic organisms but there are some pathogens that are able to build protective shields, called spores, around themselves. These spores can withstand chemicals, heat, and unfavorable conditions. When conditions are favorable, they can shed their spore covering and prosper. There are also some resistant viruses that can survive heat and harsh chemicals. Only through prolonged exposure (hours) to some specific chemical solutions, can these viruses' lives be broken down and killed. Therefore, to be sterilized, all forms of life, including spores and resistant viruses, must be killed.

When sterilization is not possible, disinfection must be applied. This process is the chemical destruction of as many pathogens as possible and the inhibiting of growth of any remaining organisms. The assistant attempts to either sterilize or disinfect each and every item used in the dental operatory.

When working with chemicals, the assistant must read the manufacturer's directions. The chemicals should be EPA- and American Dental Association (ADA)-accepted products. These products can be purchased in a variety of forms from powder packs to small vials to large liquid containers. Some are mixed with distilled water, others are activated, and still others are diluted in precise measurements to fulfill disinfecting or sterilizing duties. The manufacturer indicates what proportion ratio of product and amount of time to use to sterilize or disinfect. Sterilization requires hours; disinfection can occur in minutes.

Shelf or active life, the amount of time the solution is effective, is also indicated. Some chemicals need an **activator** to become active and then are effective for a specific amount of days. The activator is added, and the container is marked for the expiration date. Each time the chemical is used, it must be checked for effectiveness. Sodium hypochlorite, common household bleach, when mixed in a 1:10 solution can be an effective disinfectant; but because it is not a stable product, it must be mixed daily for use.

Some chemicals have a built-in indicator—color changing—that shows when the effectiveness of the product is gone. Other chemicals need an indicator strip, which is dipped into the solution to attest to the chemical's active life. Any indication of weakness or loss of effectiveness requires a new solution to be prepared and used.

The mixing ratio of chemicals is important also. In one ratio, the chemical may be effective as a disinfectant, while in another ratio, it is used as a holding solution. Reading the manufacturer's directions and using the measuring cup or device included helps assure compliance with the necessary requirements for preparation. Use distilled water when the need for water dilution is necessary as some chemicals lose effectiveness in hard water.

Chemicals differ in their use, but the assistant should treat all chemicals with respect. Avoid spills and splashing chemicals on the body and clothing. Flush any affected areas with water and check the manufacturer's directions for precautionary tactics to be used. Never place fingers into solutions, but use transfer forceps to manipulate in these liquids. Always read directions and move in a controlled manner, avoid mixing and preparation in a rush. When the assistant is done with a solution or when a solution has expired, check for disposal methods. Disposal procedures are listed on the package also.

It usually is not the responsibility of the assistant to choose the type of sterilizing product used in the dental office; but the assistant has the responsibility to read the directions, use it in a proper manner, test the effectiveness periodically, and record the test results.

Maintain a solution log sheet when preparing disinfecting and sterilizing solutions. These log sheets may be made up in the office or acquired from various manufacturers. The assistant should record the dates of solution activation and expiration and test strip applications and dates with pass-fail results in the log sheet. The assistant making the solutions and tests may initial the procedure for future reference.

The procedure the assistant follows when working with sterilizing and disinfecting solutions begins with assembling the following: necessary chemicals, measuring instruments, spray bottle, chemical sterilizing holder, and a marker or pen and paper to record times.

Because of the nature of the product being used, the assistant dons protective attire. Utility gloves are a must. A mask to protect from vapors and eyeglasses to protect from vapors and sprays are suggested. The assistant must mix the spray solution according to the manufacturer's directions.

After the mixing is completed, the date is marked on the container so active life can be anticipated. Mixing procedures and dates are noted in the solution log book or the office infection control manual.

Fill spray bottles for office use. The bottles are cleaned out and checked for proper working condition and then filled with the chemical solution. The proper spray must be placed into the properly marked spray bottle. If a new chemical is being used or the spray bottle contents are being changed, the assistant must clean the old spray chemical out, fully clean the bottle, and relabel the spray bottle for the new contents. Expired solution may be aspirated into the evacuation lines for disposal and rinsing of the evacuation system.

To use the disinfectant, the assistant first sprays the surface, wipes up any matter or dirt present, and disposes of the paper towel. A 4 x 4 gauze pad may be used, but towels are less expensive and cover more. After the surface has been wiped off, the assistant resprays and permits the solution to remain in a wet pool for the manufacturer's recommended time, usually from 2 to 10 minutes. Any pool solution remaining after this time may be blotted up with a clean towel, and the towel is placed into the disposal container (Figure 3–14).

Chemicals to be used as sterilizers are carefully prepared according to the manufacturer's directions. Glass or plastic solution containers are washed, dried, and then filled to three-quarters full to permit space for placement of items to be sterilized. A clean strip of white adhesive tape may be placed on the lid of the container to mark the time of insertion of items so proper timing for sterilization is assured. Once the timing cycle has begun, no new items may be added without restarting the cycle. When the disinfecting and sterilizing period is over, the instruments are drained,

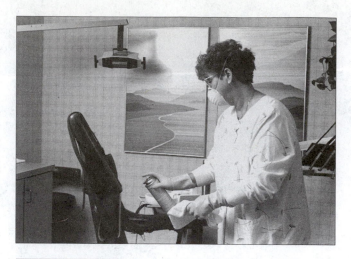

FIGURE 3–14 The assistant has the responsibility to properly disinfect with the spray-wipe-spray technique.

rinsed, and dumped onto sterile toweling and then patted dry (Figure 3–15).

Lids are kept on the container to prevent dust contamination and evaporation. All items placed into the chemical sterilizing solutions must be dried so that the solutions are not weakened. When the instruments are removed from the chemical solution, they should be rinsed with sterile water to remove chemical aftertaste, dried with sterile toweling, bagged or wrapped, and placed in a dustproof storage area.

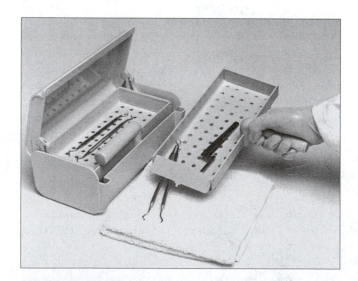

FIGURE 3–15 Instruments can be sterilized if placed in a properly mixed, active chemical solution for the prescribed time, usually 10 hours. (Courtesy of Palmero Dental Manufacturing Company.)

PROCEDURE 10

Using Chemicals as Disinfectants and Sterilizers

1 Assemble the Necessary Items

2 Don PPE

3 Prepare Disinfectant Spray

4 Record Active Life

5 Fill the Spray Bottle

6 Prepare Chemical Solutions for Sterilization

7 Use the Disinfecting Spray

8 Use the Chemical Sterilizer

9 Storage and Disposal of Chemicals

10 Clean Up the Area

1 Assemble the Necessary Items

The assistant gathers the necessary items to prepare for disinfection and sterilization: concentrated chemical solutions, distilled water, activation chemical, chemical solution log book, spray bottles, chemical solution sterilizer, indicator tapes, PPE, and marking pen.

2 Don PPE

Personal protection equipment is worn by the assistant. Eyeglasses are necessary to prevent splatter of chemicals into the eyes. Utility gloves are needed for protection of the hands, and if the chemicals are vaporous, a mask should be donned.

3 Prepare Disinfectant Spray

Each chemical solution is different. The assistant must follow the manufacturer's directions. If the solution needs dilution, distilled water is used because hard or soft tap water may cause the neutralization of the chemicals.

Some chemicals require an activator to become effective. The proportions, ratios, and directions for preparation are important. The same chemical at one ratio is considered a sterilizer, while diluted into another ratio, the same chemical may be considered a disinfectant. Follow the manufacturer's directions.

Each chemical label should indicate the contents of the bottle; and manufacturer's safety data sheets can direct the care, storage, mixture, properties, and disposal of the contents.

4 Record Active Life

The expiration date of the solution should be marked on the master bottle. Any smaller bottles of the solu-

tion must be labeled with the name of the contents. The name of the chemical and the date should be obvious. The procedure should be recorded in a solution log book, giving the solution name, the date of preparation, the expiration date or active life, and the initials of the person who prepared the solution.

5 Fill the Spray Bottle

The spray bottle to be filled is washed out and the condition of the bottle is checked. Any leaking areas or loose connecting tops indicate the bottle needs to be replaced.

Once the bottle is filled and the top is secured, the action is tested. The marked bottle is placed in the operatory or proper storage place. Hot storage areas should be avoided because heat breaks down the chemicals faster.

6 Prepare Chemical Solutions for Sterilization

Chemicals to be used as sterilizers are prepared according to the manufacturer's directions. The containers to hold the solution are washed and dried. The container is filled with the new sterilizing solution to the fill line or at least three-quarters full to permit the placement of articles. The date of placement may be marked on a tape and placed on top of the container. Solutions should be changed frequently.

7 Use the Disinfecting Spray

When using the chemicals as a disinfectant, the assistant should spray-wipe-spray. The disinfectant being used must contain a detergent to remove the debris and organic matter or another spray must be used to clean the surface before disinfection.

The disinfectant is sprayed on the surface and wiped off with a disposable towel, which is dropped into the contaminated container. The area is resprayed, and the solution is permitted to remain on the surface for the manufacturer's recommended exposure time (2 to 10 minutes). At the end of the cycle any small pools of solution may be blotted off with a clean paper towel.

8 Use the Chemical Sterilizer

When using the chemicals as a sterilizing solution, the assistant cleans the articles and pats them dry so the solutions will not be diluted. The articles are submerged totally into the solution. (Any surface not covered will not be sterilized.) The articles are permitted to remain covered by the solution for the prescribed exposure time (usually 10 hours). When the articles are submerged, the time is written on the tape on top of the container. No new articles may be added to the solutions without starting a new cycle.

After the prescribed time has been met, the articles are raised in the sterilizing tray and permitted to drain. They are then rinsed with water to remove the chemical aftertaste. The articles are transferred to a sterile towel and patted dry. The items are taken to their proper storage area using sterile transfer forceps. The area is cleaned up and the towels are placed in the trash container.

9 Storage and Disposal of Chemicals

The chemicals are stored according to the manufacturer's directions. Generally, they are placed in cool, dark areas. The bottles are rotated in stock, using the older ones first. When preparing to use chemicals, the assistant checks the expiration dates to be sure the chemical is effective.

Old chemicals must be disposed of following the manufacturer's directions and according to the local EPA regulations. If the purchased chemicals were ADA and EPA approved, they can be disposed of in the local sewage system. Some local restrictions, such as proximity to a water treatment plant, may be of concern to local environmental agencies. A good way to dispose of expired chemical sterilizing and disinfecting solutions is to aspirate them into the evacuation lines at cleanup.

10 Clean Up the Area

When the chemicals are prepared, the assistant cleans up the area. All spills and liquids in the area are wiped up. The floor is wiped of any drips. All wipe up towels may be placed into the trash container.

The assistant washes, dries, and removes the utility gloves. The PPE equipment is put away, and the hands are thoroughly washed and dried.▲

T H E O R Y   R E C A L L
Chemicals as Disinfectants and Sterilizers

1. What are spores?

2. Chemicals used in the dental office should bear acceptance seals from which two organizations?

3. If disinfection and sterilization chemicals need dilution, what substance is used?

4. When speaking of immersion time, which process takes hours to complete—disinfection or sterilization?

5. What is shelf or active life?

6. What is the active life of sodium hypochlorite?

7. What is the purpose of built-in indicators in disinfecting and sterilizing solutions?

8 Why is the mixing ratio important in preparing disinfecting and sterilizing solutions?

9. What are some rules of conduct a dental assistant should use when working with chemicals?

10. What is the dental assistant's responsibility in the preparation of chemicals?

Now turn to the Competency Evaluation Sheet for Procedure 10, Using Chemicals as Disinfectants and Sterilizers, located in Appendix C of this text.

Cleanup of Operatory and Equipment Techniques

After the patient has left, the assistant flushes all tubing lines. Handpieces should be operated for at least 30 seconds to move water through the hoses. Suction should be performed on a half gallon of disinfecting and deodorizing solution to clean and freshen these lines. The handpieces and suction tips are removed and placed with the tray of dirty instruments to be taken to the sterilizing room. If the handpieces cannot be sterilized by autoclave or dry heat, they must be disinfected. All soiled barrier shields and loose objects are gathered with the dirty instruments and removed. The assistant makes a preliminary wipe up of all loose debris and returns to the sterilizing area to complete the cleanup.

When all items have been assembled in the sterilizing area, the assistant removes the latex exam gloves, records the treatment, and takes the chart to the front desk or designated area. Upon returning to the sterilizing area, the assistant returns to wash hands and don the utility gloves for sterilizing and disinfecting.

The assistant reenters the operatory and disinfects the area with the spray-wipe-spray technique. All surfaces are sprayed with a disinfectant, wiped clean with a towel or 4 × 4 sponge, and sprayed again. The sprayed solution should remain on the surface for the manufacturer's allotted time, usually 2 to 10 minutes. Particular attention is given to the operatory light. Handles are cleaned thoroughly and the front light panel is wiped off. Sprays are not aimed directly at electrical switches or connections. Towels saturated with disinfectant are used in these areas. After all surfaces, handles, switches, tubing, and equipment have been disinfected, the assistant replaces any barrier covers and places the contaminated towels into the disposal bag or container and returns to the sterilizing area to clean up the used articles.

The first attention to the tray is to the sharp objects. These are removed from the tray and disposed of in a sharps container (Figure 3–16). Never should the hands be used to loosen the sharps. Always use pliers or special appliances to remove sharps and place them in the sharps container.

All paper and disposable products, such as cotton rolls, plastic suction tips, cups, paper points, prophy angles, and pumice cups are discarded into the disposal container. This container is lined with a marked, leakproof bag and is kept covered at all times. A foot lever control for closing is good to use as the hands need not touch the container at any time during the disposal.

Handpieces and ultrasonic scaler handpieces must be heat sterilized. Manufacturer's cleaning and lubricating directions must be followed for these expensive items. Most modern handpieces can be scrubbed with soap and water to remove gross debris and matter, patted dry, and lubricated (if required) before sterilization. After cleaning, the handpieces are placed in paper sleeves and placed in the autoclave or chemical vapor sterilizer. If the handpiece requires lubrication after the sterilizing process, a separate clean lubricant is used to condition the instrument. Handpieces are never placed in cold sterilizing solutions.

Eyeglasses, face shields, hand mirrors, light curing processing shields, and larger articles are disinfected and placed aside. The assistant then carefully removes the instruments from the tray and if not using a cassette load program, places them in a holding solution or a cleaning solution. Instruments must be cleaned before they are sterilized. The assistant may use a hand brush to brush off debris and blood from the instruments and then rinse them. After the rinse, the instruments are placed on paper toweling and patted dry. They are then placed into the ultrasonic cleaner for a more thorough cleansing before proper sterilizing.

The counter tops are sprayed, wiped clean, and sprayed with disinfectant again. The floor space is checked and cleaned if needed. The sink is wiped out and all disposable toweling is placed in the disposal bag or container. The gloves are washed, disinfected, removed, and placed on a drying rack until next use (Figure 3–17). The assistant washes hands as a final precaution.

Once the instruments and equipment are sterilized, they may be returned to the operatory for future use. Cabinet drawers and storage places must be periodically cleaned and disinfected. The cleaning for this procedure is done on an office schedule and recorded in the office manual. If there is obvious contamination, debris, or dirt, the drawer must be cleaned, washed, and disinfected, no matter what time the schedule dictates.

Proper and correct sterilizing and disinfecting techniques are required to lessen the chances of infection in the dental office.

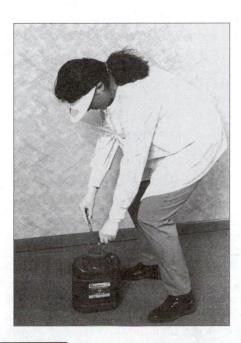

FIGURE 3–16 When disposing of sharp items, care must be taken to avoid a finger stick or cut. Any unfortunate incident should be reported at once to the dentist or infection control officer.

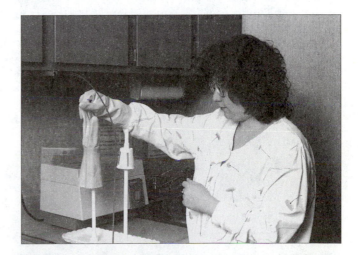

FIGURE 3–17 The assistant places the utility gloves on the rack to drip dry until the next use. Contamination to patient and operator is lessened.

74

PROCEDURE 11

Cleanup of Operatory and Equipment Techniques

1. **Clean Up the Operatory**
2. **Gather Items for Sterilization**
3. **Don PPE**
4. **Disinfect the Operatory**
5. **Remove the Sharps**
6. **Remove the Disposables**
7. **Prepare the Handpieces**
8. **Prepare the Instruments**
9. **Sterilize the Instruments**
10. **Clean Up the Area**

1 Clean Up the Operatory

The assistant begins the operatory cleanup by flushing the lines. The handpieces are run for at least 30 seconds to remove any contaminated back flow from the previous patient. The handpieces and all suction and spray tips are removed from the lines and placed on the tray to be taken for sterilization.

The evacuation lines are washed out by aspirating water or expired disinfectant solution. This solution cleans out the lines, which helps keep them fresh and odor free. Some commercial evacuation powders and solutions are available to be used to **deodorize** and flush the lines.

2 Gather Items for Sterilization

All removable items are placed on the tray and removed to the sterilizing room for conditioning. The patient's records, x-rays, and items are also removed. Any instrument present for the procedure must be considered contaminated regardless if it was used or not. All items are sterilized. If using a cassette load system, the used items to be sterilized are replaced into their proper position in the cassette for ultrasonic cleaning and sterilization.

3 Don PPE

The assistant removes the exam gloves, washes and dries the hands, and records the patient's treatment on the chart and places them in the appropriate place. Utility gloves and eyeglasses are donned for the cleanup procedure.

4 Disinfect the Operatory

After donning PPE, the assistant returns to the operatory area. All surfaces are disinfected with a spray-wipe-

spray technique. Particular attention is given to the areas known to be used, such as lamp handles, drawer openers, and chair levers. Barriers are checked and replaced if needed. A quick check is made to be certain the room is ready for the next patient.

5 Remove the Sharps

In the sterilizing area, the assistant removes and disposes of the sharps first. Recapped needles are removed by grasping the sheath and rotating the needle from the syringe. The entire assembly is deposited directly into the sharps container. If resistance is found, the assistant removes the needle with pliers or a mechanical device. (Do not use fingers.) All other sharp objects, such as blades, are taken apart using a mechanical device and placed directly into the center of the sharps container. All removal of sharps is done in an outward motion to avoid stabbing self.

6 Remove the Disposables

Disposables are carried to and placed in the designated contaminated bag by their ends or loops. Any article present during the procedure is considered contaminated. Used disposable items are placed in marked bags, the unused items are resterilized before reusing. Large items are disinfected.

7 Prepare the Handpieces

The handpieces are sterilized following the manufacturer's directions. These are expensive items and need proper care. The manufacturer may recommend washing with detergent to remove gross debris, patting dry, and placing into an autoclave bag or sleeve for sterilization in an autoclave, dry heat sterilizer, or chemical vapor sterilizer. Some handpieces require lubrication before and some after sterilization. All lubricating materials must be kept separate to avoid cross contamination. The assistant must read the directions before sterilizing the handpieces.

8 Prepare the Instruments

Instruments that have been removed from the operatory must be precleaned and sterilized before reuse. They may be placed in a holding solution for a short time, but all must be precleaned before sterilization and disinfection. A brush and water or an ultrasonic cleaner may be used to remove gross debris. The instruments must be patted dry and wrapped or prepared before sanitation processing. Toweling used to prepare the instruments is disposed of in the contaminated container.

9 Sterilize the Instruments

The instruments and items are sterilized according to the method chosen in the facility. All sterilizing processes must be completed to the fullest. No short cuts may be allowed.

10 Clean Up the Area

The area is cleaned up after the processing is completed. The counter tops, floor, surfaces, and sink are wiped up of spills and spots. The towels are placed in the contaminated bag.

The PPE is removed. Utility gloves are washed, dried, disinfected, and removed. To permit the gloves to air dry and prevent a moisture buildup and messy, contaminated area, the gloves may be placed on a drip rack until the next use. The hands are washed and dried.▲

THEORY RECALL

Cleanup of Operatory and Equipment Techniques

1. Why are the handpieces operated for 30 seconds during the cleanup procedure?

2. How are the suction lines cleaned during the cleanup procedure?

3. What must be done to handpieces that cannot be autoclaved or dry heat sterilized?

4. How long is the sprayed solution required to stay on the surfaces for disinfection?

5. What item is given attention first during the disposal of objects on the contaminated tray?

6. What must be done to the instruments before sterilization?

7. Where are the disposable towels and paper products from the contaminated tray placed?

8. What attention is given to floor space during cleanup procedures?

9. What is done to the utility gloves when all work has been completed in a cleanup procedure?

10. How does the assistant handle the sterilized instruments that have not been wrapped or placed in sleeves or envelopes?

Now turn to the Competency Evaluation Sheet for Procedure 11, Cleanup of Operatory and Equipment Techniques, located in Appendix C of this text.

HAZARD AND FIRE CONTROL

Chemical and Vaporous Hazard Management

There are many different chemicals used in the dental office. Some are hazardous to the skin, mucous membranes, and surface materials. The assistant must be careful when working with any chemical or liquid.

To comply with OSHA standards, any product considered hazardous is labeled. If the assistant desires to make smaller supply bottles of a chemical for the operatory use or other areas, the smaller bottle must bear a label with the contents identified. If hazardous, the cabinet must also be labeled to warn personnel (Figure 3–18).

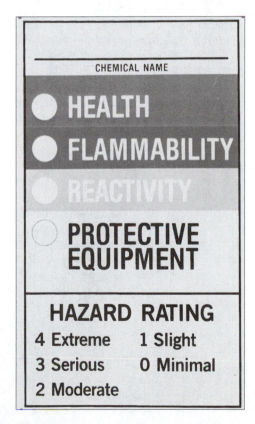

FIGURE 3–18 Labels can identify possible hazards. Products are marked indicating levels of care needed. Blue denotes a health hazard. Red indicates burning susceptibility. Yellow shows chemical stability, and white indicates protective equipment is needed. (Photo courtesy of Lab Safety Supply, Inc., Janesville, WI.)

The manufacturers supply the dental office with material safety data sheets (MSDS). These papers identify the product, its hazards, the care that must be given the product, and the disposal of the product. All MSDS must be maintained in an office manual, and each employee must know the location of the manual and how to interpret the sheets (Figure 3–19).

The assistant must be aware that hazardous products are not always in large gallon jugs. Any size liquid vials may be very caustic or harmful to people. Small liquids, such as acid etch liquids or monomers, can harm skin and mucous membranes if not used properly. Solid liquids, such as mercury, give off harmful vapors. The assistant must be careful of all products.

There are general rules to observe when working with chemicals:

▶ Always know the identity of the material and its qualities in use.
▶ Always wear protective equipment, such as gloves, eyeglasses, and masks.
▶ Keep an MSDS file for reference.
▶ Always investigate contents of new products.
▶ Keep bottles and jars capped when not in use.
▶ Know first-aid procedures for contact with hazardous materials.
▶ Have good ventilation when using chemicals.
▶ Keep flames and heat sources away from chemicals.
▶ Store products according to the manufacturer's directions.
▶ Clean up any messes immediately; dispose of items properly.

When working with vaporous hazard materials, such as mercury, monomers, nitrous oxide, solvents, and other vaporous materials, the assistant must keep the area well ventilated. Eyeglasses and masks are worn to protect mucous membranes. Caution must be taken not to work too long a period with these types of chemical vapors. Manufacturers' recommendations should be followed for these materials also.

Power Equipment Hazard Management

MODEL TRIMMER. In many dental offices, a model trimmer is a standard piece of laboratory equipment (Figure 3–20). This device is a large, round abrasive wheel encased in a metal frame that forcefully rotates when electrical power is turned on. The function of the machine is to grind or trim down gypsum models and products. Because of the abrasive nature of the wheel, water must be circulated onto the surface at all times of use. The water keeps the wheel from becoming clogged and losing its effectiveness.

There are two hoses attached to the trimmer. The smaller one supplies the water to the unit and the larger hose empties the water and gypsum trimmings into the sink.

When using the model trimmer, the assistant must follow some rules for managing the hazards of this power machine. The assistant must:

▶ Wear safety glasses when working on the trimmer.
▶ Pull back long hair to avoid trapping in the trimmer.
▶ Roll up sleeves and remove bracelets.
▶ Keep electrical cord out of the way and behind the trimmer.
▶ Plug in just before use.

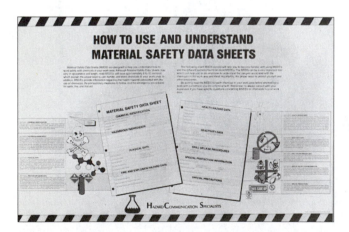

FIGURE 3–19 Material safety data sheets (MSDS) can provide much information about a product. OSHA requires that dental personnel understand how to use these sheets and that an MSDS file be maintained for all products used. (Photo courtesy of Lab Safety Supply, Inc., Janesville, WI.)

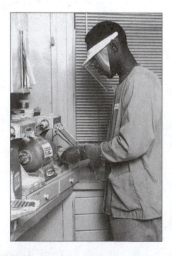

FIGURE 3–20 The assistant observes safety rules when working on a trimmer machine or any power-driven appliance.

▶ At turn-off time, remain with trimmer until all wheel circulation is completed.

▶ Always have a sufficient supply of water circulating on the abrasive wheel.

▶ Never trim any other product but gypsum materials.

▶ Use moderate, firm pressure when holding models to wheel.

▶ Keep models on trimmer tray for stability.

▶ Concentrate on the job at hand.

▶ Always leave the wheel clean; run water on the wheel until clear.

▶ Brush and clean wheel only when stopped and unplugged.

DENTAL LATHE. Another large piece of power equipment in the dental office operated by the assistant is the dental lathe. This machine is used to finish and polish dental appliances and equipment. The source of power is electrical and the force is determined by the horsepower of the motor.

There are two drive shafts, one on either side of the dental lathe motor. Various grinding, abrasive wheels, brushes, and polishing apparatus are placed upon these shafts. The assistant must be sure to apply these appliances correctly and test for stability before turning on the lathe.

There are two speeds, fast and slow. The machine should be started in "slow" to be sure all is functioning well before the speed is increased, if needed.

The assistant should follow all rules set for power equipment:

▶ Always wear eyeglass protection; tie hair back; remove jewelry.

▶ Check electrical cord; place it behind the lathe.

▶ Check the sturdiness of any attached apparatus.

▶ Start in slow speed; increase speed later, if needed.

▶ Remain nearby until the motor is completely stopped.

▶ Clean only when the motor is stopped and unplugged.

▶ Concentrate on the job at hand.

General Hazard Management

No matter where the assistant may be in the dental office, there are possible general hazards. Many of these hazards are the result of careless handling by the office staff. Some general care should be taken by all members of the dental team:

▶ Avoid clutter by picking up and putting things away.

▶ Close all drawers and file cabinet shelves and drawers.

▶ Keep electrical cords behind appliances.

▶ Read directions before using equipment and materials.

▶ Maintain a watchful eye for any hazards that may occur.

With cooperation of all employees and an awareness of hazards and their management, the office should be a safer place to work.

Heat and Flame Hazard Management

Some sources of heat and flame hazards in the dental office are the sterilizers (autoclave and dry heat), hot oil and glass bead endodontic sterilizers, and laboratory Bunsen burner flames.

When working around heat sources, the assistant must keep all clutter and materials away from the source of heat. Electrical cords to the heating units should be checked periodically for frays and condition. Cords should always be kept behind the appliance and not where they could catch and drag the equipment with it.

The assistant should practice manipulating the equipment at a slow speed until he or she is comfortable with the use of the items. Never act in a rushed or quick manner when working with hot materials.

In the case of oil or glass bead sterilizers, the assistant must make sure they are placed in a level position where they will not be knocked over or tumble and spill their contents.

Bunsen burners and alcohol torches should be used with care. All tubing must be kept as short as functionally effective, and the assistant should be aware of the position of the main gas shutoff if a need should arise. Tubing should be kept untangled and checked for wear. Combustible materials should not be placed around the flame areas.

The dental assistant should know the location of the fire extinguisher and how to operate it. There are three basic types of extinguishers and the assistant should take time to become familiar with the units in the office (Figure 3–21).

Most offices purchase a general use fire extinguisher, which suffocates the flame. The assistant should know how to get the extinguisher from the wall to the site, how to aim (six inches before the source), how to release the safety pin, and how to trigger or release the fire extinguishing material. Practice and simulated fire drills help an assistant become competent in heat and fire hazard management.

The best fire prevention is to be prepared. Review the fire exit plan for the facility; know the location, type, and use of the first extinguishers; rehearse practice drills; know the emergency phone number for help; and always remain calm.▲

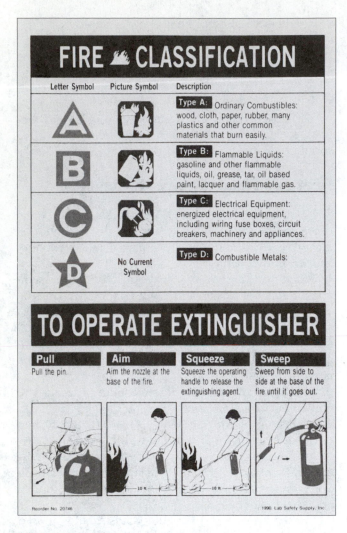

FIGURE 3-21 This fire chart shows extinguisher types and uses. The assistant should become familiar with the position and use of the extinguisher before an actual emergency. (Photo courtesy of Lab Safety Supply, Inc., Janesville, WI.)

THEORY RECALL

Hazard and Fire Control

1. If the assistant makes up a small supply bottle from a large chemical bottle, what must the assistant do?

2. What does the manufacturer supply to the dental facility that tells about the contents and safety features of the item?

3. In what size bottle will the assistant find a hazardous chemical?

4. List six rules an assistant should follow when working around chemicals.

   a. _____

   b. _____

   c. _____

   d. _____

   e. _____

   f. _____

5. What PPE should be worn when working with chemicals?

6. What piece of PPE must the assistant wear when working with a trimmer?

7. In what speed should the assistant start the dental lathe when using it?

8. Where should the electrical cord be placed when working with the power appliance?

9. List two sources of heat hazards found in the dental facility.

   a. _____

   b. _____

10. What is the best preparation for a fire emergency?

For additional activities related to this lesson, turn to Assignment Sheet 3.1, Hazard and Fire Control, located in Appendix B of this text.

POST TEST

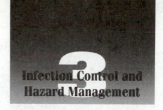

Total possible points = 100 points
80% needed for passing = 80 points

Total points this test _____ pass _____ fail _____

MATCHING: Write the letter from column B that best describes or matches the word in column A. Each question is worth 2 points for a total of 20 points.

Column A

_____ 1. State Dental Practice Act
_____ 2. disinfection
_____ 3. autoclave
_____ 4. EPA
_____ 5. HIV
_____ 6. OSHA
_____ 7. HBV
_____ 8. sterilization
_____ 9. cavitation
_____ 10. deodorize

Column B

a. human immunodeficiency virus
b. bubbling, imploding action
c. agency concerned with worker safety
d. process of lessening odors
e. process of destroying all life forms
f. agency controlling dental profession
g. hepatitis B virus
h. process to destroy pathogens
i. a machine that sterilizes
j. agency that enforces clean air, water;
  conservation and recovery act

MULTIPLE CHOICE: Circle the correct answer. Each question is worth 4 points for a total of 80 points.

1. Which of the following methods is the most effective way to preclean instruments?
   a. autoclave   b. steel brush   c. holding solution   d. ultrasonic cleaner

2. What type of gloves does the assistant wear when cleaning up and sterilizing or disinfecting?
   a. latex   b. surgical rubber   c. plastic overgloves   d. utility gloves

3. What is the usual time required for instruments to be submerged in chemical solutions in the sterilization process?
   a. 1 hour   b. 2 hours   c. 5 hours   d. 10 hours

4. HIV and HBV are infections that
   a. are caused by easily detected viruses.   c. make use of universal precautions a necessity.
   b. are cured with a vaccine.   d. are not considered a serious health problem.

5. Maintaining an area as free of microorganisms as possible is called
   a. asepsis.   b. universal precautions.   c. antisepsis.   d. sepsis.

6. Hepatitis B inoculation requires three injections completed during what time span?
   a. 1 month   b. 2 months   c. 3 months   d. 6 months

7. What are spores?
   a. disposable shoe coverings   c. combination dental bur and brush
   b. protective capsules covering germs   d. chemical indicators

8. Chemicals used in dental facilities should show acceptance seals from:
   (1) ADA, (2) EPA, (3) OSHA, (4) CDC, or (5) SDPA.
   a. all of the above   b. 1 and 2   c. 1, 2, and 3   d. 1, 2, 3, and 4

9. Clothing used in barrier attire for the professionals should be
   a. moisture resistant.   b. waterproof.   c. fire resistant.   d. a, b, and c.

10. The final evaporation time in the autoclave is usually
    a. 30 seconds.   b. 4 to 5 minutes.   c. 10 minutes.   d. 20 minutes.

79

11. Which temperature is needed to sterilize instruments in two hours in the dry heat sterilizer?
    a. 120°F   b. 320°F   c. 340°F   d. 100°C

12. Etched ultrasonic beakers should not be used when they are scratched because
    a. they are unsightly.
    b. they discolor articles.
    c. they break easily.
    d. they interfere with solution action.

13. What is used to transfer sterile instruments from the autoclave to the dental unit drawers?
    a. dry, sterile transfer forceps
    b. transfer forceps held in disinfectant solution
    c. fingers
    d. utility gloves

14. What must be destroyed before an article can be considered sterile?
    a. all life   b. all pathogens   c. all germs   d. all viruses

15. Which of the following is *not* considered a necessity for sterilizing in an autoclave?
    a. a tilted jar   b. do not overcrowd   c. open the hinges   d. set all articles flat

16. Which solution is *not* used to aspirate and cleanse evacuation lines?
    a. an x-ray fixer   b. chlorinated water   c. expired disinfectant   d. tap water

17. What is the active life of sodium hypochorite as a disinfectant?
    a. 1 day   b. 1 week   c. 1 month   d. as indicated by color

18. Which of the following may be used as an effective barrier for infection control of equipment: (1) aluminum foil, (2) latex tubing, (3) plastic wrap, or (4) clear sheathing?
    a. 1, 3, and 4   b. 1, 2, and 3   c. all of the above   d. none of the above

19. Which of the following is *not* needed for a hand-wash technique?
    a. antimicrobial soap lotion   b. sterile towel   c. cuticle or orange stick   d. running water

20. What substance is placed in the reservoir of the autoclave?
    a. distilled water   b. disinfecting oil   c. alcohol   d. disinfectant

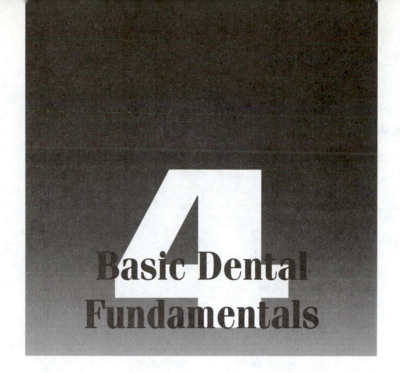

4 Basic Dental Fundamentals

▶ OBJECTIVES

Upon completion of this unit, the student will achieve a score of 80% or better on the Post Test covering the following material.

1. Identify kinds, types, numbers, names, and identification of teeth, as well as tooth and gingival tissues.
2. Identify divisions of the mouth and various surfaces of the teeth. Demonstrate the method to abbreviate and combine surface names.
3. Explain the method of numbering teeth for the Universal, Palmer, and Federation Dentaire Internationale systems.
4. Discuss and demonstrate the methods for dental charting of existing mouth conditions, using both anatomical and geometrical charts.
5. Identify the different types and kinds of hand and rotary instruments and explain the function of each.
6. Demonstrate various methods of passing and transferring hand instruments, including pen, palm, and palm-thumb grasp.

▶ KEY TERMS

abrasive	deciduous	mesial
alveolar	dentin	molar
apical	distal	occlusal
arch	enamel	papilla
bicuspid	foramen	periodontium
buccal	gingiva	permanent
canine	incisor	primary
cementum	interproximal	proximal
central	lateral	pulp
cervix	lingual	quadrant
condense	mandibular	roots
crosscut	mandrel	rotary
crown	maxillary	shank
cuspid		

TOOTH ANATOMY

Amounts and Types of Teeth

The three main reasons we have teeth are to chew (masticate) our food, to aid in speaking (articulate), and to look good (esthetics).

We have four different kinds of teeth in our mouth:

incisors—cutting teeth used to bite and cut food

canines or **cuspids**—(eye teeth) used to tear and break off food

bicuspids or premolars—used to break up and mash food

molars—used to grind and pulverize food

Our teeth are situated in jawbones. The lower jaw is a strong, solid bone called the mandible; therefore, when speaking of anything in the lower jaw, we use the term **mandibular**.

Our upper jaw is composed of two bones called maxilla, right and left; therefore, when speaking of anything in the upper jaw we use the term **maxillary**.

We have two sets of teeth, **primary**, or **deciduous** teeth, which are also called baby teeth. As adults we have secondary teeth, which are called **permanent** teeth. During our lifetime we receive 20 deciduous teeth and 32 permanent teeth (Figure 4–1).

In the 32 permanent or secondary teeth, we receive:

8 incisors—4 maxillary and 4 mandibular
4 canines or cuspids—2 maxillary and 2 mandibular
8 premolars or bicuspids—4 maxillary and 4 mandibular
12 molars—6 maxillary and 6 mandibular

32 total permanent or secondary teeth

In the 20 deciduous or primary teeth, there are no bicuspids and no third molars; therefore, we receive 12 less teeth (Figure 4–2).

8 incisors—4 maxillary and 4 mandibular
4 canines or cuspids—2 maxillary and 2 mandibular
8 molars—4 maxillary and 4 mandibular

20 total deciduous or primary teeth

There are no premolars or bicuspids in the deciduous dentition. When these teeth erupt, they replace the primary molars. Secondary or permanent molars do not replace any teeth.

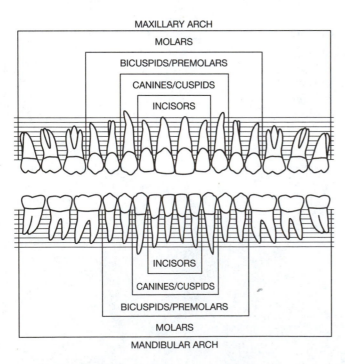

FIGURE 4–1 Adult dentition showing arrangement of incisors, cuspids, premolars, and molars (32 teeth).

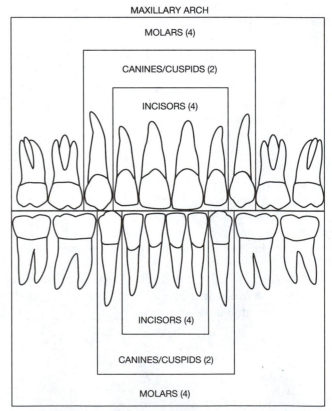

FIGURE 4–2 Deciduous dentition showing arrangement of incisors, canines, and molars (20 teeth).

Each arch has a right and left side. The midline, an imaginary vertical line through the center of the face, divides the mouth into four parts called **quadrants** (Figure 4–3). The four quadrants are:

maxillary right quadrant
maxillary left quadrant
mandibular left quadrant
mandibular right quadrant

In each quadrant of the permanent set of teeth (dentition), there are eight teeth. They are named from the midline (center of the face) moving toward the posterior:

1 **central** incisor—anterior or front tooth
1 **lateral** incisor—anterior or front tooth directly next to the central
1 cuspid or canine—eye tooth, situated at the corner of the mouth
2 premolars or bicuspids—shorter, stubbier teeth; fourth and fifth back; have two cusps or prominences
3 molars—large grinding teeth in back; sixth, seventh, and eighth teeth back from the midline

In each quadrant of the primary teeth (dentition), there are five teeth (Figure 4–4):

1 central incisor—anterior or front tooth
1 lateral incisor—anterior or front tooth directly next to the central incisor
1 cuspid or canine—eye tooth at corner of mouth
2 molars—grinding teeth in back of mouth; fourth and fifth from the midline

A person having only secondary teeth is considered an adult patient and is said to have permanent dentition. A person having only primary teeth is considered a child patient and is said to have a deciduous dentition. A person having primary and secondary teeth at

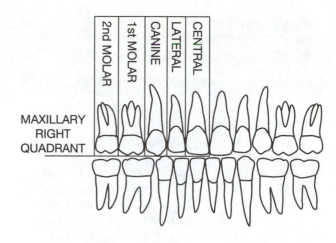

FIGURE 4–4 Deciduous maxillary right quadrant with each tooth identified (5).

the same time (between the ages of 6 and 14) is said to have a mixed dentition.

Besides being divided into quadrants, the teeth may be typed also as anterior or posterior (Figure 4–5). Anterior teeth are the ones in the front of the mouth from and including canine to canine. They are longer and more slender teeth and single rooted. Incisors and cuspids or canines are the anterior teeth.

Posterior teeth are the shorter, thicker teeth in the back of the mouth. Bicuspids or premolars have single roots, except for the first maxillary bicuspid or premolar, which has two root canals causing splitting into two small roots at the apical third of the tooth. Mandibular molars have two roots, and the three rooted maxillary

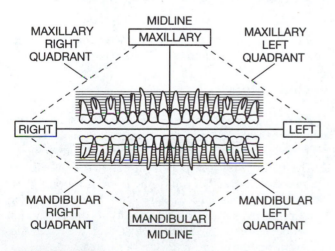

FIGURE 4–3 The imaginary vertical line in the center of the face divides the mouth into four quadrants.

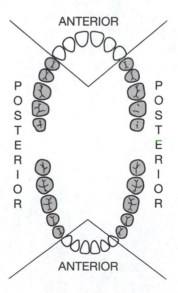

FIGURE 4–5 Adult dentition showing anterior (white) and posterior (shaded) division.

molars need one extra for a total of three roots. The bicuspids and the molars make up the posterior teeth.

There are some general rules when dealing with the identification of the teeth:

▶ **Roots** will normally tip or slant distally.
▶ Teeth get larger and bulkier when moving posteriorly, except for the central or lateral and the third molar, which undergoes growth pressures and many times is wrinkled, multirooted, and irregularly shaped.
▶ Maxillary bicuspids or premolars have two well-defined cusps (therefore, the name bicuspid), while the mandibular bicuspids or premolars' **lingual** cusp is not as developed or large, therefore, looking more like a molar (thus the term premolar).
▶ Maxillary molars have a general diamond or round shape when looking down on the occlusal surface, while the mandibular molars are more box shaped or rectangular in form.
▶ Mandibular molars have two roots—**mesial** and **distal**. The maxillary molar needs one more root to hold on; therefore it has three roots—mesial, distal, and lingual.

Tooth Tissues

Each tooth has a **crown** portion and a root section and is made up of four tissues—**enamel**, **dentin**, **cementum**, and **pulp**.

Enamel is the very hard, white covering over the crown of the tooth. It is composed mostly of inorganic material (98 percent) and is shaped into prismatic rods. The matrix, which holds the rods together, is the organic matter of the tissue. The function of the enamel is to protect the tooth (Figure 4–6).

Dentin is a hard tissue, but it is softer than enamel. It is composed of very small S-shaped tubules and is yellow in color. Dentin is found in the crown and the root section of the tooth. It gives shape to the tooth and registers sensation to thermal and pain conditions. There are two kinds of dentin—primary and secondary. The primary dentin is the original tooth tissue,

while the secondary dentin appears after the tooth has erupted. Secondary dentin is formed as a reaction to pain, stress, abrasion, or injury to the tooth. Secondary dentin grows throughout our lives.

Cementum is the tissue that covers and protects the root section of the tooth. It is yellowish-white and has a porous, rough, textured surface to permit the periodontal fibers to attach. Cementum too can rebuild its tissue, forming secondary cementum. Injury, abrasion, trauma, and stress can stimulate the growth of secondary cementum.

The pulp is the most living tissue of the tooth. It is composed of nerve, blood, and lymph tissues. The function of the pulp is to register sensation and to nourish and supply life to the tooth. The pulp is encased within the walls of the hard dentin tissue. The body of the pulp is situated in the larger open area of the dentin called the pulp chamber, while the ends of the pulp extend out through the pulp canals in the root section. The pulp exits the tooth through the **apical foramen** (opening) at the tip of the root.

Tooth Shapes (Morphology)

Each tooth has its own distinctive characteristic, which is determined by cusps, roots, grooves, and linear ridges. Anatomical landmarks found on a tooth are:

cusps—round mounds or hilly growths
ridges—linear elevations in a tooth, particularly on the sides or margins
pits—small depressions in the surfaces of the teeth
fissures—developmental grooves between lobes
grooves—linear depressions running between cusps; give distinct character
lobes—bumps or lumps arising from a surface; when these lobes arise from the lingual side of the maxillary anteriors (a distinctive feature), they are called cingulum

Each tooth has a different characteristic, making it unique in its pattern and identifiable (Figure 4–7).

Periodontium

The tissues surrounding the teeth are considered the **periodontium**. There are three major types—**alveolar** plate, periodontal ligaments, and **gingiva** (Figure 4–8).

The tooth "sits" in a pocket in either the maxilla or the mandible bone. On top of the bone is a bony plate called the alveolar process or plate. This buildup of bony plate gives support and stability to the tooth and disappears when the tooth is lost and the jawbone undergoes attrition and chewing pressures.

Within this socket area there are periodontal ligaments, which are bundles of fibers that hold and support the tooth in the jawbone. These fibers circulate in

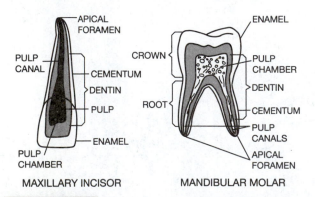

FIGURE 4–6 Tooth tissues of maxillary incisor and mandibular molar.

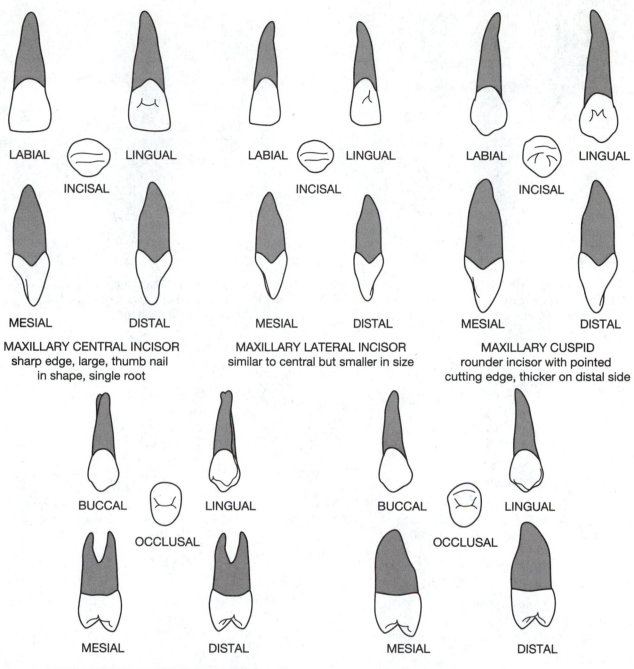

LABIAL   INCISAL   LINGUAL

MESIAL   DISTAL

MAXILLARY CENTRAL INCISOR
sharp edge, large, thumb nail
in shape, single root

LABIAL   INCISAL   LINGUAL

MESIAL   DISTAL

MAXILLARY LATERAL INCISOR
similar to central but smaller in size

LABIAL   INCISAL   LINGUAL

MESIAL   DISTAL

MAXILLARY CUSPID
rounder incisor with pointed
cutting edge, thicker on distal side

BUCCAL   OCCLUSAL   LINGUAL

MESIAL   DISTAL

MAXILLARY FIRST BICUSPID (PREMOLAR)
two-cusped tooth, cusps are pointed shape,
has small two-rooted root section (or two canals in root)

BUCCAL   OCCLUSAL   LINGUAL

MESIAL   DISTAL

MAXILLARY SECOND BICUSPID (PREMOLAR)
smaller, less bulky than the first bicuspid,
singular root with one canal

FIGURE 4–7A Tooth identification.

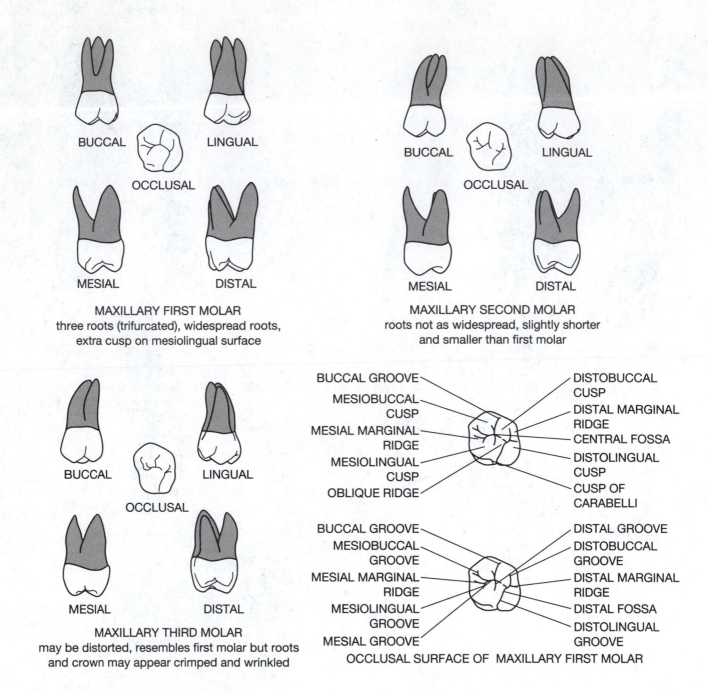

BUCCAL   OCCLUSAL   LINGUAL

MESIAL   DISTAL

MAXILLARY FIRST MOLAR
three roots (trifurcated), widespread roots,
extra cusp on mesiolingual surface

BUCCAL   OCCLUSAL   LINGUAL

MESIAL   DISTAL

MAXILLARY SECOND MOLAR
roots not as widespread, slightly shorter
and smaller than first molar

BUCCAL   OCCLUSAL   LINGUAL

MESIAL   DISTAL

MAXILLARY THIRD MOLAR
may be distorted, resembles first molar but roots
and crown may appear crimped and wrinkled

BUCCAL GROOVE
MESIOBUCCAL CUSP
MESIAL MARGINAL RIDGE
MESIOLINGUAL CUSP
OBLIQUE RIDGE

DISTOBUCCAL CUSP
DISTAL MARGINAL RIDGE
CENTRAL FOSSA
DISTOLINGUAL CUSP
CUSP OF CARABELLI

BUCCAL GROOVE
MESIOBUCCAL GROOVE
MESIAL MARGINAL RIDGE
MESIOLINGUAL GROOVE
MESIAL GROOVE

DISTAL GROOVE
DISTOBUCCAL GROOVE
DISTAL MARGINAL RIDGE
DISTAL FOSSA
DISTOLINGUAL GROOVE

OCCLUSAL SURFACE OF MAXILLARY FIRST MOLAR

FIGURE 4–7B Tooth identification (continued).

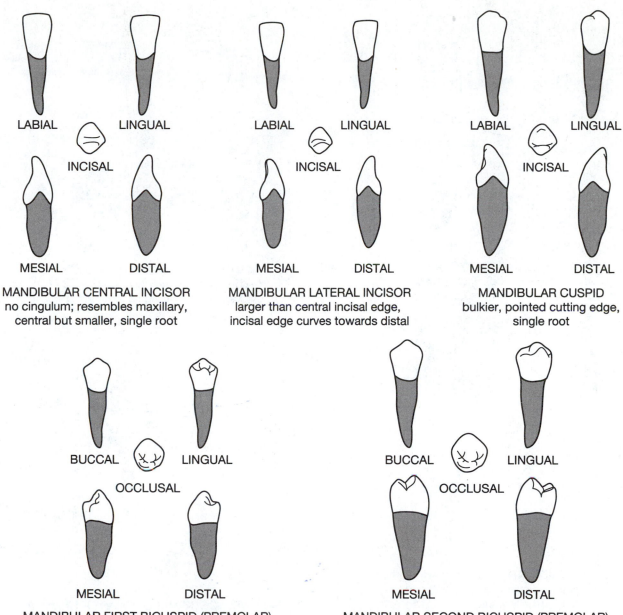

LABIAL   LINGUAL
INCISAL
MESIAL   DISTAL

MANDIBULAR CENTRAL INCISOR
no cingulum; resembles maxillary,
central but smaller, single root

LABIAL   LINGUAL
INCISAL
MESIAL   DISTAL

MANDIBULAR LATERAL INCISOR
larger than central incisal edge,
incisal edge curves towards distal

LABIAL   LINGUAL
INCISAL
MESIAL   DISTAL

MANDIBULAR CUSPID
bulkier, pointed cutting edge,
single root

BUCCAL   LINGUAL
OCCLUSAL
MESIAL   DISTAL

MANDIBULAR FIRST BICUSPID (PREMOLAR)
lingual cusps smaller than buccal cusps, single root,
smaller than second premolar,
occlusal view may appear as bell shape

BUCCAL   LINGUAL
OCCLUSAL
MESIAL   DISTAL

MANDIBULAR SECOND BICUSPID (PREMOLAR)
larger than first bicuspid, lingual cuspid may split
or look like two buccal cusps, single root,
sometimes looks like a three-cusped tooth

FIGURE 4–7C Tooth identification (continued).

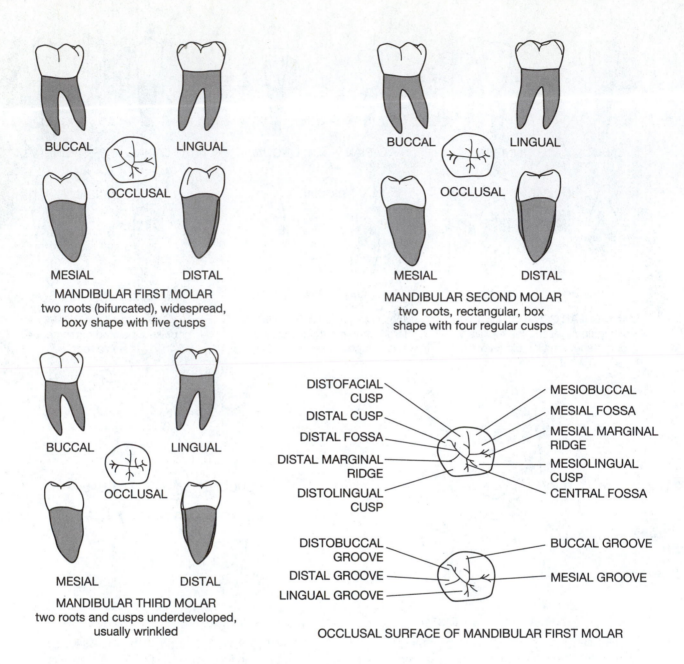

BUCCAL **LINGUAL**

OCCLUSAL

MESIAL **DISTAL**

MANDIBULAR FIRST MOLAR
two roots (bifurcated), widespread,
boxy shape with five cusps

BUCCAL **LINGUAL**

OCCLUSAL

MESIAL **DISTAL**

MANDIBULAR SECOND MOLAR
two roots, rectangular, box
shape with four regular cusps

BUCCAL **LINGUAL**

OCCLUSAL

MESIAL **DISTAL**

MANDIBULAR THIRD MOLAR
two roots and cusps underdeveloped,
usually wrinkled

DISTOFACIAL CUSP — MESIOBUCCAL
DISTAL CUSP — MESIAL FOSSA
DISTAL FOSSA — MESIAL MARGINAL RIDGE
DISTAL MARGINAL RIDGE — MESIOLINGUAL CUSP
DISTOLINGUAL CUSP — CENTRAL FOSSA

DISTOBUCCAL GROOVE — BUCCAL GROOVE
DISTAL GROOVE — MESIAL GROOVE
LINGUAL GROOVE

OCCLUSAL SURFACE OF MANDIBULAR FIRST MOLAR

FIGURE 4–7D Tooth identification (continued).

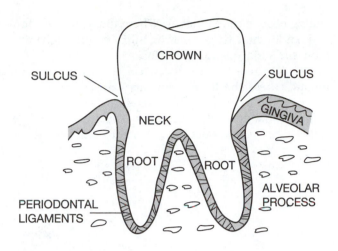

FIGURE 4–8 Periodontium is composed of gingiva, periodontal ligaments or fibers, and the alveolar process.

all ways and are angled in each direction, holding and supporting the tooth. The roughness of the cementum and bone permit the attachment of the fibers and the anchorage and flexibility needed for the chewing stresses.

The last major tissue of the periodontium is the gingiva or gums, which are the covering tissues. The gingiva covers the bone and ligaments and part of the tooth. It acts as a protector for the underlying tissues. There is usually a margin around the crown **cervix** or neck. This is called the gingival margin.

Some of the gingiva is attached and some is free. The area between the two is called the gingival sulcus. The sulcus is an opening or an unattached area around the crown of the tooth, especially in the cervix area. This opening or unattached area is 2 to 3 millimeters in size and the area of concern in sulcus brushing.

The interdental papilla is the area where the gingival tissue mounds up between the teeth in the **interproximal** area. The height and physical condition of the **papilla** indicate much about the general oral health of the patient.▲

THEORY RECALL

Tooth Anatomy

1. What are the three main reasons or functions for teeth?

   a. _____

   b. _____

   c. _____

2. List the four types of teeth and the function of each.

   a. _____

   b. _____

   c. _____

   d. _____

3. What do the terms mandibular and maxillary signify?

   _____

4. What are the names for the teeth adults develop? children?

   _____

5. What teeth do adults develop that children do not?

   _____

6. What is the section of mouth called when an arch is divided in two?

   _____

7. List three anatomic landmarks of a tooth.

   a. _____

   b. _____

   c. _____

8. Name the three major tissues that make up the periodontium and the function of each.

   a. _____

   b. _____

   c. _____

9. What is the area between the attached and loose gingiva called?

   _____

10. What is the interdental papilla?

   _____

For additional activities related to this lesson, turn to Assignment Sheet 4.1, Tooth Anatomy, located in Appendix B of this text.

TOOTH SURFACES

It is very important for a dental assistant to know the names of the surfaces of the teeth and the terminology associated with their use. Tooth surface knowledge is necessary to assist with charting the teeth, posting treatment and charges, completing insurance forms, as well as a general understanding of the dental world. There are six sides to a tooth, but only five are visible in the crown views of the teeth (Figure 4–9).

The top, or chewing surface, which is the working part of the teeth, is called incisal in anterior teeth and **occlusal** in posterior teeth. Where the teeth are long and slender and have edges that cut like scissors, the

cutting edge is called incisal. Where the teeth are short and stubby and have grinding surfaces that pulverize food, the surface is called occlusal.

The surfaces of the teeth on the inside of the mouth, where the tongue touches, are called lingual. *Lingus* is the Latin word for tongue.

The surfaces of the teeth that touch the face are called facial. Some dentists use other names for these

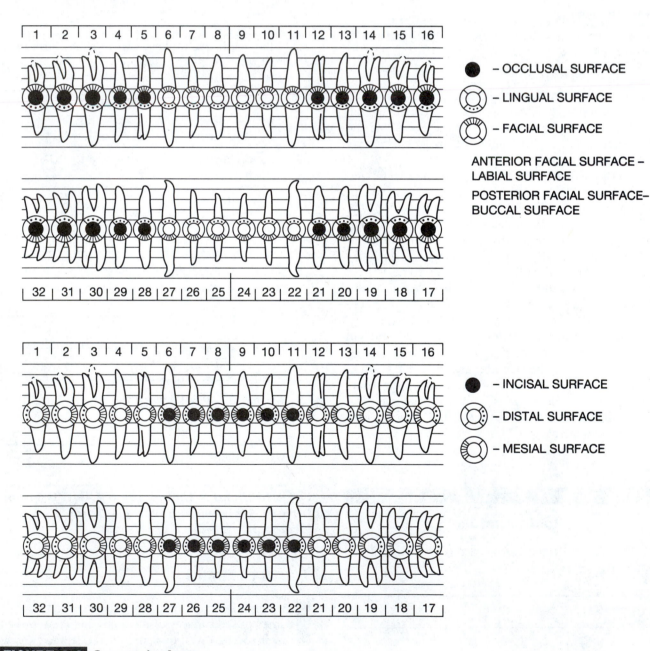

● – OCCLUSAL SURFACE

⊙ – LINGUAL SURFACE

⊙ – FACIAL SURFACE

ANTERIOR FACIAL SURFACE – LABIAL SURFACE

POSTERIOR FACIAL SURFACE– BUCCAL SURFACE

● – INCISAL SURFACE

⊙ – DISTAL SURFACE

⊙ – MESIAL SURFACE

FIGURE 4–9 Geometric charts.

surfaces, such as labial and **buccal**. Because the Latin word for lip is *labium*, the surfaces of the anterior teeth that touch the lips are called labial. The surfaces of the posterior teeth that touch the cheek are called buccal, named after the buccal cheek muscle they touch.

The teeth meet and touch each other side by side (**proximal**). The side of the teeth closer to the middle of the face (midline) is called mesial. The side of the teeth closer to the back of the head is called distal, because this side is farther or more distant from the midline. When the teeth are proximal, or side by side, the distal of the front tooth touches the mesial of the next tooth back, except in the very center of the mouth (midline) where mesial touches mesial.

The sixth surface of the tooth is the apical, which is the bottom of the tooth or the apex. This surface term is not frequently used, except perhaps in an apical abscess, apical foramen, or root canal treatment.

The names of the tooth surfaces apply to both arches. The inside surfaces of the maxillary permanent and deciduous teeth are the lingual surface and the inside surfaces of the mandibular teeth are also called lingual. The surfaces of the primary teeth are the same as the secondary teeth surfaces.

Surface Abbreviations

When speaking of a singular tooth surface, the following terms and abbreviations are used:

incisal (I)—cutting edge of anteriors
occlusal (O or Occ)—grinding surface of posterior
lingual (Li)—surface that touches tongue
labial (La or Lab)—surface of anterior teeth touching lips
buccal (B or Buc)—surface of posterior teeth touching cheek
facial (F)—surface of all teeth touching cheek
mesial (M)—side surface of tooth closer to midline
distal (D)—side surface of tooth farther from midline

Many times more than one surface is involved in the concern or procedure. When uniting one surface to another surface, the *-al* of the first surface is dropped and the letter *o* is inserted to hold the two terms together. For example, a restoration involving the distal and occlusal surfaces is called a disto-occlusal restoration.

As other surfaces are added to the restoration, only the final surface keeps the *-al* at the end of the word. The preceding surfaces drop the *-al* and add the letter *o*. For example, a restoration involving the mesial, occlusal, and distal surfaces is a mesio-occluso-distal restoration (Figure 4–10).▲

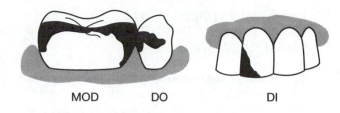

| MOD | DO | DI |

MOD – MESIO-OCCLUSO-DISTAL
DO – DISTO-OCCLUSAL

DI – DISTO-INCISAL

FIGURE 4–10 Restorations involving more than one surface. Class II MOD and Class IV DI.

THEORY RECALL

Tooth Surfaces

1. For which dental assisting procedure is knowledge of tooth surfaces necessary?

2. What is the working or cutting surface of the anterior teeth called?

3. What is the grinding surface of the posterior teeth called?

4. What are the surfaces of the teeth that touch the tongue called?

5. What part of the teeth are called facial surfaces?

6. What is the term for where the teeth touch together side by side?

7. What is the side of the tooth closer to the midline of the face called?

8. What is the side of the tooth farther from the midline called?

9. What are the abbreviations for the occlusal, buccal and distal surfaces?

10. How would a restoration involving the mesial, occlusal, distal, and lingual surfaces be abbreviated? How would it be written?

For additional activities related to this lesson, turn to Assignment Sheet 4.2, Tooth Surfaces, located in Appendix B of this text.

TOOTH NUMBERING SYSTEMS

Universal Numbering System

Historically, teeth have been numbered in various ways. Dentists used the method they learned in dental school. Not all schools agreed upon one proper way and so conversation and record-keeping could be confusing. In 1968, the American Dental Association adopted the Universal numbering system as an official method of tooth numbering.

This system simply begins numbering permanent teeth by starting with the maxillary right third molar as tooth #1 and counts around the **arch** to #16, the maxillary left third molar. The system drops down to the mandibular left third molar, which is #17, and moves along the lower arch to the mandibular right third molar #32 (Figure 4–11). The same course is followed for the primary teeth, but the letters A–T are used instead of numbers.

THE PALMER METHOD. One of the more popular methods before the adoption of the Universal numbering system was the Palmer method of numbering teeth. While many professionals use the Universal numbering system, orthodontists still do much of their work

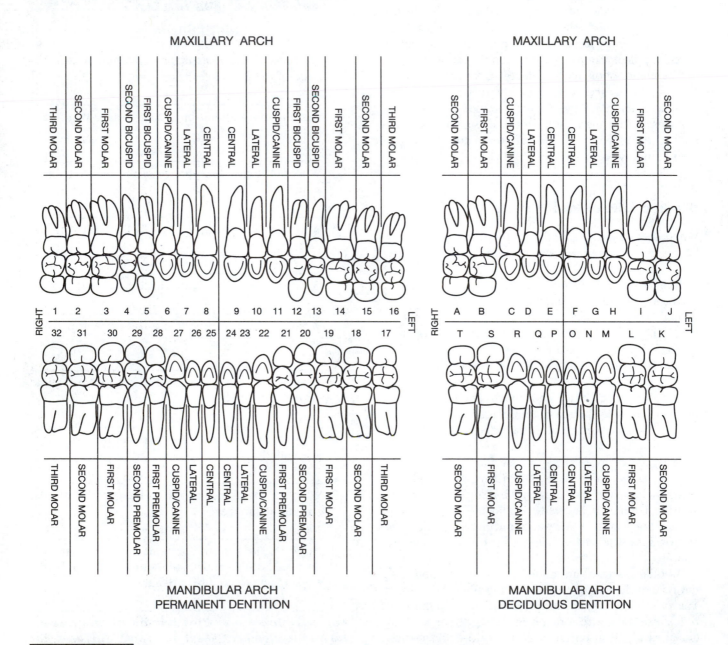

FIGURE 4–11 The Universal numbering system of the permanent dentition.

using the Palmer method. In this system, the central incisors are #1 because they are the first teeth away from the midline. The laterals, the second teeth away from the midline, are numbered 2 and so on. Brackets around the number are used to designate in which quadrant the tooth is located. For example, the permanent maxillary right central is 1⌋ and the permanent mandibular left central is written as ⌈1 The deciduous teeth are marked with letters from A–E and bracketed in the same way (Figure 4–12).

Since brackets are not part of the typewriter or computer keyboard, recording the Palmer method is not possible; so another method has been developed for the computer age.

THE FEDERATION DENTAIRE INTERNATIONALE SYSTEM. The Federation Dentaire Internationale system is a two-digit method of numbering the dentition. This method keeps the Palmer numbers for each tooth but prefixes another number to replace the brackets and designate the quadrant. The maxillary right quadrant has a prefix of 1; the maxillary left is 2; the mandibular left is 3; and the mandibular right is 4. Therefore, the maxillary right permanent central incisor is numbered 11, and the mandibular left permanent central incisor is 31.

The primary dentition numbering is not patterned off the Palmer method. All teeth have numbers. In the Palmer method, the deciduous teeth are lettered from A–E; but in the Federation Dentaire Internationale system, the primary teeth have numbers from 1–5, with #1 being the central, the closest to the midline.

Prefixes are added to the 1–5 numbers to designate the quadrants. The prefix 5 signifies the maxillary right quadrant; 6 is for the maxillary left, 7 is the mandibular left, and 8 denotes the mandibular right quadrant. Therefore, the maxillary right deciduous central is #51 and the mandibular left deciduous central is #71 (Figure 4–13).

The assistant uses the method of numbering the teeth that the dentist prefers. Practice and use makes the assistant comfortable and efficient in the use of the tooth numbering system.▲

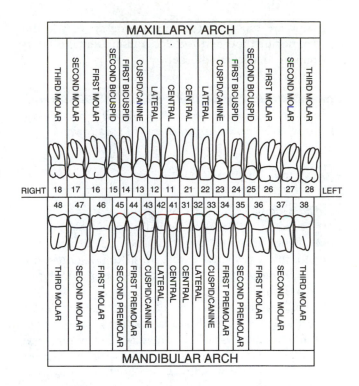

FIGURE 4–13 The Federation Dentaire Internationale system of numbering the permanent dentition.

Tooth Numbering Systems

1. In what quadrant does the Universal numbering system start its numbering?

   _____

2. How are deciduous teeth identified in the Universal numbering system?

   _____

3. Why are the permanent central incisors numbered 1 in the Palmer method?

   _____

4. What is used to designate the quadrants in the Palmer method?

   _____

5. What does the Federation Dentaire Internationale system use to replace the brackets of the Palmer method?

   _____

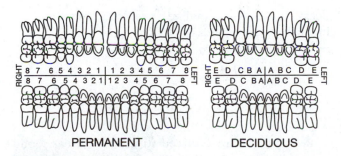

FIGURE 4–12 The Palmer method of numbering the permanent dentition.

6. How are the deciduous numbering systems in the Palmer method and the Federation Dentaire Internationale system different?

For additional activities related to this lesson, turn to Assignment Sheet 4.3, Tooth Numbering Systems, located in Appendix B of this text.

CHARTING TEETH

The dental assistant's services may be very valuable to a dentist or dental hygienist during the dental examination. By working as a team, the operator and assistant are able to make notations on a chart and graphically show all the existing conditions of the mouth.

To participate in this process, the assistant must know the charting code, abbreviations, and system used in that particular office. There is no truly universal method of charting, but the process is similar in most offices. If an assistant is knowledgeable in the method of charting, it is easy to adjust from office to office.

The first rule in charting is to make all entries neat, legible, and correct. Many offices use colors to code conditions. Red signifies carious lesions, also known as decay or cavities. Blue indicates restorations, and green is often used to show existing restorations of a new patient.

Colored marks are drawn on a patient's chart, which shows a full-mouth dentition outline. Many charts present both the secondary and primary dentition and may be used to chart an adult or a child.

The outline on the charts may be drawn anatomically or geometrically. Anatomically-drawn charts have two to three lines of tooth drawings, showing the natural shape and anatomy of each tooth in the arch (see Figure 4–14A for an example). Geometric charts designate a line for each arch showing a circle divided into five sections, corresponding to the tooth surfaces (see Figure 4–14B for an example).

The colored marks are placed and shaped on the chart in a manner to resemble what the operator has indicated as existing. Some marks are used to signify past or future treatment. Usually, it is safe to say that if the work needs to be done, the notation is in red. If the work has been completed, or no attention is necessary, the notation is in blue.

Some codes used in charting are:

indicates a missing or unerupted tooth	blue X marked through drawing of entire tooth
indicates an impacted tooth	red circle is placed around entire tooth
indicates an extraction is needed	red diagonal line drawn through entire tooth
indicates direction of impaction or drifting	blue arrow drawn close to area
indicates full crown	blue outline drawn on crown surface only; stripe for gold
indicates fractured tooth TOOTH ROOT	red jagged line drawn through fractured surface or root
indicates ¾ metal crown FACIAL LINGUAL	drawn on crowned area only
indicates porcelain fused to metal 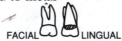 FACIAL LINGUAL	facial side not filled; blue stripe on cervical third
indicates root canal treatment MOLAR INCISOR	filled in canal area— red to be done, blue if finished
indicates abscess	red open circle placed at apex of root
indicates fixed dental bridge	root of missing teeth crossed out; crowns of the bridge circled together
decay or caries—red outline in affected surface area	filled in red

Restorations are outlined in affected areas. Solid blue indicates amalgam, striped indicates gold, and clear or dotted blue indicates an anterior composite restorative (white) material.

Brackets are drawn to cover area affected by partial appliances. Missing teeth are indicated by roots crossed out.

Full arch dentures are indicated by half-moon of entire arch and a large X is drawn over the teeth in that arch.

Procedure

The operator begins the charting procedure by examining the #1 tooth (maxillary right third molar). If it is present, the operator relates the existing conditions found on this tooth. If there are no notations to be regarded, the operator indicates, "#1—all right" and proceeds to #2 tooth. A mesio-occlusal restoration may be present, and the operator relates this information by saying "a large MO amalgam restoration," or "an MO amalgam restoration extending distally and buccally on the occlusal surface." With practice and usage, the operator and assistant can develop their conversations to a point where the patient's chart records are an exact duplication of mouth conditions.

Each tooth is examined fully and recorded in sequential order. All significant information is placed on the patient's chart and these become permanent records. See Figure 4–14A for an anatomic chart recording and Figure 4–14B for a geometric chart.

Some abbreviations that may be used in charting and posting of dental treatment are:

AM	amalgam	In	inlay
Br	bridge	M	missing
BWX	bitewing x-rays	P	prophylaxis
Comp	composite	PFM	porcelain fused to metal
CRN	crown		
Ext	extraction	PJC	porcelain jacket crown
FMX	full-mouth x-rays		
G	gold	Rem	removable
GF	gold foil	RCT	root canal treatment
GI	gold inlay		
IMP	impression	Temp	temporary
Impac	impaction		

One other classification the assistant needs to know for charting and posting treatment is cavity classification. All cavities are classified in two ways. A cavity may be simple, which means the decay affects only one tooth surface. A compound carious lesion (cavity) means the decay affects two surfaces. A complex carious lesion is a cavity involving more than two tooth surfaces.

Cavities are also classified according to Dr. G. V. Black's six divisions, which are sorted by the method and equipment needed for treatment:

Class I—one surface (dig a hole and fill it)
Class II—two or more surfaces of a posterior tooth (use a matrix to restore a proximal wall)
Class III—proximal wall of anterior tooth (need clear matrix)

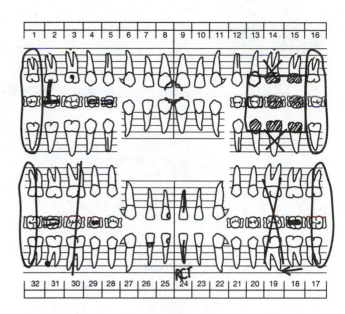

Maxillary right third molar—impacted
Maxillary right second molar—MODB amalgam restoration
Maxillary right first molar—amalgam restoration facial view
Maxillary right second bicuspid—MO caries
Maxillary right first bicuspid—DO caries
Maxillary right central incisor—MI fractured tooth
Maxillary left central incisor—MI fractured tooth
Maxillary left second bicuspid—part of fixed bridge PFM crown
Maxillary left first molar—missing replaced by crown pontic
Maxillary left second molar—full gold crown part of fixed bridge
Maxillary left third molar—fully impacted
Mandibular left third molar—partially impacted (distally)
Mandibular left second molar—MO amalgam restoration and drifting mesially
Mandibular left first molar—missing
Mandibular left central incisor—needs root canal treatment
Mandibular right central incisor—mesial caries
Mandibular right canine—gingival white restoration on facial view
Mandibular second premolar—Occlusal amalgam restoration
Mandibular first molar—needs extraction
Mandibular second molar—DO caries, abscessed distal root
Mandibular third molar—partially impacted (distally)

FIGURE 4–14A **Example of completed anatomic dental chart.**

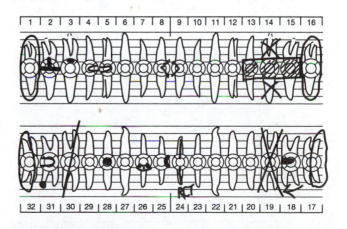

FIGURE 4–14B **Example of same charted conditions using a geometric chart.**

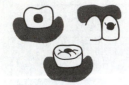

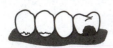

CLASS I
BUCCAL ⟩ FISSURES
LINGUAL ⟩ MOLARS

LINGUAL OF INCISORS

SIMPLE ONE SURFACE OF
POSTERIOR OCCLUSALS

CLASS II
PROXIMAL WALLS OF
POSTERIOR TEETH

CLASS III
PROXIMAL WALLS OF
ANTERIOR TEETH

CLASS IV
PROXIMAL AND INCISAL
WALL OF ANTERIORS

CLASS V
GINGIVAL THIRD NEAR
CERVIX OF TOOTH
ANTERIOR OR POSTERIOR

CLASS VI
INCISAL AND CUSP EDGES

FIGURE 4-15 Cavity classification according to Dr. G. V. Black's system.

Class IV—proximal wall and incisal edge of anterior (need crown form or build up)

Class V—gingival caries (involvement of gingival tissue at gingival third of tooth)

Class VI—abrasions of incisal and occlusal edges (all others)▲

THEORY RECALL

Charting Teeth

Use the anatomic and geometric charts (Figures 4–14A and 4–14B) as a reference, to answer the following questions:

1. Which tooth is missing and not replaced?

_____

2. In which quadrant is the fixed bridge located?

_____

3. What is the name of the tooth that needs to be extracted?

_____

4. What does RCT on tooth #24 mean?

_____

5. What class of restoration is used on tooth #27?

_____

6. On which surface of the maxillary right first molar is the restoration?

_____

7. Which way (mesially or distally) is tooth #18 drifting?

_____

8. What is the meaning of the striped area of tooth #15?

_____

9. What do the zigzag lines indicate on teeth #8 and #9?

_____

10. Is the mouth used in the charting exercise an adult, deciduous, or mixed dentition?

_____

For additional activities related to this lesson, turn to Assignment Sheet 4.4, Charting Teeth, located in Appendix B of this text.

OPERATIVE HAND INSTRUMENTS

Although there are many kinds and types of hand instruments in the dental office, the new assistant need not panic in fear of learning the names and uses of all. Dental hand instruments are divided into families or grouped according to their work task.

Most hand instruments are made of metal; but there are some plastic, disposable and composite, working instruments. When sterilizing hand instruments, the assistant should check first to see what method the manufacturer recommends. Most of today's instruments are able to be sterilized by all methods, but there are a few carbide-coated or brass-plated ones that may rust when placed in a wet situation. The assistant may "read" the handle of the instrument. Most companies engrave their name, code number, or the name of the instrument and material composition on the handle. If "stainless" is etched on the shaft, all methods of sterilization may be performed. Some manufacturers may engrave a trade name for stainless or may state the metal type. If the assistant is unsure of the company's coding, a call to the manufacturer or dental dealer may provide the information needed.

Most dental hand instruments are approximately six inches long and divided in three parts—the shaft, the shank, and the blade or nib.

The shaft is the handle of the instrument and may be smooth, rough, or serrated. It may be round, six- or eight-sided, or oversized for comfort, control, and less fatigue.

The shank is the neck of the instrument and connects the handle and the blade or nib. It may be straight or angled for better access.

The blade or nib is the working end of the instrument. It is shaped or formed with a particular purpose or function in mind and is used to perform a certain procedure.

Hand instruments are grouped according to their function or use. Some groups are basic, cutting, plastic filling, and miscellaneous functions.

Basic Setup Instruments

The assistant prepares for every procedure by placing the basic setup on the tray. This grouping includes a mouth mirror, one or two explorers, and cotton or college pliers.

MOUTH MIRRORS. Mouth mirrors come in sizes 3 to 6. They may have a regular or magnified reflection. They also may be

▶ disposable or reusable (after sterilization),
▶ double sided (back to back),
▶ regular or front surfaced for less distorted reflection, or
▶ plain or cone-stemmed.

The heads of the mouth mirrors are made to be replaceable when they become scratched or ineffective. These mirror heads come in a simple or cone socket style. The cone socket mirror heads have an edge or a "lip" extending out before the threads on the neck of the mirror head, while the simple stem has only a threaded end on the neck of the mirror head. Cone socket heads must be used in cone socket handles and likewise for the simple socket ones.

Mouth mirrors are used for vision, reflection, retraction of the tongue, protection of mouth tissues, percussion and mobility testing, and many other functions in the mouth.

EXPLORERS. Explorers may be single ended or double ended, which means both ends have a working part. Some double-sided instruments come in sets, one end for the right side and the other end for the left side.

Explorers come in various shapes. Some may have a very small head point, while others have a large half circle. All explorers have one thing in common, the explorer end is a very thin, flexible, sensitive tip that snags or catches on a minute piece or area of roughness (Figure 4–16). The function of the explorer is to indicate decay or tooth surface irregularities by catching or snagging in that particular area.

COTTON OR COLLEGE PLIERS. Cotton or college pliers are used to transport materials to and from the mouth, pick up in small places, and any other practice for which the dentist might find them useful. These pliers

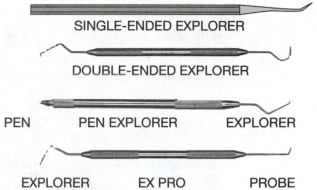

FIGURE 4–16 Explorers may be single ended or have another explorer tip, writing pen, or periodontal probe on the other end. (Photo courtesy of Hu-Friedy.)

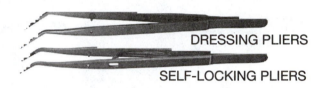

FIGURE 4–17 College or dressing pliers may be plain or self locking for secure holding. (Photo courtesy of Hu-Friedy.)

may be plain or self locking and most have serrated tips to assist with picking up and carrying paper, cotton, and gauze items (Figure 4–17).

Cutting Instruments

Since instruments are placed on the setup tray in the order of their use, the cutting instruments are placed second, after the basic setup, in a tooth preparation appointment.

Instruments in this family are chisels, hatchets, hoes, gingival margin trimmers, spoon excavators, and sometimes the discoid-cleoid and some carvers. These instruments all have sharp edges or beveled edges and are used to cut or break off hard tooth tissue or spoon out decay. With the advent of ultra high-speed rotary instrumentation, fewer hand instruments are used; and those that are chosen soon become the dentist's "pets." The assistant should become familiar with the chosen cutting instruments through use and acquainted with all in the cutting family (Figure 4–18).

chisels—used to push or break away decayed enamel
hatchets—used to make grooves and form retention lines
hoes—used to pull away decayed enamel
gingival margin trimmers—used to break away side walls (hence the curved blade)

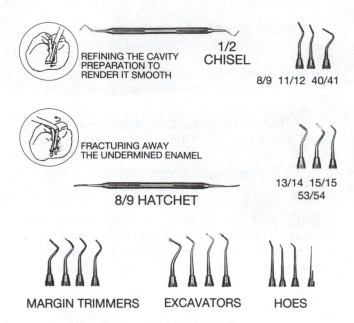

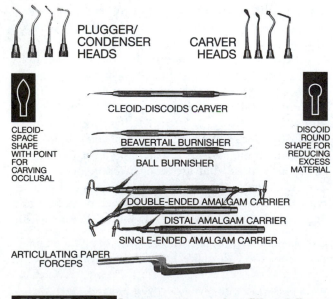

FIGURE 4–18 Cutting instruments. (Photo courtesy of Hu-Friedy.)

spoon excavators—used to scoop out decayed tissue
discoid/cleoid—used to cut and dig out decayed tissue
or carve restorations

Plastic Filling Instruments

Plastic filling instruments (PFIs) are used to condense, carve, and smooth the restoration while it is in a soft condition. Members of this family include condensers, burnishers, and carvers (Figure 4–19).

FIGURE 4–19 Instruments used to fill and finish a restoration. (Photo courtesy of Hu-Friedy.)

AMALGAM CARRIERS. Amalgam carriers are used to carry increments of plastic (form or shape) amalgam to the prepared site. These carriers may be double ended or single ended. They may have a curved or straight shank and the holes or the carrier areas come in different sizes. Carriers may be metal, teflon, or a combination of both materials (Figure 4–19).

CONDENSERS. Condensers are used to pack in and **condense** restorative materials into a preparation. The heads come in different sizes and angles. The surface of the head may be smooth or serrated. The condenser is used while the material being placed into the restoration is in a soft and pliable condition, called a plastic condition (Figure 4–19).

BURNISHERS. Burnishers are used to smooth out and pressure material into the preparation while in a plastic state. The heads of the burnisher come in ball, oval, football, and round shapes. A popular burnisher has a flat end coming out on one side; this is called a beaver-tail burnisher. Burnishers may also be used to smooth out and shape solid metals, such as a matrix band or crown form (Figure 4–19).

CARVERS. Carvers are used to cut and shape the restorative material. The discoid/cleoid carver is a popular double-sided instrument. One side has a pointed end (cleoid), which is used to carve occlusal anatomy. The other side has a disc type end (discoid) shape used for reducing excess material. The dentist may alternate ends until the desired shape is completed.

There are other carvers in various shapes and sizes. The dentist probably will have a few favorites that he or she will use frequently.

There are hard plastic carvers that are used on composite restorations, because the dentist does not want to chance discoloring the anterior material with any metal rub off (Figure 4–19).

Miscellaneous

There are other hand instruments used in the dental office and laboratory; still others are used in specialty procedures. Some instruments are used rarely. If the assistant is knowledgeable in the preparation instruments, unfamiliar ones can be learned during usage.▲

THEORY RECALL

Operative Hand Instruments

1. How are instruments divided into families or groups?

   _____

2. What information may an assistant read on an instrument handle?

   _____

3. List the three working parts of an operative hand instrument.

   a. _____

   b. _____

   c. _____

4. How may the shaft or handle of an instrument be supplied?

   _____

5. List three groups of hand instruments.

   a. _____

   b. _____

   c. _____

6. In what condition may cotton plier tips differ?

   _____

7. How are instruments arranged on the dental tray?

   _____

8. When working with plastic filling instruments, what does the term plastic signify?

   _____

9. In what forms or shapes may a burnisher be purchased?

   _____

10. Which end of the discoid/cleoid instrument is pointed?

   _____

For additional activities related to this lesson, turn to Assignment Sheet 4.5, Operative Hand Instruments, located in Appendix B of this text.

TRANSFER OF INSTRUMENTS

To be able to participate in the transfer of instruments, the assistant must first be knowledgeable of the various types of instruments used in dentistry. Although each dentist has a few favorites that are used more often than others, dental instruments are designed and manufactured for a specific purpose, tooth, or area. The new assistant should take some time to become familiar with those used in the office.

One way instruments may be grouped into types is according to the manner in which they are passed and received. The two basic groups are pen grip and palm grip instruments, but there are modifications of these grips. Instruments held in the hand like a pencil are called pen grasp, those held in the palm like scissors are called palm grasp. Some examples of each are:

Pen grasp	**Palm grasp**
mouth mirrors	anesthetic syringe
explorers	dental dam clamp holder,
scalers, curettes	punch
excavators, hatchets	elevators
burnishers	pliers
condensers	forceps
	scissors

Before attempting to pass instruments, the assistant should be aware of some general rules to the procedure:

▶ Never pass instruments over the patient's face. The passing zone is close to the face, but below the patient's view.

▶ Always await a signal from the operator before taking or presenting any instrument. The operator usually has a signal, such as a flick of the wrist or a code word, that will indicate the time for action.

▶ To avoid moving the dentist's hand and eyes from the site, keep the passing zone close to the face, a few inches below the chin.

▶ Arrange the instruments on the tray in sequential order and in the proper position for the type of passing. Pen grasp instruments are placed on the tray with the working end away from the assistant. Palm grasp instruments are placed with the working end toward the assistant.

▶ Pass the instrument so the working area is facing the work site, aimed at its particular arch. For example, before releasing the mouth mirror for viewing the upper arch, spin the mirror head around so it is facing upward.

▶ Double-ended instruments are to be placed on the tray in the order of planned use. Be prepared to reverse the working ends on the tray setup as needed.

▶ Use the left hand for passing and receiving when assisting a right-handed operator. The assistant's right hand holds the syringe or HVE.

▶ Be alert and watch the procedure. With time, a new assistant will be able to anticipate and be prepared in advance of the transfer.

P R O C E D U R E   1 2

Transfer of Instruments

1 Prepare for the Procedure

2 Perform the Pen Grasp Transfer

3 Perform the Palm Grasp Transfer

4 Perform the Palm-Thumb Grasp Transfer

5 Perform Alternating Transfers

6 Cleanup Procedures

1 Prepare for the Procedure

To perform this exercise, the assistant needs an assortment of instruments and a partner to share the transfer duties. The assortment should include:

single-ended and double-ended pen grasp instruments
  —mirror, explorer, PFI
palm grasp instruments—scissors, forceps, or rubber
  dam clamp holder
palm-thumb grasp instruments—chisel used in modified grasp
latex exam gloves

The assistant washes hands and dons exam gloves during the transfer exercise. The instruments are arranged in the proper sequence and position for transfer before starting the procedure.

2 Perform the Pen Grasp Transfer

The assistant uses the left hand to pick up the instrument at the end of the shaft with the thumb and forefinger (working tip away). Allow the working end to slant down and carry the instrument to the transfer zone parallel to the dentist's instrument (Figure 4–20A).

If not exchanging, place the instrument into the waiting hand of the operator, who accepts the instrument into a writing or pen position. Rotate the working part toward the work site. Release. If exchanging, bring instrument toward the transfer zone. On signal, the operator withdraws the used instrument. Align the new instrument parallel with the used one. Extend the small finger of the left hand and grasp the used instrument from the underside (Figure 4–20B). Rotate the

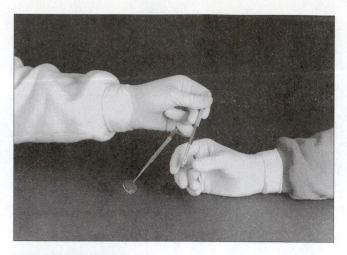

FIGURE 4–20B Assistant extends little finger under old instrument and grasps it, removing it from the operator's hand.

hand toward the operator, taking the used instrument and leaving the new one. Use fingertips to spin the working part toward the work site (Figure 4–20C). Return the used instrument to the tray and place it in the proper order and position for future use.

3 Perform the Palm Grasp Transfer

There are two types of palm grasps, one in which the entire palm is used, such as with a rubber dam clamp holder. The other palm grasp involves the thumb's use more, such as extraction forceps or chisel use. The assistant passes and receives the palm grasp instruments in the same manner, but the reception given the instrument is either a full palm or a palm-finger grasp.

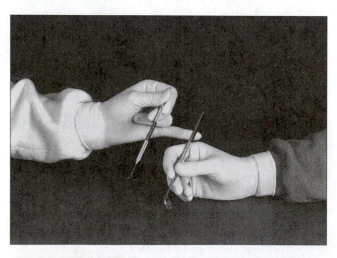

FIGURE 4–20A Assistant grasps new instrument away from the working end and positions it parallel to the old instrument.

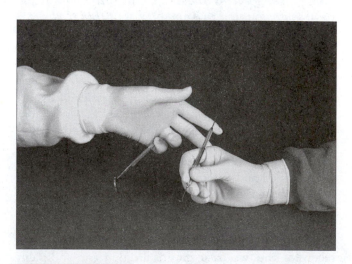

FIGURE 4–20C Assistant rotates new instrument into the operator's hand with working part aimed toward the operative site. The old instrument is returned to the tray.

Palm grasp instruments are arranged with the working end toward the assistant. Grasp the neck of the instrument, behind the working area and pick up the instrument (Figure 4–21A). Carry the instrument (handles out toward the operator) to the transfer zone. If not exchanging, place the instrument into the palm of the operator.

If exchanging, parallel the new instrument with withdrawn used instrument, extend the little finger, and grasp used instrument from top side (Figure 4–21B). Rotate the hand toward the operator, and place the instrument into the palm of the operator's hand (Figure 4–21C). Return the used instrument to the tray, and place in the proper order and position.

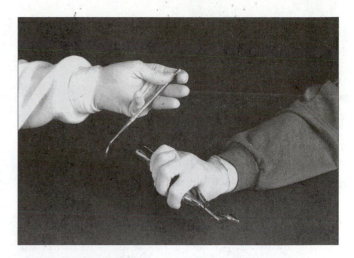

FIGURE 4–21C The assistant takes the old instrument and rotates the new one into the operator's palm, making sure the working side is toward the site.

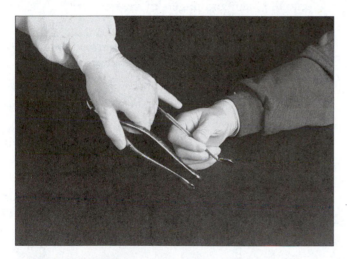

FIGURE 4–21A The assistant grasps the instrument behind the working end and positions it parallel to the operator's instrument.

4 Perform the Palm-Thumb Grasp Transfer

Instruments to be used in the modified palm-thumb grasp are passed to the operator in a similar pattern as other palm grasp instruments except the handle or shank of the tool is placed onto the finger area instead of into the palm. In this manner, the operator may flip the instrument over against the thumb and use the tool in a wedging manner (Figure 4–22).

5 Perform Alternating Transfers

After demonstrating the ability to transfer in each specific manner, the assistant follows the orders of the

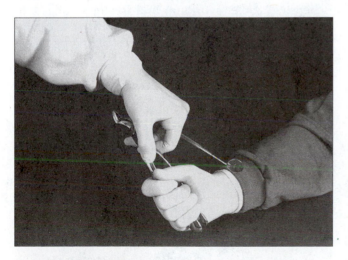

FIGURE 4–21B The assistant removes the operator's instrument and places new instrument into operator's palm.

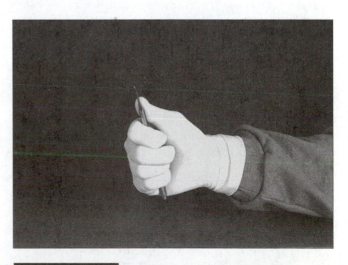

FIGURE 4–22 Instruments held in a palm-thumb grasp are used in a push-pull pattern.

partner student or instructor and passes requested instruments in random order, alternating the grasp styles.

6 Cleanup Procedures

All instruments assembled for the exercise are taken to the sterilization room for processing. The exam gloves are removed and utility gloves are donned. The operatory practice area is disinfected and cleaned up. The instruments are placed in the ultrasonic cleaner, patted dry, placed in sterilization bags, and sterilized. When this procedure is finished, all equipment is returned to the proper place.

The utility gloves are washed, dried, disinfected, and removed. The hands are washed. Practice and use will develop good teamwork and effortless dentistry.▲

T H E O R Y   R E C A L L

Transfer of Instruments

1. To be able to participate in transfer of instruments, what should the assistant know?

   _____

2. Name two basic groups of instruments that are determined by the manner of their transfer. Give two examples of each type.

   a. _____

   b. _____

3. List at least four rules the assistant should follow when transferring instruments.

   a. _____

   b. _____

   c. _____

   d. _____

4. How does the assistant pick up an instrument for a pen grasp transfer?

   _____

5. What finger is used to receive a used instrument when transferring a new instrument?

   _____

6. Where is the used instrument placed after the transfer is completed?

   _____

7. List the two types of palm grasps. How is the reception different in each?

   a. _____

   b. _____

8. What type of instrument may be used in the palm grasp with the open palm?

   _____

9. Is the working end of the palm grasp instrument placed toward or away from the operator when placed on the tray?

   _____

10. In what modified manner may the operator use the instrument passed in the palm grasp manner into the palm and fingers of the operator?

   _____

Now turn to the Competency Evaluation Sheet for Procedure 12, Transfer of Instruments, located in Appendix C of this text.

DENTAL ROTARY INSTRUMENTS

Dental burs are **rotary** instruments used to cut, reduce, finish, and polish teeth, restorations, and dental appliances. There are three parts to a dental bur: the head, which is the working part; the shaft, which is the body of the bur; and the neck, which unites the head and **shank** (Figure 4–23).

Composition

The shank and neck are made of steel, but the head may be steel or carbide metal. Carbide burs are more expensive, cooler working, and longer lasting than steel burs and are used more frequently in the operatory. Steel burs are used mainly for laboratory work.

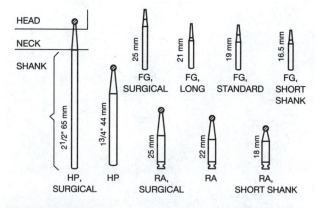

FIGURE 4–23 Assorted sizes and types of dental rotary instruments (burs).

Manufacturers designate carbide burs by etched rings on the shaft, different neck shape, or color coding.

Steel burs and carbide may be sterilized in the autoclave, or dry heat, chemical or oil sterilizers; but some carbide burs will lose their cutting efficiency when placed in a chemical disinfecting solution. Manufacturers' recommendations should be checked before sterilizing carbide burs.

Bur Numbers

The head is the working portion of the dental bur and the shape and size of the head determines the bur's number (Figure 4–24). The larger the number, the larger the head. All dental burs from #$\frac{1}{4}$ to 9 have round shaped heads and are used on single-surfaced cavities, anterior interproximals, opening pulp chambers in endodontics, and drilling for pin retention holes.

Burs numbered from 33$\frac{1}{2}$ to 39 are inverted cone burs, which are used to perform undercuts in restorations. This type of cut helps retention of the restorative material in the finished restoration.

Burs #56 to 58 are plain fissure straight burs, which are used to make parallel wall and floor preparations. If the dentist requires a faster working bur of the same shape, a **crosscut** straight fissure bur can be used. These burs have extra cuts on the blade edges, which provide more abrasiveness and faster cutting. The numbers for the crosscut straight fissure bur are 556 to 558.

If the dentist requires slightly divergent parallel and floor preparations, a tapered fissured bur may be used. These burs are numbered from 169 to 171 for the plain style and 699 to 703 for the crosscut tapered fissure bur.

The end cutting bur, one with cutting blades only on the end of the head is numbered 957 to 958. This bur is used for shoulder preparations of full crowns.

There are other burs with other shapes and functions. The dentist will choose a few favorites and call upon these more often, but the assistant should be familiar with all types. Use a dental catalog as a source of information and study guide.

Types of Handpieces

The dental bur can only function when placed in a handpiece. Handpieces are classified by the amount of rotations per minute they are capable of performing. Slow handpieces rotate from 150 to 40,000 rpm and are used for exacting and finishing work. They may be belt driven motor or air turbine operated under compressed air. They require an insertion of a long, shafted bur (SHP), contra angle handpiece (CAHP), right angle handpiece (RAHP), or prophy angle snap or screw in head to function. Some manufacturers are making a slow handpiece with an attached contra angle head now.

High-speed handpieces operate at 150,000 to 800,000 rpm and are driven by compressed air. The high-speed handpiece heads may be standard size or miniature and may contain a fiber optic light system for better viewing. The handle may or may not be a swivel type, and there are a variety of bur changing methods from auto push-pull to types that need bur chuck releasing devices to change friction grip (FG) burs. The type of handpiece employed determines the dental bur shank to be used (Figure 4–25).

A dental bur with a long, smooth-ended shaft (SHP) may be placed directly into the slow handpiece open-

INVERTED CONE

33 $\frac{1}{2}$
34
35
36
37
38
39

ROUND

1/4, 1/2, 1, 2, 3, 4, 5, 6, 7, 8, 10

ASSORTED TYPES

END CUTTING

957

WHEEL

14

ROUND NOSE TAPER

1171, 1172

ROUND NOSE CROSSCUT CYLINDER

1557, 1558

PLAIN FISSURE STRAIGHT

56, 57, 58, 59,

TAPERED FISSURE

169, 170, 171, 169L, 170L, 171L

CROSSCUT FISSURE STRAIGHT

557, 558, 558L

TAPERED CROSSCUT FISSURE

699, 700, 701, 702, 703, 701L

FIGURE 4–24 The shape of the bur's head determines the number of the bur. The insert end of the bur determines the type of bur.

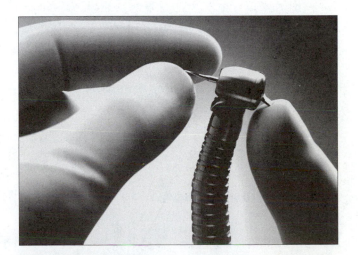

FIGURE 4–25 Handpieces are expensive dental items and must be carefully maintained. (Courtesy of Midwest Dental Products Corporation.)

ing; then the knob at the other end of the handpiece is tightened to hold the bur in place. This type of bur is used mostly for dental laboratory procedures.

A right, contra angle or prophy handpiece may be put into the opening of the slow handpiece and tightened into place. The contra angle and right angle (RA) handpieces have a latch opening and closure. The closure requires a notched latch (LH) or RA bur to be placed into these handpieces and locked into place. Attachments may be purchased to convert a slow latch handpiece into a friction chuck type handpiece that uses the friction burs (FG) in slow motion.

Prophy angles may be disposable or may be sterilized for future use. Some angles use screw-in cups and brushes; others use snap-on appliances. Prophy cups and brushes may also be purchased for a right angle handpiece.

High-speed handpieces have heads that hold a smooth shafted friction grip (FG) bur and are used for gross removal of tooth tissue. Because of the intense heat generated by the friction, they should be water cooled while functioning. These handpieces may or may not require a bur releaser attachment to loosen and tighten for bur placement. Some shanks of the FG bur are shortened and are called short shank. There are miniature friction burs that may be used in smaller heads.

Diamond Rotary Instruments

Diamond rotary instruments are often mistakenly called diamond burs because their shapes, shafts, and functions are similar to dental burs. The head of the diamond is not made with knife edges or biting teeth. The diamond instrument is steel shafted and headed. Pulverized, industrial diamonds are either electroplated or bonded to the head surface. The surface of the diamond head may be coarse, medium, fine, or ultra fine grit. Manufacturers color code these to designate their degree of abrasiveness. The degree of grit helps to determine if the diamond instrument is to be used for cutting, trimming, finishing, or polishing. The diamond rotary instruments follow the manufacturer's numbering system and may be purchased in any of the handpiece shafts. They may be called white, black, or blue diamond points or stones.

The most often used diamond rotary instruments are round, flame, football, tapers, wheels, cylinders, and cones, although there are others. See Figure 4–26 for a chart of common selection of these items.

The diamond rotary instrument generates much friction heat and must have a water stream on its surface while in operation to cool the work site and keep the stone from clogging. Commercial **abrasive** blocks can

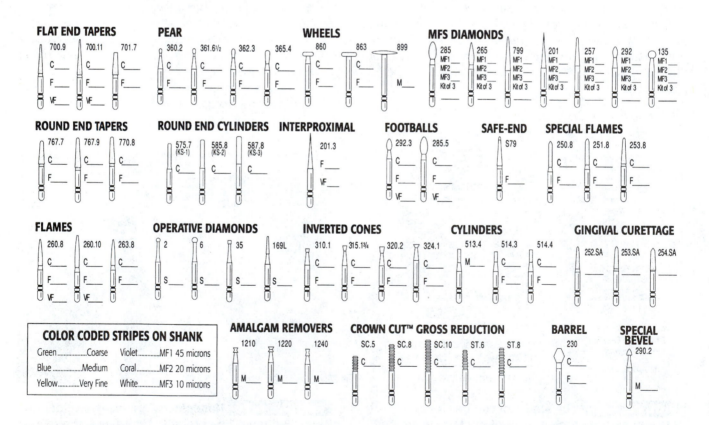

FIGURE 4–26 Diamond rotary instruments are used for gross tooth removal.

be used to unclog diamond rotary instruments by operating the handpiece while running the instrument over the surface of the block. Running the points over the surface of a pencil rubber eraser may help unclog some diamonds. Most diamonds may be sterilized in the customary manner, but the manufacturer's recommendations should be checked before processing.

Dental Stones

Some burs have finishing and polishing heads instead of cutting edges. These are stones and vary in shape. They follow the manufacturer's numbering system and come in all shafts (Figure 4–27).

The rough heads of the stones may be impregnated with chemicals to assist with the finishing of a specific material. White stones (aluminum oxide) are used for finishing composites, porcelain and enamel. Green and brown stones (silicon carbide) are used to finish porcelain, gold, amalgam, and composites.

Surgical Burs

Other rotary instruments are surgical burs that are used to reduce, drill, and bisect teeth and trim bone. These burs have long shafts and large heads, since they are used not on small teeth but on the alveolar processes, impacted molars, and maxillary and mandibular bones.

Mandrels

Mandrels are rotary instruments used for cutting, finishing, and polishing, depending on which disk is attached.

Mandrels come in all shafts and have either a snap head, pin head, or screw head onto which some disk, wheel, or cup is placed. Round or oval abrasive or rubber disks may be attached to the mandrel's head and used in the mouth or in the dental laboratory.

The disks used in the mandrel may be made of silica, carborundum, cuttlefish bone, garnet, emory, and other abrasive materials. They may be abrasive on one or both sides and come in different diameters of $1/2$, $5/8$, $3/4$, or $7/8$ inch. The rubber disks may be impregnated with minerals or chemicals to aid in polishing. Some mandrels have permanently attached wheel tops. These are called mounted mandrels (Figure 4–28).

P R O C E D U R E   1 3

Dental Rotary Instruments

1 Assemble Equipment and Materials

2 Demonstrate Background Knowledge of Dental Burs

3 Demonstrate Ability to Place Burs in Handpieces

4 Explain Operative Procedure Function of Burs

5 Explain Sterilizing and Care Instructions for Burs

6 Demonstrate Knowledge of Diamond Instruments

7 Demonstrate Knowledge of Dental Rotary Stones

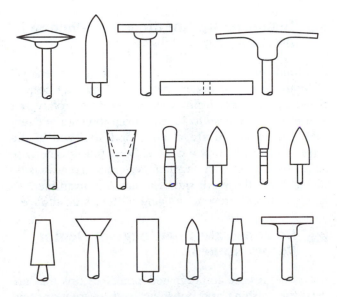

FIGURE 4–27 Dental stones come in assorted shapes, grits, and colors.

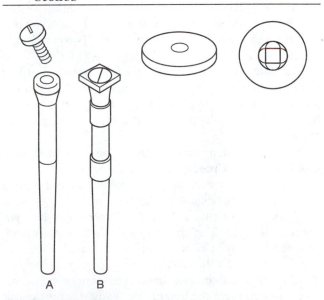

FIGURE 4–28 Disks, wheels, and cloths of various grits and materials may be placed in an (A) screw type or (B) snap-on type mandrel.

8 Demonstrate Knowledge of Surgical Burs

9 Demonstrate Knowledge of Mandrels

10 Demonstrate Knowledge of Handpiece Sterilization

11 Clean Up the Area

1 Assemble Equipment and Materials

To complete the competency evaluation exercise, the dental assistant must assemble the following items:

slow- and high-speed handpieces
contra angle handpiece and right or prophy angle handpieces
assortment of burs
ultrasonic cleaner
sterilizing bag or block
stiff bur brush
dental stones assortment
mandrel with disks and wheel assortment

2 Demonstrate Background Knowledge of Dental Burs

The dental assistant must be able to identify the three main parts of the dental bur—the head or working part, which gives the number to the bur; the neck, and the shank, which indicates the type of handpiece to use and the composition material of the rotary instrument.

3 Demonstrate Ability to Place Burs in Handpieces

Each bur must be securely placed in the proper handpiece using the correct method. The straight handpiece bur (SHP) is inserted into the opening of the slow-speed straight handpiece as deeply as possible. The turning knob on the opposite end is rotated until the bur is tightly held in the handpiece.

The latch bur (LT) is placed into a contra angle handpiece, which has been placed onto the slow-speed straight handpiece. After insertion, the latch is flipped closed, which hooks the bur securely inside the head.

The friction grip bur is placed into the head of a high-speed handpiece or a special attachment on a slow handpiece contra angle. A chuck inside the head is loosened for insertion of the bur and retightened to hold the bur in place. Each handpiece has its own method of controlling the internal chuck. Some manufacturers supply a special appliance called a bur releaser to place on the handpiece to open and close the chuck. Other handpieces have auto chucks or power levers to complete the action. The assistant must check the manufacturer's suggested method to place burs in the handpiece. *All burs placed into handpieces must be checked for security and function before use.

4 Explain Operative Procedure Function of Burs

Each bur is designed for a specific function. The dental assistant should have a general knowledge of the bur's operative function so instrument selection may be anticipated. The bur's functions are:

round ($\#^1/_4$ to #9)—opening pulp chambers, drilling for retention holes, single-surface cavities, anterior interproximals
inverted cone (#33^1/$_2$ to #39)—undercut in restoration preparation
straight plain fissure (#56 to #58)—parallel wall and floor preparations
straight fissure, crosscut (#556 to #558)—same as plain only more cutting edges
tapered fissure bur (#168 to #171)—slightly diverges parallel wall cuts
tapered fissure bur, crosscut (#699 to #703)—more cutting edges than plain
end cutting (#956 to #958)—shoulder preparations for crowns

5 Explain Sterilizing and Care Instructions for Burs

Dental burs are precleaned before sterilization. This may be accomplished either by rubbing their surfaces with a stiff brush and disinfectant solution or inserting them into a bur block run in the ultrasonic cleaner for five minutes. After cleaning, the burs may be autoclaved, chemiclaved, or oil or dry heat sterilized. All burs placed out for a procedure are sterilized, regardless of whether or not they were used.

6 Demonstrate Knowledge of Diamond Instruments

Diamond rotary instruments are used for gross removal of tooth tissue and dental materials. They may be prepared in any form from wheel to point to rotary bur shape. They are easy to identify from their surface texture and color and are cleaned and sterilized in the same manner as carbide or steel burs, unless otherwise suggested by the manufacturer. Water should always be directed into the work site of a diamond instrument to lessen heat and prevent clogging of the rough surface.

7 Demonstrate Knowledge of Dental Rotary Stones

Rotary stones are impregnated points or tips that are used for finishing and polishing teeth restorations and dental appliances. The color of the surface denotes the chemical, which is used for a specific purpose or material, that is embedded into the surface. Dental stones and burs are sterilized in the same manner unless otherwise directed by the manufacturer.

8 Demonstrate Knowledge of Surgical Burs

Surgical burs have larger heads than the average tooth bur but operate in a similar pattern and function. Since surgical burs are used on the larger bone areas, the heads of the surgical burs must cover more surface and have deeper penetration. Surgical burs are sterilized in the same manner and are kept in sterilized envelopes until used in a procedure.

9 Demonstrate Knowledge of Mandrels

Mandrels are long, metal shaft inserts for slow handpieces or shorter LT shafts for contra angles. They are used to hold rubber polishing wheels and abrasive disks. The heads of the mandrels where the wheels and disks are attached may be a screw or a snap connector. Each uses its own type. Some mandrels are premounted before purchase and used until the edges

are rough or worn through. Most head items are disposed of after the procedure, but the mandrels and any reusable heads are cleaned and sterilized before the next use.

10 Demonstrate Knowledge of Handpiece Sterilization

Dental handpieces must be sterilized between each patient. Manufacturer's directions determine the care and sterilizing procedure to follow for the specific handpiece; but general handpiece care, lubrication, and sterilization methods may be attempted in most cases (Table 4–1).

11 Clean Up the Area

All materials and equipment used in the experiment are cleaned and sterilized before being replaced in their proper storage area. When processing soiled rotary instruments, the assistant must always wear personal protective equipment, such as gloves and eyeglasses. After sterilization of the equipment, lubrication and storage procedures may be performed without PPE.▲

TABLE 4–1

General Handpiece Maintenance Chart

*Always check manufacturers' recommendations for specific instructions.

Low- and High-Speed Handpieces

1. Wearing protective gloves, flush handpiece over the cuspidor bowl after each use by operating appliance for 20 seconds to flush out internal debris.

2. Disassemble handpiece from line.

3. Remove bur or cup. Use disinfectant or detergent-saturated sponge to wipe off the external surface. Rinse under hot tap water. Swab off turbine lines.

High-Speed Handpieces only

4. Preclean internal surfaces by inserting an aerosol lubricant tip into the drive air tube and press for 1 or 2 seconds. On power lever handpieces spray air drive with lever down, and chuck with lever up.

5. Reassemble handpiece to turbine line.

6. Insert bur or blank bur. *Never operate handpiece without inserting bur.* Run for 30 seconds to remove internal debris and excess lubricant. Remove from line. Wipe handpiece with disinfectant-soaked sponge. Use sponge to wipe turbine lines.

7. Clean fiber optic handpiece in same manner, followed by rubbing both ends of handpiece with alcohol-saturated cotton applicator to remove residue film.

8. Bag handpiece in sterilization bag (not plastic). Cycle through autoclave or chemiclave. Do not sterilize over 275°F or 135°C.

Some manufacturers suggest that after sterilizing, the handpiece should be lubricated again in the same manner. If doing so, use another marked or labeled aerosol spray can and tip that is kept exclusively for processed sterilized handpieces.

CONTRA ANGLE HANDPIECE

1. While wearing protective gloves, wipe off external debris with a disinfectant-soaked sponge. Insert handpiece head with latch opened into small jar of handpiece cleaning solvent solution. Operate handpiece in forward motion for one minute; reverse the procedure by running the handpiece in solvent for one minute using a backward motion.

2. Use clean tissue to wipe off excess solvent. Hold tissue over the head of the handpiece, and operate the motor for a few seconds to remove excess solvent. Remove handpiece.

3. Wipe off excess solvent. Bag or wrap contra angle for sterilization, and complete the process.

4. If the manufacturer recommends lubrication after sterilization, remount the handpiece and insert it into marked or labeled clean handpiece lubrication oil. Always use only sterilized handpieces in this solution to avoid contamination. Operate the handpiece in both forward and backward motion for lubrication.

5. Wipe off any excess. Operate a few seconds with tissue covering head to collect excess spray. Wipe clean and store for operative procedure.

RIGHT ANGLE HANDPIECE

1. Repeat contra angle handpiece maintenance steps 1 and 2.

2. Disassemble handpiece with manufacturer's supplied wrench. Wrap or bag handpiece sections for sterilization. Complete the process.

3. After sterilizing handpiece sections, apply petroleum jelly to the gear assembly parts. Reassemble. Rebag for operatory procedures. To avoid recontamination, always keep jar of petroleum jelly marked or labeled "clean" and use only on sterilized handpieces.

T H E O R Y   R E C A L L

Dental Rotary Instruments

1. List four functions of dental burs.

   a. _____

   b. _____

   c. _____

   d. _____

2. What are the three parts of the dental bur?

   a. _____

   b. _____

   c. _____

3. What determines the number of the dental bur?

   _____

4. What is the difference between a crosscut bur and a plain bur?

   _____

5. Name the following bur shanks:

   HP_____

   LT_____

   FG_____

6. Why aren't diamond rotary instruments considered burs?

   _____

7. Why is a stream of water placed on the surface of the diamond instrument while it is operating?

   _____

8. What are the uses for dental stones?

   _____

9. Why do surgical burs have larger heads than regular dental burs?

   _____

10. What is attached to the head of a mandrel? What is the main use for these attachments?

   _____

Now turn to the Competency Evaluation Sheet for Procedure 13, Dental Rotary Instruments, located in Appendix C of this text.

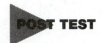

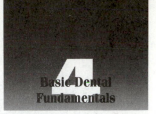
POST TEST

Total possible points = 100 points
80% needed for passing = 80 points

Total points this test _____ pass _____ fail _____

MATCHING: Write the letter from column B that best describes or matches the word in Column A. Each question is worth 3 points for a total of 30 points.

Column A	Column B
_____ 1. round bur	a. cutting tooth
_____ 2. mesio-occluso-distal	b. three-rooted tooth
_____ 3. deciduous	c. 17
_____ 4. maxillary molar	d. nourishes tooth
_____ 5. mandibular left third molar	e. forceps
_____ 6. pulp tissue	f. Class V
_____ 7. central incisor	g. MOD
_____ 8. high-speed bur	h. primary
_____ 9. gingival restoration	i. 6
_____10. palm grasp instrument	j. FG

TRUE OR FALSE: Write true or false in the blank before the statement. Each question is worth 2 points for a total of 10 points.

_____ 1. In the Federation Dentaire Internationale numbering system, deciduous teeth are numbered with letters of the alphabet.

_____ 2. The deciduous first and second premolars are replaced by permanent first and second molars.

_____ 3. One of the functions of surgical burs is finishing and polishing of restorations.

_____ 4. The maxillary first premolar contains two root canals and bears into two roots at the apical third of the tooth.

_____ 5. When examining and charting teeth, the operator begins in the lower right quadrant.

MULTIPLE CHOICE: Circle the correct answer. Each question is worth 4 points for a total of 60 points.

1. When dividing the mouth into four areas, the teeth in one of these areas is said to be in what type of division?
   a. quadrant   b. arch   c. semi-circle   d. proportional

2. The surface of the teeth that touches the tongue are
   a. labial.   b. lingual.   c. occlusal.   d. facial.

3. Which of the following tissues gives bulk and shape to a tooth?
   a. enamel   b. dentin   c. pulp   d. cementum

4. Which of the following is *not* a use for the dental rotary stone?
   a. finishing   b. smoothing   c. removing decay   d. polishing

5. During the charting procedure, placing a blue stripe line through the crown area signifies
   a. amalgam was used.   c. composite was used.
   b. porcelain was used.   d. gold was used.

6. In the Federation Dentaire Internationale system, which tooth is #55?
   a. the permanent right maxillary central incisor   c. the permanent mandibular left second molar
   b. the deciduous right maxillary second molar   d. the deciduous mandibular left central incisor

7. Which type of rotary bur does the slow-speed handpiece require?
   a. FG   b. HP   c. surgical   d. latch type

8. How are instruments arranged on the dental tray?
   a. largest are first
   b. most commonly used one in front
   c. in order of use
   d. cutting in back, reflecting in front

9. A dental chart showing the teeth as they generally appear is said to be
   a. geometric. b. anatomic. c. geographic. d. surface.

10. In the Universal numbering system, the maxillary right central incisor is
    a. #3. b. #8. c. #12. d. #20.

11. The area between the attached and loose gingiva is
    a. papilla. b. occlusal. c. rugae. d. sulcus.

12. When accepting a used instrument in an instrument transfer, which finger does the assistant use?
    a. thumb b. longest finger c. index finger d. smallest finger

13. During charting procedures, a circle placed around the entire tooth indicates
    a. decay. b. restoration. c. an impacted tooth. d. a permanent retainer.

14. When the instrument to be used is placed in the full, open hand, the transfer is said to be a
    a. pen grasp. b. palm grasp. c. palm-thumb grasp. d. open grasp.

15. The lateral incisor teeth are considered
    a. anterior teeth. b. posterior teeth. c. occlusal teeth. d. new teeth.

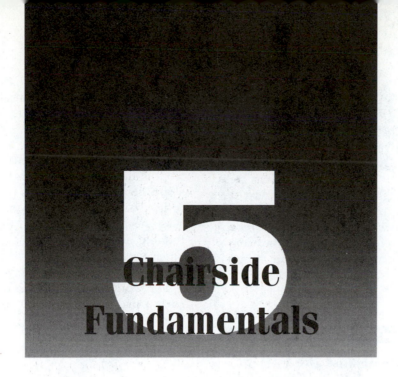

5 Chairside Fundamentals

▶ OBJECTIVES

Upon completion of this unit, the student will achieve a score of 80% or better on the Post Test covering the following material.

1. Discuss proper procedure for preparing, positioning, and dismissing patient for dental treatment.
2. Demonstrate correct method for rinsing and evacuating mouth fluids during dental procedures.
3. Demonstrate method for preparation, delivery, reception, and care of local anesthetic syringe and materials.
4. State the use of various cements and liners and demonstrate method of preparation and cleanup for cavity varnish, zinc phosphate cement, zinc oxide eugenol material, calcium hydroxide, glass ionomers, polycarboxylate cements, and resin cements and liners.
5. Explain the purpose of the Tofflemire matrix retainer and demonstrate how to choose the proper bands and wedges, prepare the retainer, and supply all materials necessary for the placement of an artificial wall.

▶ KEY TERMS

amalgamator	eugenol	lute
anesthesia	evacuation	matrix
aspirate	gauge	ora-evac
biodegradable	homogeneous	retractor
cartridge	HVE	saliva ejector
confirmation	infiltration	supine
calls	injection	topical
consistency	intensity	vasoconstrictor

PREPARING AND DISMISSING THE PATIENT

Preparation for a patient does not begin when the patient arrives for an appointment. Preparation begins the day before. In an office where there is more than one assistant, the receptionist pulls the charts for the patients scheduled for the next day and makes **confirmation calls** to ensure that the patients are aware of their appointments. The receptionist makes up a day schedule listing the next day's appointments by name, time, and procedure planned. A copy is displayed in each operatory and sterilizing room.

PROCEDURE 14

Preparing and Dismissing the Patient

1 Prepare for the Appointment

2 Prepare the Patient

3 Take the Health History

4 Prepare for the Procedure

5 Adjust the Operatory Light

6 Clean up and Dismiss the Patient

7 Cleanup Procedures

Preparing the Patient

1 Prepare for the Appointment

The chairside assistant obtains the charts and plans out the coming day by preparing as much as possible. Trays may be set up in advance, covered to protect from dust and contamination, and then placed in a holding area, away from the sterilizing room. The assistant makes sure all materials, laboratory work, records, and items necessary for the appointments are at hand. The operatory room is disinfected and prepared with all necessary materials and equipment assembled before the patient is summoned.

2 Prepare the Patient

The assistant escorts the patient to the waiting dental contour or lounge chair, which has been placed in the lowest level in an upright position. The chair may or may not be unlocked and swiveled to permit easier access for seating. If it is the custom to unlock and pivot the chair, the assistant is sure to lock the chair into position whenever the patient is entering or leaving the chair.

The right arm of the chair is raised to accommodate the patient, who sits and places his or her feet up on the chair. When the patient sits back in this resting position, the assistant lowers the armrest and adjusts the covered headrest for the patient's comfort.

The contour dental chair is placed in certain positions for work in a specific quadrant. When planning work in the upper arch, the chair back is lowered into a **supine** position, which is placing the patient on his or her back with the knees on a level with the nose. With the headrest adjusted, the patient will be comfortable and the dentist may place his or her legs under the chair and approach the patient from behind and beside in a close area (Figure 5–1).

For work in the lower arches, the contour chair back is placed at a 30 to 40 degree angle to the floor.

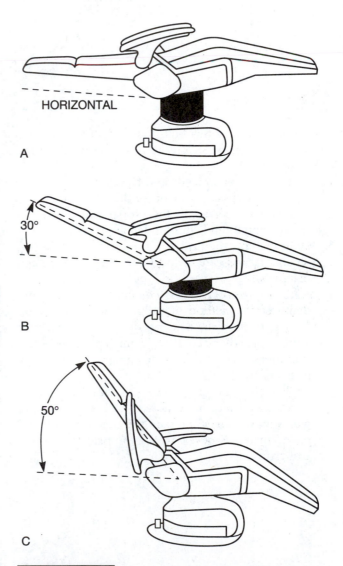

FIGURE 5-1 The dental chair is adjusted to provide good visibility and proper working conditions. (A) Maxillary position. (B) Mandibular position. (C) General position.

In this position, the patient is in a comfortable, seated position and the dentist approaches the patient from the front. When work is being completed in the entire arch, the patient is placed in the seated position and readjusted as needed. Raising and lowering the chair is done to accommodate the dentist's preference and comfort. *Caution:* The chair should not be moved without first notifying the person in the chair.

Occasionally, the patient will be carrying packages or a purse. The assistant should offer to take these and place them within view of the patient but out of the operative work area.

After the patient and chair are positioned, the assistant drapes or bibs the patient. If surgery is scheduled, or an appointment that might produce some spraying or messing, such as impression or prophylaxis, the patient is first covered with a long, plastic, disinfected drape. A paper or plastic backed towel is placed around the patient's neck. To avoid cluttering and crowding around the patient's face, the assistant places the alligator clip on the furthest bib end and brings the chain rope around the back of the patient's neck to attach on the near side. The chain should not be placed on bare skin; but if it cannot be avoided, the assistant should warm the metal chain by friction rub in the hands before attaching. The patient is asked to don eyeglasses if wearing no eye protection. There is always a possibility of chemical or foreign body invasion of a patient's eyes during dental treatment.

The assistant unwraps the instruments and places a clean cup, **HVE** (high vacuum evacuator) tip, and saliva ejector tip into position while the patient is observing. In this manner, the patient is assured that the equipment and materials being used for the appointment are fresh and sterile.

Some effort at light conversation may be started to make the patient feel at ease but is not forced if the patient declines to talk. If the patient does participate and mentions a particular fact, the assistant may jot it down on the chart and make reference to the incident at a following visit. This helps start conversation later, makes the patient feel important, and establishes a patient-office bonding.

A tissue swipe is offered to the patient. Patients are encouraged to remove lipstick to avoid smearing and most patients like to have a swipe handy to use as a napkin when rinsing the mouth. An alert assistant may observe how the patient is holding the tissue. Some very nervous patients will twist and tangle the tissue, showing signs of stress and anxiety. The assistant should monitor the emotional state of this patient closely.

3 Take the Health History

The assistant inquires into the patient's health history. If this person is a returning patient, the assistant questions

if there have been any changes made in the person's health since the last visit. Particular attention is given to any addition or cessation of medications during this time. The assistant must show a genuine interest in the patient during this questioning, as many people may be reluctant to discuss health problems, particularly if the interviewer seems busy or disinterested. New patients will have filled out a health history form and it may take a longer period of time for questioning. The assistant must inquire and then inform the dentist of any unusual remarks and record the conditions on the patient's chart. Many times the dentist too inquires about the patient's health.

4 Prepare for the Procedure

The stools for the dentist and the assistant are arranged around the dental chair. The dentist's stool is placed near the head of the patient and the dentist adjusts the final position after sitting. The assistant's chair is opposite the dentist, raised slightly higher (approximately 6 inches) than both the dentist and the patient for visibility. It is positioned slightly out from the patient's elbow. Each person adapts or slides the chair into the best position for comfort and visibility (Figure 5–2). The work tray or table is brought into the work area.

The assistant then washes hands and dons PPE. The operative lights are adjusted to focus into the patient's mouth. The **intensity** of the light beam may be adjusted; but in most instances, a normal setting is made and change is called upon only when needed.

5 Adjust the Operatory Light

The light is turned on when the lamp is positioned in a low angle, focusing at the patient's neck. The lamp

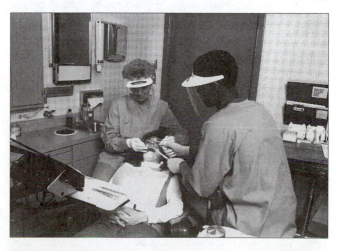

FIGURE 5–2 The assistant is positioned six inches higher than the dentist for increased viewing and access.

is raised slowly so the beam is controlled and stopped before it reaches the patient's eyes. The lamp is held back from the patient's face about a yard's length or as much as needed to permit room for the operator and assistant to work.

With the patient seated and prepared and the equipment and materials at hand, the procedure is ready to begin when the dentist wishes to start.

Dismissing the Patient

6 Clean Up and Dismiss the Patient

When the operative procedure has been completed, the patient is dismissed. The assistant wipes the patient's face. There should be no impression material, blood, or anything on the patient's face when the patient is released. The work tray or table is moved out of the way, and the bib or drape is removed. The assistant should caution the patient that the chair is being lowered and review any postoperative instructions with the patient, making sure that the instructions are fully understood.

When the chair reaches the lowest position, the assistant raises the armrest and assists the patient to rising. If any packages or a purse were put away before the appointment, the assistant retrieves them and returns them to the patient. The assistant then gives the patient the charge slip and escorts or directs him or her to the front desk for rescheduling.

7 Cleanup Procedures

The assistant returns to the operatory, gathers all contaminated materials, equipment, and items and removes them to the sterilizing room. At this time, the exam gloves are removed and the hands are washed. The patient's records are updated and the chart is taken to the front desk or wherever appointed by office protocol. The assistant returns to the sterilizing room, dons utility gloves, disinfects the operatory, and sterilizes the instruments. When all disinfection and sterilization is completed, the utility gloves are washed, disinfected, removed, and placed to dry. The hands are washed; and the assistant can move on to the next patient, beginning the greeting and seating procedure again.▲

THEORY RECALL
Preparing and Dismissing the Patient

1. When does the preparation for a patient's appointment begin?

2. In dental offices with more than one assistant, who pulls the charts for the coming day?

3. What duties may the chairside assistant perform to prepare for the patient's appointment?

4. Who escorts the patient to the operatory?

5. Where is the chair back placed when preparing to work on the upper arch? the lower arch?

6. What must the assistant do with a patient when raising or lowering the chair?

7. When reviewing the patient's health history, particular attention is given to what item?

8. Where is the operatory light positioned during an operative procedure?

9. When will the assistant review the postoperative instructions with the patient?

10. When does the assistant record the procedure on the patient's chart?

Now turn to the Competency Evaluation Sheet for Procedure 14, Preparing and Dismissing the Patient, located in Appendix C of this text.

EVACUATE AND RINSE

Removal of saliva and mouth moisture is an essential part of the dental assistant's duties. Operating in an area full of debris and liquids is quite difficult. Excess moisture and materials may cause a patient discomfort and trigger a gagging reflex. Even a small drop of moisture may limit viewing because the light reflection from the drop obscures the area. Retained mouth moisture may also affect the chemical setup time of some restorative materials.

The dental assistant may help with removal of fluids by correctly placing and using an **evacuation** device. There are two common types used in the dental office—a **saliva ejector** tip and an HVE. The saliva ejector tip is placed in the mouth to gently **aspirate** during treatment. The tip remains there, gently removing fluids. A dental assistant may occasionally reposition the tip during treatment to clear a troublesome area. The tip of the saliva ejector is smaller than the HVE tip. It is rounded and bendable at the end and is made of soft plastic. Some are white and opaque, while others are clear or lightly tinted. They are supplied 100 to a bag and are inexpensive, so they are considered disposable. They should never be used from patient to patient.

The second type of moisture removal appliance is the HVE. This tip is larger than the saliva ejector tip and is inserted into a handle, which has a knob or dial on the side that can be turned to regulate suction force. Use of this system permits the patient to be placed in a supine position, eliminates the cuspidor use, and accommodates aspiration of the water coolant of the high-speed rotors. Some solid debris can be aspirated as the opening is much larger than the saliva ejector. The tip of the HVE is larger all over and stronger. It can withstand the pressure of the cheek so it may be used also as a cheek **retractor**. HVE tips may be made of white, opaque plastic or stainless steel. Disposables may be purchased, or they may be reused after total cleaning and sterilization.

Evacuation systems need attention at cleanup. All lines and tubes must be flushed, cleaned, and sanitized. **Ora-evac** (oral evacuation) system solutions are available for purchase from dental supply houses. These concentrated liquids or powder packages are mixed into a solution that is aspirated into the hoses between patients and at the end of the day. When purchasing an ora-evac solution, one should check to see if it has EPA approval. Some common properties of these solutions are that they keep systems free from organic waste by dissolving gross debris, are nonfoaming, **biodegradable**, pleasantly scented, and concentrated for easy use. Failure to flush hoses with water, followed by oral-evacuation cleaning solution causes odors, clogging, and, finally, uselessness.

All evacuating systems have screen traps to serve as a safety container to capture any large aspirated item (Figure 5–3). These traps must be cleaned regularly, either by removal and thoroughly washing or by installing a disposable type and replacing at frequent intervals.

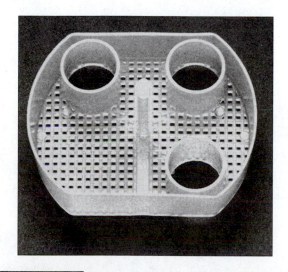

FIGURE 5-3 **Disposable traps and screens for evacuation systems are changed at frequent intervals. (Courtesy of Pinnacle Products.)**

PROCEDURE 15

Evacuate and Rinse

1 Prepare for the Procedure

2 Demonstrate Use of Saliva Ejector

3 Prepare HVE Tip

4 Assist with HVE in Maxillary Quadrants

5 Assist with HVE in Mandibular Quadrants

6 Assist with HVE in Anterior Region

7 Monitor Mouth Area

8 Demonstrate Use of Triple Syringe

9 Cleanup Procedure

1 Prepare for the Procedure

Saliva ejector and HVE aspirating tips are assembled with the tray setup and are not placed into their position until the patient has been seated. In this manner, the patient is aware that the tips are new and not left over from the previous patient.

2 Demonstrate Use of Saliva Ejector

The procedure for using a saliva ejector is to place the tip into the evacuating hose, bend the tip to a hook shape and "hang" the suction end over the mandibular incisors opposite the work site, where it will not obstruct the view. Occasionally, the tip may be moved by the dentist or dental assistant to aspirate accumulated liquids and then returned to the original site. Since the tip cannot "hang" in the maxillary arch, there are some limitations to its use. It also lacks much force in evacuation.

3 Prepare HVE Tip

HVE tips require practice before use. The assistant holds the tip, which is placed into a vacuum handpiece, in a palm-thumb grasp, much like one would hold a knife for stabbing. If the procedure is to be short, the handpiece may be held in a pencil grip also. The thumb of the dental assistant operates the knob or dial, which regulates the force of evacuation (Figure 5–4). The tip portion is positioned in the mouth with the opening always facing the water flow. The tip does not need to touch the teeth but only be close to the area for effectiveness. Scraping the tip on the teeth may make a noise and irritate the patient.

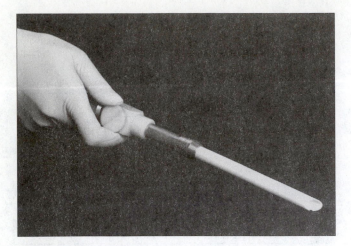

FIGURE 5–4 The assistant regulates the evacuating force by using the thumb knob or sliding bar found in the evacuation handle.

4 Assist with HVE in Maxillary Quadrants

To aspirate the maxillary quadrants, the assistant inserts the tip into the mouth, gently retracting the cheek. The opening of the HVE is placed facing the source of moisture and distal to the work site. The tip is held parallel to the lower arch for the maxillary left arch and at a 45 degree angle to the floor of the mouth for the maxillary right quadrant. The tip is held approximately ¼ inch below the occlusal plane of the maxillary teeth. If the tip opening is too high, it cannot function properly as the teeth will be situated between the flow and the opening (Figure 5–5A).

5 Assist with HVE in Mandibular Quadrants

The mandibular arches are aspirated in the same manner. The tip opening is toward the moisture source. The tip is parallel to the floor, and the opening is placed ¼ inch above the occlusal plane, distal to the work site (Figure 5–5B).

6 Assist with HVE in Anterior Region

Aspiration in the anterior region is completed in the same manner. The opening of the tip faces the source of water flow. The tip is placed ¼ inch away from the incisal edge, but the tip is not parallel to the floor. Now the tip works with the operator, distal to the work site, but not in direct conflict with the point of view. Care must be taken not to slide or scrape over the teeth and irritate the patient (Figure 5–5C).

7 Monitor Mouth Area

Occasionally, a piece of cheek tissue or tongue may become aspirated and cause a loud noise. The assistant needs only to gently twist the tip in a rotating manner and the suction will disappear easily. Pulling away only makes more noise and irritates the tissue. The assistant remains alert and prepared to alternate into any area that may be accumulating moisture.

8 Demonstrate Use of Triple Syringe

Another duty of the dental assistant closely related to evacuation is the rinsing of the patient's mouth. The

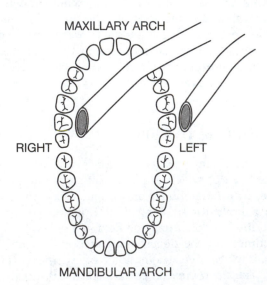

FIGURE 5–5A Position of evacuation tip for the maxillary arch. The opening of the tip always faces the source of moisture.

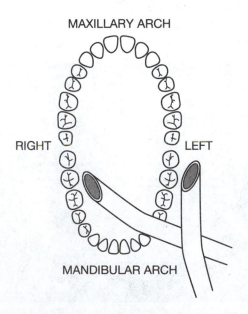

FIGURE 5–5B Position for the HVE tip in mandibular arch. The tip is always held slightly above or below the occlusal plane of the teeth.

Practice in the use of the air, water, and spray syringe will make an assistant proficient in its use. When using the syringe with a new patient, hold up the syringe and test it in view of the patient. This prepares the patient for its use and avoids arousing a patient's fear of a new item.

When using the syringe in the mouth, the assistant retracts the cheek, gently cupping it to hold in the water flow. In the anterior region, the assistant may gently pull the lower lip out to make a cup to catch any flow over of moisture from the syringe. Ideally, the dentist and the assistant may work as a team during the evacuation and rinse procedure. The assistant may gently retract the lip or cheek to catch the flow from the dentist's syringe or rotor and evacuate with the other hand. This saves the patient from the urge to empty the mouth or an uncomfortable feeling of fullness.

9 Cleanup Procedure

When completed with the procedure, the patient is dismissed and the assistant cleans up, disinfects, and sterilizes in the usual manner. The tips of the evacuation systems and the spray rinse system are inserted into containers of water and ora-evac rinsing solutions. These solutions are aspirated into the system to clean the hoses so odors and matter do not accumulate. After the suction of the fluids, the tips are removed and taken to the sterilizing room. The handles are disinfected. Barriers may be replaced on the handles, if needed. If the tips are disposable, they are placed in the contaminated disposal bag. If the tips are to be reused, they are cleaned and sterilized. The evacuation traps are not changed at every patient seating but are usually cleaned daily.

All equipment is cleaned and sterilized and the area is cleaned up. The materials are replaced. The utility gloves are washed, disinfected, dried, and removed to a drying rack. The hands are washed.▲

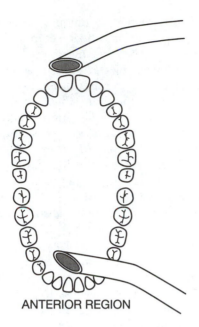

ANTERIOR REGION

FIGURE 5-5C Position for the HVE tip in the anterior region. The assistant works on the opposite surface to the water source.

dental assistant uses a triple flow syringe to rinse, dry, blow away, or spray. The triple syringe has two buttons on the handle; one is for water, one for air, and both for spray flow. The tips of the syringe may be purchased either in disposable plastic or a metal tip, which is removed, cleaned, and sterilized before use on another patient (Figure 5–6). The handle must be disinfected after each use or covered with barrier material.

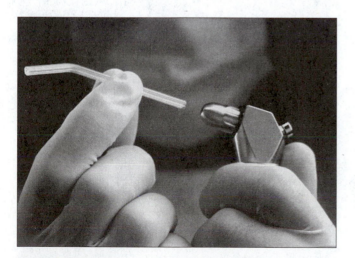

FIGURE 5-6 Disposable tips for the triple syringe assure cleanliness. The internal surface of metal tips cannot be adequately precleaned before sterilization. (Courtesy of DW Technology/Sani-Tip.)

T H E O R Y   R E C A L L

Evacuate and Rinse

1. List two reasons why it is important to evacuate the mouth of fluids and debris during a dental procedure.

   a. _____

   b. _____

2. What is the difference between a saliva ejector tip and a high vacuum evacuator tip?

   _____

3. What must be done to all evacuation lines at cleanup?

_____

4. Name three common properties of the ora-evac system solutions.

   a. _____

   b. _____

   c. _____

5. When ordering ora-evac system solutions, one should check to see if the solution is approved by whom?

_____

6. Where is the tip of the saliva ejector placed during operation?

_____

7. List three general rules to observe when using the HVE tip in the mouth.

   a. _____

   b. _____

   c. _____

8. What is the name of the syringe used in the dental office to rinse the mouth?

_____

9. What three functions does the syringe in question 8 perform?

   a. _____

   b. _____

   c. _____

10. What may the assistant do with the cheeks or lip when using the syringe to rinse the mouth?

_____

Now turn to the Competency Evaluation Sheet for Procedure 15, Evacuate and Rinse, located in Appendix C of this text.

ADMINISTRATION OF LOCAL ANESTHESIA

Local anesthesia is administered in the dental office to permit painless dental procedures. This type of **anesthesia** produces a deadened or painfree area where the dentist may perform sensitive operative tasks with relatively no discomfort to the patient. To assist in the administration of local anesthesia, the dental assistant must be aware of the various types of anesthetics, techniques, and the proper method to prepare an anesthetic setup and to deliver and receive the anesthetic syringe.

Before the dentist injects local anesthetic solution into the selected site, the area is prenumbed with a **topical** anesthetic. Topical anesthetics are supplied in gel, ointment, spray, or liquid form. These preparations are used to produce a loss of sensation in the gingival tissue, so the patient does not experience much pain when receiving the local anesthetic injection. The topical anesthetic is applied to a dried off selected site. (See Figure 5–7 for specific areas.) When the area undergoes maximum anesthesia, it is ready for **injection**.

Local anesthesia is completed by injecting a solution into a specific area to anesthetize a nerve. The solution is placed near the nerve, which absorbs the anesthesia and becomes senseless to pain. It is interesting to note that in local anesthesia, the patient will not perceive pain but will retain the feeling for pressure. Many patients may complain that they still "feel" after anesthesia, but in reality are not sensing pain but pressure.

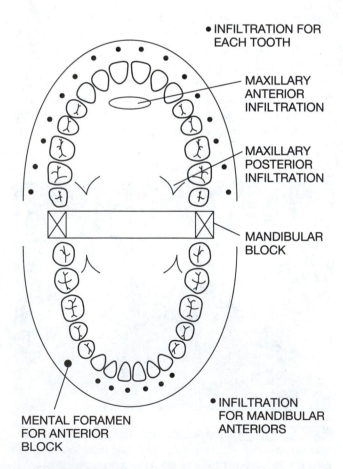

FIGURE 5–7 Topical anesthesia sites for painless local injections.

The dentist is careful not to inject the solution into a blood vessel as this may cause complications from the sudden rush of medication to the heart and brain. To avoid puncturing and injecting into the blood vessels, the dentist uses an aspirating injection syringe. This type of syringe has a harpoon, or barbed hook, on the end of the plunger that goes up and down inside the barrel of the syringe. After the injection, the dentist draws back with the plunger and aspirates a small amount. If blood is present, the dentist moves the needle off that site to avoid the vessel.

To prepare an anesthetic syringe for a procedure, the assistant obtains a sterile syringe, disposable needle, and an anesthetic **cartridge**. The anesthetic syringe may be an aspirating or nonaspirating style. The two are similar, except for the harpoon on the end of the aspirating syringe plunger. The syringe is composed of a threaded needle nose where the needle is attached, a long barrel where the solution cartridge is placed, a finger grip where the dentist grasps the instrument, and a finger ring on the end, which the dentist uses to push or pull on the plunger inside the barrel (Figure 5–8). Hidden inside the handle part, under the finger grip, is a spring that helps with the insertion of the cartridge. All these pieces may be taken apart and lubricated in the spring part when the syringe becomes stiff or hard to operate. A regular maintenance schedule for the care of this instrument should be kept.

The disposable needle, which fits on the front of the syringe, is in a protective plastic sheath. These needles come in two lengths and assorted **gauges** (thicknesses). The length of the needle to be used, either 1 inch or 1⅝ inches, is usually determined by the type of injection expected. Short needles (1 inch) are used in **infiltration** of local anesthesia mostly in the maxillary arch. The longer, 1⅝-inch needles are used to perform the deeper injections for the block anesthesia of the mandibular arch. The dentist may choose either length.

The gauge of the needle is numbered. The most popular sizes are 25, 27, and 30. The higher the number, the thinner the needle. (The assistant can remember this by assuming that if it takes 5 needles of 25 gauge to fill a hole and 7 needles of 27 gauge to fill the same hole, then the 25 gauge must be larger.) The needle is covered by a plastic sheath and a protective cap or cover on the syringe attachment end. The plastic sheath covering the needles is color-coded so the assistant will know what size gauge is inside. In many offices, the 25 or 27 gauge is popular. The dentist has the final selection and chooses the preferred gauges and needle length.

The cartridge is a long, slender, glass vial that holds the anesthetic solution. A rubber diaphragm is held on by an aluminum cap on one end and a rubber plunger on the other end (Figure 5–8B). In some brands, the color-coded rubber plunger or printed wrap around shows the type of solution and if any **vasoconstrictor** (epinephrine) has been added and if so, what concentration. One color indicates none added, another color indicates 1 drop of vasoconstrictor to 50,000 drops of solution, and still another color denotes 1 drop of vasoconstrictor to 100,000 drops of solution. Each brand of anesthetic has its own color code and method of identification.

Vasoconstrictors, such as epinephrine, are added to the anesthetic solution to hold the solution in the injection site for a long period. With the blood vessels constricted, the blood does not remove the solution from the injection site so rapidly and the area does not need as much anesthetic solution. There are a few cautions with the vasoconstrictors. Some high blood pressure and heart patients and persons who react to some drugs cannot be given the anesthetic solution containing vasoconstrictors, so the assistant must always review the patient's health history and receive orders from the dentist before loading the injection syringe.

Anesthetic cartridges are supplied 100 in a sealed can or sealed sterile pouch. They are sterile when opened and the assistant must try to keep them in this condition. Some offices have cartridge containers that keep the solution clean and dust free, but the assistant should wipe the diaphragm end off with alcohol before placing it into the syringe. Disinfectants are not used on the aluminum caps because some solution brands may cause corrosion.

The supply of cartridges must be kept out of sunlight and at room temperature. The temperature of the solution at injection time should be close to body temperature. There are some cartridge holders that are electrically heated and regulated to keep the solution near 97°F. Cartridges should never be frozen as the expansion extrudes the plunger and ruins the sterilized condition as well as the solution. One can tell if

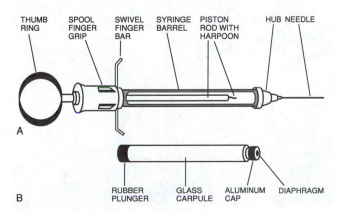

THUMB RING   SPOOL FINGER GRIP   SWIVEL FINGER BAR   SYRINGE BARREL   PISTON ROD WITH HARPOON   HUB NEEDLE

A

RUBBER PLUNGER   GLASS CARPULE   ALUMINUM CAP   DIAPHRAGM

B

FIGURE 5–8 **(A) Anesthetic syringe, barrel, and needle. (B) Anesthetic cartridge.**

the cartridges have been frozen if the plunger is extruded and there are large air bubbles present in the solution quality.

The assistant must also check for expiration dates and rotate the stock so the solutions are always effective. Older anesthetic solutions tend to become dark and sometimes clouded. When preparing to load the syringe, the assistant should always check the physical condition of the cartridge for cracks as well as for the clearness of the solution, the condition of the plunger, and the size of the bubbles. Small bubbles are expected.

P R O C E D U R E 1 6

Assisting with Local Anesthesia Administration

1 Complete the Preparations

2 Load the Syringe

3 Assist with Topical Anesthesia

4 Assist with Local Anesthesia Injection

5 Dismiss the Patient

6 Cleanup Procedure

1 Complete the Preparations

The setup for local anesthetic administration is:

▶ basic setup—mirror, explorer, cotton pliers
▶ 2 gauze squares (2 × 2)
▶ 2 cotton-tipped applicators
▶ topical anesthetic of choice
▶ anesthetic syringe
▶ anesthetic cartridges
▶ anesthetic needles
▶ triple syringe for rinse
▶ HVE for evacuation

The assistant checks with the dentist for orders of desired cartridge and syringe, washes hands, and gathers the necessary materials and equipment.

2 Load the Syringe

The desired cartridge is obtained and checked for cracks, bubbles, plunger condition, and overall appearance. An alcohol sponge is used to wipe off the diaphragm end on the cartridge before insertion into the syringe.

The assistant removes the syringe from the sterilized package and pulls back on the finger ring, inserting the cartridge into the barrel with the plunger end first, then dropping the cap end in (Figure 5–9). The

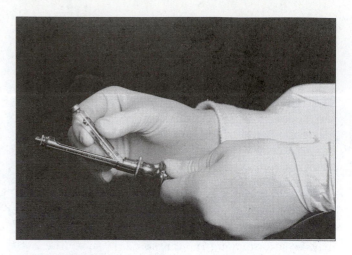

FIGURE 5–9 The anesthetic cartridge is placed into the syringe barrel and the harpoon is engaged.

finger ring pressure is released and the plunger moves down the barrel to meet the cartridge.

The protective cap is removed from the short end of the needle and this point end is screwed into the end of the syringe being careful to insert the needle into the center of the diaphragm (Figure 5–10).

If using an aspirating syringe, the assistant engages the harpoon or barbed hook by a quick press or "hit" on the finger ring. The assistant tests to see if the plunger is engaged (Figure 5–11).

The assistant replaces the sheath onto the needle and the prepared syringe is placed on the tray and covered in preparation for injection.

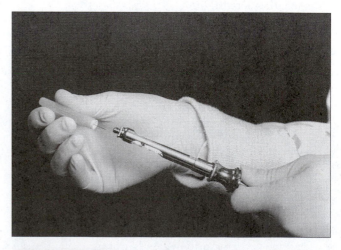

FIGURE 5–10 The needle tip is inserted into the center of the diaphragm and securely attached.

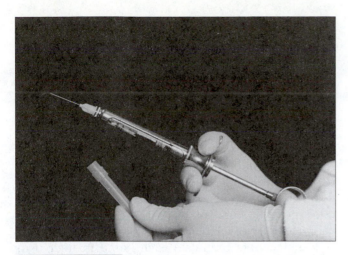

FIGURE 5-11 The syringe is tested for effectiveness.

3 Assist with Topical Anesthesia

After the patient has been escorted into the disinfected operatory and seated and draped, the assistant reviews the patient's health history. Particular attention is given to changes in medications, any allergies, and any past experiences with local anesthesia. The assistant washes hands, dons PPE, and rinses and evacuates the patient's mouth. A 2 × 2 gauze pad is used to dry off the proposed injection site, and the assistant places an applicator with the ointment or liquid topical solution on the site. If more ointment or topical liquid is desired, the assistant uses a new applicator to apply additional anesthesia. The applicator is permitted to remain on the site, and the dentist is summoned.

4 Assist with Local Anesthesia Injection

When the dentist gives the appropriate signal, the assistant receives the used applicator, picks up the syringe, and passes it below the patient's chin (out of sight). The dentist slips a thumb into the thumb ring and grasps the syringe at the finger rest. As the dentist takes the syringe, the assistant holds onto the sheath and guards the patient's arms against flinging or raising into the area.

After the injection is finished, the syringe is lowered and the assistant may retrieve it by grasping the syringe over the barrel, away from the needle end. The assistant brings the syringe back to the tray and then recaps by inserting the needle into the sheath laying on the tray. After the needle has been inserted into the sheath, the assistant tilts the syringe up on the sheath end and presses down to snap it into place. The syringe remains covered on the tray until further use or the appointment is over. An alternate method to maintain an anesthetic syringe is in a needle holder

(Figure 5-12). This holding device can be used for storing the syringe and for passing and receiving the syringe with the dentist.

The assistant monitors the patient's respirations and general health. If there is an increase in breathing rate or any adverse reaction, the assistant should notify the dentist. The anesthetized patient should not be left alone. The assistant performs the appointed duties for the scheduled appointment, ready to repass the anesthetic syringe if requested.

5 Dismiss the Patient

When the appointment is finished, the patient is cleaned up and dismissed. Before the patient is given the charge slip and assisted from the chair, the assistant cautions the patient about not biting on the numbed lip. Some offices give stickers to remind the patient.

6 Cleanup Procedure

After the patient is gone, the assistant gathers the contaminated instruments and materials and takes them to the sterilizing room where the latex gloves are removed and the hands are washed. The treatment rendered and the type and amount of local anesthesia used are marked on the patient's chart, which is taken to the front desk.

The assistant dons utility gloves and disinfects the operatory. The assistant removes the needle encased

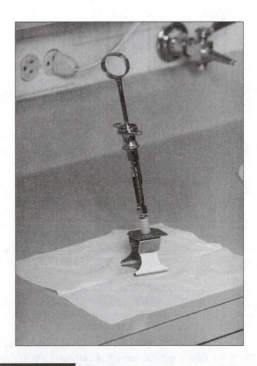

FIGURE 5-12 Needles are recapped with one hand or by using a mechanical device.

in the sheath and disposes of both in the sharps container. The syringe is cleaned and sterilized. Any punctured or unused solution is discarded.

The disposables are placed in the correct containers, and the instruments are cleaned and prepared for sterilization. The large items are disinfected and the area is cleaned up. The utility gloves are washed, disinfected, and removed. The hands are washed.▲

THEORY RECALL
Administration of Local Anesthesia

1. Before the administration of local anesthesia, what is done to the injection site?

_____

2. What are the lengths of the anesthetic needles? Which is used for a mandibular block injection?

_____

3. What do the different colors of the rubber plungers in a cartridge denote?

_____

4. List four things an assistant should examine a cartridge for when preparing to load a syringe.

   a. _____

   b. _____

   c. _____

   d. _____

5. What does the assistant monitor after the injection of the anesthesia?

_____

6. Where does the assistant grasp the syringe to retrieve it after injection?

_____

7. How does the assistant replace the sheath onto the needle after the injection?

_____

8. What does the assistant caution the patient to do after receiving local anesthesia?

_____

9. Where is the needle and sheath placed after use?

_____

10. When is the local anesthetic procedure recorded on the patient's chart?

_____

Now turn to the Competency Evaluation Sheet for Procedure 16, Assisting with Local Anesthesia Administration, located in Appendix C of this text.

PREPARING DENTAL LINERS AND CEMENTS

There is a large assortment of materials that may be used to line or prepare a tooth for a restoration or to **lute** (stick together). Many of these materials serve dual or triple purposes when dispensed and mixed in different ratios or methods. They may serve as a luting agent (cement); or in a tackier **consistency**, they may be used as a protective base under a restoration. In an even stiffer consistency, some may be used as a restoration. The operative procedure, the depth of the preparation, the pulpal involvement, and the type of restorative material help to decide the choice and use of the material.

Manufacturers formulate each brand in their own particular manner and package the material in kits or units. Some manufacturers may supply the particular cement in a paste system while others may package the same cement in a powder and liquid mixture. Some cements may be treated to be radiopaque (to show up on x-rays); some may need to be light cured to set up. Others may be supplied in shaded powders, and so on. Many of the materials are now being prepared and supplied in capsule form, which is activated by squeezing in special pliers and mixing them on an **amalgamator** (Figure 5–13). This method is expensive, but it saves time, is regulated in dosages, and helps prevent cross-contamination, which may occur when dispensing materials from bottles and jars.

The dentist selects the materials to be used in the operative procedures. The assistant must learn how to order, store, prepare, and clean up after each type. The best source of information about dental materials is supplied from the manufacturer in the manufacturer's safety data sheets (MSDS), which specify what

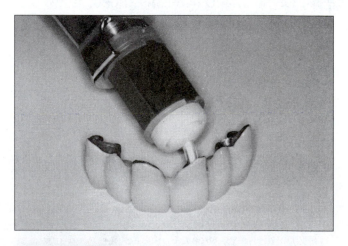

FIGURE 5-13 Capsule mixes offer sanitary, measured portions ready to be mixed. Cross-contamination is decreased with the use of separate, disposable capsule mixes. (Courtesy of ESPE America.)

type of hazard and safety precautions need to be observed. When opening a new material, the assistant should read the enclosed directions and specifications. In this manner, the assistant will know how to work with the item.

Table 5–1 offers specific rules per mix but there are some general rules to follow when working with liners and cements:

▶ Always follow the manufacturers' directions for storage, ratios, and preparation. Use the scoops and droppers supplied by the manufacturers.
▶ Never mix one manufacturer's brand with part of another manufacturer's brand, such as powder from one and liquid from another.

▶ Keep materials and containers as clean as possible. Prevent cross-infection by using overgloves during preparation, or opening and closing bottles and units using a gauze barrier.
▶ Always recap or close jars immediately to prevent liquid evaporation or contamination of materials.
▶ Check all expiration dates before use. Rotate stock.
▶ Use level scoops when measuring. Hold droppers upright to obtain the correct size of drops. (End openings are calibrated to provide the right amount.)
▶ Fluff powders and shake liquid before use.
▶ Clean up as soon as possible. Have cleanup sponge at hand while working. Soak or wash clean immediately. Don't scratch glass slab to remove materials. Soak in water and suggested chemical solutions for cleaning.

TABLE 5–1
Procedure Steps for Preparing Dental Liners and Cements

To prevent cross-contamination when mixing cements, the assistant should don overgloves or use a protective barrier, such as a gauze square, when opening, closing, or dispensing materials. All items should be disinfected at cleanup.

CAVITY VARNISH—VARNAL, COPAL, HANDI-LINER, CONTACT DENTIN SEALANT, AND BARRIER
Use: protective sealant under restorations

1. Remove cap from bottle. Insert pliers with small cotton pellet or small squeezie into liquid. Remove. Recap bottle.
2. Touch pellet against side of sterile cotton roll to absorb excess liquid.
3. Pass plier with pellet to dentist.
4. Receive plier; pass air syringe.
5. Repeat procedure for second application, using clean cotton pliers.

ZINC PHOSPATE MATERIAL—HYBOND, FLECK'S, AND AMES CEMENT
Use: cement, base or temporary restoration

1. Fluff powder bottle. Remove cap. Insert scoop and level off for accurate amount. Place on paper pad. Recap bottle.
2. Use spatula to divide powder into two halves. Divide one-half into fourths and one-fourth into eighths.
3. Shake bottle, invert, and dispense recommended drops. Hold bottle perpendicular to glass slab to get correct size of drops.
4. Draw smallest amount of powder into liquid and spatulate over large area in figure-eight motion for desired consistency (one minute mixing time).
5. Hold slab near operative site for dentist's use. Wipe instruments with wet sponge.

ZINC OXIDE EUGENOL MATERIAL—WONDERPAK, ZOE–B&T, CAVITEC, INTERVAL, AND IRM
Use: cement, base, and temporary restoration

1. Dispense zinc oxide onto paper pad using scoop measurer or clean spatula.
2. Divide powder into halves. Divide one-half into fourths.
3. Dispense liquid with dropper onto paper pad near powder piles.
4. Using a disposable or stainless steel spatula, draw largest amount of powder into liquid mass. Incorporate more powder as needed to get desired consistency (approximately one minute).
5. Pass prepared material to dentist.
6. Clean instruments with alcohol sponge. Dispose of paper mixing page.

CALCIUM HYDROXIDE MATERIAL—PRELINE, LIFE, ALKALINE, DYCAL, HYPO-CAL, AND DROPSIN

Use: sedative base and pulp capping

Paste method:

1. Dispense approximately 1 mm of paste from each tube onto paper pad.

2. Use small ball burnisher to mix both pastes together until homogeneous.

3. Pass loaded ball burnisher to dentist. Hold pad nearby for refill.

Powder and liquid method:

1. Use spatula to dispense small amount of powder onto paper pad.

2. Use dropper to place distilled water drop onto paper pad.

3. Incorporate small amount of powder to water until desired consistency.

4. Load ball burnisher. Pass to dentist. Hold pad nearby for refill.

GLASS IONOMER MATERIAL—KETAC–CEM, FUJI CEMENT, VITREBOND, BASELINE, AND EMKA

Use: cement, base, and selected restorations

1. Uncap bottle of selected powder. Insert scoop or spatula to obtain powder. Place powder on paper pad.

2. Remove lid. Dispense desired drops of liquid near powder on paper pad. Recap immediately.

3. Incorporate powder into liquid in small mixing area (approximately one minute) until desired consistency is obtained.

4. Pass material to dentist. Wipe instruments with damp sponge to remove cement.

POLYCARBOXYLATE CEMENT—HYBOND, DURELON, AND TYLOK–PLUS

Use: cement, base, and temporary restoration

1. Fluff powder. Uncap and use scoop to obtain powder. Level off for desired amount. Place on paper pad. Divide into halves.

2. Shake bottle. Uncap and dispense recommended amount of drops or use calibrated syringe to obtain amount of liquid on pad.

3. Incorporate powder into liquid quickly until desired consistency is reached.

4. Pass material to dentist. Wipe off instruments with wet sponge. Soak dried up material in 10 percent sodium hydroxide solution.

RESIN CEMENT—RESIMENT, TIMELINE, COMSPAN, AND DUAL CEMENT

Use: luting agent for inlays, onlays, bridges, endo posts

1. Pass acid-etch material and brush to dentist for tooth preparation.

2. Place cement materials onto mixing pad in close proximity.

3. Receive brush and pass triple syringe for water bath and dry of preparation.

4. Mix resin material to creamy, homogeneous mixture. Pass instrument.

5. Hold mix pad and material near work site for refill.

6. Receive luting instrument. Hold visible light source near preparation (if needed).

7. Wipe instruments; clean in ultrasonic; sterilize. Dispose of brush and paper pad page.

PROCEDURE 17
Preparing Dental Liners and Cements

1 Assemble Equipment and Materials

2 Prepare Cavity Varnish

3 Prepare Zinc Phosphate Material

4 Prepare Zinc Oxide Eugenol Material

5 Prepare Calcium Hydroxide Material

6 Prepare Glass Ionomer Material

7 Prepare Polycarboxylate Cement Material

8 Prepare Resin Cement

9 Cleanup Procedure

1 Assemble Equipment and Materials

Dental liners and cements require various working items, from paper pads to assorted spatulas. Each material has a separate requirement, which is listed with the exercise. Exam gloves should be worn throughout the exercise to prepare the assistant for actual mixing and preparation situations.

2 Prepare Cavity Varnish

The equipment needed is:

cavity varnish bottle
2 sterile cotton pliers
cotton rolls
small cotton pellets or squeezies

Cavity varnish is used in restorative preparations to seal and protect the dentin tubules. Copal varnishes, containing organic solvents, must be used only under amalgam restorations because the solvent material in the varnish prevents resin setup. Universal varnishes without the organic solvent may be used under all restorations. These liners are supplied in a paste or liquid form and may be applied to the dentin walls by brush or mixing tip.

The cap is removed from the bottle. A pair of sterile cotton or college pliers holding a cotton pellet or squeezie is gently dipped into the varnish solution and passed to the dentist. If the pellet contains too much solution, it is touched against a sterile cotton roll, which removes the excess. The cap is replaced immediately to prevent evaporation of the solvent solution and a thickening of the varnish.

If the varnish becomes too thick, the assistant may add a small amount of replacement varnish solvent, which can be purchased from the supply house. A second application of varnish is generally used. The procedure is repeated after the first coat dries and the dentist is ready for the second application. The cotton pellets or sponge squeezies are disposed of at the end of the appointment, and the cotton pliers are cleaned and sterilized in the usual manner.

3 Prepare Zinc Phosphate Material

Equipment and materials needed are:

glass slab
flexible stainless steel spatula
timer
shade guide
powder and liquid
scoop and liquid measurer

Zinc phosphate cement may be used as a permanent cement for crowns, inlays, and other dental appliances. The material possesses a good holding power and is used to lute (stick together). When used under porcelain crowns, a proper shade is selected to maintain the translucency of the crown. There are two types of powder grains—Type I and Type II. Type II is used for most procedures, but Type I may be chosen for fine detailed luting.

To use as a cement, zinc phosphate is mixed to a thin creamy consistency on a cooled dry glass slab, because heat is given off during the chemical union of the materials. The slab absorbs much of this heat, thereby saving thermal trauma to the tooth.

Since the crushing strength of zinc phosphate is better than other types of cement and it contains no **eugenol** to retard composite setting, this material may be used as a base in large restorations where tooth structure has been lost. After a medicated protection or seal has been painted in the preparation, a thicker mixture of zinc phosphate may be placed before the restorative material is inserted. The zinc phosphate acts as a thermal insulator absorbing heat or cold that may be given off from the restoration's exposure to food and drink.

To prepare zinc phosphate, the assistant fluffs the powder bottle and inserts the scoop to retrieve the amount specified by the manufacturer. The scoops of powder are leveled off and placed on the glass slab. The powder pile is divided into sections from halves to quarters to eighths. A small amount of powder may be placed on the corner of the slab and presented to the dentist. The dentist dips used instruments into the powder to prevent material from sticking.

The assistant shakes and inverts the bottle to drop the specified amount of drops of liquid on the slab, or if needed, inserts a dropper into the bottle to obtain the solution and places the required drops on the slab.

The smallest amount of powder is drawn and spatulated over a wide area into the liquid. More powder is drawn and spatulated in until a creamy mixture is obtained within a two-minute mixing time limit (Figure 5–14). The material should begin setting at that time and obtains final set within six to eight minutes.

Zinc phosphate mixed for base consistency is prepared in the same manner changing only the powder

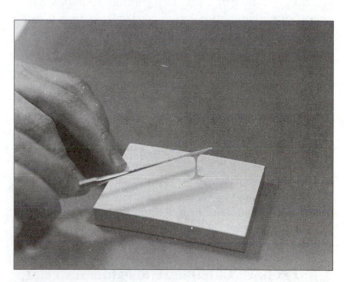

FIGURE 5–14 The materials are mixed to a creamy consistency for cement use. (Courtesy of ESPE America.)

and liquid measure to give more density to obtain a puttylike consistency. A temporary restoration mixture may be prepared by adding still more powder for a stiffer density. Manufacturers' directions indicate the ratio for cement, base, or temporary restoration use.

Cleanup is completed by placing the slab and instruments in cool water to soak, followed by a baking soda water bath to remove the cement material without scratching the slab.

4 Prepare Zinc Oxide Eugenol Material

Assemble the following:

zinc oxide powder
eugenol liquid
treated paper pad
spatula (disposable or stainless steel)
scoop and dropper
alcohol sponge
orange solvent for cleanup

Zinc oxide and eugenol (ZOE) is an old standard dental material used as a temporary cement, sedative base, or temporary restoration. Later, additives (EBA) to the powder and liquid of the formula have increased the strength of the material so it may be used as a permanent cement with gold castings. Because of the eugenol's (oil of cloves) nature-preventing setup, ZOE may not be used under composite restorations.

Since ZOE does not give off heat, it may be mixed on a treated paper pad that prevents oil leakage. The powder is dispensed by a measuring scoop or clean spatula, placed on the pad, and divided in half with one of the halves divided again. Liquid drops are set on the pad nearby. The large amount of powder is incorporated into the liquid and mixed in a wiping motion over a large area until the desired consistency is reached within one minute (Figure 5–15). Cement consistency is creamy; base consistency is tacky; and the temporary restoration consistency is quite stiff. The powder/liquid ratio is determined by the manufacturer. Setup time is usually approximately five minutes but may hasten under humid conditions.

Cleanup is accomplished by obtaining a clean spatula or instrument, inserting between the pad pages, and loosening the top dirty page, which is discarded. The instruments are wiped with an alcohol sponge and cleaned and sterilized in the usual manner. Orange solvent solution may be used for stubborn, dried-on ZOE material.

5 Prepare Calcium Hydroxide Material

Equipment and materials needed are:

calcium hydroxide pastes or powder and distilled
  water

paper pad
spatula
small ball burnisher
sponge
timer

Calcium hydroxide material may be used as a sedative base under any restoration and is frequently used where pulp exposure has occurred in the preparation procedure. This material provides an immediate therapeutic effect and helps to promote the growth of secondary dentin for a more permanent protection. It is applied in a thin layer by using a small ball burnisher instrument and is covered with another, stronger base material that provides bulk and thermal protection.

Calcium hydroxide is supplied in two forms: two pastes, which require equal amounts to be mixed together, or a powder, which may be united with water to make a paste for coverage. The two-paste system is more popular and used frequently in the dental office. The materials are mixed on a paper pad and completely blended in approximately one-half minute. Cleanup is done with soap and water with normal instrument sterilization. Calcium hydroxide may also be supplied premixed in a syringe. It is expressed when needed by twisting the dispensing end.

6 Prepare Glass Ionomer Material

Equipment and materials needed are:

powder and liquid
paper pad
measuring scoop wand
spatula
timer

There is more than one type of glass ionomer material. The finer grained cement powder (Type I) was formulated to be used as a luting agent for crowns

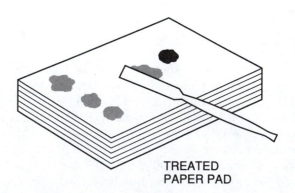

TREATED
PAPER PAD

FIGURE 5–15 The larger portion of powder is first drawn into the liquid eugenol when mixing ZOE.

and bridges because of its chemical bond of the metal to the tooth structure. It is particularly useful in orthodontic cementation because of the slow fluoride release of the material.

Type II glass ionomer cement has a greater crushing strength and is capable of bonding directly to the enamel and dentin tissues. These Type II cements, supplied in shaded, coarser grained powders are used in selected restorations (Class V erosion, small Class III, and pediatric restorations).

Glass ionomer base cement is formulated to act as a supportive, protective base under all stress-bearing restorations. The material chemically bonds to the tooth tissues; releases fluoride, which prevents secondary decay; strengthens tooth structures; withstands acid-etching; and is radiopaque for future reference in x-rays.

When preparing the glass ionomer cement, the assistant should fluff the powder and dispense and section the manufacturer's recommended amount of scoops onto a treated paper pad or cool glass slab. Paper pads are preferred for cleanup use, but glass slabs may be used to retard setting time. *Caution:* The assistant should avoid inhaling any powder fumes and be careful not to dispense the material close to the patient's face.

The specified amount of drops are placed onto the pad or slab near the powder piles. The bottle is capped immediately to prevent evaporation. The powder piles are drawn into the liquid one at a time and mixed over a small area until the final consistency is obtained. Cement consistency is creamy and glossy. Base consistency is tacky and stiffer, while restorative consistency is quite stiff. Mixing time is less than one minute, while the setting time is approximately five minutes.

Cleanup is completed by removing the top paper and disposing of the used sheet (Figure 5–16). In-

struments are washed up immediately or soaked in water before ultrasound cleansing.

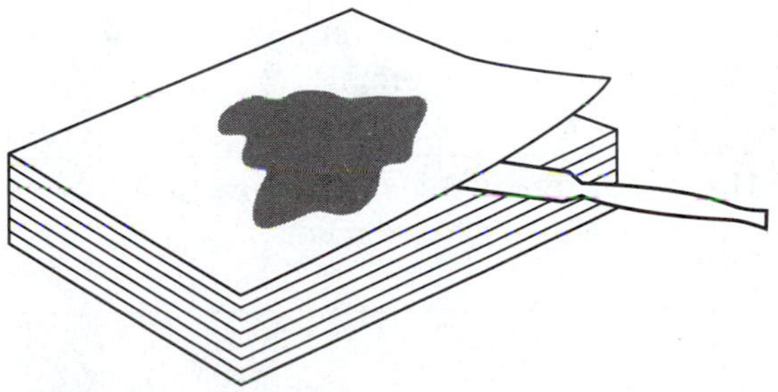

Glass ionomer cements are also available in a premeasured capsule and may be activated and mixed in the amalgamator following the manufacturer's directions.

7 Prepare Polycarboxylate Cement Material

Equipment and materials needed are:

powder and liquid
treated paper pad or cool glass slab
spatula
measuring scoop and liquid measurer or calibrated
   dispenser
timer

Polycarboxylate cement, also known as zinc carboxylate cement, is used generally for cementation of inlays, onlays, and orthodontic bands and brackets because of the bonding ability of the material and the kindness of the material to the pulp. In a stiffer consistency, it may be used as an insulating base under restorations and in a harder mass, may be used as a temporary restoration.

The assistant fluffs the powder and dispenses the selected amount of scoops onto a paper pad or cool glass slab. Manufacturer's specifications should be followed; but, generally, when preparing cement, one scoop of powder is measured out for three drops of liquid. The liquid may be placed on the pad or slab near the powder. Drops are obtained by inverting the plastic squeeze bottle or dispensing drops from a calibrated syringe (Figure 5–17). The powder is incorporated into the liquid and quickly (in 20 to 30 seconds)

FIGURE 5–16 Soiled top sheets of a mixing pad are removed by using a clean spatula and inserting under the used leaf.

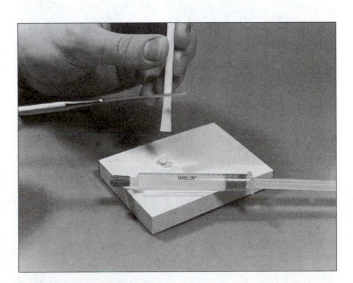

FIGURE 5–17 Liquid used for mixing some cements may be dispensed from a syringe. (Courtesy of ESPE America.)

mixed to the cement consistency. The cement will have a glossy appearance while effective. Cement that loses the gloss must be discarded and a new batch must be made. When making polycarboxylate cement for use as a base, the assistant uses the same procedure but decreases the liquid ratio to two drops or two-thirds a calibrated mark on the dispensing syringe. The consistency is glossy but tacky and stiff.

Setup time is usually five minutes and cleanup is done immediately by wiping the spatula with a wet cloth or soaking dried up material in a 10 percent sodium hydroxide solution. The paper pad sheet is removed and disposed of at cleanup.

8 Prepare Resin Cement

Some very fine resin cements have been developed for use as a luting agent for inlay, onlays, bridgework, and endodontic posts. These cements maintain pulp vitality, may be shaded to complement translucency of the prosthesis, and may be radiopaque treated to be observed on x-rays. Some also help promote secondary dentin formation. They resist acid-etching, which is required in the resin makeup. Some are auto cured in two stages, mixing and placing in 90 seconds with final cure of three minutes, while others need a visible light curing session for immediate final set (Figure 5–18).

They may be supplied in a two-paste system, powder and liquid set, or syringe. The manufacturer may supply the acid-etch gel or liquid with the unit.

To assist with resin cementation, the assistant passes the acid gel brush to the dentist for tooth tissue preparation. During the etching session, the assistant places

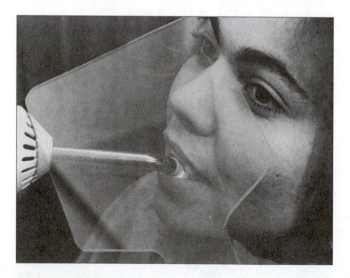

FIGURE 5–18 Some restorative materials require a light curing process for final set. Care of the eyes is done with a protective shield or special eyeglasses. (Courtesy of Premier Dental Products Co.)

the resin cement materials on the mixing pad in close proximity. Then the assistant passes the triple syringe for water bath and blow dry of the preparation and prepares the material by mixing the materials to a **homogeneous** creamy mixture, which is passed on a small instrument. The pad is held in the working area for refill. The assistant holds a sponge for cleaning instruments as needed. If the visible light system is needed for setup, the assistant receives the cement instrument and holds the light in place, using the light shield for protection against eye irritation.

Cleanup is done immediately. Brush tips and paper pad pages are discarded. Instruments are washed up, placed in ultrasonic cleaner, and sterilized for future use.

9 Cleanup Procedure

All materials and equipment are cleaned up and replaced in their proper positions. Disposable papers and spatulas are placed in the trash. The area is cleaned and wiped. The assistant removes the practice latex gloves and washes hands.▲

THEORY RECALL
Preparing Dental Liners and Cements

1. List three purposes some dental cements may serve in dental procedures.

   a. _____

   b. _____

   c. _____

2. What three factors help to determine the choice of material to use?

   a. _____

   b. _____

   c. _____

3. Why are manufacturers supplying more cement materials in capsule form?

   _____

4. List four general rules to follow when working with dental liners and cements.

   a. _____

   b. _____

   c. _____

   d. _____

5. For what three purposes may zinc phosphate cement be used?

   a. _____

   b. _____

   c. _____

6. Why is zinc phosphate cement mixed on a glass slab?

   _____

7. Under what restorative materials may calcium hydroxide be used?

   _____

8. For what purpose is Type I glass ionomer material used?

   _____

9. In which restorations may Type II glass ionomer material be used?

   _____

10. What type of growth do materials that release fluoride help?

   _____

Now turn to the Competency Evaluation Sheet for Procedure 17, Preparing Dental Liners and Cements, located in Appendix C of this text.

PLACEMENT AND REMOVAL OF THE TOFFLEMIRE RETAINER

Whenever a wall or sides of a tooth are destroyed either from decay or in cavity preparation, an artificial wall must be erected before a proper restoration can be placed. After the preparation has been completed and lined with medication, the dentist places a band around the tooth. This **matrix** band gives support and provides resistance when the amalgam or restorative material is being packed in. The band remains around the tooth until an initial carve has been made. The dentist carefully removes the matrix band and then does a final carving and adjustment.

Matrix bands may be held in position around the tooth by a matrix band retainer. There is an assortment of retainers, but the most popular is the Tofflemire type. The assistant should have a knowledge of the loading of this matrix band retainer as well as any other type the dentist may prefer.

Since the placement of a matrix occurs during the appointment for a Class II restoration, the setup needed for the assembling and operation of a Tofflemire retainer is added to the restoration equipment.

PROCEDURE 18

Placement and Removal of the Tofflemire Retainer

1. Complete the Preparations
2. Prepare Matrix Retainer
3. Position Band in Retainer
4. Insert Band into Retainer
5. Stabilize Band in Retainer
6. Adapt Band Size
7. Adapt Loop Shape
8. Pass Matrix Retainer and Band to Dentist
9. Pass Wedge Holder and Wedge to Dentist
10. Removal of Tofflemire Retainer and Matrix Band

1 Complete the Preparations

To assist with a posterior restoration involving the loss of a proximal wall, the assistant adds the following Tofflemire matrix retainer materials to the restoration setup:

Tofflemire matrix retainer
assortment of bands
assortment of wedges
wedge holder

(*This exercise may be completed on a prepared typodont preparation.)

2 Prepare Matrix Retainer

When the dentist is ready for the matrix placement, the assistant prepares the matrix retainer by rotating the outer knob counterclockwise to retract the spindle pin head toward the handle. When the tip is free of the slot and there is room for the insertion of the band ends, the assistant ceases the rotations.

3 Position Band in Retainer

The assistant selects the stainless steel band ordered by the dentist, but may anticipate the choice by observing the preparation and the tooth involved. There are premolar and molar bands (Figure 5–19A). Some have a bump or two bumps on one side. These bumps permit larger coverage. These are used when gingival involvement requires a deeper wall replacement.

Tooth observation is important because sometimes a small molar may do better with a premolar band and likewise a large premolar may adapt better in a molar band. Generally, though, the bands are presized correctly.

4 Insert Band into Retainer

The band is prepared for placement into the matrix retainer by turning the wing tips toward the gingiva (Figure 5–19C). This action places the smaller side of the band closer to the cervix of the tooth, which is smaller than the broad contact surfaces of the teeth.

The assistant positions the matrix retainer for insertion of the band. The matrix retainer is placed so the slot in the head faces the gingiva, permitting closer adaptation of the band to the tooth.

The loop side coming out from the retainer head is inserted into one side of the gate located in front of the head. When the assistant inserts the band through the front or one of the side gates, the loop turns for closer adaptation (Figure 5–19B).

When the band comes out the front slot, it is in position for anterior teeth. When the band comes out the gate on the side of the attaching arm, it is in position to be placed on a maxillary left or mandibular right tooth. When the band is placed through the gate on the side of no attachment, the band is prepared to be placed on a maxillary right or mandibular left tooth (Figure 5–20).

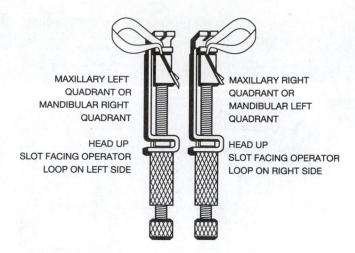

FIGURE 5–20 Matrix band retainer gate selections and position for band placement for each quadrant.

The tips of the band are pressed together and inserted into the slot in the head of the retainer, extending a small amount (approximately 1/16 inch).

5 Stabilize Band in Retainer

The band is stabilized in the holder by turning the outer knob clockwise, causing the spindle pin head to press against the band ends, which are inside the retainer head.

6 Adapt Band Size

The tightening or rotating of the head, which is caused by twisting the inner knob, lengthens or shortens the size of the loop.

7 Adapt Loop Shape

To help open the band to form the loop, the assistant turns the inner knob to tighten the band slightly.

If the loop is not fully opened or needs adaptation, the assistant takes the handle of a mouth mirror, inserts it into the band loop, and contours the band to a loop shape.

8 Pass Matrix Retainer and Band to Dentist

When the band is placed securely in the retainer in the proper position, the assistant passes the retainer and band to the dentist, who positions it around the tooth, extending slightly above and below the preparation. A burnisher may be requested by the dentist to smooth and contour the band closer to the surface.

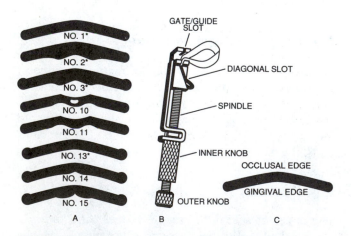

FIGURE 5–19 (A) Assorted matrix strips or bands. (B) Tofflemire retainer with matrix band sizes and shapes. (C) The curved band wings face toward the gingiva so the longer edge makes a larger circle to better conform to the width of the crown.

9 Pass Wedge Holder and Wedge to Dentist

A plastic or wood V-shaped wedge or two are passed to the dentist following matrix placement. The wedge not only stabilizes the band on the tooth but also contracts the band close at the embrasure area of the tooth, permits a better restoration, and avoids overhanging restorations (Figure 5–21).

The assistant passes a wedge in a wedge holder to the dentist after the matrix has been placed.

10 Removal of Tofflemire Retainer and Matrix Band

When the restorative material has been placed and roughly carved, the dentist signals for the removal of the matrix. The assistant passes the wedge holder or pick ups to the dentist who removes the wedges and places them into the assistant's waiting hand. While holding one finger on the matrix band, the dentist carefully releases the tension on the holding knob of the retainer. The retainer becomes free and the dentist deposits it in the assistant's hand. Using the pick ups, the dentist gently teases the matrix band out of the interproximal space.

The assistant accepts the band and wedge holder or pick ups and passes a carver, burnisher, articulating paper, or the instrument of the dentist's choice. The restoration is completed.▲

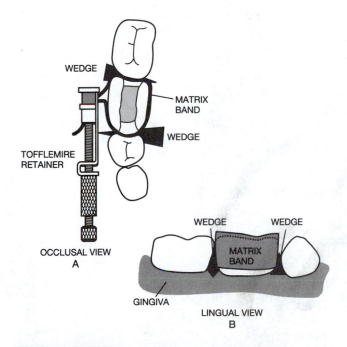

OCCLUSAL VIEW
A

LINGUAL VIEW
B

FIGURE 5-21 **(A) Tofflemire retainer with matrix band and wedges in place for a Class II restoration. (B) Wedges are used to stabilize the band and prevent overhanging restorations.**

Placement and Removal of the Tofflemire Retainer

1. What is the purpose of a matrix band?

_____

2. What keeps a matrix band in place?

_____

3. How does the assistant prepare the matrix band retainer for a placement of a matrix band?

_____

4. What two assessments are made to help with the selection of a proper matrix band?

    a. _____

    b. _____

5. In what direction are the wing tips of the matrix band placed before positioning?

_____

6. In what direction is the head slot of the matrix retainer placed in relation to the gingiva?

_____

7. How is the band stabilized in the matrix retainer?

_____

8. Out of what gate side would the loop be placed for a maxillary right quadrant restoration?

_____

9. What does the assistant pass to the dentist after the band has been placed around the tooth preparation?

_____

10. What is the purpose of the plastic or wood wedge?

_____

Now turn to the Competency Evaluation Sheet for Procedure 18, Placement and Removal of the Tofflemire Retainer, located in Appendix C of this text.

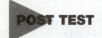
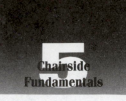
Total possible points = 100 points
80% needed for passing = 80 points

Total points this test _____ pass _____ fail _____

MULTIPLE CHOICE: Circle the correct answer. Each question is worth 4 points for a total of 60 points.

1. What must be done with the evacuation lines after operatory use?
   a. dispose of properly
   b. flush, rinse, sanitize
   c. detach and autoclave
   d. wipe lines with alcohol

2. Why is the aspirating type of anesthetic syringe used during injection of local anesthesia?
   a. to test for patient breathing
   b. to test for location of needle
   c. to test patient sensitivity
   d. to determine correct solution

3. The HVE tip should be placed on which side of the work site during a procedure?
   a. mesial
   b. apical
   c. occlusal
   d. distal

4. Calcium hydroxide material is used as
   a. restoration.
   b. an insulating base.
   c. permanent cement.
   d. a sedative base.

5. How does the assistant sanitize the anesthetic carpules before use?
   a. by autoclaving
   b. with an alcohol swipe
   c. with a disinfectant swipe
   d. by chemiclaving

6. Type I glass ionomer material is used for which purpose?
   a. luting
   b. base cement
   c. restoration
   d. instrument cleanser

7. Where is the operatory light placed during an operative procedure?
   a. opposite the work site
   b. straight down from the ceiling
   c. horizontal to the work site
   d. approximately 36 inches directly out from the mouth

8. Copal varnish can be used as a sealant under which restorations?
   a. amalgam
   b. composite
   c. both
   d. neither

9. The gauge of an anesthesia needle is indicated by
   a. the color of the sheath.
   b. the length of the sheath.
   c. the diameter of the sheath.
   d. none of these choices.

10. The dental triple syringe used at chairside is capable of what three uses?
    a. water, air, and oil spray
    b. water, air, and moist spray
    c. water, oil, and air
    d. oil, air, and water spray

11. When placing a patient in the dental chair for a maxillary procedure, into which position should the chair be placed?
    a. horizontal
    b. chair back 30 to 40 degrees to the floor
    c. upright
    d. supine

12. In relation to the operator's stool, the assistant's stool should be placed:
    a. 6 inches higher than the operator
    b. 6 inches lower than the operator
    c. even with the operator
    d. 12 inches lower than the operator

13. Instruments should be placed on the dental tray in which fashion?
    a. reflective in back, cutting in front
    b. random order
    c. in order of use
    d. light ones in front, heavy in back

14. Which is not a function of capsulated cement mixes?
    a. premeasured amount
    b. prevent cross contamination
    c. cheaper cost
    d. fast, easy use

15. Which is not a function of the Tofflemire matrix retainer and band?
     a. prevents overhanging restoration   c. makes the area more visible
     b. provides an artificial wall   d. helps hold material

MATCHING: Write the letter from column B that best describes or matches the word in column A. Each question is
          worth 4 points for a total of 40 points.
          Column A   Column B
_____ 1. seals dentin tubules in preparation   a. calcium hydroxide
_____ 2. promotes secondary dentin growth   b. homogeneous mixture
_____ 3. dental materials information   c. MSDS
_____ 4. cement consistency   d. decreases blood flow
_____ 5. proper two-paste mix   e. block anesthetic
_____ 6. common maxillary anesthetic injection   f. creamy mixture
_____ 7. common mandibular anesthetic injection g. copal varnish
_____ 8. vasoconstrictor   h. infiltration anesthetic
_____ 9. injection preparation   i. glass ionomer
_____ 10. tooth tissue bonding cement   j. topical anesthetic

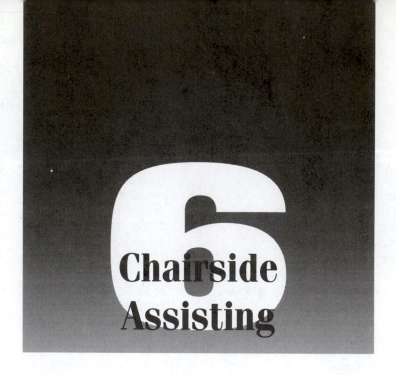

6 Chairside Assisting

OBJECTIVES

Upon completion of this unit, the student will achieve a score of 80% or better on the Post Test covering the following material.

1. Describe the duties and responsibilities of the dental assistant with the preliminary examination of the dental patient.
2. Demonstrate the method for obtaining a chairside full-mouth alginate impression to construct study models for a dental patient.
3. Discuss procedures the dental assistant may use to assist the operator in the performance of the dental prophylaxis.
4. Describe the method to deliver topical fluoride treatment in the dental office.
5. Discuss the pros and cons, preparation, and application of dental sealants for newly erupted teeth.
6. Describe methods and procedures to use for brushing and flossing technique instruction for the dental patient.
7. Discuss information and useful methods for diet and nutrition counseling of the dental patient.
8. Demonstrate the method for chairside dental dam application for the dental patient.
9. Describe the duties and responsibilities of the dental assistant while assisting with anterior restorations.
10. Describe the duties and responsibilities of the dental assistant while assisting with amalgam and composite posterior restorations.
11. Describe the procedure and techniques for the finishing and polishing of amalgam restorations.
12. Discuss the methods for assisting with the in-office bleaching of teeth.
13. Discuss the methods and procedures necessary for the preparation, demonstration, instruction, and monitoring of home bleaching of teeth.

KEY TERMS

activator	ingested	restorations
amalgam	interproximal	scaling
calcification	inversion	sealant
calculus	irreversible	sulcus
cariogenic	isolation	symmetry
cavitation	modification	systemic
composite	multitufted	temporo-
embrasure	palpation	mandibular
evacuate	preliminary	joint (TMJ)
fluoride	prophylaxis	topical
holistic	reproduction	ultrasonic
increment		

THE PRELIMINARY EXAMINATION

The **preliminary** examination is one of the most important appointments in the dental office. It is through this visit that the future tone and treatment is set. The relationship of the patient and the office personnel may be determined early in the examination. The future treatment plan is built on the facts and data obtained through this visit.

The patient is scheduled to arrive 15 to 30 minutes earlier than the expected time of treatment. This period allows for time to gather necessary information and to complete a thorough health history.

The assistant helps during the preliminary examination, welcoming and seating the new patient. The patient's health history is reviewed and the assistant gives an explanation of the planned future treatment, thereby eliminating much anxiety and nervousness that may be associated with a visit to the dentist. Returning patients are warmly remembered and an update of their physical and dental health is taken and recorded.

Throughout the appointment, the assistant aids the dentist in gathering the data necessary for planning what treatment is needed. Efficient and troublefree procedures give the patient a sense of assurance in the office and the dentist's skills.

PROCEDURE 19

Assisting with the Preliminary Examination

1 Complete the Preparations

2 Complete the Health History

3 Complete Vital Signs

4 Don PPE

5 Record Physical Exam Findings

6 Assist with Oral Tissue Examination

7 Record Findings of Neck and TMJ Examination

8 Assist with Oral Exam and Charting of Teeth

9 Complete Exam as Requested by Dentist

10 Cleanup Procedures

1 Complete the Preparations

The equipment needed for a preliminary exam follows:

▶ basic setup
▶ forms, records, and charting pens
▶ periodontal probe
▶ dental floss
▶ vital signs equipment
▶ impression equipment
▶ radiograph equipment
▶ miscellaneous equipment as needed

The assistant greets the new patient and escorts him or her to the operatory area. The rest room location and a quick walking tour may also be given to acquaint the patient to the facility. The patient is seated and made comfortable in the dental chair. The operatory preparations are completed.

2 Complete the Health History

The examination begins with a thorough health history. Most offices have the new patient fill out a health history questionnaire at the time of registration in the office, but the assistant must review the form with the patient to be sure the patient understands the questions and answers them fully. Particular attention is given to current treatment, allergies, and any medications or prescriptions the patient may be taking. The assistant should maintain an interested attitude throughout the history (Figure 6–1).

3 Complete Vital Signs

Many offices will have the trained assistant take and record the patient's blood pressure and any other vital signs the doctor sees as necessary. This procedure is performed to help detect hidden health problems and many times identifies high blood pressure patients who seldom or irregularly see a medical doctor but visit a dentist more frequently.

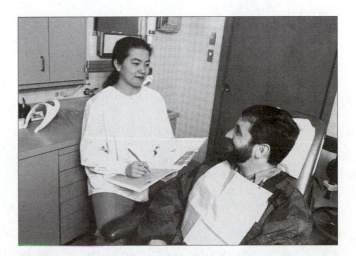

FIGURE 6–1 The assistant provides privacy and expresses a genuine interest while reviewing the health history.

4 Don PPE

When the interview and health history are completed, the assistant summons the dentist and reviews the findings. The assistant then dons the PPE and takes position on the assistant's stool.

5 Record Physical Exam Findings

The assistant records any findings that the dentist may dictate during the physical exam. The dentist starts the exam with an appraisal of the patient's general health. The dentist views the outward signs, such as condition of eyes, fingernails, and skin texture. The face is appraised for **symmetry** and any growths or eruptions. The lips are examined for any cracking or blisters, which may indicate vitamin deficiency or herpes infection. Mouth odor may indicate poor hygiene or diabetes.

6 Assist with Oral Tissue Examination

The dentist examines the tissues of the oral cavity before progressing to the teeth. Dentures and removable appliances are checked while in position and then removed to determine the tissue condition of the affected area. The lips are extended and raised to view the frenum and contour. The tongue is raised to examine the floor of the mouth and the sides of the tongue. The dentist may require a gauze pad to hold onto the slippery organ. **Palpations** of the cheek and mucobuccal folds will be taken as well in the hard and soft palate and throat area. Attention is given to the salivary glands.

7 Record Findings of Neck and TMJ Examination

The dentist checks the outside of the face and neck as well. Palpations under the chin and down the neck are taken to check the lymph glands and nodes. The **temporomandibular joint (TMJ)** is tested by observing the patient close down and open up. A stethoscope may be used to listen for irregularity in the TMJ function.

8 Assist with Oral Exam and Charting of Teeth

When the dentist is satisfied that all conditions regarding the tissues and outward areas of the oral cavity have been noted and recorded, the dentist may request a mouth mirror to begin an examination of the teeth and gingiva. Charting of each tooth and surrounding tissues can be completed using teamwork and an understanding of the charting codes.

Throughout the clinical exam, the dentist may request an exchange of mirror, explorer, and periodontal probe. Dictated findings should be recorded neatly and legibly by the assistant. The assistant may be asked to either pass or use the triple syringe to spray and dry a particular area. The dentist may wish a specific tooth section dried to avoid a water reflection obstructing the view of the tooth surface.

The assistant may also be requested to pass dental floss for the dentist to check **interproximal** areas for decay and overhanging restorations.

9 Complete Exam as Requested by Dentist

At the completion of the health history and the physical and clinical exam, the dentist may order the assistant to complete or assist with taking alginate impressions for study casts, radiographs, photos, pulp vitality testing, and whatever seems necessary for a complete and thorough exam. Each procedure is recorded on the patient's chart.

10 Cleanup Procedures

When the examination has been completed, the assistant removes the contaminated equipment from the operatory to the sterilizing room. The exam gloves are removed, hands are washed, and all procedures previously completed are noted on the patient's chart, which is returned to the front desk.

The assistant dons utility gloves, flushes and deodorizes lines, disinfects the operatory area, cleans and disinfects or sterilizes all equipment, and cleans up the sterilizing area. The gloves are washed, dried, disinfected, and removed. The hands are washed.▲

THEORY RECALL

The Preliminary Examination

1. Why is the first dental examination so important?

   _____

2. What type of equipment will the assistant need to set up for a preliminary examination?

   _____

3. How may the assistant acquaint the new patient with the facility?

   _____

4. The dental examination begins with what procedure?

   _____

5. Why is the patient's blood pressure taken in the dental office?

   _____

6. What are the assistant's duties during the physical examination of a patient?

_____

7. What may an offensive mouth odor represent?

_____

8. What does the dentist check under the chin and down the neck?

_____

9. What instruments may the dentist request during the examination of the teeth?

_____

10. Why may the assistant pass or use the air syringe to dry the mouth?

_____

Now turn to the Competency Evaluation Sheet for Procedure 19, Assisting with the Preliminary Examination, located in Appendix C of this text.

ALGINATE IMPRESSIONS

Many times in a preliminary examination, a dentist requires an alginate impression to be taken. Alginate is a colloid material, originally taken from seaweed. When mixed with water, the alginate forms a gel, which will solidify, much like making instant, no cook pudding.

There are two kinds of alginate impression materials—**irreversible** and reversible. If the material is made into gel using heat, then cooled into a set state, and then can be reheated to gel again, it is considered reversible. If the material is turned into gel state by the addition of liquids and then sets up and cannot be used again, it is said to be irreversible. The most popular type of impression material used for study models in the dental office is irreversible alginate.

Alginate impression material may be purchased in individual packets or in a bulk can. It comes in different setting times—regular and fast set. Alginate may be flavored and either regular or heavy bodied. Some alginates have an antimicrobial agent added to reduce microorganisms present in the impression. The assistant should always read the manufacturer's directions when using alginate and follow the prescribed dosages and mixing techniques.

An impression is a negative **reproduction** of a person's dentition. What is a cusp or bump on a tooth becomes a dent in the impression material. These dents are filled with a wet gypsum substance, which hardens and makes a positive reproduction of the patient's teeth. Therefore, after the impressions are taken, poured up, and trimmed, the dentist has an exact physical reproduction of the patient's mouth to study and work on.

PROCEDURE 20

Assisting with Alginate Impressions

1	Complete the Preparations
2	Prepare the Trays
3	Mix the Alginate
4	Load the Mandibular Tray
5	Assist with the Insertion and Removal of the Impression Tray
6	Freshen the Patient's Mouth
7	Mix the Second Alginate Impression Material
8	Load the Maxillary Tray
9	Assist with the Insertion and Removal of the Impression Tray
10	Freshen the Patient's Mouth
11	Assist with Bite Registration
12	Dismiss the Patient
13	Prepare the Impressions
14	Cleanup Procedures

1 Complete the Preparations

Assemble materials and equipment. The materials and equipment needed for alginate impressions of the mouth follow:

▶ basic setup
▶ alginate impression material and measuring devices
▶ two flexibowls (one for each arch)
▶ two spatulas (wide blade)
▶ assortment of trays (adhesive if using disposable)
▶ beading wax
▶ baseplate wax or bowl of hot and bowl of cool water (for bite registration)
▶ disinfectant spray and paper towels
▶ plastic bag (for completed impressions)
▶ plastic drape, swipes, and basin for patient

The patient is covered with a large plastic drape to protect the clothing from drips of impression material and also as a precaution against any accidents caused from a severe gagging reaction. The patient is offered tissue swipes to use as napkins and a basin is placed nearby.

The assistant dons PPE, if not already on. When gathering and preparing, the assistant uses overgloves to prevent contamination in the operatory area.

The patient is prepared for the procedure by explaining to them what is to be done. Any mouth appliances, such as removable bridgework, are removed and the patient's mouth is rinsed, either by a spray or by offering a mouthwash to use. A light coat of petroleum jelly may be applied to the patient's lips to prevent cracking from the stretching movements.

2 Prepare the Trays

The properly sized tray is picked out by testing for size in the patient's mouth. Trays are not inserted straight into the mouth but are placed inside by a rotation movement. The side of the tray is inserted and then the rest of the tray is rounded into the open mouth.

Once in place, the assistant checks that all the teeth are covered by the tray within a 2-mm enclosure. If the tray is too large or too small, the appropriate size is inserted.

Beading wax may be added to assist with the fit and to provide comfort for the patient by covering sharp edges and holding in the alginate material. All trays tested in the patient's mouth are considered contaminated and must be sterilized, even if they were not used for the procedure.

If a disposable plastic tray is used instead of the metal perforated tray, the assistant must paint or spray on an adhesive material to ensure that the alginate remains in the tray throughout the impression procedure (Figure 6–2).

3 Mix the Alginate

If the bulk can of alginate is used instead of the individual package, the can is shaken to mix all the powder material, which may have settled during storage. The top of the can is slowly and carefully removed to prevent alginate powder from puffing out.

The prescribed amount of scoops of alginate are taken from the can. Most manufacturers indicate on the can or envelope how much alginate is needed for a full arch or partial impression. The scoops are leveled off for an accurate amount. Water at room temperature or slightly cooler is placed into the measuring device supplied by the manufacturer. The assistant fills the vial to the prescribed line according to the amount of scoops used and the manufacturer's recommendation.

The water is added to the alginate and the assistant mixes the two together. When the powder particles are wet, the assistant blends them into a creamy, smooth mixture by stirring and pressing the mixture against the side of the bowl. The assistant also moves the bowl around in the hands to offer a more thorough mixture (Figure 6–3).

4 Load the Mandibular Tray

There is no rule regarding which tray is used first. The assistant may choose to do the mandibular first because there is less of a gagging reflex present. While the maxillary impression is setting up, the assistant may permit the patient to hold the tray until the setting reaction is completed. While the patient is holding the tray, the assistant may use the remaining alginate to fill in the tongue space of the mandibular tray. If the assistant feels the patient is unable to hold the tray in a secure manner, the assistant may hold the tray stationary until the final set and at a later time make up a tongue spacer for the mandibular tray.

All trays are loaded from the posterior edge and are filled in more than one **increment** to avoid air bubbles. The alginate is carried to the tray on the blade of

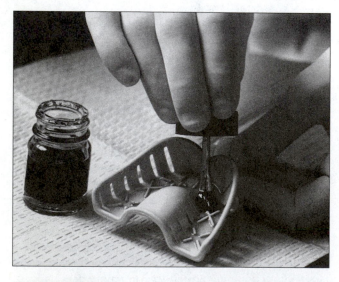

FIGURE 6–2 Adhesive is sprayed or painted on the plastic tray to help retain the alginate material.

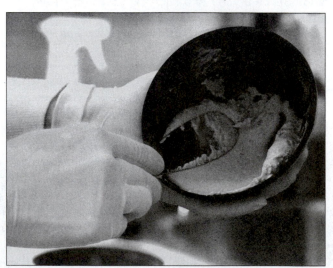

FIGURE 6–3 After moistening the alginate powder, the assistant finishes the mixing by pressing the material against the side of the bowl, which is rotated with the other hand.

the spatula and then scraped off into the tray, which is filled only to the top. The assistant then uses a wet finger to smooth off the top of the alginate, and removes overhanging alginate from the side.

5 Assist With the Insertion and Removal of the Impression Tray

The filled tray is placed into the mouth in a rotating motion. The side of the tray is inserted and the tray is revolved around until it is completely in the mouth (Figure 6–4).

The assistant moves the tray over the teeth, making sure not to touch the teeth until in position. After the tray is centered over the teeth, the assistant seats the tray by pressing the tray onto the teeth from the posterior to the anterior region, forcing the air out in front of the tray (Figure 6–5). Once the tray is centered on the teeth, the assistant inserts a finger into the vestibule of the mouth and circulates around, releasing any trapped tissue or turned in lip. The patient is requested to raise the tongue to seat the lingual side of the tray when the lower impression is taken.

The patient is monitored at all times. The assistant watches for any gagging reflex or choking pattern. If a patient is having difficulty breathing, the assistant encourages the patient to bend over and take short breaths.

A finger is reinserted to press and contour the alginate around the edges of the tray and to feel if the material has set up. The assistant may test the alginate remaining in the bowl to determine if the material has set but must remember that the mouth is warmer and sets up faster than the bowl.

Once the alginate has set, the assistant breaks the suction hold on the tray by gently twisting on the handle of the tray. If the suction remains, the assistant in-

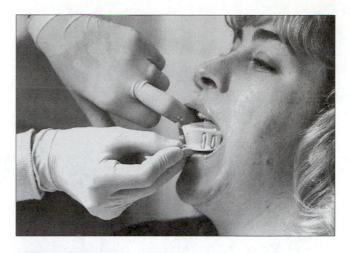

FIGURE 6–5 When the tray has been inserted into the mouth, it is centered over or under the chewing surfaces and then "seated" by pressing from the rear to the front.

serts a finger into the vestibule and under the edge of the tray in a pinching motion with the handle to get a final release of suction (Figure 6–6). The assistant will hear and feel the suction give way and then slowly and gently rotate the tray out of the mouth. The impression is rinsed under tap water, sprayed with disinfectant, and wrapped in a paper towel that has been moistened with disinfectant (Figure 6–7).

6 Freshen the Patient's Mouth

The patient is cleaned up by wiping off the face and either spraying the mouth with the water syringe or offering the patient some mouthwash for rinsing. Once the mouth is freshened, the assistant compliments the patient and explains the next impression step.

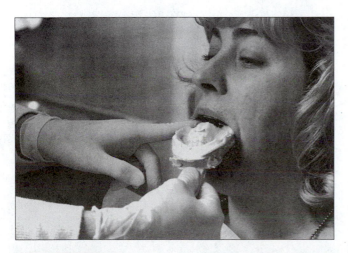

FIGURE 6–4 The impression tray is inserted into the mouth by rotating the tray into the opening.

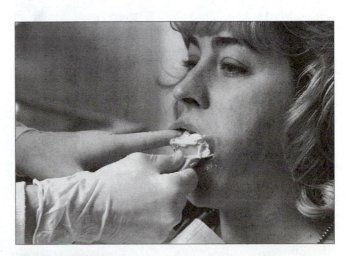

FIGURE 6–6 To release the tray suction, the assistant inserts a finger along the tray edge and twists the tray away from the tissues.

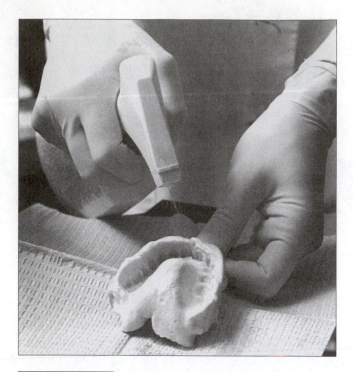

FIGURE 6-7 The impression is removed from the mouth, rinsed under tap water, and sprayed with a disinfectant before placing it in the bag.

7 Mix the Second Alginate Impression Material

A second batch of alginate is mixed using a new bowl and spatula. The amount of powder and water is determined from the manufacturer's recommendation. The measuring and mixing procedure is the same as for the first mix.

8 Load the Maxillary Tray

The other tray is filled from the posterior area and in more than one increment. The spatula brings the alginate to the tray and fills it to the top. The assistant smooths off the top of the alginate with a wet finger and wipes off the overhanging alginate from the sides of the tray.

9 Assist with the Insertion and Removal of the Impression Tray

The tray is inserted into the patient's mouth in a rotating motion. Once inside, the tray is centered under the teeth edges and then pressed up onto the tooth surfaces from the posterior area to the anterior area. The assistant inserts a finger and frees any trapped tissue or lip and monitors the patient for gagging and coughing.

The material is allowed to set while the tray is held stationary in the mouth. The assistant inserts a finger to pressure contour the alginate around the edges until the alginate has set. The release, removal, rinse, and wrap are the same in this arch as in the other.

10 Freshen the Patient's Mouth

The patient is cleaned up in the same manner as the first impression. The patient is complimented and the bite registration procedure is explained.

11 Assist with Bite Registration

The doubled sheet of baseplate wax is removed from the hot water and placed into the mouth. The assistant makes sure the occlusal area of the premolars and first molars are covered and asks the patient to bite down. The assistant contours the wax around the teeth and then asks the patient to release and open. The wax bite registration is removed and placed in cold water to set up. This wax bite form will be used later in the trimming of the gypsum models that are made when the impressions are poured up in plaster or stone material.

Another method to obtain a registration of the bite is by using a syringe apparatus that may express a silicone mass. The material is squeezed directly onto the occlusal surface of the lower teeth or into the interproximal spaces of the closed jaw. After the setting is complete (approximately two minutes), the transparent silicone bite register is kept with the impressions and used in the trimming and articulation processes.

12 Dismiss the Patient

The patient is cleaned up. All impression material is washed off the face. The mouth is refreshened and the drape is removed. The patient is dismissed if no other procedure or treatment is to be performed.

13 Prepare the Impressions

The wrapped impressions are unwrapped and resprayed with disinfectant. The assistant inserts a finger or instrument handle into a plastic bag, without touching the bag, and makes an opening for the insertion of the sprayed impressions and bite registration, which has been spray disinfected (Figure 6–8). The finger or handle is removed and the assistant does not close the bag until after hands are washed and the case is sealed for the laboratory.

14 Cleanup Procedures

The assistant cleans up the operatory and removes disposables and contaminated materials to the sterilizing room. The latex gloves are removed, and the assistant washes hands.

When the hands are clean, the assistant returns to the operatory, records treatment on the patient's chart

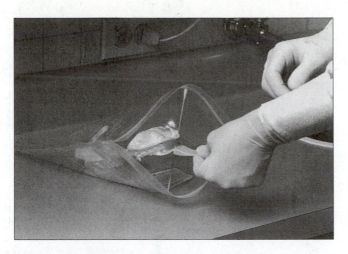

FIGURE 6-8 The impressions and bite registration are carefully placed into the propped-open plastic bag. After the gloves are removed, the bag is closed by touching the outside only.

and takes it to the desk or appropriate place. The bag of impressions and bite registration is closed from the outside and taken to the lab for further work.

The assistant returns to the sterilizing area, dons utility gloves and PPE, and returns to the operatory to disinfect all equipment. In the sterilizing room, the instruments and materials are disinfected, washed, and prepared for sterilizing. The utility gloves are washed, dried, and disinfected. The assistant washes hands.▲

T H E O R Y   R E C A L L

Alginate Impressions

1. What is alginate material that turns from a gel to a solid state and cannot be returned to a gel state called?

2. Why is an impression considered a negative reproduction?

3. If the assistant already is wearing PPE and needs to gather material for impression taking, what does the assistant do?

4. How is the patient prepared for taking an impression?

5. What must be done to a disposable tray before placing alginate material?

6. Why is the alginate placed on the tray in more than one increment?

7. If a patient is having trouble breathing during an impression taking, what may the assistant suggest?

8. What does the assistant do with the impression and tray after it is removed from the mouth?

9. What tooth surface must the assistant be sure to include in a bite registration?

10. What does the assistant do to the impressions before bagging them?

Now turn to the Competency Evaluation Sheet for Procedure 20, Assisting with Alginate Impressions, located in Appendix C of this text.

DENTAL PROPHYLAXIS

The dental prophylaxis appointment is the backbone of the dental practice. Prophylaxis, the **scaling** and polishing of the teeth, and the ensuing examination are performed on all new patients and periodically on the regular patients. It is this appointment that not only determines the future treatment necessary but also establishes the complexion of the relationship between the patient and the staff.

During the dental prophylaxis, the dental assistant may assist the dentist or dental hygienist in many ways. The first type of assistance given is in the preparation for the appointment. The assistant dons the heavy utility gloves to make everything ready.

The dental operatory is disinfected and prepared. The assistant cleans, with a spray-wipe-spray method, all surfaces and items too large to be sterilized. Protective barrier shields are placed on the equipment (chairs, handles, syringe tubing, x-ray, and any other item desired). The utility gloves are washed, disinfected, and removed. The hands are washed, and the assistant assembles the necessary items.

The assistant may greet and seat the patient, review the health history, and generally prepare the patient for the procedure. Throughout the treatment, the assistant may aid the operator by passing instruments, rinsing and evacuating the mouth, and recording charting notes. Home-care instructions may be given by the assistant.

PROCEDURE 21

Assisting with Dental Prophylaxis

1 Complete the Preparations

2 Assist with Mouth Rinse and Evacuation

3 Assist with Scaling of Teeth

4 Assist with Polishing of Teeth

5 Assist with Flossing of Teeth

6 Assist with Charting, Notations, and Instructions

7 Dismiss the Patient

8 Cleanup Procedures

1 Complete the Preparations

The setup needed for a dental **prophylaxis** follows:

▶ disposable items—swipes, drinking cup, gauze sponges, cotton rolls, bib, saliva ejector tip, and HVE tip and handle
▶ basic instruments—mouth mirror, explorer, and pick ups
▶ dappen dish with wetting solution
▶ hand and **ultrasonic** scalers (if used)
▶ prophy angle, handpiece, prophy cup, and brushes
▶ prophylaxis polish, premeasured or individual cup
▶ prophy tip (air polisher, if used)
▶ dental floss and aids
▶ hand mirror
▶ pen and marker for patient's chart

The patient's chart and records are gathered. The latest x-rays are placed on the viewer. All items are cleaned up, and a final evaluation of the cleanliness and preparations are taken.

The patient is brought into the operatory and comfortably seated in a reclined position. A drape and bib are placed on the patient's neck. The patient is offered a swipe and the sundry items are placed out in full view. The patient is warned of any movement as the chair and light are moved into operative position. The patient's health history is reviewed for any health hazards or possible cautions to be taken.

The assistant washes hands and dons the mask, eyeglasses or shield, and latex exam gloves, summons the dentist, and sits on the assistant's stool.

2 Assist with Mouth Rinse and Evacuation

The dental assistant may rinse the patient's mouth of debris and **evacuate** the moisture practically at the same time. When the mouth has been rinsed, the prophylaxis begins.

3 Assist with Scaling of Teeth

Scaling or removal of tartar and **calculus** buildup is the first procedure aspect. The assistant passes a mirror and a scaler of choice to the operator. With teamwork and observation, the assistant will become familiar with the routine and be prepared to anticipate the next item. See Figure 6–9 for a sample of scaling instruments.

The assistant passes and receives instruments intermittently as called for or signaled. It may be helpful for the assistant to hold a piece of gauze near the operative site where the operator may clean off the instrument of use. Occasionally, there may be a need for rinsing and evacuation of the mouth throughout the scaling process. This function may be performed by the assistant, or the syringe may be passed to the operator for use.

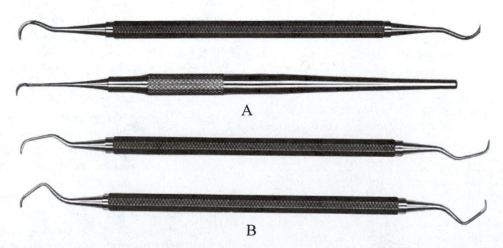

A

B

FIGURE 6–9 (A) Scalers and (B) curettes are used to remove hard deposits from the teeth. These instruments must be kept sharp to be effective. (Courtesy of Hu-Friedy.)

Some operators may choose to use ultrasonic scalers instead of, or along with, the hand instruments. The ultrasonic scalers work on the same principle as the ultrasonic instrument cleaner. The **cavitation** caused by the sonic waves breaks up and removes stain and calculus buildup. The ultrasonic tip is inserted into the handle, which holds water (Figure 6–10). When the machine is activated, the water in the handle causes the bands of the tip to vibrate the tip in microscopic movements, removing teeth accumulations. The rapid vibrations of the tip need to be cooled so a fine stream of water is jetted onto the tip. This machine needs to be "tuned" before use, which is merely an adjustment of the power vibration and the flow of water onto the tip. The dials are turned until a fine spray mist hits the ultrasonic tip and a hum is heard.

Operators who choose to use these tips feel there is less tension, noise, and irritation than with the hand scaling, making it more comfortable for the patient. Because of the water flow need for cooling, there is more moisture to be removed through evacuation by the assistant.

When the teeth have been scaled (scraped clean of hard materials and stain), they are rinsed. The mouth is evacuated and air dried with the triple syringe. This procedure may be performed by the assistant.

4 Assist with Polishing of Teeth

Polishing of the teeth is the next step in the prophylaxis appointment. Prophylaxis paste is put into a small paste cup or an individual cup of paste is opened and the operator scoops a small amount of the paste into the rubber cup or small brush on the prophylaxis angle. Prophylaxis paste comes in bulk jar sizes or in small individual cups. It may come in assorted flavors and grits, fluoridated or nonfluoridated. This paste contains pumice, which is a gritty, abrasive powder that helps remove stains and material from the crowns of the teeth. The operator selects the prophylaxis paste of choice for the appointment.

The operator, who has scaled the teeth with the ultrasonic tip, now polishes the patient's teeth using a polishing tip. This insert is placed into the handle, which has been emptied of the ultrasonic tip. When engaged, the new insert forces a fine abrasive mixture of soda and water through the tip. This forced powder stream cleans the tooth surface and removes stain without the sound or tension of the handpiece rotation. Many patients enjoy this method but some dislike the aftertaste and feel of gritty powder. The sand polisher does not need to be "tuned" but may need a small adjustment of powder flow regulation.

When the operator finishes polishing the teeth, the assistant passes or uses the syringe to rinse the patient's mouth of polish and saliva.

5 Assist with Flossing of Teeth

Once the teeth have been scaled and polished, the operator passes dental floss through the teeth and around any permanent appliances. The assistant may pass the floss to the operator. Bridge cleaners, flossing aids to insert floss under and around fixed appliances, and stimulators for pocket areas may be called upon by the operator, and the assistant passes them as needed or signaled.

6 Assist with Charting, Notations, and Instructions

At this point the operator may perform other examination or charting procedures or may release the care of the patient to the assistant, who cleans up the patient and gives home-care instructions. The assistant demonstrates and instructs the patient with the proper method of brushing and flossing the teeth and might discuss diet and nutrition in relation to healthy teeth. This is not an easy procedure and must be done with extreme patience and understanding. The patient must practice the techniques until they have been mastered. If this is a returning patient, the assistant must review the procedure and reevaluate the effectiveness of the patient's habits.

7 Dismiss the Patient

After demonstrating a good command of the brushing and flossing techniques, the patient is excused and given another appointment, if necessary.

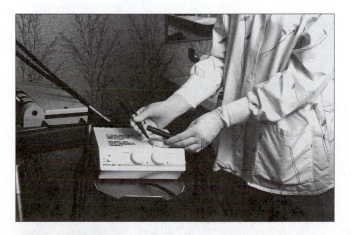

FIGURE 6–10 An ultrasonic unit can remove hard deposits without the trauma, noise, and effort caused by hand instruments. With a change of tips, the machine can polish the tooth surfaces.

8 Cleanup Procedures

The instruments and contaminated items are taken to the sterilizing room where the assistant removes the exam gloves, washes hands, and records the treatment on the patient's chart. The assistant then dons the utility gloves, returns to the operatory, and disinfects the room with the spray-wipe-spray technique. Barriers are replaced as needed, and the room is readied.

The assistant returns to the sterilizing area, disposes of the contaminated articles; cleans, prepares, and disinfects or sterilizes the instruments. The area is cleaned up. The utility gloves are washed, disinfected, and removed. The assistant washes hands.▲

THEORY RECALL
Dental Prophylaxis

1. After the mouth has been rinsed and checked, what is the first procedural aspect of a prophylaxis?

   _____

2. What will help the assistant become familiar with the routine and better be able to anticipate the next item?

   _____

3. When should the assistant pass or receive an instrument?

   _____

4. Why should an assistant hold a piece of gauze near the work site during a prophylaxis appointment?

   _____

5. What principle does the ultrasonic scaler work on as compared with the ultrasonic cleaner?

   _____

6. Why is water jetted onto the tip of the ultrasonic prophylaxis piece?

   _____

7. What do we mean when we say the teeth have been scaled in a prophylaxis appointment?

   _____

8. What procedure follows scaling in a prophylaxis?

   _____

9. Name some of the various differences between different prophylaxis pastes.

   _____

10. What is the next procedure after polishing in a dental prophylaxis?

    _____

Now turn to the Competency Evaluation Sheet for Procedure 21, Assisting with Dental Prophylaxis, located in Appendix C of this text.

TOPICAL FLUORIDE PROTECTION

Many times the dentist recommends a **topical fluoride** treatment after the dental prophylaxis has been completed, particularly if the patient is a child who has developing teeth. Fluoride applied to the teeth to help make the enamel surfaces stronger and more resistant to decay is called topical. **Ingested** fluoride placed in city water supplies or from natural sources is considered **systemic** fluoride. A combination of the two types of fluoride helps reduce decay.

The ideal time to apply fluoride to the crowns of the teeth is when they have just been cleaned of any debris and plaque and polished. The dentist chooses the type of fluoride and either delivers the treatment or assigns it to the hygienist or, in some cases, to the trained dental assistant. In either case, the assistant may be of great assistance in the topical fluoride application.

Topical fluoride may be delivered to the tooth surfaces in four different consistencies—foam, gel, liquid, or paste. It is supplied in many flavors and colors to appeal to children.

Each fluoride has its limitations and restrictions, and the assistant should read the manufacturer's direction regarding storage, active life, preparation, and delivery.

A saliva ejector is placed in the mouth to eliminate moisture, and the medication is applied by either swabbing the crowns of the teeth with the fluoride solution or by placing a tray filled with fluoride gel onto the teeth.

The medication is allowed to remain on the teeth for a prescribed time, usually about four minutes. During this period, the assistant periodically empties the mouth of saliva and moisture by evacuating with the HVE tip. Children are given books to read or look at during this time because engaging in conversation is quite difficult with the mouth so full. The assistant may tell a favorite story or two while waiting for the exposure time. Young children may sit longer when entertained.

When the time has expired, the trays and cotton rolls are removed, and the procedure is carried out in the other arch if a double tray system was not used. When all the crowns of the teeth have received the topical fluoride treatment and the mouth has been emptied, the patient is dismissed. The patient (and the patient's companion) are advised that the patient is not to eat or drink for at least 30 minutes to permit final absorption of the medication.

The treatment is recorded on the patient's chart, and the contaminated materials and equipment are removed to the sterilizing area. The assistant then performs an operatory cleanup to complete the topical fluoride appointment.

There are some topical fluoride rinses developed that are effective to strengthen tooth surfaces and resist decay. These may be prescribed by the dentist to be used in the office setting or by the patient at home. These rinses are always used after the teeth have been cleaned or brushed and flossed.

PROCEDURE 22

Assisting with Topical Fluoride Application

1 Complete the Preparations

2 Assist with the Prophylaxis and Coronal Polish

3 Assist with the Isolation of the Mouth

4 Assist with the Topical Fluoride Application

5 Dismiss the Patient

6 Cleanup Procedures

1 Complete the Preparations

The setup for the topical fluoride treatment follows:

▶ prophylaxis setup
▶ cotton rolls
▶ cotton swabs
▶ topical fluoride treatment medication and appropriate equipment
▶ commercial trays and liners (if needed)
▶ evacuation devices (HVE or saliva ejector tips)

The assistant will be wearing the personal protective equipment of the prophylaxis appointment or will don such wear before assisting with this procedure.

2 Assist with the Prophylaxis and Coronal Polish

The teeth will have been cleaned or the assistant will assist with the cleansing of the tooth surfaces. No matter which form of fluoride is delivered to the site, the area must be precleaned.

3 Assist with the Isolation of the Mouth

The surfaces to receive the fluoride medication must be isolated with cotton rolls. The assistant passes the rolls, which are placed between the teeth and the cheek and tongue. The crowns of the teeth are air dried by the assistant, using the triple syringe warm air spray. A gentle stream of air is passed over the surfaces to remove or dry up any moisture that may in-

terfere with the fluoride absorption. A saliva ejector is placed in the mouth to help relieve the patient's accumulation of saliva and moisture throughout the treatment.

4 Assist with the Topical Fluoride Application

The fluoride is either painted on the surfaces with a wet cotton swab, polished on the surfaces with a rubber cup, or delivered by tray. Fluoride trays are made of a soft material and are supplied in sizes. They may be made for one arch or come in a set, which makes application of the entire mouth in one step (Figure 6–11). Some trays require liners to hold solutions, while others accommodate the gel material without liners. If the tray is used, it is first measured to find the correct size.

Fluoride applied to the teeth is allowed to remain on the teeth for the prescribed time, during which the assistant helps evacuate the mouth. Moisture is removed from the mouth during fluoride treatment so the patient will be comfortable and does not swallow any of the fluoride medication.

After the prescribed time has passed, the mouth is emptied and the procedure is repeated for the other areas of the mouth until all tooth crowns and surfaces have received the topical fluoride medication.

5 Dismiss the Patient

The patient is advised to not eat or drink for 30 minutes to allow the fluoride to be absorbed. The patient is cleaned up and dismissed.

6 Cleanup Procedures

The assistant removes the latex exam gloves, washes hands, records the treatment on the patient's chart,

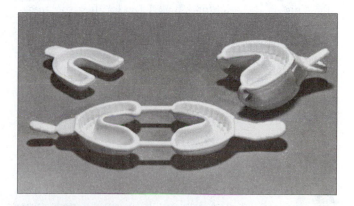

FIGURE 6–11 Fluoride applications can be given in a disposable single or double tray. (Courtesy of Sultan Dental Products.)

and takes the chart to the prescribed place. Utility gloves and equipment are donned. The assistant disinfects the operatory and prepares and sterilizes the equipment. The utility gloves are washed, dried, disinfected, removed, and placed to dry. The hands are washed.▲

► T H E O R Y   R E C A L L

Topical Fluoride Protection

1. What is the purpose of applying fluoride?

    _____

2. What is the difference between topical fluoride and systemic fluoride?

    _____

3. When is the ideal time to apply topical fluoride?

    _____

4. In what forms are topical fluoride treatment medications supplied?

    _____

5. Where can the assistant find information about the use and care of topical fluoride medications?

    _____

6. Why are saliva and moisture removed from the mouth during a topical fluoride application?

    _____

7. Why does the assistant discuss the treatment with the patient prior to performing the application?

    _____

8. Why does the assistant don overgloves when mixing and preparing topical fluoride medicine?

    _____

9. How is the mouth isolated?

    _____

10. What is the patient advised to do after the treatment is finished?

    _____

Now turn to the Competency Evaluation Sheet for Procedure 22, Assisting with Topical Fluoride Application, located in Appendix C of this text.

APPLICATION OF SEALANTS

Another preventive treatment used to preserve and protect children's teeth is the application of sealants. A **sealant** is an epoxy resin type of material that is painted over the cleaned surfaces of a tooth and then allowed to auto-cure or set up by special lights.

There are pros and cons to the use of this material. Some dentists feel that the placing of sealants protects the pits and fissures of developing teeth until **calcification** has fully occurred and the patient has become mature enough to establish a good home cleansing, brushing, and flossing technique. Other dentists dislike the false sense of security that patients get and feel there is too easy a chance for the sealant to wear away or chip off and become more of a detriment than a preservative.

If the dentist decides to place a sealant on a tooth or several teeth, the assistant may be of assistance in this appointment. Many times the sealant is applied immediately after a prophylaxis while the teeth are clean and free of plaque and matter. Sealants are never placed over decayed teeth or on teeth that have just been treated with fluoride; therefore, the prophylaxis paste used to polish the teeth in a prophylaxis must be nonfluoridated if a sealant procedure is to follow.

► P R O C E D U R E   2 3

Assisting with Sealant Application

1 Complete the Preparations

2 Assist with Coronal Polish

3 Assist with Isolation of the Teeth

4 Assist with Acid-Etching of the Teeth

5 Assist with Rinsing and Repacking

6 Assist with Sealant Placement

7 Assist with Examination of Sealant

8 Assist with Finishing of Sealant

9 Dismiss the Patient

10 Cleanup Procedures

1 Complete the Preparations

The setup for a sealant appointment (if completed with a prophylaxis) follows:

► **isolation** material, either dental dam or cotton rolls
► etching material with dappen dish and applicator
► sealant material and equipment
► curing lamp (if needed)
► explorer
► finishing burs and handpiece
► articulating paper

If the assistant is wearing personal protective equipment during the prophylaxis appointment, the clinical attire is the same. If not, PPE is donned after the materials and equipment have been gathered and placed in the disinfected operatory.

2 Assist with Coronal Polish

The teeth to receive the sealant material are thoroughly cleaned. If the patient has just received a prophylaxis, the sealant is applied. If not, the assistant helps with the cleaning of the selected teeth.

The assistant dons overgloves to prepare and measure out the sealant materials and equipment so that the supply bottles are not contaminated. After all materials are on the tray and ready to use, the assistant may remove the overgloves and proceed with the sealant duties.

3 Assist with Isolation of the Teeth

The patient's clean tooth or selected teeth are isolated. This may be accomplished by placing a dental dam or by packing cotton rolls around the area receiving the sealant. The selected tooth is then air dried with a gentle spray from the triple syringe. All moisture is removed before the etching process.

4 Assist with Acid-Etching of the Teeth

The assistant passes an applicator or brush containing acid-etch solution which is painted on the occlusal surface of the tooth. The acid is permitted to remain on the surface for the manufacturer's recommended time period, usually about one minute.

5 Assist with Rinsing and Repacking

At the end of this period, the tooth is spray bathed with the water from the syringe and the mouth is emptied of cotton rolls. The acid-etched tooth should have a dull, whitish look; if this condition is not present, the tooth is repacked with cotton rolls and re-etched. Once the tooth shows evidence of an etched condition, the dentist repacks the area with cotton rolls or dries the dental dam and applies the sealant. Cotton rolls should be replaced by positioning the new dry rolls over the used wet rolls and removing the older ones from the bottom. In this manner, no saliva or debris comes into contact with the etched surface, and the sealant adheres better.

6 Assist with Sealant Placement

The assistant passes the sealant material to the dentist. The choice of the type of sealant is the dentist's responsibility, but the assistant must read the manufacturer's direction to become familiar with its properties and use.

Sealants are either self-curing or need a visible white light to complete the chemical conditioning to get hard. If the dentist wishes to use a self-cure material, the assistant mixes two pastes together and passes the mixture to the dentist on an applicator. The assistant then holds the remaining mixture near the work site for the dentist to obtain as needed. After a period of time, the mixed resin gets hard.

Another type of sealant requires the presence of a curing lamp to set up. The sealant material is placed on the clean, nondecayed, isolated tooth. The assistant places the lamp tip near the site and exposes it for the manufacturer's recommended time, usually a few seconds. Excessive use of this lamp may cause eye problems. It is wise for the operator and the assistant to wear tinted glasses during this procedure or to hold a special light-curing shield between the source of light and the eyes. The patient may be supplied safety eyeglasses and recommended to close the eyes also.

7 Assist with Examination of Sealant

After the prescribed time has passed, the dentist checks the effectiveness of the sealant with an explorer (Figure 6–12). If the process was successful, the finishing process begins. If not, the procedure is repeated until done correctly. The isolation is removed from the tooth, and the assistant lightly rinses the mouth.

8 Assist with Finishing of Sealant

The assistant hands the dentist a handpiece containing a small round abrasive finishing bur, which is used to remove any overfilled areas. Articulating paper may be placed for the patient to bite to check the occlusion,

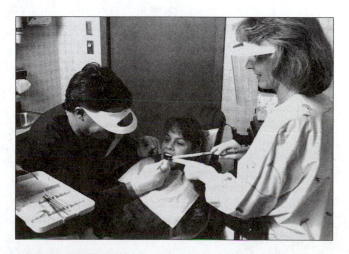

FIGURE 6–12 By testing the surface of the tooth with an explorer, the dentist can determine if the sealant covers all areas for protection.

and finishing is repeated until the tooth is properly finished.

9 Dismiss the Patient

The patient is cleaned up. The bib is removed, and the chair is lowered after cautioning the patient about the movement. Personal property items are returned. The patient is dismissed.

10 Cleanup Procedures

The contaminated materials are taken to the sterilizing room. The exam gloves are removed and the hands are washed. The treatment procedure is recorded on the patient's chart, and the chart is taken to the desk.

The utility gloves are donned. Sterilization is completed and the area is cleaned up. The gloves are washed, disinfected, and removed. The assistant washes hands.▲

THEORY RECALL
Application of Sealants

1. What is a sealant?

_____

2. What is an advantage to placing a sealant? a disadvantage?

_____

3. What type of prophylaxis paste is used if a sealant procedure is to follow?

_____

4. How is the tooth isolated for the sealant procedure?

_____

5. How long is the acid permitted to remain on the tooth receiving the sealant?

_____

6. What color does the acid-etched tooth display after etching?

_____

7. What are the two types of sealants?

_____

8. How does the dentist check for a successful sealant product?

_____

9. When is the isolation removed from the sealant application site?

_____

10. What does the dentist use to finish the sealant?

_____

Now turn to the Competency Evaluation Sheet for Procedure 23, Assisting with Sealant Application, located in Appendix C of this text.

BRUSHING AND FLOSSING TECHNIQUES INSTRUCTION

After the operator has finished the prophylaxis, the assistant may continue with the appointment. One of the duties a dental assistant may perform in a prophylaxis appointment is instructing the patient in home care. Teaching the correct method of brushing and flossing is easier to do when the patient understands why proper home cleansing is important. When the patient learns that home care can eliminate dental decay and periodontal problems, they will perform this task more readily.

PROCEDURE 24
Brushing and Flossing Techniques Instruction

1 Complete the Preparations
2 Explain Plaque Buildup
3 Demonstrate the Patient's Plaque
4 Demonstrate Brushing Technique
5 Demonstrate Flossing Technique
6 Demonstrate Use of Interproximal Stimulators and Aids
7 Review all Techniques
8 Dismiss the Patient
9 Cleanup Procedures

1 Complete the Preparations

Brushing and flossing instruction may be given while the patient is seated in the dental chair or may take place in a specially designed room for patient education.

The assistant will need the following items for instruction:

▶ typodont, brush, and floss
▶ interdental aid, stimulators
▶ dentifrice
▶ hand mirror
▶ disclosing tablets or solution, tissues
▶ video aids, chalkboard, and chalk

2 Explain Plaque Buildup

The dental assistant begins instruction by explaining that plaque, an invisible thin coating, adheres to the teeth. This film contains protein matter and bacteria, which live off the sugars and debris of the mouth. As the bacteria feed, they give off an acid that attacks the surface of the teeth, causing tooth decay. The dental assistant also explains that dental plaque can, if permitted to remain on the teeth, absorb calcium salts from saliva or mouth fluids and turn from a soft mass into a hard substance, which irritates the periodontal tissues. If this hard substance (calculus) remains and grows in size, it will irritate the soft, swollen tissues of the mouth and place pressure on the bones holding the teeth. Pressure destroys bone, and soon the teeth become loose. Periodontal pockets will form. Halitosis (bad breath) develops, and eventually tooth loss occurs.

3 Demonstrate the Patient's Plaque

One way to demonstrate the presence of plaque is to apply a disclosing solution to the teeth. This procedure will not be effective immediately following a prophylaxis because the teeth are clean. It is better to be done and observed when the patient first arrives.

Disclosing solutions vary in type and form. The most common is the red dye disclosing material, which can be supplied in tablet or solution form. Patients chew on a tablet or a few drops of solution are dripped into the mouth. The plaque is stained and becomes visible as a dark red mass. Some soft tissues of the mouth are also colored, but this redness washes away in a short period of time.

Another disclosing agent is a fluorescent solution that is dripped in the mouth. It shows a yellow plaque accumulation when the patient holds a special light, similiar to a black light, to the mouth for viewing. There is no noticeable staining of soft tissues with this solution.

Some dental offices combine disclosing solutions, such as a blue dye and a red dye, showing harder, old accumulations and newer, soft masses. In any case, dyes are a very effective tool to encourage patient participation in a home-care project.

4 Demonstrate Brushing Technique

The choice of a toothbrush is the next item of discussion in a home-care demonstration. There are many kinds and styles of toothbrushes, with newer types coming on the market every day. The handles of the brush are usually made of plastic, while the bristles can be of a natural boar hair material or of a synthetic type. The bristles may be rigid to soft, **multitufted** or single groups of tufts, or cut straight or wavy crested. The dentist will select the type of brush that the patient will need, or the office will have a supply of the kind that is preferred in that practice. Many dentists prefer the softer, multitufted, straight-edged type; but the main concern is to have a brush that the patient is able to handle and will feel comfortable using.

There are some fine electric toothbrushing machines on the market. Some are bristled, and some are cupped. A few brush in an up and down motion, others rotate with single or double heads. A dentist may prefer one brand or type over another and may recommend such a machine for a patient. Using the electric machine takes practice as much as the hand-held, regular toothbrush. In fact, the patient must learn to work with the moving force of the bristles and circulate the head of the machine around the mouth to cleanse all surfaces. Again, the importance is to get the surfaces of the teeth clean, with whatever appliance the patient prefers to use. All toothbrushes or toothbrush heads must be discarded and changed when they become worn.

Toothpaste is another dental product chosen by an individual's preference. There are many fine kinds of toothpaste. Most contain fluoride, which has been proven to help retard decay. They all contain some abrasive, detergent, and flavoring ingredients. Some toothpastes contain properties that lessen sensitivity to temperature changes, lighten teeth, or remove smokers' tartar. They are supplied in pumps, tubes, powders, and drops—whatever mechanism entices people to buy and use them. The dentist selects the type of toothpaste or dentifrice the patient should use and the assistant instructs in the brushing technique.

There is no one correct way to brush the teeth. Many techniques have been developed but no method is effective unless it is one that the patient understands and feels comfortable with. The main priority is to encourage the patient to establish a routine where all the surfaces of the teeth are cleaned each and every brush time. The dental assistant may demonstrate or suggest a method.

One popular way to clean the teeth with a brush is to **sulcus** brush, which is done by placing the toothbrush at a 45 degree angle to the sulcus (gingival attachment area), wiggling, and then brushing away from the sulcus (Figure 6–13A). A routine pattern is established in which the patient begins at one part of the mouth (usually the maxillary molar) and brushes, then moves along repeating the process in each new section, rotating around the teeth, both maxillary and mandibular (Figures 6–13B and C). When moving through the anterior region, the brush may be tilted vertically to accommodate the smaller areas and the curve of the jaw, (Figure 6–13D). This is especially true of the mandibular area, which is small and curved. The brushing process is repeated on the inside of the teeth (lingual) and then the chewing surfaces are brushed in a circular motion to clean the pits and fissures of the occlusal chewing surfaces (Figure 6–13E). The last step demonstrated is a gentle brushing of the tongue. This area is cleansed to remove bacteria and help restore cleanliness to the entire mouth.

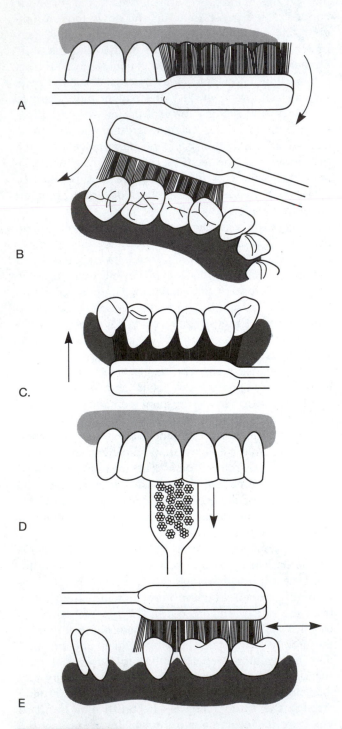

A

B

C.

D

E

FIGURE 6–13 The brush is wiggled into the sulcus area and then brushed away from the gingiva.

After demonstrating the procedure, the dental assistant asks the patient to perform the technique. The assistant may don overgloves or exam gloves and assist with in-mouth instruction. The patient's method must be evaluated for cleansing of all surfaces and for a pattern establishment. If the patient finds this method difficult but can demonstrate an effective one that does the cleaning job, the assistant should encourage this technique. The important factor is that the patient is getting the teeth clean. Patience and understanding is needed when teaching this skill. Not all patients learn easily and not all people have the same dexterity the assistant may have. Even when the patient has learned a correct method to brush the teeth, there may be a need for reinforcement at times. Reevaluation should occur periodically or if there is an obvious lack of hygiene. Patients may monitor their progress at home by using disclosing solutions to find any areas missed by brushing and then adjusting their method to correct this site.

5 Demonstrate Flossing Technique

Flossing the teeth removes debris and plaque from the surfaces between the teeth. Floss may be purchased in either waxed or unwaxed condition. Many dentists prefer the unwaxed because no residue is left behind in the interproximal (between the teeth) surfaces when flossing has been completed. Other dentists prefer a waxed type for easy insertion between the teeth.

Floss may be purchased as flavored, colored, or impregnated with fluoride or baking soda. It may be thick or thin. There is even a flat, tape style and a super floss that is very thick and may be used to remove plaque from gap areas. The choice of the proper type of floss is for the dentist to make, but some offices routinely order the type they prefer to recommend.

The flossing technique begins with a string of floss about 18 inches long. The floss is wrapped around the long or middle finger of each hand tightly enough to stay on but not tight enough to cut circulation to the finger (Figure 6–14A). The pointer fingers or thumbs of each hand are used to guide the floss between the teeth (Figure 6–14B). The working area of exposed floss to be inserted between the teeth is kept 1 to 1½ inches long. Too long a space may lessen control and make it more difficult to hold tension.

Once the patient has mastered holding the floss, he or she may attempt to begin flossing by gently wiggling or working the floss between the teeth (Figure 6–14C), wrapping the floss around one side of the tooth and then "scraping" the plaque off with an upward or downward motion of the floss (away from the gums) (Figures 6–14D and E). The floss is wrapped around the surface on the other side of the tooth and it

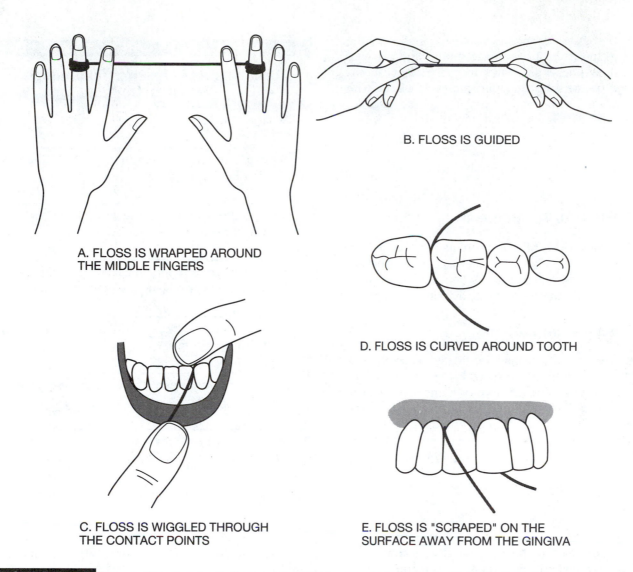

A. FLOSS IS WRAPPED AROUND
THE MIDDLE FINGERS

B. FLOSS IS GUIDED

C. FLOSS IS WIGGLED THROUGH
THE CONTACT POINTS

D. FLOSS IS CURVED AROUND TOOTH

E. FLOSS IS "SCRAPED" ON THE
SURFACE AWAY FROM THE GINGIVA

FIGURE 6–14 Proper flossing techniques can help to prevent decay and gingival problems.

too is "scraped" clean of plaque. Each time the patient moves to a new area, the floss is wrapped and rotated on the fingers to permit a fresh piece to be inserted between the teeth. Again, the main principle of the flossing technique is to help the patient establish a routine pattern that will include all the interproximal surfaces of the teeth.

The assistant may suggest starting the flossing procedure in the same manner as the brushing technique, starting with the maxillary molar area and rotating around to the other side. The patient then drops down to the mandibular area and flosses from molar to molar. Flossing of the teeth is a complex, difficult task for a beginner. The assistant should assure the patient that the process will become easier as experience grows. In fact, many people become so efficient at flossing they can do it anywhere, including while watching the late news on TV.

6 Demonstrate Use of Interproximal Stimulators and Aids

Because very few mouths are perfectly formed, the assistant may find a particularly difficult or troublesome area, such as a gapping or overlapping site. There are other appliances and items designed to help cleanse the mouth. Interproximal stimulators, either rubber tip or wood points, can be used to stimulate in pocket areas where the tissue has been irritated. These devices are inserted into the interproximal area near the gingiva and rotated gently to massage the tissues.

Water pics and irrigating devices are also sold for home use. These machines have a reservoir or tank of water, which may be slightly flavored with mouthwash. When activated, the motor sends jets of water out a thin wand and gently but forcibly flushes out debris and matter from pockets and from around bridgework. Patients are instructed to bend over the sink area, insert the tip into the mouth and wave or aim the tip at pocket areas and under fixed appliances.

Bridge cleaners are thin, stiff pieces of plastic with a large loop on the end. Floss is inserted into the loop, which is drawn under the bridge by gently threading the cleaner point under the bridge (Figure 6–15A). Once the floss is through, it is scraped back and forth to clean the area under the bridge (Figure 6–15B).

7 Review All Techniques

The assistant reviews all the techniques before preparing for dismissal. If any questions occur, they are answered and fully explained. When the patient feels comfortable with the procedures, dismissal is planned.

8 Dismiss the Patient

Each and every patient must be treated as an individual. The assistant must work with the patient to discover the best possible method for home care that will ensure proper brushing and flossing techniques. The patient may be given a supply of floss, aids, and brushes for home care when dismissed. A followup appointment is made to reevaluate progress.

9 Cleanup Procedures

The assistant gathers the contaminated items and materials, removes them to the sterilizing room, and removes the overgloves used during patient assistance. The hands are washed and the procedure is marked on the patient chart, which is taken to the assigned place. PPE is donned. The area is sprayed with disinfectant in the usual manner, and all contaminated objects are disposed of or cleaned and disinfected or sterilized. When the PPE is removed, the assistant washes hands.▲

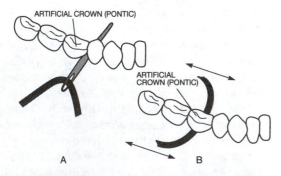

FIGURE 6–15 (A) The bridge threader is inserted under the artificial tooth. (B) The floss is drawn through and then gently moved back and forth to clean the area.

THEORY RECALL

Brushing and Flossing Techniques Instruction

1. What is plaque?

2. Why is it better to demonstrate a disclosing solution before the prophylaxis?

3. What is the main priority to have a patient do in the toothbrushing technique?

4. What is the most important factor that the patient must perform in brushing the teeth?

5. What service does flossing do in the dental home-care cleansing plan?

6. Name a reason a dentist may prefer waxed dental floss? unwaxed?

7. What does the patient do with the floss when placing it between the teeth?

8. How are the interdental stimulators used?

9. What device could a patient use to thread dental floss under a bridge or some other permanent appliance?

10. What two points should the assistant remember when working with a patient in toothbrushing and flossing technique instructions?

Now turn to the Competency Evaluation Sheet for Procedure 24, Brushing and Flossing Techniques Instruction, located in Appendix C of this text.

DIET AND NUTRITION COUNSELING

Another method to control decay and provide good dental health is through proper nutrition. The dental assistant may be able to discuss this subject with a patient. Many times the value of proper eating habits is started during the patient's prophylaxis appointment. The dentist may feel that the patient may need some instruction in this area and ask the assistant to counsel the patient.

Many offices have a preventive dentistry room prepared to handle diet counseling as well as instruction in brushing and flossing. Some offices take a **holistic** health (entire body) approach to patient care and have lend-lease libraries on all types of health subjects, as well as dentistry. When the patient is brought from the operatory to this setting, two things are accomplished. First, the operatory area is freed for productive operatory work and, more importantly, the patient is placed in an atmosphere of patient care and concern.

Lecturing and faultfinding cannot establish a good relationship. The subject must be placed in a positive manner. The counselor and patient must form a teamwork approach and a mutual understanding.

PROCEDURE 25

Diet and Nutrition Counseling

1 Complete the Preparations

2 Explain the Decay Process

3 Review Brushing and Flossing Techniques

4 Demonstrate and Display Cariogenic Foods

5 Demonstrate Diet Modification

6 Dismiss the Patient

7 Cleanup Procedures

1 Complete the Preparations

To perform the diet and nutrition counseling session, the following items are needed:

► patient education booklet
► sugar, bowls, and a spoon
► list of cariogenic food
► nutritional foods chart
► chalkboard, chalk

The patient must feel comfortable and not rushed. Many offices have an educational room where the patient may be taken for privacy and for a warmer atmosphere.

2 Explain the Decay Process

The session may begin with an explanation of the decay process, showing the interrelationship between teeth, bacteria, and sugar (food). One way to visualize this process is by drawing three interweaving circles. One represents teeth, the second represents bacteria, and the third represents sugar (food). The area where the three meet may be defined as possible decay. Showing the patient that we do not care to eliminate

the teeth circle and that we cannot eliminate the bacteria circle, we can show the patient that the only control we have is with the sugar (food) circle (Figure 6–16).

3 Review Brushing and Flossing Techniques

At this time, the assistant may demonstrate brushing and flossing techniques to show the patient how bacteria may be lessened. Although we cannot totally eliminate bacteria in the mouth, we can decrease their numbers and disturb the decay-making process when these functions are completed.

4 Demonstrate and Display Cariogenic Foods

The greatest control over the sugar (food) supply to the mouth bacteria is through diet counseling. The assistant may explain to the patient how sugar is the primary food of bacteria. Most patients are very surprised to find how much hidden sugar is in the foods they eat. One way to illustrate the fact that refined sugar is placed in so many common foods is to have a bowl of sugar or box of sugar cubes handy and then ask the patient to name a favorite food. There are many charts available with sugar contents listed (Figure 6–17). The assistant may look up the food and dip out the hidden teaspoons of refined sugar in that food. After the patient sees the pile grow and grow, the assistant may start to suggest substitute foods.

Some foods are considered **cariogenic**, which means decay starting or enhancing. These are sugary, sticky foods that adhere to the teeth and leave a sugar substance on the plaque buildup. Many of the favorites

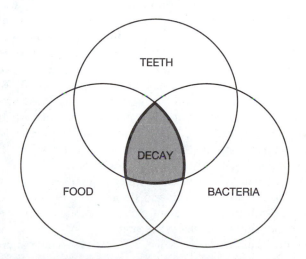

FIGURE 6–16 **The three elements needed for decay are teeth, food, and bacteria.**

HIDDEN SUGAR CONTENTS IN COMMON FOODS

FOOD SOURCE	SERVING SIZE	APPROXIMATE TEASPOONS
cola drinks	6 ounces	3½–4
cider	1 cup	6
chocolate milk	1 cup	6
angel food cake	4-ounce piece	7
cheese cake	4-ounce piece	2
coffee cake	4-ounce piece	4½
fruit cake	4-ounce piece	5
chocolate cake (iced)	4-ounce piece	10
sponge cake	4-ounce piece	2
cherry pie	⅛ of pie	14
pumpkin pie	⅛ of pie	10
custard	½ cup	4
sherbet	½ cup	6–8
jello	½ cup	4
honey	1 tablespoon	3
jam	1 tablespoon	3
apple butter	1 tablespoon	1
ice cream cone	1	3½
malted milk shake	10-ounce glass	5
fudge	1-ounce square	4½
Lifesaver	1	½
hard candy	4 ounces	20
chocolate bar	average size	3–7
donut	1	3
donut	1 glazed	6
applesauce	½ cup	2
fruit cocktail	½ cup	3

FIGURE 6–17 Many foods contain more sugar than expected. Eliminating excessive sugar consumption can help to lessen decay.

Nutrition Facts

Serving Size About 3 Tbsp (37g)
Servings Per Package About 2.5

Amount Per Serving	As Packaged	Per Cup Popped
Calories	170	30
Calories from Fat	110	20

	% Daily Value**	
Total Fat (12g, 2g)*	19%	3%
Saturated Fat (3g, 0.5g)	15%	3%
Polyunsaturated Fat (0.5g, 0g)		
Monounsaturated Fat (3g, 0.5g)		
Cholesterol (0mg, 0mg)	0%	0%
Sodium (320mg, 50mg)	13%	2%
Potassium (80mg, 15mg)	2%	0%
Total Carbohydrate (17g, 3g)	6%	1%
Dietary Fiber (5g, less than 1 gram)	21%	2%
Insoluble Fiber (4g, less than 1 gram)		
Sugars (0g, 0g)		
Protein (3g, less than 1 gram)		
Vitamin A	60%	10%
Vitamin C	0%	0%
Calcium	0%	0%
Iron	4%	0%

FIGURE 6–18 Nutritional labeling found on the food containers can help the patient determine which foods to choose for a good diet.

of our population are these types of foods. People cannot and will not go without sugar in their living habits, so the assistant must be realistic and suggest pleasant foods to be eaten at sugar-craving times.

5 Demonstrate Diet Modification

Candy bars, cakes, and puddings are considered cariogenic, while popcorn, apples, and vegetable sticks can serve as substitutes. Sugarless gum may be chewed instead of gum coated with powdered sugar. The assistant may have a supply of some sample nutrition labels from miscellaneous foods (Figure 6–18). By demonstrating a method to observe the carbohydrate and sugar content of food in a container, the patient may be better able to judge and substitute foods with less sugar content. Most offices have a list of cariogenic foods and another list of substitute foods that can be given to a patient for quick reference.

If a patient is willing and desires to attempt a diet **modification**, the assistant may encourage the patient to make out a diet diary keeping a record of what the patient eats and drinks for a few days. The patient must be counseled to keep an accurate record of what the patient eats and not what the patient thinks the assistant wants the patient to eat.

When the patient returns with the diet diary, the assistant and the patient return to the educational room and evaluate the diary. The sugar foods are circled in one color and the substitute foods are circled in another color. This provides a graphic display of the patient's efforts.

6 Dismiss the Patient

There will be return visits and reinforcement talks, but once a patient has learned and accepted a diet modification, most patients become happy and satisfied patients with less decay and a better general health outlook.

The patient is dismissed with a supply of diet sheets, lists of cariogenic foods, and food modification substitutes. Another appointment is made for followup counseling and encouragement.

7 Cleanup Procedures

The assistant picks up the area and replaces equipment. The counseling appointment is written on the patient's chart, along with notes of concern or interest for the next visit. Hands are washed. ▲

THEORY RECALL

Diet and Nutrition Counseling

1. What value does good nutrition have on decay and health?

_____

2. What two feelings must the counselor and the patient establish in a diet and nutrition counseling meeting?

_____

3. What lesson begins the diet and nutrition counseling session?

_____

4. How can one visualize the decay process? What do the three circles represent?

_____

5. How may one find out how much hidden sugars are in food?

_____

6. How can an assistant help a patient visualize the amount of hidden sugar in a favorite food or drink?

_____

7. What is a cariogenic food?

_____

8. What is one of the first steps to accomplish when attempting a diet modification?

_____

9. How can the assistant point out cariogenic and substitute foods on a patient's diet diary?

_____

10. What outlook can the patient expect once the patient has learned and accepted a diet with less refined sugar?

_____

Now turn to the Competency Evaluation Sheet for Procedure 25, Diet and Nutrition Counseling, located in Appendix C of this text.

DENTAL DAM APPLICATION

Dental dam (formerly called rubber dam) application may be performed by the dentist for a multitude of dental procedures, such as:

▶ to provide the dentist with more visibility and access because it eliminates tongue and tissue clutter and resistance
▶ for endodontic procedures to establish sterile conditions and safety from swallowing small instruments
▶ to help maintain a dry field so moisture does not interfere with the bonding or setting up reactions of the restorative materials
▶ to be effective in pediatric dentistry as they provide safety, moisture, tongue, and patient control
▶ to be useful in general dental procedures as a barrier and effective measure against contamination. See Figure 6–19 for applied dental dam.

For whatever reason, a dentist may choose to use a rubber dental dam, the presence and assistance of a dental assistant will be of great value. In this procedure four hands are a blessing.

Dental dam material is supplied in rolls six inches wide or in prepared squares or sheets— 5 χ 5, 6 χ 5, or 6 χ 6 inches. The material can be purchased in five thicknesses—thin, medium, heavy, extra heavy, or special heavy weights. The latex material is colored light or dark latex, blue, green, or designer's colors.

Dental dam frames are used to hold the dam material around the mouth. These U-shaped frames may be made of stainless steel, plastic, or radiolucent nylon. There are also some accordion styled, boxed shape, or strap frames or holders, but the U frames are the most popular. These U shapes hold the material in place and somewhat off the face; they are easy to work around and can be easily sterilized between patients.

Dental dam napkins are placed under the frame between the dam material and the patient's face. These treated paper tissues are slightly larger than the frame, with a large hole in the middle to permit access

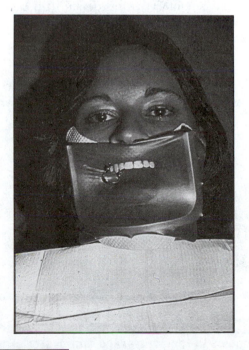

FIGURE 6–19 Dental dam application can help to ensure a safe, dry, and sterile field for dental procedures. (Courtesy of Hygienic Corporation.)

to the mouth. The napkin is used for comfort, to absorb moisture and to prevent any irritation from the latex material.

Holes are punched into the dam material to isolate the tooth or teeth. Each tooth requires a hole. In order to know the location to punch a hole, the assistant should use a dental dam stamp or a template to mark the material. The dental dam stamper is moistened on an ink pad and then pressed onto a sheet of dam material. The assistant who chooses to use a template places the dam material on top of the template and then presses a pencil into the holes to mark the sites. Both the stamper and the template come in a 5 × 5- or 6 × 6-inch size.

There are a few things an assistant must consider when marking the dam material for the punch holes. The marks for the holes must match the anatomy of the mouth. If a tooth is missing, has rotated, or is out of alignment, then the assistant must not mark the hole for that tooth or make adjustments for the tooth's irregularity. The misaligned or rotated tooth requires the assistant to move slightly off target of the template or stamp mark toward the position of the errant tooth. No hole should be placed for missing teeth.

To be sure the dental dam fits the deeply posterior anchor teeth and yet has enough material left to fit the frame, the assistant may scoot the material a little off center toward the side of the working site. This allows for a little more flexibility in the work area while still fitting throughout the mouth.

After the marks have been made for the hole placement, the assistant takes the dental dam punch and positions the stylus or stage into the proper position (Figure 6–20). There is a series of five indentations,

from very small to large, on a round stage, which can be rotated for selection. The smaller the tooth, the smaller the hole indentation selection. Once the assistant has determined which indentation to use, the stage is rotated until the selected indentation comes into position. The assistant should test the accuracy of the positioning by squeezing the punch to see if the punch and the indents match perfectly. If these two parts do not meet in exact position, a ragged or uneven hole may be punched. These types of punched holes rip very easily and can cause much trouble while adjusting the dental dam.

The dentist gives the orders for which teeth to isolate, but a general rule is to isolate one tooth deeper than the work site and two teeth in front of the site. Only the tooth receiving an endodontic treatment is exposed in a root canal procedure, because the dentist is trying to maintain a sterile field as well as protect the patient.

To hold the dam material onto the teeth, the dentist uses dental dam clamps. There are different kinds and sizes of clamps. These devices are made of a stainless steel, chrome metal, or a disposable synthetic one which has been tempered to a spring condition, much like a hairpin or paper clip. A special clamp forceps is used to spring the clamp open, carry the clamp to the site, position the jaws of the clamp around the tooth and then release it onto the tooth (Figure 6–21).

Dental dam clamps are made to match the anatomic shape of a specific tooth. Since the maxillary molars are rounded diamonds and the mandibular teeth are more boxed shaped, the assistant chooses the shape clamp that fits the exact molar tooth. With practice and use, the assistant should look at the jaw shape of

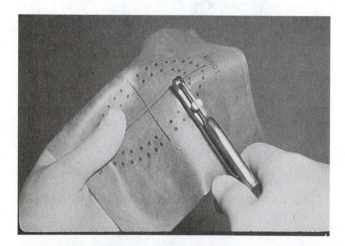

FIGURE 6–20 The assistant uses the punch to make holes in the premarked dam material. Preparing the dam material before the appointment can save valuable chair time. (Courtesy of Hygienic Corporation.)

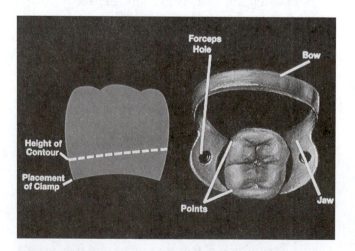

FIGURE 6–21 Dental dam clamps are manufactured to fit a specific tooth. The clamp must touch in four areas to be stable when placed on a tooth. (Courtesy of Hygienic Corporation.)

the clamp to determine which fits the tooth being anchored. Some offices have boxed sets that mark and indicate which clamp fits in which area. In either case, the assistant passes and receives clamps until one is chosen that anatomically fits the anchor tooth.

To assist with stabilizing the dam material in the mouth, the dentist attaches tie off lines called ligatures. These are pieces of dental floss that are pressed between the teeth and then tied off to help hold the material down onto the teeth. Sometimes a dentist uses a small piece of dam material and presses it between the teeth or does it with the ligatures. A latex stabilizing cord called a "widget" has been developed in three different thicknesses to replace ligature tying. Small pieces of the cord are inserted into the inter-proximal spaces, much like dental floss. These dispos-able cords wedge the dam material and tooth without trauma to the tissue or enamel (Figure 6–22).

P R O C E D U R E   2 6

Assisting with Dental Dam Application

1 Complete the Preparations

2 Assist with Dental Dam Application Preparation

3 Assist with Clamp Selection

4 Pass Dental Dam Materials

5 Assist with Dental Dam Inversion

6 Assist with Removal of Dental Dam

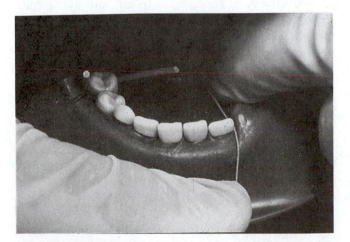

FIGURE 6–22 Stabilizing cords can be used to hold the dam in place. Many times the cord is so effective that a clamp is not needed. (Courtesy of Hygienic Corporation.)

---

7 Clean Up Patient

8 Cleanup Procedures

1 Complete the Preparations

To prepare for dental dam application, the assistant sets up the equipment and materials needed. Such a setup would include:

- basic instruments—mirror, explorer, pliers
- dental dam material
- dental dam frame
- dental dam template or stamp and pad, pen
- dental dam punch
- dental dam clamps
- dental dam clamp forceps
- dental dam napkin
- scissors
- dental floss or rubber wedges
- lubricant or shaving soap
- blunt instrument for inverting dam material
- saliva ejector
- sandpaper strips (optional for clearing interproxi-mal areas)

After the patient is seated and prepared, the assis-tant explains the procedure to allay any fears or ap-prehensions. The assistant dons PPE and summons the dentist.

2 Assist with Dental Dam Application Preparation

The patient's mouth is rinsed and air dried. The assis-tant may place a light coat of cocoa butter or petro-leum jelly over the lips for the patient's comfort. The dentist examines the site to be isolated. Special atten-tion is given to the interproximal areas to determine if the dental dam material will be able to correctly pass between the teeth in question. If there are overhang-ing **restorations** or rough areas, the dentist may call for sandpaper strips to smooth the spaces. *Any anes-thetic injection needed for the dental procedure is completed before dam placement.

3 Assist with Clamp Selection

Once the mouth is ready to receive the dam material, the dentist tests various clamps to find the one that fits properly. The assistant should have tied a piece of dental floss around the test clamp, so the clamp may be retrieved easily if aspirated or swallowed (Figure 6–23). The clamp should have been loaded into the dental dam clamp forceps and passed to the dentist in a palm grasp transfer with the working area of the clamp facing the gum line.

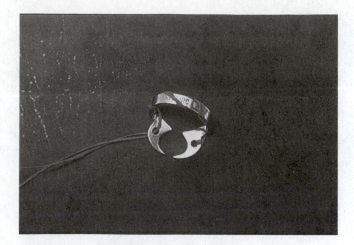

FIGURE 6–23 Dental floss ligatures are tied to the wing of the dental dam clamp. This is a safety precaution to guard against an accidental swallowing. (Courtesy of Hygienic Corporation.)

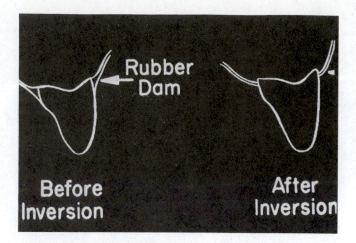

FIGURE 6–24 The illustration shows how the inversion of the dam material protects against leakage. (Courtesy of Hygienic Corporation.)

4 Pass Dental Dam Materials

If the passed clamp is a proper fit, the assistant prepares the prepunched dam material by rubbing a lubricant of petroleum jelly, cocoa butter, or shaving soap around each punched hole. The dam material is placed over the clamp in the forceps and gathered into a mass in the center. The clamp is replaced and the dam material is slipped over the clamp and tooth on the anchor tooth and then on the other teeth to be isolated.

The dental dam napkin is then slipped over the material mass and spread out over the face. The dam material is opened up and placed over the napkin. The dental dam frame is then secured by holding the frame under the material and drawing the dam material up and around the little spikes on the side of the frame. A final adjustment of the frame and material may be made after the dam material has been stabilized and ligated.

The assistant may pass dental floss to the dentist or may assist by wiggling the floss interproximally to secure the dam material around the teeth. The floss may be tied around a tooth to help hold the material in place or the assistant may pass small pieces of latex stabilizing cord to be inserted interproximally to hold the dam material in position around the teeth.

5 Assist with Dental Dam Inversion

The dam material is then inverted around the crowns of the teeth. The assistant may use the syringe to spray a warm jet of air on the tooth and material while the dentist may use a flat instrument to turn under (invert) the edge of the material into the sulcus of each isolated tooth (Figure 6–24). This action seals the isolation and

keeps moisture from seeping through the dam and causing slipping of the material and contamination of the site.

A saliva ejector is used to relieve the moisture from the patient's mouth. It is placed under the frame and material, but over the napkin. The assistant hooks the saliva ejector on the side opposite the work site. Occasionally, throughout the work procedure, the assistant may be required to use the HVE to relieve the patient's moisture accumulation.

6 Assist with Removal of Dental Dam

When the procedure has been finished and the dam material is to be removed, the assistant aspirates all material and moisture from the dental dam site and passes scissors to the dentist to cut and assist with removing the ligatures. The dam material is then pulled gently away from each tooth and the material between the teeth is snipped until there is nothing holding the dam material interproximally.

The assistant removes the saliva ejector from the patient's mouth and hands the dental dam clamp forceps to the dentist who engages the clamp and forces it open to release the hold on the anchor tooth.

Once the assistant has received the clamp forceps holding the clamp, the dam material can be wiggled off the teeth, and the frame and material are taken from the mouth and face.

7 Clean Up Patient

The assistant then removes the napkin, sprays, rinses, and evacuates the mouth gently massaging the gingival area to increase circulation. The assistant holds the removed dam material up to the light to see if any small pieces are missing or broken off. Any piece of material not present in the dam must be located and removed before the patient is released.

At this time, the patient's work may be completed, such as finishing of a restoration, or the patient may be cleaned up and dismissed. The assistant gathers the equipment and materials to be removed to the sterilizing room. Any clamps exposed to the work site are sterilized, even if they were not used in the mouth. The clamps and any other equipment set out are considered contaminated since they may have been exposed by splattering or sprays.

8 Cleanup Procedures

All contaminated items are removed to the sterilizing room. Exam gloves are removed and hands are washed. The completed operative procedures are marked on the patient's chart, which is taken to the front desk or appropriate area. The assistant dons utility gloves, disinfects the operatory, flushes lines, and returns to the sterilizing area to clean, disinfect, and sterilize equipment. The area is cleaned up. Utility gloves are washed, dried, disinfected, and removed. Hands are washed.▲

THEORY RECALL
Dental Dam Application

1. List three reasons for a dental dam application.

   a. _____

   b. _____

   c. _____

2. Dental dam frames are supplied in what materials?

3. What does the assistant use to locate the position for placement of holes in dental dam material?

4. What considerations must an assistant make when determining hole placement?

5. What is the importance of making a clean cut in hole placement?

6. What appliance holds the dental dam material on an anchor tooth?

7. For what problem is the used dental dam examined after removal from the mouth?

8. What procedure is it when the dental dam material is turned in and tucked into the sulcus of the teeth? Why is this done?

9. Once the dental dam is in place, what is used to remove the patient's mouth moisture?

10. What does the assistant do to the patient when the dental dam is removed?

Now turn to the Competency Evaluation Sheet for Procedure 26, Assisting with Dental Dam Application, located in Appendix C of this text.

ANTERIOR RESTORATIONS

Anterior restorations may be in any cavity classification except Class II (proximal walls of posterior tooth). Since the anterior teeth are involved, the dentist will restore the tooth with a white or tooth-shaded material. The final choice of restorative material depends on many factors, from patient age and habits, to size and placement of carious lesions.

The choice of bases and liners beneath the restoration is determined by the type of material in the restoration. Some bases and restorative materials do not work together.

To be of value in the anterior restoration, the assistant must be able to assist with local anesthesia, dental dam placement, cavity preparation, bases and liner use, restorative mixture and placement, and restoration finishing and polishing. The routine for anterior restoration is similiar throughout the dental world, but the dentist will have a particular style and pattern to the procedure. With careful attention and practice, the assistant will become familiar with the procedure and feel comfortable and knowledgeable.

PROCEDURE 27
Assisting with Anterior Restoration

1 Complete the Preparations

2 Assist with Local Anesthesia

3 Assist with Dental Dam (If Used)

4 Assist with Cavity Preparation

5 Assist with Cavity Base and Liners or Etch

6 **Assist with Preparation of Restorative Materials**

7 **Assist with Placement of Restorative Materials**

8 **Assist with Finishing of Restoration**

9 **Dismiss the Patient**

10 **Cleanup Procedures**

1 Complete the Preparations

The materials and equipment needed for an anterior restoration are:

▶ basic setup
▶ local anesthetic setup
▶ dental dam setup
▶ basic sundry products—gauze, floss, cotton rolls, matrix strip, pellets, applicators, saliva ejector tips, HVE tip
▶ slow- and high-speed rotors, handpieces, burs, disks, mandrels, bur changer, stones
▶ cutting and preparation hand instruments
▶ bases, liners, and varnish with mixing equipment, as needed
▶ shade guide
▶ restorative material and equipment
▶ matrix and wedges (Class III)
▶ finishing instruments—rotors, handpieces, burs, stones, disks, abrasive strips
▶ * for Class IV and VI—clear crown form, scissors, articulating paper
▶ * for Class V—gingival matrix, retraction clamp

The assistant greets and escorts the patient to the operatory area. The patient is seated, bibbed or draped, and fitted comfortably into the dental chair in a position regulated by the upcoming treatment. The assistant reviews the patient's health history, noting and highlighting any changes.

After washing hands, the assistant dons PPE. Mask and eyewear or shield are placed first and then the gloves are drawn on.

2 Assist with Local Anesthesia

The assistant checks the proposed treatment plan and begins topical anesthetic application by rinsing the patient's mouth, drying the injection area, and then placing topical anesthetic liquid, foam, ointment, or cream on the site.

When the dentist is ready to inject the local anesthetic solution, the assistant receives the topical applicator and passes the anesthetic syringe, while watching and guarding for unpredictable movement from the patient. The assistant continues to monitor the patient's reaction to the anesthetic after the syringe has been received and the needle has been covered using a one-handed technique.

3 Assist with Dental Dam Application (If Used)

After the anesthetic has been given, the assistant helps with the placement of the dental dam, if needed. The lubricated, prepared dam material, premeasured clamp, and frame are passed to the dentist. The assistant helps with the placement of the dental dam napkin and the ligature tie offs or stabilizing cord insertion. The saliva ejector tip is situated into position, opposite the work site area.

4 Assist with Cavity Preparation

The cavity preparation is begun by passing the mirror and high-speed rotor with bur. Hand instrument transfers and rotor and bur changes are completed at the dentist's request. The assistant should be prepared to exchange, rinse, and evacuate the mouth and keep the work site visible by cleaning the mouth mirror with a warm air spray from the triple syringe and locating the ora-evac tip at the work site to remove excess moisture and spray.

5 Assist with Cavity Base and Liners or Etch

When the dentist is satisfied with the preparation, a signal for the mixing of a base lining material is given. The exact type is determined by the proposed restorative material and the size and shape of the preparation. The assistant passes cotton rolls for isolation of the preparation (if no dental dam is present), measures and mixes the material according to the manufacturer's recommendation, and passes a ball burnisher to the dentist, who takes small increments into the preparation.

The assistant holds the mixing slab with material close to the site so the dentist may refill the ball burnisher tip for more applications. A piece of gauze is also held close to the site so the instrument tip may be wiped off if needed.

If the material to be used requires a pre-etching of tooth tissue, the assistant carefully opens the bottle and moistens the brush or pellet to pass to the dentist. At the end of the timing period for the etching process, the assistant passes or uses the air and water syringe to flush and dry the etched preparation.

6 Assist with Preparation of Restorative Materials

The dentist signals when to prepare the anterior restorative material. The assistant activates a restorative capsule and prepares it for syringe placement (Figure 6–25), or measures and mixes the required material according to the manufacturer's recommendations. If the restoration preparation needs an artificial wall, a greased clear mylar matrix strip is passed.

7 Assist with Placement of Restorative Materials

A plastic filling instrument is given to the operator, while holding the prepared material near the site. The dentist carries the material to the tooth and signals for the matrix strip holder and wedge (if Class III) when the preparation has been filled.

If the anterior restorative material needs to be light cured, the assistant holds the light tip at the site and exposes the material for the proper amount of time (Figure 6–26). As a safety precaution, the assistant should also hold a light shield or don specially tinted glasses for this part of the procedure. The patient may be advised to close eyes for the timing session.

8 Assist with Finishing of Restoration

After the timing session is over and the matrix strip or form has been removed, the assistant must be prepared to pass and receive finishing instruments. The dentist may call for hand instruments, such as a carver, or may wish to use a slow-speed rotor with burs, points,

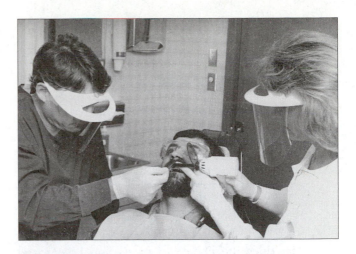

FIGURE 6–26 The light-curing tip is placed close to the clear matrix strip during the curing process.

stones, or disks. The assistant will become more familiar with the dentist's pattern after a few sessions.

The assistant is prepared to pass the slow-speed handpiece with acrylic burs and finishing stones and measuring results with articulating paper until the finishing process in completed.

9 Dismiss the Patient

When the restoration has been finished and polished, the patient's dental dam is removed and the patient is cleaned up and dismissed. The assistant rinses the mouth, wipes the patient's face, restores appliances, cautions the patient for movement, and lowers the chair for release.

At this time, the assistant may give postoperative instructions, such as not to bite the lip and not to eat or drink for a certain length of time. The patient is escorted from the room and returned to the front desk to make a followup appointment, if needed.

10 Cleanup Procedures

The assistant returns to the operatory and gathers contaminated materials and equipment to take to the sterilizing area. The latex exam gloves are removed, the hands are washed, and the assistant records treatment on the patient's chart. The type and quantity of anesthesia, type of base liner and restorative material, as well as classification of restoration are noted and dated. The chart is taken to the front desk or appropriate place. The assistant returns to the sterilizing area and dons utility gloves and PPE. The operatory area is disinfected, lines are flushed, and all disinfection is completed. The instruments and materials are cleaned and prepared for sterilization. The area is cleaned up and

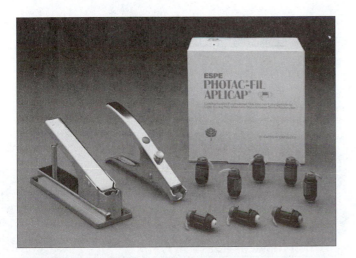

FIGURE 6–25 The materials and instruments needed for the capsule mixes are shown here. The capsule is activated in the activator on the left and then placed into the syringe handle on the right. (Courtesy of ESPE America.)

the gloves are washed, disinfected, and removed. The assistant washes hands.▲

Anterior Restorations

1. Anterior restorations can be present in any cavity classification except which one?

_____

2. The dentist bases the choice of anterior restorative material on what factors?

_____

3. What does the choice of bases and liner to be placed in the restoration depend on?

_____

4. What does the assistant check before applying topical anesthetic material?

_____

5. During a cavity preparation, how can the assistant aid the dentist in maintaining visibility?

_____

6. Where does the assistant hold the prepared liner and base mixes during placement?

_____

7. After the preparation is overfilled with the restorative material, what does the assistant pass to the dentist?

_____

8. If the restorative material needs to be light cured, what does the assistant do?

_____

9. What does the dentist use to finish an anterior restoration?

_____

10. What treatment items may be noted and recorded on a patient's chart?

_____

Now turn to the Competency Evaluation Sheet for Procedure 27, Assisting with Anterior Restoration, located in Appendix C of this text.

AMALGAM POSTERIOR RESTORATION

Posterior restorations can be in Class I, II, or V classification. The restorative material used may be **amalgam**, **composite**, or gold foil Class V restorations. The most common material has been amalgam; but with the recent improvements in strength and adhesion, the use of composite restorations is increasing.

The basic preliminary procedures, such as anesthesia, dental dam, and cavity preparation, are the same. The restorative process is adapted to the particular technique required by the material to be used. Cavity bases and liner selection depend on the restorative material used, and the finishing and polishing technique is different for each.

Composite restorations are completed in the original appointment. The restoration is finished and polished before the patient is released, but the amalgam restoration must have at least 24 to 48 hours to fully harden before polishing. Patients receiving amalgam restoration require an amalgam finishing and polishing appointment at a later date.

Posterior restorations, which involve replacement of proximal walls (Class II), require auxiliary equipment, such as matrix bands and wedge holders, to replace the original sides. Composite restorations, particularly the light-cured type, require clear or mylar strips and wedges (Figure 6–27), which permit the curing light ray penetration, while the amalgam restorations need stainless steel precut or prerolled strips. Both strips may be hand held, clipped on, or placed in a matrix retainer when they are placed to encircle the prepared tooth.

Wedges are used in the **embrasure** areas, after matrix replacement. These devices stabilize the matrix, prevent restorative material forming overhangs, maintain contact areas, and provide embrasure room. Wedges may be made of wood or plastic material.

The restorative procedure consists of removing decay, preparing, inserting, finishing, and polishing of the restoration.

Assisting with Amalgam Posterior Restoration

1 Complete the Preparations

2 Assist with Local Anesthesia

3 Assist with Dental Dam Placement

4 Assist with Cavity Preparation

5 Assist with Cavity Preparation Dressings

6 Assist with Matrix Placement (If Needed—Class II)

7 Assist with Amalgam Placement

8 Assist with Carving Restoration and Matrix Removal

9 Assist with Dental Dam Removal

10 **Assist with Final Carving**

11 **Dismiss the Patient**

12 **Cleanup Procedures**

1 **Complete the Preparations**

The setup for an amalgam posterior Class II restoration (two or more surfaces) follows:

▶ basic setup
▶ local anesthetic setup
▶ dental dam setup (if needed)
▶ basis sundry setup—gauze, cotton rolls, pellets, swipes, floss, applicators, HVE tip, saliva ejector tip
▶ cavity preparation instruments—excavators, hoes, hatchets, chisels
▶ high- and slow-speed rotors, handpieces, burs, bur changer
▶ base, liner, and varnish with mixing materials and placement instruments
▶ matrix—matrix retainer, wedges, wedge holder or hemostat, scissors
▶ amalgam materials, amalgamator, squeeze cloth, amalgam well or dappen dish, carrier
▶ placement and carving instruments—condenser, plugger, carver, discoid-cleoid, burnisher, articulating paper and holder

The setup listed is the same for an amalgam posterior restoration in the Class I classification with the exception of the matrix and materials necessary for wall replacement. Class I is merely preparing a one surface tooth preparation and placing a restoration.

The patient is greeted and escorted into the operatory. After seating, draping, and positioning for the procedure, the assistant reviews the health history. The assistant dons the PPE, placing the mask and eyewear on first and then dons latex gloves.

2 **Assist with Local Anesthesia**

After checking the proposed treatment plan, the assistant rinses the patient's mouth, dries the injection site, and then applies topical anesthetic in the form of a gel, ointment, or liquid.

The dentist is summoned, and signals for the local anesthetic syringe. The assistant passes and then guards against sudden movements. After the injection, the assistant receives the syringe and replaces the cap onto the needle using a one-handed technique or capping device.

3 **Assist with Dental Dam Placement**

If a dental dam is to be used, the assistant passes the prepared, lubricated, punched dam material and clamp holder with the clamp. The dental dam napkin is placed between the dam material and the patient's face and the frame is passed and situated. The assistant helps with the placement and tie off of ligatures or stabilizing with cords and the saliva ejector is placed under the dam opposite the work site.

4 **Assist with Cavity Preparation**

The cavity preparation is begun with the passing of a mirror and high-speed handpiece with bur. The assistant maintains visibility throughout the procedure by cleaning the mirror with air streams and evacuating the work site with the HVE tip. The assistant also passes and receives instruments and rotors at the dentist's signal (Figure 6–27).

5 **Assist with Cavity Preparation Dressings**

When the preparation is finished, the assistant passes a cotton pellet or one saturated with a commercial preparation cleaner to wash and clean the preparation. A dry pellet is then passed to absorb moisture. The assistant mixes the liner, varnish, and base the dentist requires and passes the initial increment on the instrument. Excess amounts are held close to the work site for the dentist's use.

If a light-cured base or liner is being used, the assistant also holds the light tip near the curing material and holds up the barrier shield or dons tinted glasses. The patient may be advised to close the eyes during this procedure.

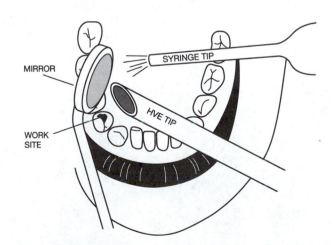

FIGURE 6–27 The assistant maintains visibility by air drying the mirror and evacuating the moisture. The evacuation tip is kept distal to the work site.

6 Assist with Matrix Placement (If Needed—Class II)

Once the base has set or cured, the assistant passes the Tofflemire matrix retainer with band to the dentist. After the matrix placement, the assistant passes the wedge in a wedge holder or hemostat. The dentist places the wedge and returns the holder to the assistant.

7 Assist with Amalgam Placement

At the dentist's signal, the assistant begins preparing the amalgam restorative material. There are two common ways of assembling the amalgam alloy and mercury. One way is to center the proportioner over the capsule opening and eject the needed amount of doses into the container with the pestle. The lid is screwed on tightly and the entire capsule is placed into the mechanical amalgamator for blending (trituration). The other method is to activate a prepared capsule by either turning the capsule top or squeezing the container with **activator** pliers, which releases the mercury for the mixing procedure. Once activated, the capsule is placed into the amalgamator for trituration. The amount of time needed for the blending of the metals is specified by the size of the load and the manufacturer (Figure 6–28). The assistant must read the directions of the materials to be used before setting the amalgamator timer.

If no dental dam has been used, the tooth is isolated with cotton rolls. The assistant passes the cotton rolls to the dentist.

When the amalgam material has been mixed or activated, the assistant removes the capsule from the activator and places it into the syringe for use. If mixing on an amalgamator, the mixture is removed from the capsule and placed while in a movable (plastic) shape into the amalgam squeeze cloth, well, or dap-

pen dish for loading into the amalgam carrier. The assistant fills the carrier in small increments to avoid air entrapment. The loaded amalgam carrier is passed to the dentist and then alternate passing of the carrier and condenser or plugger is done until the preparation is overfilled.

8 Assist with Carving Restoration and Matrix Removal

After the restorative material has been placed, the assistant passes and receives carving and finishing instruments at the dentist's signal. The assistant operates the HVE tip near the site to aspirate any amalgam shavings.

The assistant aids with the removal of the matrix by passing the wedge holder or hemostat and receiving the wedge. The assistant passes the explorer to the dentist and then receives the matrix retainer while passing the college pliers to the dentist to remove the band. When the band is released, the assistant receives the band and passes the discoid/cleoid or instrument of the dentist's choice for finishing the carving anatomy of the restoration.

9 Assist with Dental Dam Removal

If a dental dam was placed, it is carefully removed at this time. The assistant passes the scissors for cutting the dam and then passes the clamp holder to receive the clamp, frame, and napkin. When the dental dam is returned, the assistant checks to see if any pieces are missing.

The mouth is rinsed and the patient's gingiva is lightly massaged.

10 Assist with Final Carving

The dentist completes the final carving. The assistant passes the carver and then holds the articulating paper in the holder over the occlusal site for testing (Figure 6–29). The patient is instructed to gently tap the teeth together. Additional carving and testing are done until the dentist is satisfied with the restoration.

11 Dismiss the Patient

The restoration is wiped off with a wet cotton roll, which the assistant passes to the dentist. The assistant may rinse the patient's mouth and clean up the patient's face.

The patient is cautioned about the lowering of the chair movement, and the assistant gives the patient postoperative instructions before dismissal. An appointment is made for the final finishing and polishing of the restoration.

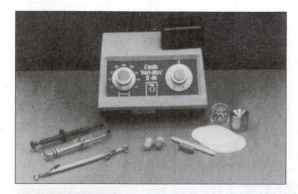

FIGURE 6-28 Assembled amalgam materials. (Courtesy of Anderson and Burkard, *The Dental Assistant*, 3E, © 1995, Delmar Publishers.)

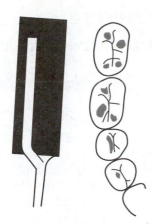

FIGURE 6-29 The articulating paper is placed on the occlusal surfaces. The patient bites down. When the paper is removed, the high spots are indicated by the marks.

12 Cleanup Procedures

After the assistant gathers the contaminated materials and removes them to the sterilizing room, the latex gloves are removed and the hands are washed. The assistant then records the treatment of type and quantity of local anesthetic, type of base, liner, or varnish, and class and material of restoration on the patient's chart and returns the chart to the front desk or appropriate place.

The assistant then dons the utility gloves and PPE to clean and disinfect the operatory area. The sharps are disposed of in the sharps container. The disposables are placed into the contaminated trash container. The large items, such as eyeglasses and shields are disinfected and the instruments are cleaned and prepared for sterilization. The area is cleaned up. The utility gloves are washed, disinfected, and removed. The assistant washes hands.▲

THEORY RECALL

Amalgam Posterior Restoration

1. What is the most common material used for posterior restorations?

_____

2. In regard to timing, what is the difference between the finishing and polishing of a composite and an amalgam restoration?

_____

3. If the dentist requires a dental dam for the procedure, when is it placed?

_____

4. If a light-cured base or liner is used, what are the duties of the assistant in this part of the procedure?

_____

5. After the matrix has been placed, what does the assistant pass to the dentist?

_____

6. If no dental dam has been applied, what is used to isolate the preparation?

_____

7. What does the assistant do while the dentist carves the restoration?

_____

8. What instrument does the assistant pass to the dentist to retrieve the matrix band?

_____

9. When does the assistant give postoperative instructions to the patient?

_____

10. What does the assistant do to the patient before lowering the chair?

_____

Now turn to the Competency Evaluation Sheet for Procedure 28, Assisting with Amalgam Posterior Restoration, located in Appendix C of this text.

COMPOSITE POSTERIOR RESTORATION

Restoring a posterior tooth with a composite material follows the basic procedure of an amalgam restoration except for a few steps. The anesthesia, dental dam placement, and cavity preparation procedures are completed in the same manner; but the placement of composite differs from amalgam.

Calcium hydroxide, glass ionomer, or polycarboxylates may be used under the restoration to protect, soothe, and insulate; but zinc eugenol and copal varnishes cannot because these items hamper the chemical setting up of the composite mixture.

A clear mylar strip or form and clear wedges are used with the composites, especially if the restoration is filled with a light-curing material. Some reflecting wedges have been constructed to relay or carry the prismic light into the inner areas for the curing and setting purpose (Figure 6–30).

Composite restorations can be completed using various types of materials and each type demands its own special mixture, placement, and setup (polymerization). Some composite resins require a mixture of liquid and shaded powder stirred until thickened to restoration consistency. Others are composed of two pastes mixed,

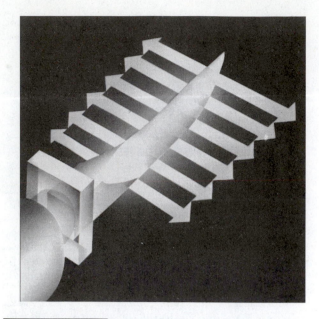

FIGURE 6-30 The Cure-Thru® wedge not only permits the light to enter the preparation site but helps to reflect it in the area. (Courtesy of Premier Dental Products Co.)

placed in the preparation, and allowed to auto-set. Still others require a pre-etch to ensure proper bonding.

Composite restorations may be finished and polished at the original appointment. There is no waiting for hardening as is required by amalgam. To avoid darkening or discoloring the restoration, finishing, polishing, and placement are completed using special nonmetal instruments and composite stones.

PROCEDURE 29

Assisting with Composite Posterior Restoration

1 Complete the Preparations

2 Assist with Local Anesthesia

3 Assist with Dental Dam Placement (If Requested)

4 Assist with Cavity Preparation

5 Assist with Cavity Protective Dressings

6 Assist with Etching of Cavity Preparation

7 Assist with Placement of Restorative Material

8 Assist with Dental Dam Removal (If Used)

9 Assist with Finishing and Polishing of Restoration

10 Dismiss the Patient

---

11 Cleanup Procedures

1 Complete the Preparations

The setup for a light-cured composite requiring a pre-etch placement is:

▶ local anesthetic setup
▶ dental dam setup (optional)
▶ basic sundry setup—gauze, cotton rolls, pellets, swipes, floss, HVE tip applicators, saliva ejector tip
▶ cavity preparation instruments—excavators, hoes, hatchets, chisels, high- and slow-speed rotors, handpieces, burs, bur changer
▶ base, liner, and dentin sealant materials and instruments
▶ clear mylar matrix and clear wedges
▶ composite materials—etch materials and instruments
▶ restorative materials and instruments
▶ shade guide (if needed)
▶ placement and carving instruments—nonmetallic
▶ finishing and polishing instruments—points, burs, disks, abrasive strips, articulating paper, dappen dish with pumice paste, prophy cup

The patient is greeted and escorted into the operatory. After seating, draping, and positioning for the procedure, the assistant reviews the patient's health history.

The assistant dons the PPE, placing the mask and eyewear on first and then washes hands and dons latex exam gloves.

2 Assist with Local Anesthesia

After checking proposed treatment plan, the assistant rinses the patient's mouth, dries the injection site, and then applies topical anesthetic in the form of a gel, ointment, or liquid.

The dentist is summoned and signals for the local anesthetic syringe, which the assistant passes in one hand while accepting the used applicators in the other hand. The assistant guards against sudden movement, receives the syringe, and replaces the needle cap using a one-hand technique or a capping device.

If a shade must be determined for the composite material, it is taken before the placement of the dental dam. The wet guide is held against the tooth with the artificial light turned away.

3 Assist with Dental Dam Placement (If Requested)

If a dental dam is to be used, the assistant passes the prepared, lubricated, punched dam material and clamp holder with the clamp. The dental dam napkin is placed between the dam material and the patient's face and the frame is passed and stabilized. The assistant helps with the placement and tie off of the ligatures, and the saliva ejector is placed under the dam opposite the work site.

4 Assist with Cavity Preparation

The cavity preparation is begun with the passing of a mirror and high-speed handpiece with bur. The assistant maintains visibility throughout the procedure by cleaning the mirror with air streams and evacuating the work site with the HVE tip. The assistant also passes and receives instruments and rotors at the dentist's signal.

5 Assist with Cavity Protective Dressings

When the preparation is completed, the assistant passes a cotton pellet or one saturated with a commercial preparation cleaner to wash and clean the preparation. A dry pellet is then passed to absorb and dry moisture.

The assistant mixes the desired sealant and base and passes the instrument to the dentist, holding any excess close to the area for refill. If a light-cured material is used, the assistant dons tinted glasses or obtains a shield and holds the light tip close to the material for the proper time period.

6 Assist with Etching of Cavity Preparation

The assistant passes a brush or applicator tip containing the acid-etch material to the dentist who applies the bonding acid. The assistant passes or sprays the air from the syringe into the area for spreading the solution and drying. If the dentist is satisfied with the etch process, the assistant passes a wet pellet for wash and spray or passes the air syringe for drying. If the etching process needs to be repeated, all steps are done again.

7 Assist with Placement of Restorative Material

At the dentist's signal the assistant mixes the composite material according to the manufacturer's directions. If a matrix is needed, the assistant passes the clear strip for placement before the restorative material. When the composite is mixed, the assistant passes the placement instrument (or syringe) to the dentist and holds the prepared material nearby for instrument refill. The assistant holds the light tip and shield near the newly placed material and exposes the light for the prescribed time (usually 30 seconds). The fill and light-curing processes are repeated over and over until the dentist is satisfied with the overfilled preparation and returns the filling instrument (Figure 6–31).

8 Assist with Dental Dam Removal (If Used)

If a dental dam was used for this procedure, it is removed. The assistant passes the clamp holder and receives the clamp holder and clamp. Scissors are passed, and the dam, napkin, and frame are received. The assistant checks for any missing parts to the dam material, rinses the patient's mouth, and lightly massages the area.

9 Assist with Finishing and Polishing of Restoration

The restoration is finished when the assistant hands a mirror and the slow handpiece containing a composite bur to the dentist. The assistant places the articulating holder with paper on the occlusal surface for testing restoration height. The assistant washes the testing marks off with water and dries the area with the evacuation tip. Throughout the finishing process, the assistant must be ready to maintain visibility by spraying and evacuating, and changing burs, disks, stones and rubber cups at the dentist's signal.

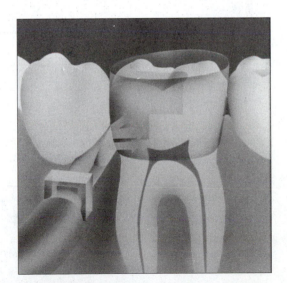

FIGURE 6–31 An illustration of how the clear matrix and wedge permit light entrance and polymerization of the material. (Courtesy of Premier Dental Products Co.)

10 Dismiss the Patient

The patient's mouth is rinsed and face is wiped off. The assistant cautions the patient about the lowering of the chair and reminds the patient not to bite or chew on the numbed lip. The drape and bib are removed, and the patient is given postoperative instructions and dismissed.

11 Cleanup Procedures

The assistant gathers the contaminated materials and removes the articles to the sterilizing room, where the latex gloves are removed and the hands are washed. The treatment is recorded on the patient's chart, and the chart is taken to the front desk or appropriate place.

The assistant returns and dons utility gloves and disinfects the operatory area. The sharps and disposables are placed in the correct containers, and the instruments are cleaned and prepared for sterilization. The area is cleaned up; the gloves are washed, disinfected, and removed. The assistant washes hands.▲

THEORY RECALL

Composite Posterior Restoration

1. The procedure for a composite posterior restoration is similar to an amalgam restoration in what steps?

_____

2. Name three base materials that may be placed under a composite restoration.

   a. _____

   b. _____

   c. _____

3. What type of matrix and wedges are used with a light-cured composite?

_____

4. Which material—composite or amalgam—may be finished and polished at the original appointment?

_____

5. To avoid discoloring the composite restorative material, what type of instruments does a dentist use?

_____

6. After passing the etching solution to the dentist, what does the assistant pass to the dentist?

_____

7. What directions does the assistant follow when mixing the composite restorative material?

_____

8. How often does the assistant hold the curing light tip next to the work site?

_____

9. What duty does the assistant perform when the dentist wishes to check the occlusion height of a new restoration?

_____

10. What instruments does the dentist use to finish and polish the composite restoration?

_____

Now turn to the Competency Evaluation Sheet for Procedure 29, Assisting With Composite Posterior Restoration, located in Appendix C of this text.

FINISHING AND POLISHING OF AMALGAM RESTORATIONS

The final finishing and polishing of an amalgam restoration is usually completed at least 24 to 48 hours after the initial placement. The material is given enough time to harden and adjust. Older amalgam restorations may have accumulated tarnish and rough surfaces through attrition and use. Smoothing and polishing the amalgam material may extend the life of the restoration and help improve gingival health (Table 6–1).

The purpose of this appointment is to provide a more natural and functional restoration through a recontouring, smoothing, and polishing process. A smooth and functional restoration is much more serviceable, esthetic, natural, and healthy to the patient. The plaque-free maintenance, functional stability, tissue health, and overall general appearance are enhanced by finishing and polishing the restoration to a smooth and shiny appearance.

*In some states, the expanded-duty dental assistant is permitted to perform the finishing and polishing procedure and acts as operator in this process.

PROCEDURE 30

Assisting with Finishing and Polishing of Amalgam Restorations

1 **Complete the Preparations**

2 **Assist with Evaluation of Restoration**

3 **Assist with Occlusal Adjustment**

4 **Assist with Isolation (If Requested)**

5 **Assist with Contouring of Restoration Surfaces**

TABLE 6-1

Finishing and Polishing Amalgam Restorations

RECONTOURING

Purpose—to remove excess restorative material, shape for function, and provide esthetic use, simulate tooth anatomy

INSTRUMENTS	AREA OF USE	METHOD OF USE
amalgam knife, file	overhangs and excess buildups	use chipping action in motions away from gingiva
abrasive discs (slow speed)	embrasure areas, Class V	use abrasive side toward material
polishing strips	interproximal areas	use smooth surface for entering, slide back and forth in horizontal motion
brown abrasive point, cup	on excessive areas	short contacts with enamel, do not use if metal shaft shows
small, round finishing bur	on occlusal surface	retrace original grooves, fossae, do not overdefine

SMOOTHING

Purpose—to provide smooth surface, lessen tarnish and plaque buildup

INSTRUMENT	AREA OF USE	METHOD OF USE
large, round finishing bur	remove tarnish surface	use on restorative material only, not on enamel, motion is from middle to edge
white stone	restoration surfaces	use as bur, but may extend onto enamel
abrasive green point, cup	restoration surfaces	light pressure for no heat buildup

POLISHING

Purpose—to provide attractive restoration and nonabrasive areas, esthetic value for patient

INSTRUMENT	AREA OF USE	METHOD OF USE
prophy cup/brush with pumice/water mixture	all areas of tooth	short contact uses, wet mix, avoid heat
whiting or tin oxide mix	all areas of restoration	keep mixture wet
abrasive green/yellow band point	restoration surfaces	slow speed, short applications, avoid use if worn
waxed dental tape or floss	interproximals	carry pumice into interproximals, up-down sawing motion
toothpaste	all areas	slow speed, short contacts

6 **Assist with Smoothing and Polishing of Restoration**

7 **Assist with Interproximal Surfaces**

8 **Assist with Final Evaluation**

9 **Cleanup Procedures**

1 **Complete the Preparations**

The setup needed for this appointment follows:

▶ basic setup
▶ sundry items—pellets, gauze, applicator, floss or tape, cotton rolls

▶ slow handpiece, contra angle, burs, stones, disks, abrasive strips
▶ amalgam knife, file
▶ articulating paper and holder
▶ dappen dishes with pumice, tin oxide
▶ HVE tip and saliva ejector tip
▶ dental dam and equipment (if desired)

After the operatory and equipment are ready, the patient is greeted, seated in the dental chair, and offered safety glasses. If a period of time has passed between appointments, the assistant reviews the patient's health history. The assistant dons the PPE and summons the dentist.

2 Assist with Evaluation of Restoration

The assistant passes the mirror and explorer to the dentist, who checks the integrity of the restoration, making sure the margins are tight and the restoration is firm and in good condition. Proximal contacts are checked for effectiveness and function. (See Figure 6–32 for an example of overhanging restoration and an occlusal buildup of amalgam.) The dentist evaluates and prepares to contour, finish, and polish. Since finishing and polishing an item is a matter of going from large scratches to the very smallest, the dentist performs the most abrasive procedure first.

3 Assist with Occlusal Adjustment

The assistant passes or holds the articulating paper on the occlusal surface for contact testing. If the testing shows any premature occlusion, the assistant passes the slow handpiece and small, round finishing bur or amalgam knife or file to the dentist for recontouring the surface. The assistant is prepared to pass or wipe the occlusal markings with a wet pellet at the dentist's signal and then pass or hold articulating paper for retesting and recontouring as needed. The assistant should be ready to flush and aspirate the work site throughout the procedure because heat is generated through the friction of the finishing bur.

4 Assist with Isolation (If Requested)

A dental dam may be applied, isolating the teeth to be finished. This material serves as a protection for collection of amalgam shavings, polishing materials, or debris and works as a fluid and tongue control. If a dental dam is to be placed, it is performed in this sequence. The assistant aids with the placement of the dam.

5 Assist with Contouring of Restoration Surfaces

The assistant passes the slow handpiece with a large finishing bur to the dentist who finishes the occlusal surfaces of the teeth. Dental floss may be passed to check the contact points and the assistant may pass the handpiece with an abrasive disk for interproximal finishing. The safe or smooth side of the disk is positioned to touch the adjacent tooth structure, while the abrasive side is placed upon the amalgam material. The disks are used in their sequence of coarseness, usually from the darker coarse ones to the lighter, finer ones.

An abrasive rubber point may be used to decrease amalgam buildup. Rubber abrasives are used in the order of their coarseness from most abrasive to least abrasive. Snofu, a popular brand of rubber abrasives are color coded. Brown are coarsest, green are finer, and green with a yellow band are finest in abrasiveness. Figure 6–33 shows an example of a few types of abrasive items to use in polishing and finishing.

6 Assist with Smoothing and Polishing of Restoration

A large, round finishing bur or white stone may be used to remove the top surface that is heavily tarnished. The bur head is applied with a slow speed and in short strokes so as not to build up heat. The operator moves from midcenter to the margin edges of the restoration, avoiding the enamel surface. The white stone is used in the same manner but may extend onto the tooth surfaces.

When the tooth has been contoured and smoothed, the dentist may want to polish the tooth surfaces. The assistant passes the slow handpiece with a rubber cup or brush of pumice and then tin oxide for the dentist

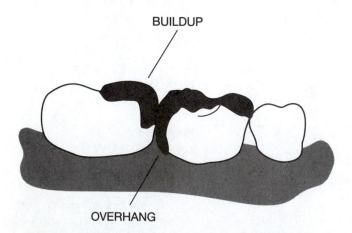

FIGURE 6–32 Restorations with a buildup or overhang of materials must be finished and polished to correct anatomic size and shape.

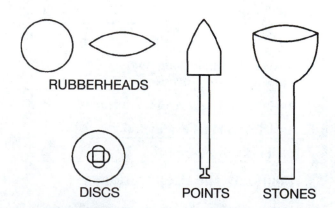

FIGURE 6–33 Rubber wheels, points, mounted stones, and disks may be used to finish and polish restorations.

to polish the restoration surfaces. Toothpaste may be the final abrasive mixture used to polish the restoration. Throughout the polishing procedure, the assistant rinses, evacuates the mouth, maintains visibility, and controls heat buildup.

7 Assist with Interproximal Surfaces

The assistant passes dental floss or an abrasive strip to the dentist, who checks the interproximal contact points and surfaces. A dappen dish of a slurry of pumice and liquid (water or mouthwash) may be placed near the site for the dentist to drag or pull dental floss or tape through the interproximals to smooth the area (Figure 6–34). The assistant keeps rinsing and evacuating the area through the procedure.

8 Assist with Final Evaluation

The assistant passes an explorer to the dentist who makes a final evaluation of the restoration finish. If the dentist is satisfied, the area is cleaned, rinsed, and dried. The isolation, either dental dam or cotton roll, is removed at this time. Another check of the occlusal function is made with articulating paper. If the dentist is satisfied with the restoration, the patient is cleaned up and dismissed from the operatory. If not, the procedure is redone, beginning at the necessary stage.

9 Cleanup Procedures

The assistant cleans up the operatory area, removes the latex gloves, washes hands, and records the treatment on the patient's chart, returning the chart to its appropriate place.

The assistant returns to the sterilizing area, dons utility gloves and disinfects the operatory. The instruments are cleaned and prepared for sterilization. The area is cleaned up and the gloves are washed, dried, disinfected, and removed; the hands are washed.▲

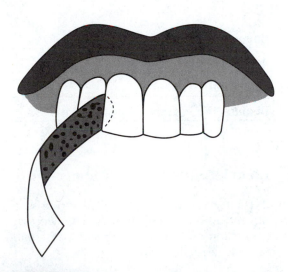

FIGURE 6–34 The coarse side of the abrasive strip is placed next to the restoration or surface needing smoothing. The smooth or safe side is placed next to the unaffected tooth.

THEORY RECALL

Finishing and Polishing of Amalgam Restorations

1. When is the final finishing and polishing of the amalgam restoration completed?

   _____

2. What is the purpose of the finishing and polishing appointment?

   _____

3. What does the assistant pass to the dentist for checking the integrity of the restoration?

   _____

4. In the finishing and polishing procedure, the dentist goes from large to small scratches by using which abrasive first?

   _____

5. What does the articulating paper test indicate to the dentist?

   _____

6. What is passed through the teeth to check contact points?

   _____

7. What does the assistant pass to the dentist to begin the polishing of the restoration?

   _____

8. In what order should the impregnated points be used in smoothing and polishing restorations?

   _____

9. Where is the abrasive strip used in the refining of a restoration?

   _____

10. What may the assistant place on the dental floss used interproximally for polishing the restoration?

    _____

Now turn to the Competency Evaluation Sheet for Procedure 30, Assisting with Finishing and Polishing of Amalgam Restorations, located in Appendix C of this text.

TOOTH BLEACHING APPOINTMENTS

Surface bleaching of teeth has been attempted for some time, but only since about 1989 has this procedure become a standard part of dental office services. There are two modern methods to whitening teeth: they are in-office bleaching and home bleaching. Patients may take advantage of one or the other or both techniques in their quest for brighter smiles.

Bleaching tooth surfaces can be accomplished most easily on teeth that have been stained from habits or foods, such as tobacco or coffee and tea stains. Yellow-, brown-, or orange-colored teeth will lighten a shade or two, while the deeper-toned stains may require more treatments and have limited success. Results vary from case to case. Patients should be cautioned not to expect too drastic a change as disappointment may easily result from not reaching expectations.

A minimum of three appointments is required for the completion of this treatment. During the first visit, the patient is advised of the benefits, responsibilities, and cost of the processing. The dentist is careful not to raise the patient's expectations too much. Patients with severe periodontal problems must have this condition treated first. Those with large and numerous resin or porcelain restorations are cautioned that these restorations may not bleach as well as the tooth surface and may need replacement due to color mismatch. Patients under 13 years of age are requested to wait until an older age.

When the patient makes the decision to complete the process, an alginate impression and bite registration are taken and an appointment is made for the office bleach session and instruction in the home regimen. The patient is released until that time.

Between the first and second appointments, the impressions are poured into a stone study cast; a clear, acrylic tray is constructed using the cast as a model. The tray is trimmed very closely to the gingival sulcus (approximately 3 mm) so when gel is inserted and expressed upon the teeth, the gel will not spread upon the gingival tissues and cause irritation.

The patient returns for the second appointment and receives the office bleaching procedure, which is followed by a training session in the home bleaching process. The office bleaching procedure involves placing a bleaching gel on the polished tooth surface for a specified period of time, followed by rinsing and drying. The placement of the bleaching gel may be accomplished by painting the gel directly on the facial surface or immersing the teeth in gel that has been placed in a bite tray fabricated upon the patient's stone study model.

Because of the oxidizing property of the gel, protection for adjacent tissue surfaces must be provided by dental dam placement or by covering the gingiva with a protective shield.

Upon completion of the office bleaching process, the assistant may instruct the patient in the procedure for home care. The patient is taught how to apply the gel to the teeth for the prescribed time and method.

The third appointment is merely to verify the results and monitor the progress and treatment.

PROCEDURE 31

Assisting with Tooth Bleaching Appointments

Visit 1

1 Complete the Preparations

2 Assist with Examination and Consultation

3 Take Photographs

4 Assist with Impressions

5 Cleanup Procedures

Visit 2

6 Complete the Preparations

7 Assist with Coronal Polish of Teeth

8 Assist with Gel Placement

9 Review Instructions for Home Care

10 Dismiss the Patient and Clean Up

Visit 3

11 Complete the Preparations

12 Assist with Assessment

13 Take Photographs

14 Dismiss the Patient and Clean Up

Visit 1

1 Complete the Preparations

The assistant may help in the initial tooth bleaching appointment by preparing the materials necessary for the consultation and impression visit. The equipment and materials needed follow:

▸ basic setup
▸ hand mirror and shade guide
▸ literature and photo examples of the bleaching process

▶ alginate impression material and equipment
▶ bite registration for trimming of models
▶ photographic camera and equipment

The patient is greeted and seated for the appointment. The dentist may prefer to talk with the patient in a consultation room until the decision for acceptance is made and then transfer to the operatory for the impressions and bite registration; or, the consultation and impression taking may both be completed at chairside.

2 Assist with Examination and Consultation

During the consultation, the dentist examines the teeth for general condition, sensitivity, marginal leakage, and existing restorations. The treatment process is explained. The patient may be shown home education books or videos of the bleaching treatment. A moistened shade guide is placed against the patient's teeth in a natural light source. The matching shade number is recorded. The projected shade number may be moistened and shown to the patient. All findings and notations are recorded on the patient's chart.

3 Take Photographs

If the decision to accept the tooth bleaching regimen is made, the assistant takes photographs of the original tooth colors. This task is usually accomplished in a standard setting using the same background and lighting for each and every photo session. In this manner, the color differences will be more apparent.

A previously prepared identification card with patient's name and date may be placed around the patient's neck with a pair of alligator clips. The assistant inserts cheek retractors into the patient's mouth and requests the patient to hold them while a full face view photograph is exposed. Some dentists may also request side view photographs to be taken with the same method.

4 Assist with Impressions

The patient is seated in the dental chair. PPE is donned and the dentist is summoned for the impressions if the dental assistant is not permitted by state law to take alginate impressions. Those trained assistants who are allowed, may take an alginate impression of each arch and a wax bite registration, which will be used as patterns for the gel bite trays.

5 Cleanup Procedures

The patient is cleaned up and dismissed. An appointment for the second visit is made at this time. The assistant cleans up, disinfects, and sterilizes in the usual manner.

In the time period between the first and second visits, the impressions are made into stone study casts; a custom vinyl tray covering the crown areas of the teeth is fabricated.

Visit 2

6 Complete the Preparations

When the patient returns for the second visit, the assistant assembles the following equipment and materials for the office bleaching session and the instruction and demonstration of the home bleaching process:

▶ basic setup
▶ hand mirror
▶ patient's bite tray and carrying case
▶ prophy handpiece, cup or brush and pumice
▶ bleaching dam material
▶ bleaching material
▶ gauze

The patient is escorted to the operatory, seated, draped, and offered safety eyeglasses for protection from oxidizing chemicals. A bib is placed around the neck. The assistant dons PPE.

7 Assist with Coronal Polish of Teeth

In states where it is permissible, the dentist may request the assistant to polish or assist with the polish of the crowns of the teeth to remove any plaque or residue on the tooth surfaces that may interfere with the bleaching action of the gel. The mouth is rinsed.

8 Assist with Gel Placement

The assistant passes cotton rolls to the dentist for isolation of the teeth. A cheek retractor may be inserted into the front of the mouth to elevate the lips from the bleaching area. Liquid bleaching dam material is passed to the dentist, who covers the surrounding gingiva to protect from irritation. The tooth surfaces are air dried.

The assistant fills the patient's tray with a thin line of bleaching gel and passes the tray and gel to the dentist for insertion (Figure 6–35). An alternate method would be passing the bleaching gel syringe to the dentist for direct application to tooth surfaces. A gauze pad may be passed to remove any expressed excess of gel.

A saliva ejector is placed into the mouth to eliminate saliva buildup and moisture presence. The assistant may evacuate with the HVE tip if necessary. The bleaching process is timed (usually about 10 to 15 minutes). The

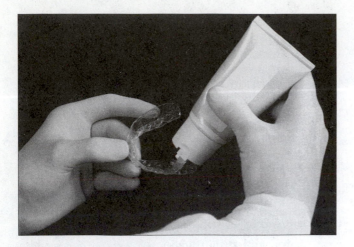

FIGURE 6–35 The bleaching tray does not extend onto the gingiva, so the gel will not come into contact with the gum area or cause irritation and blanching of tissues. The tray is filled with the gel material and inserted into the mouth for a prescribed amount of time.

tray is removed, and the mouth is rinsed. All bleaching dam material is peeled off and removed.

9 Review Instructions for Home Care

The dentist may instruct and demonstrate the home regimen or may delegate the assistant to teach the patient. The assistant reviews the dentist's prescription for home treatment, which may vary from patient to patient. Some patients are instructed to prepare and insert the tray at bedtime and remove upon awakening. Others are instructed to wear the tray during the day for one or two series of four-hour wear.

In either case, the patient is instructed to thoroughly brush and floss the teeth. The teeth are rinsed and the assistant demonstrates the procedure (minus the gel) using the patient's bite tray and study cast.

The assistant demonstrates how to express a thin line of gel into the moistened tray and insert the tray on the tooth crowns. A slight pressing or conforming of the tray to the tooth surfaces is completed with the index finger. Any gel material extruded from the tray in this conforming maneuver is wiped off with a gauze pad.

All patients are cautioned that some tingling and sensitivity may occur. Tissue whitening may be evident, but these symptoms will disappear in a few hours. If the patient suffers severe pain or sensitivity, he or she is requested to call the office immediately. The dentist may choose to prescribe fluoride mouthwashes and a mild analgesia for some patients.

The patient is told not to play with the seated tray with the fingers or tongue and to rinse the tray after removal from the mouth. Trays are to be removed for

eating. If the timed session is interrupted, the patient is instructed to rinse the tray, reinsert new gel, and continue the session.

Tobacco and food staining should be avoided by regulating the eating and smoking habits, and the bleaching gel material should not be placed in a warm place or sunlight.

Noticeable results should be seen within the first two weeks. The patient will remain on the regimen until satisfactory results are obtained. A recall appointment will be scheduled in two weeks to assess the results.

10 Dismiss the Patient and Clean Up

When the patient understands the instructions and feels confident of the ability to follow the home plan, the assistant requests removal of the tray and has the patient rinse the tray and place it in the carrying case. A quick review is made. The patient is scheduled for a recall appointment, dismissed, and sent home with the bite tray in the carrying case and a supply of gel material, syringes, or tubes.

The assistant gathers the materials, disinfects, sterilizes, and cleans up in the usual manner. The treatment is recorded on the patient's chart.

Visit 3

11 Complete the Preparations

During the third visit, the patient is recalled for a followup assessment. The assistant gathers the following material:

▶ basic setup
▶ sundry setup
▶ hand mirror
▶ shade guide
▶ photographic equipment

The patient is greeted and seated and a bib is placed around the neck. The assistant dons gloves.

12 Assist with Assessment

The dentist is handed a mirror for the exam assessment. A wet shade guide indicator is passed, and the operatory light is subdued for natural lighting. When the correct tooth shade is selected, the color is noted on the patient's chart.

13 Take Photographs

The assistant may take photographs of the recall visit using the same techniques and conditions as the first visit to ensure comparative examples.

14 Dismiss the Patient and Clean Up

If the results are satisfactory, the patient is dismissed. There may be a continuation of the bleaching process, and another appointment may be made. A recall appointment for future examination and preventive cleaning may be scheduled.

The assistant cleans up, disinfects, and sterilizes in the usual manner. The treatment is recorded on the patient's chart.▲

THEORY RECALL

Tooth Bleaching Appointments

1. What are the two methods that may be attempted to bleach teeth?

   a. _____

   b. _____

2. Which type of teeth may be bleached most easily?

   _____

3. What must patients with severe periodontal problems do before the bleaching process?

   _____

4. What may happen to large resin or porcelain restorations in a bleaching process?

   _____

5. What happens to the patient's impression during the first and second visit?

   _____

6. Why is the acrylic gel tray trimmed so closely to the gingiva?

   _____

7. What must be done to the teeth before the placement of the bleach gel?

   _____

8. In what two ways may the bleach gel be applied to the tooth surfaces?

   a. _____

   b. _____

9. What is the purpose of the shade guide's use in the bleaching visits?

   _____

10. Why are the lips elevated from the bleaching site?

   _____

Now turn to the Competency Evaluation Sheet for Procedure 31, Assisting with Tooth Bleaching Appointments, located in Appendix C of this text.

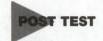

Total possible points = 100 points
80% needed for passing = 80 points

Total points this test _____ pass _____ fail _____

MULTIPLE CHOICE: Circle the correct answer. Each question is worth 2 points for a total of 100 points.

1. Offensive mouth odor may represent
   a. diabetes.   b. cancer.   c. anemia.   d. heart problems.

2. Photos are taken before and after cosmetic bleaching procedures to
   a. provide patient practice.   c. be used to choose the shade.
   b. use as a marketing tool.   d. use as a reference source.

3. The dental assistant wears overgloves when measuring and preparing alginate materials for impressions to
   a. protect from caustic materials.   c. prevent contamination.
   b. protect from materials' heat.   d. prevent material contact.

4. The last surface brushed in a toothbrushing procedure is
   a. upper occlusal.   b. lower occlusal.   c. all anteriors.   d. the tongue.

5. After placement and hardening of a composite restoration, how long does the dentist wait until the final finishing and polishing?
   a. no restrictions   b. 30 minutes   c. 2 hours   d. 48 hours

6. What are patients with large resin or porcelain restorations cautioned about when considering cosmetic bleaching of teeth?
   a. Restorations will react with bleach.   c. Restorations will be brighter than teeth.
   b. Restorations will be weakened.   d. Restorations may not match teeth.

7. Scaling of teeth consists of
   a. removing decay.   c. recording vitality.
   b. removing tartar and calculus.   d. measuring pocket depth.

8. After the impression procedure is finished, which trays are sterilized?
   a. those trays used   b. all exposed trays   c. mandibular trays   d. none

9. Interdental stimulators are used to (1) stimulate tissues, (2) remove debris and plaque, (3) clean gaps in teeth, and (4) stimulate tissue growth.
   a. 1 and 2   b. 1, 2, and 3   c. 2 and 3   d. all

10. Tooth surfaces are etched prior to the application of sealants to
    a. soften enamel.   b. soften dentin.   c. sterilize field.   d. flatten pits.

11. Which of the following methods of toothbrushing is correct for patients?
    a. Bass   c. roll/rotating
    b. Stillman   d. whichever efficiently removes patient's plaque

12. Of the three conditions needed for decay, which can the patient control?
    a. germs   b. teeth   c. food   d. none

13. In a dental dam application, why is a ligature wrapped around the arch of the clamp?
    a. for safety   c. for the stability of the clamp
    b. for easy removal   d. to indicate work site

14. Choice of base and liners under restorations is determined by
    a. the size of preparation.   c. the classification of restoration.
    b. the color of restorative material.   d. the type of restorative material used.

15. How long does the dentist wait before the final finishing and polishing of an amalgam restoration?
    a. no restrictions   b. 24 hours   c. at least 72 hours   d. at least 1 month

16. Wedges are used with matrix placement to
   a. prevent overhanging restorations.   c. indicate work site.
   b. hold preparation space open.   d. hold matrix band on tooth.

17. A needle is recapped for possible reuse by an assistant using (1) the one-handed recap method, (2) the two-handed method, or (3) a recapping device.
   a. 1 and 2   b. 1 and 3   c. 2 and 3   d. all of the above

18. Which type of glove does the assistant use when sterilizing and cleaning?
   a. latex exam gloves   b. plastic overgloves   c. utility gloves   d. linen undergloves

19. Which type of handpiece is used in the finishing and polishing of restorations?
   a. slow speed   b. high speed   c. ultrasonic   d. lab bench engine

20. Which type of tray is used to dispense and hold bleaching gel during the office cosmetic bleaching process?
   a. acrylic   b. perforated plastic   c. metal   d. water-cooled metal

21. When should the assistant pass an instrument?
   a. when the assistant feels the need   c. when signaled to pass
   b. when the assistant knows the procedure time   d. after the dentist passes the instrument to the assistant

22. An alginate impression is considered which type of reproduction?
   a. gypsum   b. negative   c. positive   d. neutral

23. How long is the patient advised not to eat or drink after an office topical fluoride treatment?
   a. 30 minutes   b. two hours   c. all day   d. it does not matter

24. Water is jetted onto ultrasonic tips to (1) clear the area, (2) cool the area, (3) soften the noise, or (4) open pockets.
   a. 1 and 2   b. 1, 2, and 3   c. 1, 3, and 4   d. all

25. Adding antimicrobial water to the alginate may be done to
   a. lessen germ activity.   b. hasten set.   c. delay set.   d. no effect.

26. Disclosing tablets and solution are used to
   a. disclose decay.   c. disclose sugar content.
   b. disclose plaque.   d. disclose overhanging restorations.

27. How does the dentist check for successful sealant application?
   a. x-ray   b. visual observation   c. explorer tip   d. finger palpation

28. What instrument is used to invert a dental dam?
   a. dental dam punch   b. dental dam clamp holder   c. blunt instrument   d. hemostat or pliers

29. Anterior restorations can be classified in what class? (1) Class I, (2) Class II, (3) Class III, (4) Class IV, or (5) Class V
   a. 1 and 2   b. 1, 2, and 3   c. 1, 3, and 4   d. 1, 3, 4, and 5

30. Cotton rolls can be used in dental procedures to (1) isolate the teeth, (2) control the tongue, (3) retract the cheek, or (4) retard moisture.
   a. 1, 2, and 3   b. 1, 2, and 4   c. 1 and 4   d. all

31. Restorative materials can be supplied in capsule forms to
   a. provide economy.   c. match colors.
   b. provide constant measurement.   d. make ordering easy.

32. If a material needs to be cured by a light-cure appliance, the assistant employs
   a. PPE.   b. a special shield or glasses.   c. no special care.   d. a special drape.

33. Articulating paper is used in the dental practice to
   a. indicate high spots.   c. indicate sterilization.
   b. make paper copies.   d. indicate supply levels.

34. Which side of the matrix band is longer?
   a. coronal   b. neither   c. gingival   d. holder side

35. The amalgam carrier is loaded in small increments to
    a. help mix materials.   b. eliminate air pockets.   c. eliminate masses.   d. help the setting time.

36. Which abrasive point is first used in finishing and polishing restorations?
    a. least abrasive   b. doesn't matter   c. most abrasive   d. none are used

37. Which instrument is used to mix and carry calcium hydroxide material?
    a. amalgam carrier   b. a large blunt instrument   c. PFI   d. a small ball burnisher

38. During the amalgam carving process, what is the duty of the assistant?
    a. to spray air on site   b. to spray water on site   c. to condense the mix   d. none

39. After finishing and contouring a restoration, the next procedure is to
    a. polish.   b. condense.   c. scale.   d. carve.

40. The crowns of the teeth are dried before fluoride application to
    a. improve visibility.   b. expose decay.   c. prevent dilution of fluoride.   d. comfort the patient.

41. Which is *not* considered a good use for ZOE?
    a. temporary restoration   c. base under amalgam restoration
    b. sedative gingival pack   d. base under composite restoration

42. After the dental dam material is removed, the assistant looks for
    a. blood.   c. excess filling material.
    b. a stretched size.   d. missing dental dam material.

43. The dentist uses dental floss before the application of the dental dam to
    a. locate loose restorations.   c. check tight areas.
    b. prevent overhanging restorations.   d. spread contact points.

44. Which of the following appliances is *not* considered to be effective in a prophylaxis procedure?
    a. an electrosurgical tip   b. an ultrasonic tip   c. a handpiece   d. an air polisher

45. Fluoride, that is drunk, is considered which type of application?
    a. systemic   b. local   c. topical   d. surface

46. When is the ideal time for the application of office fluoride treatment?
    a. when the tooth erupts   c. after prophy
    b. anytime   d. when work is completed

47. Subplaster study models are considered which type of reproduction?
    a. positive   b. negative   c. neutral   d. neither

48. If a material needs to be light cured, what precautions should the assistant take?
    a. a special drape   c. PPE
    b. a special shield or eyeglasses   d. none

49. Sealants are used in dentistry to
    a. lock in restoration.   c. seal denture edges.
    b. seal tissues under the restoration.   d. seal out decay processes.

50. Dental dam clamps are designed for
    a. a specific tooth.   b. the patient's age.   c. the work site.   d. each quadrant.

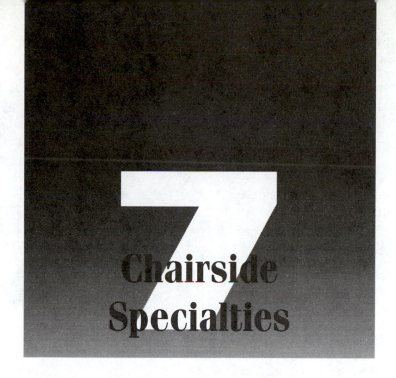

7 Chairside Specialties

◢ OBJECTIVES

Upon completion of this unit, the student will achieve a score of 80% or better on the Post Test covering the following material.

1. Describe the duties and responsibilities of the dental assistant during the preliminary examination of a pediatric patient, including the coronal polishing of teeth, application of sealants, and fluoride treatment.
2. List the various types and methods of pulpal treatment for children and the procedural application of protective covers and crowns to the affected teeth.
3. Discuss the types, purposes, and methods for application of space maintainers for a pediatric patient.
4. Demonstrate the duties and responsibilities of the dental assistant in a preliminary examination for a endodontic patient.
5. Describe the procedure for each of the multiple visits required for the endodontic treatment of root canal therapy.
6. Determine the differences between fixed and removable prosthodontic appliances, and give examples of each type.
7. Describe the duties and responsibilities of the dental assistant during the impression, preparation, try in, and final visit appointments for patients receiving either a fixed or removable prosthodontic appliance.

◢ KEY TERMS

abutment	effervescent	pediatric dentistry
acrylic	exfoliate	percussion
adjacent	extirpation	pontic
appliance	homogeneous	primary
avulsed	hyperactive	reconstruction
biomechanical	irrigation	revitalization
calcification	mallet	sealant
catalyst	medicament	secondary
caustic	misalignment	sensitivity
degenerative	mobility	transillumination
dental crown	necrotic	vitality
denture	palpate	

PEDIATRIC DENTISTRY

Pediatric dentistry is the branch or area of dentistry that involves working with the child patient. The pediatric patient age may begin at 18 months and continue until somewhere around the age of 12, when the child receives the permanent second molars. During this time span, the patient's mouth contains only **primary** teeth (up to approximately age 6); then a mixed dentition of primary and **secondary** teeth appears.

With the exception of a slight modification in the size and shape of a few instruments, the dental procedures and techniques are basically the same for the child and the adult. The main area of difference is in the handling and relationship of the child and the professional staff.

The pediatric dental assistant must be both fast and slow working with the child. All techniques and procedures must be well rehearsed and worked out so treatment flows at a rapid pace. The assistant must never give a rushed appearance or do abrupt movements to startle and worry the patient.

The assistant must respect the child as a person, listen to the child, show warmth and concern, speak softly but firmly, and initiate conversation with the child. Never make fun or ignore the child's fears for all fears are real and have a background that one may not be aware of.

Don't talk "baby talk" but place the level of conversation slightly higher than the child's. Encourage the child to take an interest by showing the operation of the triple syringe or prophy angle. Give the child a little control, such as choosing the color of bib or mouthwash flavor and explain procedures beforehand.

Dental care for a child is very necessary to:

► assure the function of the teeth for chewing, speaking, and appearance;
► help maintain the integrity of the primary teeth to avoid premature loss;
► help maintain the normal growth pattern of the jaws and teeth; and
► ensure that the child does not suffer pain or discomfort from decayed or abscessed teeth.

The first dental appointment of the child patient should include a dental examination and evaluation, polishing of the teeth, some x-rays, and perhaps a fluoride treatment with tooth brushing lessons (Figure 7–1). The exact procedure depends mostly on the age and condition of the new patient. Very young children are slowly introduced to the chair and equipment, while older children receive full evaluative treatment. Children with dental problems may receive emergency dental care.

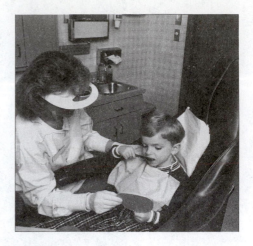

FIGURE 7–1 The dental assistant begins the child-dental profession relationship.

Fluoride Application

After the plaque has been polished off during the initial visit, the dentist may order a fluoride treatment for the child. Application of a fluoride substance is done as a topical protective measure. Fluoride in the form of a gel, foam, spray, or solution is applied to strengthen the enamel tissues of the teeth to help reduce decay of erupted and newly erupting teeth. Topical fluoride may be applied to isolated, air-dried teeth in a prepared liquid, gel, or foam fluoride treatment. After the fluoride has been placed on the surfaces of the teeth, the patient is requested to sit for one to four minutes with a saliva ejector and isolation cotton rolls, maintaining a dry field. The procedure is repeated for each arch.

Fluoride rinses may be more comfortable for a child who is able to follow directions to swish and empty the mouth. A concentrated office fluoride treatment of a two-part stannous fluoride and an acidulated phosphated fluoride (APF) system may be measured out through a pump dispenser. Each half may be swished in the mouth for one minute and emptied.

The most popular method for fluoride application is through the single or double tray procedure. Fluoride gel or foam is supplied in many flavors from bubble gum to chocolate mint. The gel or foam is dispensed into disposable, premeasured trays and placed into a dry mouth area. Single trays complete one arch application at one time, while the double-sided disposable trays may be filled and apply fluoride gel or foam to both arches at the same application. Some trays supplied by manufacturers come with tray liners, which may be placed inside the tray before the fluoride is applied. When these trays are placed in the mouth, the patient may be instructed to bite down. A pair of cotton rolls may be placed on each side in the bicuspid or midmolar area for comfort. The added pressure from the bite may force fluoride into the interproximal areas. The trays remain in the mouth for the manufacturer's recommended time period (60 seconds to 4 minutes). The child is cautioned not to swallow the saliva generated at this time, if possible.

When the trays have been removed, the patient may empty the mouth, but excessive rinsing is avoided. The assistant may wipe off any visible excessive fluoride to avoid aftertaste. The patient and parent are advised that no eating or drinking is to take place for 30 minutes to 1 hour.

Topical fluoride application may be supplemented at home with prescribed fluoride mouth rinses and the use of a fluoridated toothpaste. If the child is not exposed to drinking water containing fluoride, the dentist may prescribe a fluoride and vitamin prescription to supply the needed systemic protection.

Sealant Application

A newly erupted tooth possesses the total shape and size of the crown of the tooth but lacks the final completion of the root and **calcification** of the tissues. This hardening process is not completed until approximately two years after the tooth's eruption. During the time of final development of the tooth, the dentist may wish to protect the incomplete void areas in the deep enamel pits and fissures of the occlusal surface with a resin material, called a **sealant**. This hard plastic serves as a barrier between the tooth and plaque-forming decay that may accumulate in these vulnerable areas. The sealant material provides time for the calcification of the tooth tissue and for the child to develop a good pattern of dental hygiene practices.

Sealant resin is applied only to newly exposed, undecayed occlusal surfaces. A carious area is never covered by the material. After the crowns of the teeth have received a coronal polishing, the occlusal surface is prepared for the sealant resin by a process called etching. This processing solution or gel contains a phosphoric or citric acid, which softens and conditions the enamel tissue to accept and hold the resin seal. *Some manufacturers have developed a sealant that does not require the etching step.

Pit and fissure sealant material, which is placed on the etched surfaces of the tooth crowns, is supplied in clear, opaque, or lightly tinted colors and in self-curing or light-cured materials. The self-curing material, called auto-cured sealant, is supplied in two pastes, which are mixed together with a stirring stick. The final paste, which has a working time of approximately 1 to 2 minutes, is applied to the pre-etched occlusal surface and spread into a light covering, being careful not to leave voids or opening. When the manufacturer's recommended time has passed for curing, the sealant material is checked with the point of an explorer to determine if

the seal is hard and completely covers the area leaving no voids or openings for plaque to accumulate and build.

The visible light-curing sealant is applied with a brush or applicator tip or straw that is provided by the manufacturer. The sealant is spread onto the surface in a light coating, covering all of the area. When the application is finished, the material is cured by placing the tip of the visible light wand a few millimeters from the sealant material for the manufacturer's prescribed time (usually 10 to 20 seconds) for each surface application. An explorer point is used to test the effectiveness and hardness of the sealant after processing.

Neither type of sealant is applied in too heavy a surface as to interfere with occlusion. After the material is hard, the sealant is checked for any overpacked areas and a finishing rotary stone is used to remove any excess buildup. The sealant-prepared teeth are carefully monitored throughout the patient's following dental visits. Re-applications may be made if there is a need. The sealant placement procedure is illustrated in Figure 7–2.

PROCEDURE 32

Assisting with the Initial Exam and Preventive Techniques in Pediatric Dentistry

1 Assemble Materials and Equipment

2 Prepare the Patient

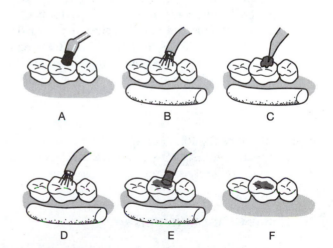

A B C

D E F

FIGURE 7-2 Sealant procedure: (A) Teeth are cleaned and polished. (B) Surfaces are rinsed and dried. (C) Isolated crown is acid-etched. (D) Acid is timed and rinsed away. (E) Sealant is painted and dabbed on surface of tooth. (F) The finished sealant protects the tooth.

3   **Don PPE**

4   **Assist with Examination**

5   **Assist with Coronal Polish**

6   **Assist with Supplemental Diagnostic Procedures (Radiological Exam)**

7   **Assist with Supplemental Preventive Procedures**

8   **Clean Up Patient**

9   **Clean Up Operatory**

10   **Clean Up Materials and Equipment**

1   Assemble Materials and Equipment

To assist with the initial examination and visit, the assistant should assemble the following:

- basic setup
- slow handpiece with prophy cup and paste, floss
- disposable items (cups, bib, napkin, gauze, cotton rolls, pellets)
- radiographic film and equipment
- fluoride with necessary equipment, or sealant and equipment
- evacuation tips
- dental dam (optional)

2   Prepare the Patient

The assistant greets the patient with a positive attitude. The child is seated in the chair and introduced to the equipment. The patient is draped, and a bib is placed around the neck. The procedure to be performed is explained. The parent is questioned regarding the child's medical history. Some offices may have had the parent or guardian fill out a preprinted questionnaire and treatment permission slip. The forms are carefully reviewed.

3   Don PPE

The assistant dons the PPE. Some children may inquire about the gear. The assistant will answer the questions honestly and sincerely but need not go into much depth.

4   Assist with Examination

The assistant may spray rinse the child's mouth and even permit the child to operate the spray syringe. The assistant clues the dentist on the conversation at hand and prepares to take notes on the patient's chart. The dentist examines the child, beginning with an appraisal of the child's general appearance, palpates the neck and throat area, and examines the lips. When entering the mouth, the dentist may appraise the mouth, lip, cheek tissues, and general dental health and care. The assistant may pass gauze for the dentist to grasp and lift the child's tongue to examine all areas. A mirror and explorer are passed so the dentist may evaluate and chart the tooth conditions. The assistant neatly and accurately records all findings of the exam. If the dentist signals for a rinse or tissue retraction, the assistant passes the syringe and assists with cheek and lip retraction.

5   Assist with Coronal Polish

Upon receiving the explorer, the assistant passes the slow handpiece with a prophy cup and paste to the dentist for coronal polishing. The dappen dish or container of paste is held near the work site for refilling and use. *In some states, the trained, expanded function duty assistant may perform the coronal polishing procedure, using a prophylaxis brush or cup and polishing the crowns of plaque and buildup.

    The assistant should be ready to pass or use the syringe for rinsing of the mouth and the HVE for evacuation of the area. The dentist may wish to re-examine tooth surfaces for caries, so the assistant may pass an explorer and dental floss at the dentist's signal.

6   Assist with Supplemental Diagnostic Procedures (Radiological Exam)

The dentist may desire to have a radiologic examination of the existing teeth as well as the erupting and forming dentition. A request for periapical, occlusal, or panoramic exposures may be ordered. The assistant assists with or, if permitted by state law, obtains these exposures.

7   Assist with Supplemental Preventive Procedures

If the dentist wishes to apply topical fluoride or occlusal surface sealants at this appointment, the assistant aids; if permitted by state law, the assistant performs these procedures following the prescribed techniques in Unit 6.

8   Clean Up Patient

Once the supplemental procedures have been completed, the assistant passes the syringe for a light spray rinse of the child's mouth. The patient's face is wiped off, and the bib and drape are removed. The patient is cautioned for the lowering of the chair and the child and parent are given any postoperative instructions. The child is dismissed.

9 Clean Up Operatory

The assistant gathers contaminated materials and equipment and takes them to the sterilizing area. The latex gloves are removed, placed in the proper container, and hands are washed. The treatment is recorded on the patient's chart, and the chart is taken to the front desk or appropriate place.

10 Clean Up Materials and Equipment

The assistant returns, dons utility gloves and PPE, and disinfects the operatory. The disposables are placed in the proper containers. The large articles are disinfected, and the instruments are cleaned and prepared for sterilizing. The area is cleaned up. The gloves are washed, disinfected, and removed; hands are washed.▲

T H E O R Y R E C A L L
Pediatric Dentistry

1. Pediatric dentistry deals with what branch of dentistry?

2. What does the term mixed dentition mean?

3. What do we mean when we say an assistant must be fast and slow in pediatric assisting?

4. State three reasons dental care for children is a necessity.

   a.

   b.

   c.

5. Why is fluoride applied to the teeth?

6. Describe the methods in which fluoride may be topically applied in the dental office.

7. What part of the final formations of the tooth is *not* present at eruption time?

8. How can the assistant make the child feel more comfortable when seating the patient?

9. The surfaces of properly etched teeth should have what appearance?

10. What two ways may the teeth receiving the sealant be isolated?

Now turn to the Competency Evaluation Sheet for Procedure 32, Assisting with the Initial Exam and Preventive Techniques in Pediatric Dentistry, located in Appendix C of this text.

PULP THERAPY AND PROTECTIVE CROWNS

Operative dentistry for the pediatric patient is similar to the adult patient, but many times pulp involvement can be treated more successfully in a child due to the larger opening in the apical foramen and the increased circulation in the pulpal chamber. There are three possible ways to perform treatment for the pulp tissue of primary teeth. These methods are pulp capping, pulpotomy, and pulpectomy.

Pulp capping involves the placing of a medication, usually calcium hydroxide, over a small pulpal exposure (Figure 7–3A). The calcium hydroxide soothes the irritated pulp and stimulates the formation of secondary dentin in the tooth. This practice is performed regularly in the normal restoration of primary and permanent teeth.

A pulpotomy is more involved than pulp capping (Figure 7–3B). If the pulp exposure is large, the dentist may choose to remove the coronal portion of the pulp and place a medication over the pulp stumps. The medication may be calcium hydroxide or, in the case of bleeding, Formo-Cresol may be used after the pulp removal. After the cotton pellet of formocresol is removed and the bleeding has ceased, the chamber receives a layer of zinc oxide and eugenol and is covered by a protective crown. If the bleeding is persistent, a cotton pellet of formocresol is left in the chamber, sealed under a temporary restoration, and reappointed in 3 to 5 days.

A pulpectomy is even more involved than a pulpotomy (Figure 7–3C). This procedure requires the removal of the pulp tissue in the crown and root. This pulpal **extirpation** is usually performed following the technique for root canal. The pulp is removed, and the canals are cleaned and irrigated and then filled with a zinc oxide eugenol paste. All procedures performed in a pulpotomy and pulpectomy are carried on with strict aseptic technique as these treatments are an invasion into the bloodstream.

Protective Crowns

Protective crowns are a useful and durable way to cover and protect primary teeth and also may serve as a temporary restorative measure for some permanent teeth situations.

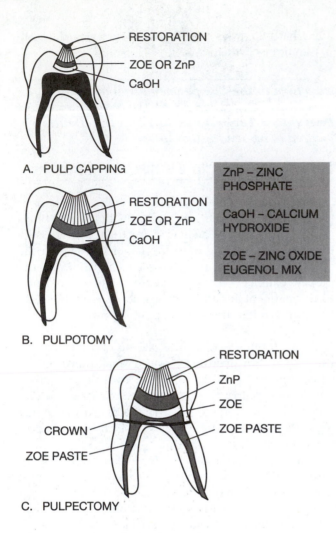

A. PULP CAPPING
- RESTORATION
- ZOE OR ZnP
- CaOH

B. PULPOTOMY
- RESTORATION
- ZOE OR ZnP
- CaOH

ZnP – ZINC PHOSPHATE

CaOH – CALCIUM HYDROXIDE

ZOE – ZINC OXIDE EUGENOL MIX

C. PULPECTOMY
- RESTORATION
- ZnP
- ZOE
- ZOE PASTE
- CROWN
- ZOE PASTE

FIGURE 7–3 Pulp cap therapy: (A) pulp capping, (B) pulpotomy, and (C) pulpectomy.

Protective crowns can be indicated:

▸ when a tooth is too broken down to hold an amalgam restoration,
▸ when a tooth crown has been fractured,
▸ where the enamel of a child's dentition is underdeveloped (hypoplasia),
▸ as a temporary restoration until development of the permanent dentition,
▸ over pulpal tissue undergoing therapy,
▸ as part of an appliance, and
▸ as a protective barrier tooth covering for a handicapped child.

Crowns may be manufactured out of different materials and in different shapes and forms. They may be made of chrome, stainless steel shapes, aluminum shells with no anatomic pattern, or preshaped resin forms. They come in assorted sizes and are measured to fit the tooth under repair. Choice depends on the child's age, the tooth condition, and the tooth position.

When the tooth receiving the crown has been prepared, it is measured with a boley gauge for the selection of a protective crown. A matching sized crown is passed and tried on for fit. Further selection may be made by selecting larger or smaller crown shapes until the properly fitting one is chosen. This final crown is scratched with an explorer when it is to be cemented in place to indicate the direction of fit.

Minor alterations to the crown shape may need to be made. The assistant is ready to pass crown and collar scissors for cutting away excess and then followed with a slow handpiece with finishing stone for smoothing rough edges. Crimping pliers may also be needed to alter the shape of the crown for better adaptations at the final fit. An explorer is used to test the final fitting.

The prepared tooth receives two light coats of varnish for protection under the crown, and the tooth is air dried. If a dental dam had been applied for preparation, it is now removed for the cementation procedure.

The zinc phospate cement is prepared, mixed to a creamy consistency, and passed to the dentist, who applies the cement to the prepared tooth. The assistant loads the prepared crown on all surfaces and passes it to the dentist for seating, which is aided by the patient biting on a bite stick for pressure adaptation.

The cement is allowed to harden. The excess is removed and the patient is cleaned up and dismissed. The protective crown remains in place to protect the tooth until it **exfoliates**, or a permanent crown is made.

P R O C E D U R E   3 3

Assisting with Pulp Treatment and Protective Covers

1 Assemble Equipment and Prepare the Patient

2 Assist with Topical and Local Anesthesia

3 Assist with Dental Dam

4 Assist with Tooth Preparation

5 Assist with Pulp Sterilization and Bleeding Control

6 Assist with Protective Cover Selection

7 Assist with Reduction of Crown Form

8 Assist with Medication of Prepared Tooth

9 Assist with Dental Dam Removal

10 Assist with Cementation of the Crown

11 Assist with Cleanup of Tooth

12 Assist with Polish of Crown

13 Cleanup Procedures

1 Assemble Equipment and Prepare the Patient

The setup for a protective crown placement is:

- anesthetic setup
- dental dam setup
- basic setup
- cavity preparation setup
- sundry setup
- assortment of crowns
- boley gauge or metric rule
- curved crown and collar scissors
- contouring and plain pliers
- fissured bur, slow handpiece, heatless stone, finishing burs
- cavity varnish
- bite stick
- articulating paper and holder
- polishing cup and pumice
- zinc phosphate cement and equipment

The patient is greeted, seated, draped, and prepared. The assistant, who has already questioned the patient's parent regarding the health history of the child, establishes communication and understanding with the child and then dons PPE.

2 Assist with Topical and Local Anesthesia

After checking the proposed treatment plan, the assistant rinses or sprays the patient's mouth, dries the injection area and places topical anesthetic on the injection site. The dentist is summoned, and the assistant passes the anesthetic syringe while receiving the used topical anesthetic applicator. The assistant receives the syringe and monitors the patient for quick movements and anesthetic reaction.

3 Assist with Dental Dam

The assistant helps with the placement of the dental dam by passing the prepared dental dam material and premeasured clamp in the clamp holder. The napkin is passed next; the assistant aids in the placement of the napkin and the frame. Ligatures are passed to the dentist and the assistant helps with their placement and tie off. The saliva ejector tip is placed under the dam, opposite the work site area.

4 Assist with Tooth Preparation

The assistant passes mirror and handpiece with bur or disk to the dentist for removal of decay and preparation of the tooth. The assistant maintains visibility and

a dry field, while exchanging handpiece, hand instruments, and rotor equipment at the dentist's request.

5 Assist with Pulp Sterilization and Bleeding Control

To assist with the control of bleeding, the assistant passes a pellet moistened with Formo-Cresol to be placed onto the bleeding pulpal site. The pellet is permitted to remain for five minutes and then removed. If the bleeding is not controlled, the dentist may decide to place a pellet into the pulpal chamber and temporarily close the tooth for a final coverage at a later date, usually one week. If the bleeding is under control, the pellet is removed and the selection of the cover is made.

6 Assist with Protective Cover Selection

When the tooth has been prepared, the assistant aids in the selection of a crown form by passing a boley gauge or rule for initial measurement and then matching sized crown to the dentist for fit. This procedure is repeated until a properly sized one is selected. At that time, the assistant passes an explorer to the dentist to mark measuring lines and surfaces. The assistant receives the explorer from the dentist, and the crown is removed for reduction.

7 Assist with Reduction of Crown Form

The curved crown and collar scissors are passed to the dentist for reduction cuts. The assistant accepts the scissors and passes a slow handpiece with finishing bur or disk stone for smoothing the cut surface. When the dentist is satisfied with the cut and returns the handpiece, the assistant passes crimping pliers to shape and contour the crown.

8 Assist with Medication of Prepared Tooth

The assistant obtains a pellet wet with cavity varnish, passes it to the dentist, and then passes or applies a gentle air spray to dry the area. The process is repeated until two coats are applied. If the dentist prefers to place pulpal medication first, the assistant mixes and prepares the medication according to the manufacturer's directions and passes some on an instrument. The excess mixture is held near the operative site for use in refilling the pulp area as needed.

9 Assist with Dental Dam Removal

The assistant passes the clamp holder to the dentist for clamp removal and receives both in time to pass scissors for cutting of dental dam and ligatures. The assistant receives the ligatures, dental dam material, napkin, and frame. While passing the triple syringe to the dentist, the assistant rinses the patient's mouth and lightly massages the area.

10 Assist with Cementation of the Crown

At the dentist's signal, the assistant mixes the zinc phosphate cement to a creamy consistency according to the manufacturer's directions. Cotton rolls are passed to the dentist for isolation of the preparation. The assistant fills the crown and passes it to the dentist, who seats the crown on the preparation. The assistant passes a wood bite stick for the patient to bite on to help complete the seating process. An explorer or excavator is passed to the dentist to wipe away any overhanging wet cement. The assistant may evacuate the mouth of saliva and moisture during the cementation.

11 Assist with Cleanup of Tooth

When the cement has hardened, the assistant passes a mirror and scaler or hand instrument to fleck off excess cement. The instrument is received and an explorer is passed for testing fit and cementation. The cotton rolls are removed and handed to the assistant who passes or holds the articulating paper holder and paper on the occlusal surface while the patient bites. If any adjustment is to be made, the dentist requests the needed finishing bur.

12 Assist with Polish of Crown

When the occlusion has been adjusted, the assistant hands the dentist the slow handpiece with a rubber cup of pumice to polish the crown. The mouth is rinsed. The patient's face is cleaned up, and the assistant may offer a hand mirror to the patient to see the new crown. The assistant gives the patient postoperative instructions and reviews them with the parent. The patient is dismissed.

13 Cleanup Procedures

The assistant gathers the contaminated materials and equipment and takes them to the sterilizing room. Latex exam gloves are removed, disposed of properly, and the hands are washed. The assistant then records treatment on the patient's chart and takes it to the front desk.

The assistant returns, dons utility gloves and PPE, and disinfects the operatory room. The equipment and instruments are cleaned and prepared for sterilization. Large articles are disinfected and the area is cleaned up. The utility gloves are washed, disinfected, and removed. The assistant washes hands.▲

THEORY RECALL

Pulp Therapy and Protective Crowns

1. What are the three possible methods to treat a damaged pulp?

   a. _____

   b. _____

   c. _____

2. What medication is placed over the exposed pulp tissue in a pulp capping? Why?

   _____

3. Why is the aseptic technique so important in a pulpotomy or pulpectomy?

   _____

4. What medications may a dentist call for the coronal area after a pulpotomy?

   _____

5. Give four examples of when a protective crown can be used in pediatric dentistry.

   a. _____

   b. _____

   c. _____

   d. _____

6. What kinds of materials are used in protective crowns?

   _____

7. After the tooth has been prepared for a protective crown, what does the assistant pass to the dentist to determine the size of the crown?

   _____

8. What material is mixed for cementation under the protective crown?

   _____

9. After the tooth is seated, what does the assistant hold on the occlusal surfaces to test for the correct height of the crown?

   _____

10. With whom does the assistant review the postoperative instructions?

   _____

Now turn to the Competency Evaluation Sheet for Procedure 33, Assisting with Pulp Treatment and Protective Covers, located in Appendix C of this text.

SPACE MAINTAINERS

Space maintainers are removable or fixed appliances that provide or hold an opening to compensate for a missing tooth. They are used to prevent drifting of teeth into the open area and causing **misalignment** and malpositioning of the remaining teeth. The appliances are placed at the tooth loss time and permitted to remain until the eruption of the underlying, new permanent tooth.

The placement need and type of space maintainer used is dependent on the age of the patient, the amount and area involved, and the condition of the existing teeth. The dentist, pediatric dentist, or orthodontist may elect to use a band and loop or band-bar, spring-activated, or distal shoe type of appliance to maintain the opening.

The most popular types are the band and loop or band-bar types (Figure 7–4, part A) in which a band is placed on the larger tooth adjacent to the opening and a bar or loop is attached to extend to the side surface of the other tooth. A protective crown may be used instead of a band if there has been excessive decay or reconstruction done on the larger adjacent tooth.

If some time has occurred since the loss of the tooth, and movement of the teeth has already happened, the dentist may use a spring-activated bar to extend within the open area (Figure 7–4, part B). This bar maintains the present amount of space and regains more of the original area by the application of spring force.

If the tooth loss occurs at the distal end of the arch and there are not two teeth to use to hold space, the dentist may apply a band with a distal shoe bar to the last distal tooth (Figure 7–4C). The shoe bar will extend distally back and down into the gingival area until the erupting tooth is guided into the proper space. After eruption of the permanent tooth, the band and shoe bar are removed. The best time to place this type of appliance is at the time of extraction of the primary second molar.

The proper application of a space maintainer can prevent serious and costly orthodontic attention in later developmental stages of a child's dentition.

P R O C E D U R E   3 4

Assisting with Space Maintainers (Visits 1 and 2)

Visit 1

1 Assemble Equipment and Prepare the Patient

2 Assist with Band Placement

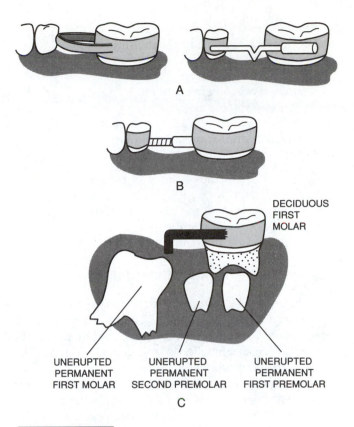

FIGURE 7–4 Examples of space maintainers: (A) band and loop or band-bar, (B) spring activated, (C) distal shoe bar.

3 Assist with Alginate Impression

4 Assist with Band and Crown Removal

5 Dismiss Patient and Clean Up

Visit 2

6 Gather Materials and Prepare the Patient

7 Assist with Try In of Appliance

8 Assist with Cementation

9 Assist with Cleanup of the Appliance and the Patient

10 Clean Up Operatory, Disinfect, and Sterilize

Visit 1

1 Assemble Equipment and Prepare the Patient

The equipment needed for visit 1 of the space maintainer procedure follows:

► basic and sundry setups
► assorted bands or primary crowns
► boley gauge or metric ruler

- band driver and band remover
- condenser or Schure instrument
- band stretcher pliers
- scaler
- adapting and contouring pliers
- crown and collar scissors
- slow handpiece with finishing disks and burs
- alginate material and equipment
- impression trays and wax rope

The patient's health history is reviewed with the parent, and then the patient is greeted and seated in the dental chair. A drape and bib are placed on the patient while the upcoming procedure is explained. The assistant dons PPE and summons the dentist.

2 Assist with Band Placement

The triple syringe may be used or passed to the dentist to rinse the patient's mouth. The excess moisture is evacuated, and an explorer and mouth mirror is passed for an examination of the general condition of the mouth and work area.

An estimated sized band or crown to be used in the space maintainer is passed to the dentist for a try in. The band driver or mallet is passed to seat the item. Bands or crowns may be removed by passing the band remover as needed. Larger or smaller bands and crowns may be called for as the sizing continues. The band stretcher or adapter and contouring pliers may be used to adapt the material for a proper fit.

If a crown is being used as an **abutment** part of the appliance, the dentist may wish to adjust the height by cutting with crown and collar scissors as needed. Any trimming of metal should be followed by a polishing or smoothing of edges with a finishing bur set in a slow handpiece.

When the correctly fitted band has been selected, the assistant passes an explorer to the dentist for scratch marking to indicate the position.

3 Assist with Alginate Impression

With the fitted band or crown in place, the assistant prepares for an alginate impression of the arch. An impression tray of approximate size is passed for testing of fit. The assistant may have previously measured the patient for tray size before summoning the dentist for the visit. If any adaptation of the tray is needed, wax may be added to the tray edges and the tray retested for fit before the impression is continued.

When the proper tray has been fitted and adapted, if needed, the patient's mouth is rinsed and air dried. The assistant mixes the alginate material to a creamy consistency and loads the tray, which is passed to the dentist for seating. The impression tray registers the positions of the units for the maintainer (Figure 7–5).

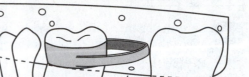
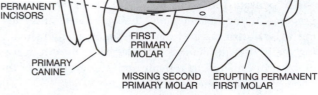

FIGURE 7–5 The impression registers the placement of all units of the space maintainer.

After the material has set, the tray is removed, rinsed, and disinfected. The assistant places the tray and impression into a plastic bag, without touching the outside of the bag. *The bag may be prepared ahead of the procedure by placing an applicator stick in the opening to keep the area free to insert without touching sides.

4 Assist with Band and Crown Removal

The assistant passes the triple syringe to the dentist to rinse after the impression and then passes the band remover or scaler to remove the band or crown from the tooth. The instrument and the band are returned to the assistant, who rinses the band, disinfects, and places it into the bag with the alginate impression.

5 Dismiss Patient and Clean Up

The patient's face is wiped off. The bib and drape are removed. The chair is lowered after cautioning the patient about the movement. The patient is dismissed.

The assistant removes the exam gloves, washes hands, writes the procedure on the patient's chart, and returns the chart to the front desk. Another appointment is made for the final setting and cementation of the space maintainer. The plastic bag, which was previously marked with the patient's name and is now holding the impression and band, is closed from the outside.

The assistant dons utility gloves and PPE. The instruments and materials are gathered and taken to the sterilization room where they are cleaned, disinfected, or sterilized. The area is cleaned up. The utility gloves are washed, dried, disinfected, and removed. The hands are washed.

Visit 2

6 Gather Materials and Prepare the Patient

The equipment needed for the second visit for a space maintainer follows:

- basic and sundry setups
- prepared space maintainer appliance
- band driver or pusher and mallet, band remover
- condenser or Schure instrument
- cementation equipment and materials
- plastic filling instrument (PFI)
- articulating paper and holder
- contouring and adapting pliers
- band stretcher pliers
- slow handpiece with finishing burs, disks, prophy cup, and pumice
- bite stick

The patient is greeted and seated. A bib is placed, and the procedure is explained. The assistant dons PPE and summons the dentist.

7 Assist with Try in of Appliance

The patient's mouth is rinsed and evacuated of excess moisture. A mirror and explorer are passed to the dentist for an examination of the general condition of the mouth and the work area. The prepared **appliance** is passed to the dentist for a try in. A band pusher is passed and received. If any adaptation is needed, pliers and band stretchers may be passed. The articulation is checked after the seating of the appliance is made.

8 Assist with Cementation

The band remover is passed to the dentist to remove the appliance from the anchor tooth. The space maintainer is checked for any roughness and is polished or smoothed.

The assistant either polishes the crown of the tooth with a prophy cup and pumice in a slow handpiece or passes the equipment to the dentist for a coronal cleaning prior to the cementation of the appliance. The mouth is rinsed, evacuated, and air dried.

Overgloves are donned, or the assistant uses gauze pads as a barrier to place the cement materials on the cool glass slab. The cement is mixed to a smooth consistency and loaded into the inner surface of the band by approaching from the gingival edge of the band (Figure 7–6).

When all inner surfaces are evenly covered, the appliance is passed to the dentist. A band pusher is passed to seat the appliance. A mallet may be called for or the dentist may wish for the patient to assist by biting on a bite stick.

The assistant receives the band pusher and **mallet** and passes an explorer or PFI for the dentist to smooth off the excess cement. A wet gauze pad is held near the site to wipe off the instrument. The cement is permitted to harden. During this waiting period, the assistant may offer the patient a book to read or perhaps a hand-held video game to play.

9 Assist with Cleanup of the Appliance and the Patient

When the cement has hardened, the assistant passes the scaler to the dentist to remove the excess set cement. The assistant aspirates the excess with the HVE tip. In some states the assistant is permitted to remove the excess cement and polish the new crown.

The explorer is passed to the dentist to check the cementation process and final fit. The assistant receives the explorer and passes the triple syringe for a final mouth rinse. The mouth is evacuated. The patient is cleaned up, and the parent is summoned.

The patient and parent are instructed in the postoperative care. The assistant demonstrates the toothbrushing technique for the appliance and area involved. The patient is dismissed.

10 Clean Up Operatory, Disinfect, and Sterilize

The assistant removes the latex gloves, washes hands, writes the procedure on the patient's chart, and returns the chart to the front desk. The utility gloves and PPE are donned and the operatory area is cleaned. All instruments and equipment are cleaned and disinfected or sterilized. The gloves are washed, dried, disinfected, and removed. The hands are washed.▲

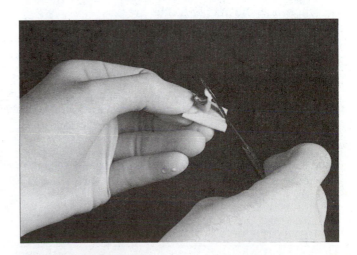

FIGURE 7–6 The inner surfaces of the band or crown are covered with the cement before being placed on the tooth.

Space Maintainers

1. What are the two types of space maintainers?

   a. _____

   b. _____

2. What is the purpose for the placement of a space maintainer?

   _____

3. How long are space maintainers kept in place?

   _____

4. List three types of space maintainers.

   a. _____

   b. _____

   c. _____

5. The most commonly used type of space maintainer appliance is which type?

   _____

6. If the space needed to be kept open is distal to all teeth in the arch, what type of space maintainer is used?

   _____

7. List two methods of coverage that may be used on the anchor tooth.

   a. _____

   b. _____

8. Which of the teeth adjacent to the missing space is chosen as the anchor tooth?

   _____

9. Of what value may the space maintainer be in the future dental development of the patient?

   _____

10. Who may place a space maintainer for a child patient, a dentist, pediatric dentist, or orthodontist?

    _____

Now turn to the Competency Evaluation Sheet for Procedure 34, Assisting with Space Maintainers, located in Appendix C of this text.

ENDODONTICS

Endodontics is the branch of dentistry that deals with the diseases, injuries, and treatment of pulpal tissue. The pulp is the vital living fibrous mass encased within the tooth. It can become injured in a variety of ways—decay, trauma, or chemical and thermal irritation. When threatened, the pulp increases the blood and lymph supply to attempt **revitalization**. This causes a swelling in the pulp chamber where there is no room for expansion. Unless the cause of irritation is removed, the process continues until the pulp tissue is seriously affected and becomes **necrotic** or dead, further increasing the irritation sources.

Various stages of inflammation, irritation, and pain occur during this process. The patient may or may not undergo pain sensation from mild to extremely severe in nature. When the dentist is consulted for a toothache, the first step in the treatment plan is to test and determine the extent of pulpal involvement and the chance of reversing the **degenerative** process (Table 7–1).

TABLE 7–1

Rationale of Endodontic Testing

Clinical examination—may detect gross carious areas, tooth discoloration, swelling, fistula drainage, tooth extension

Percussion and palpation—pressure applied to tooth causes pain reaction due to increased pressure on abscess at apex of tooth

Patient questioning—onset, type and duration of pain, thermal reactions, former treatment or accidents may indicate pulp vitality

Radiographic exam—x-ray may reveal caries and periapical involvement, resorption, cysts, fractures, abscesses, and the anatomy of the root canal available for treatment

Thermal testing—reaction to cold shows inflamed pulp, reaction to hot that lingers and later disappears indicates infected pulp, violent reaction to heat with relief when cold is applied shows abscess, no reaction to hot or cold indicates necrotic or dead pulp

Electrical vitality—stimulation of pulpal nerve fibers through the dentin tubules may indicate **hyperactive** or necrotic pulp sensitivity

Tooth mobility—pressure movement of tooth may indicate tooth expulsion due to abscess growth in periodontal socket

Transillumination—viewing with transillumination is more effective on thin anterior teeth, may show darker pulp area caused by congested pulp tissue

Anesthetic—local anesthesia may be administered to determine affected tooth, relief of pain indicates tooth with pulpal pain

Pulp tissue that has progressed to the necrotic stage must be removed. A pulpotomy, partial removal of the pulp, may be attempted in a child or very young person because of the greater amount of blood circulation available to the tooth; the older child or adult faces a removal of all the pulp tissue, which is called a pulpectomy or, more commonly, a root canal.

A root canal procedure may be accomplished in the dental office in one to three visits. The first visit is important in determining the cause and extent of the pulpal involvement and in some cases, relieving the pain. Once root canal treatment is planned, the tooth is opened, the pulp is removed, and a permanent restoration or crown cover is applied. All procedures must be carried out with a sterile technique because entering the pulp area involves entering the bloodstream.

Assisting with the Endodontic Examination

The duties of the assistant in an endodontic examination may be varied and involved. The examination is completed to locate and estimate the condition of the pulp tissue. All future treatment is determined by the findings. In many cases, the pulpal involvement is quite evident and not too difficult to determine; occasionally, a toothache can be very mysterious and require a multitude of testing before diagnosis.

P R O C E D U R E 3 5
Assisting with the Endodontic Examination

1 Assemble Equipment
2 Prepare the Patient and Don PPE
3 Assist with Clinical Examination
4 Assist with Dental Radiographs
5 Assist with Thermal Testing
6 Assist with Vitality Testing
7 Assist with Transillumination
8 Assist with Mobility Testing
9 Clean Up the Patient
10 Clean Up Operatory, Disinfect, and Sterilize

1 Assemble Equipment

The necessary equipment and materials used in an endodontic exam follow:

- basic setup
- sundry setup, including applicators
- radiographs and x-ray machine
- ice sliver
- gutta percha point; alcohol torch, match, and petroleum jelly
- vitality tester
- nonfluoridated toothpaste
- transillumination tip
- HVE tip

2 Prepare the Patient and Don PPE

The assistant greets and seats the patient, who is draped and bibbed. An inquiry into the general health history is made, especially the present medication and antibiotic reaction areas, as endodontic treatment involves the application of these items. The exam procedure is explained. The assistant dons the PPE. All materials, equipment, and procedures are performed in the most sterile technique available.

3 Assist with Clinical Examination

The assistant summons the dentist, who questions the patient regarding the toothache or problem. The dentist **palpates** the neck and gland areas looking for an infection or enlargement. The gingival area and mucobuccal fold area may also be palpated to explore for swelling.

A mirror and explorer are passed to the dentist who performs a clinical examination. The instruments may be used for a **percussion** and **mobility** test. The handle of the mouth mirror may be gently tapped on the affected tooth seeking a patient response. More than one tooth will be tapped to determine the normal patient reaction and the comparison between two teeth. Sensitivity to light pressure on tooth crowns may indicate an abscess condition exists on the root tips of the tooth. The assistant records the findings of the testing.

4 Assist with Dental Radiographs

The assistant may pass or expose a radiograph of the area, as directed by the dentist. Radiographs usually are the most significant and used diagnostic aid. The radiograph exposes the density and degree of tissue involvement in the area. Overgloves are donned to process the film. When the film has been processed, the overgloves are removed and the film is shown to the dentist. The findings are recorded.

5 Assist with Thermal Testing

The assistant may aid in the thermal testing by placing a small sliver of ice in a piece of gauze and passing it to the dentist, who holds it against the tooth (Figure 7–7). *Ice may be obtained by freezing water in empty anesthetic carpules. Reaction to cold indicates a highly irritated pulp; no reaction may mean a necrotic or dead tissue.

To test for heat reaction, which may indicate infection or abscess, the assistant passes a cotton pellet with petroleum jelly to coat the tooth surface. This protection layer prevents the hot material from adhering to the tooth. The assistant flame heats a gutta percha point until limp and passes it to the dentist to place on the cervical area of the tooth. No reaction to heat may indicate necrotic tissue. The findings are recorded.

6 Assist with Vitality Testing

The assistant may aid in the **vitality** testing of a tooth by passing cotton rolls for isolation. The area to be tested must be dry to avoid conduction of the electricity to areas other than the testing site. When the cotton rolls are placed, the assistant passes the syringe for an air dry of the tooth.

The assistant applies a nonfluoridated toothpaste to the surface of the tooth to be tested to act as a conductor for electrical impulses from the vitometer, which may be electric or battery charged. The vitality tip is passed to the dentist, who places it on the tooth surface where the paste has been applied (Figure 7–8). The assistant checks the gauge on the handle of the vitometer to make sure it is starting at zero and slowly

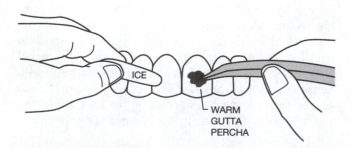

FIGURE 7–7 Application of hot and cold to a tooth may indicate degenerative stages of pulp tissue.

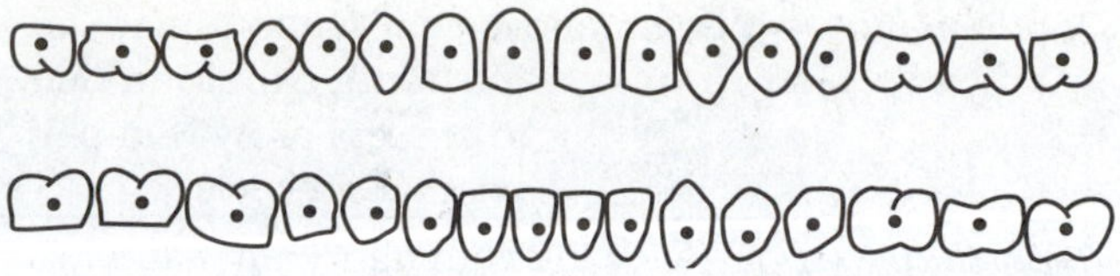

FIGURE 7–8 Position indicators for placement of vitality pulp testing tip. ⚘ No testing should be attempted on amalgam restorations. Current will be conducted through material and cause irritation and false readings.

accelerates the power until the patient gives a signal to stop. The findings are recorded. More than one tooth is checked to determine the contrast between a "normal" and an "affected" tooth. The assistant repeats the applicator dabbing of paste on another indicated tooth, rechecks the gauge at zero and accelerates again until indicated to stop. This procedure is repeated until the dentist wishes no more testing. The cotton rolls are removed, and the mouth is rinsed and dried.

7 Assist with Transillumination

The assistant may aid in **transillumination** testing by passing the illuminator tip to the dentist and activating the power. Light passing through the tooth tissue may reveal a tooth crack, restoration faults or even a dark pulpal area indicating swelling and infection. The findings are recorded. The procedure is repeated on all teeth the dentist chooses to illuminate. The assistant receives and replaces the illuminator tip.

8 Assist with Mobility Testing

Since the dentist already is using a mouth mirror, the assistant will pass another single-handled instrument, such as an explorer, to test for tooth movement. Abscessed teeth sometimes expand out of their sockets; such swelling causes the tooth to appear loose.

Two instruments are used for a mobility test instead of pressing with the fingers. Skin tissue has some "give" and does not record a true reading. One instrument is placed behind the affected tooth and another instrument is pushed against the tooth to determine if any movement is evident.

9 Clean Up the Patient

The dentist may perform all or some of the previously discussed tests to determine future treatment. When the dentist is satisfied with the examination, the patient is cleaned up and taken to the consultation room to discuss treatment. The assistant removes gloves, places them on the instrument tray, washes hands, and gathers all records and radiographs to take with the patient for the consultation.

10 Clean Up Operatory, Disinfect, and Sterilize

The assistant returns and dons utility gloves and PPE. The operatory area and equipment are disinfected. The disposables are placed in the proper containers. The transilluminator tip and vitality tip are cleaned and wrapped for sterilization. Radiographic equipment and switches are recovered. Large items are disinfected. The instruments are cleaned and prepared for sterilization. The area is cleaned up. The gloves are washed, disinfected, and removed; hands are washed.▲

THEORY RECALL
Endodontics

1. What can the series of endodontic tests indicate to the dentist?

2. What part of the health history is particularly important in endodontic examination questioning?

3. Why does the dentist palpate the neck and gland areas?

4. What tests can the dentist perform using the mirror and explorer?

5. When assisting with radiographs, what does the assistant don while processing the radiographs?

6. What two objects are used for thermal testing in an endodontic test?

   a.

   b.

7. What purpose does the nonfluoridated paste serve in the vitality test?

8. What does the assistant check before accelerating the power of the electric pulp tester?

9. Where is the patient taken when the testing is completed?

10. Where does the assistant take the records and radiographs after the exam?

Now turn to the Competency Evaluation Sheet for Procedure 35, Assisting with the Endodontic Examination, located in Appendix C of this text.

ENDODONTIC ROOT CANAL TREATMENT

When the dentist has completed a series of tests to determine the vitality of the pulp, a decision is made concerning treatment. The patient and dentist discuss the pulpal condition (diagnosis), alternatives, treatment plan, financial arrangements, and probable outcome (prognosis).

The therapy for a necrotic pulp is a root canal treatment, which is basically removing the pulpal tissue in the crown and the involved root. This treatment may be completed in a matter of one to three visits or more, depending on the severity of the pulpal infection.

The dentist opens the tooth, removes the pulp tissue, enlarges and refines or smooths the canal, removes infection, and refills the canal before placing a permanent restoration. If there is not a large amount of infection or involvement, the dentist may complete the treatment in one sitting; but when there must be more treatment for infection, the series of treatments increases. The protocol of procedures necessary for root canal treatment are:

1. local anesthesia
2. isolation of tooth
3. disinfection of site
4. opening into the canal
5. removal of pulpal tissue
6. cleaning of canal
7. canal medication
8. shaping of canal
9. filling of canal
10. tooth restoration

Except on rare occasions, such as fractured or **avulsed** (knocked loose) teeth treatment, the sequence of procedures in root canal therapy usually occurs over a two- to three-visit series. Some of the actions may not be required at each session, while others are necessary throughout. The exact treatment given depends on the individual patient. The following procedural outline is for a multiple visit series.

PROCEDURE 36
Assisting with Root Canal Therapy (Visits 1–3)

Visits 1 and 2

1 Assemble Equipment and Prepare the Patient

2 Assist with Local Anesthesia

3	Assist with Isolation of Tooth
4	Assist with Disinfection of Tooth and Dam
5	Assist with Opening of Tooth
6	Assist with Removal of Pulpal Tissue
7	Assist with Cleaning the Pulpal Canal
8	Assist with Medication of the Canal
9	Assist with Temporary Filling of the Canal and Tooth
10	Clean Up Patient, Area, and Instruments

Visit 3

11	Assemble Equipment and Prepare the Patient
12	Assist with Placement of Dental Dam
13	Assist with Removal of Temporary Restoration
14	Assist with Cleaning the Canal
15	Assist with Fitting of Central Core for Canal
16	Prepare Root Canal Cement
17	Assist with Cementation and Filling of Canal
18	Assist with Final Restoration and Cover
19	Clean Up Patient and Dismiss
20	Clean Up Operatory and Equipment

Visit 1

1 Assemble Equipment and Prepare the Patient

The following materials are needed for root canal visits 1 and 2:

▶ basic and sundry setup, including paper points and applicators
▶ local anesthesia and equipment
▶ dental dam material and equipment
▶ handpiece with round, high-speed FG burs
▶ 2 luer loc syringes (color-coded, sterile, disposable)
▶ hydrogen peroxide, sodium hypochlorite, Metaphen or disinfecting solutions
▶ temporary restorative material
▶ PFI instrument, spoon excavator
▶ scissors
▶ assorted reamers, files, and barbed broaches
▶ 2 locking pliers
▶ glass bead sterilizer
▶ x-ray and equipment

The operatory is cleaned and prepared. The patient is greeted, seated, and positioned in the dental chair. A pair of protective glasses is given to the patient to wear so chemical solutions used will not irritate the eyes. The patient is draped to protect clothing from **caustic** chemicals and a sterile bib is placed around the neck. The assistant dons PPE and summons the dentist.

2 Assist with Local Anesthesia

Local anesthesia is needed for all teeth that have **sensitivity**. In a fully necrotic (dead) tooth, the patient has no sensation; anesthesia is not required but will probably be given to anesthetize the periodontal tissue areas. Most patients need anesthesia for the first visit. After the removal of the nerve, anesthesia may or may not be required. The assistant may prepare the patient with the topical anesthetic before the dentist arrives in the room. The applicator is received, and the syringe is passed for the injection. The anesthetic syringe is either returned to the tray or the assistant grasps the syringe behind the needle and returns it to the tray. It is recapped using a mechanical capping instrument or with a one-handed technique.

3 Assist with Isolation of Tooth

A dental dam is placed on the patient to prevent any swallowing of small instruments or caustic chemicals, to provide better vision, and to maintain a sterile field. The assistant passes a dental dam clamp holder and clamp for measuring and fitting. When an acceptable clamp has been chosen, the assistant passes the prepared dental dam material, clamp, and clamp holder. The holder is received and the napkin is passed. The dental dam frame is then passed, and the assistant aids with the adjusting of the material to the frame. A small piece of dental floss, cord, or dental dam material is passed to be wedged or hold the material in place. A saliva ejector is placed in the mouth, under the dental dam material, opposite the work site.

4 Assist with Disinfection of Tooth and Dam

The assistant passes an applicator, moistened with Metaphen or some other suitable disinfectant, to the dentist, who paints the tooth and surrounding dam material. This disinfects the area prior to opening the tooth and entering into the bloodstream. If the dentist leaves the room to perform other treatment while the anesthetic takes effect, the assistant may sterilize the tooth and dental dam area (Figure 7–9).

5 Assist with Opening of Tooth

The applicator is received and the assistant passes the high-speed handpiece with a round bur (#6) to the

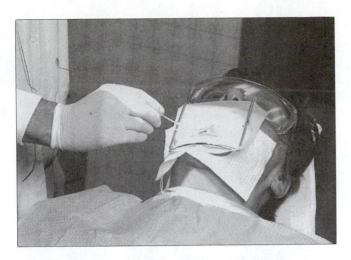

FIGURE 7-9 All parts of the exposed tooth, dam, and clamp should be disinfected before entering into the pulp.

dentist, who opens the tooth and exposes the pulp chamber. The dentist may request other burs to enlarge the opening and to gain working access to the chamber and canal. The assistant uses the HVE to evacuate all debris and accumulated moisture.

6 Assist with Removal of Pulpal Tissue

Once the tooth pulp area is open, the nerve and pulpal tissue are removed. The condition of the tissue depends on how long and how developed the infection and necrosis has progressed. The dentist inserts a barbed broach and twists to engage and remove the tissue, which may be pink or dead with flaky scab matter. The assistant holds a piece of sterile gauze near the site to receive any matter removed from the tooth.

7 Assist with Cleaning the Pulpal Canal

When the pulpal tissue has been removed, the assistant passes alternately upon request a sterile, disposable luer loc syringe with sodium hypochlorite (bleach) and a luer loc syringe of hydrogen peroxide or various endodontic hand instruments, such as a reamer or file.

The dentist performs a **biomechanical** cleansing of the root chamber and canal. The solutions are used as irrigation liquids and are important to flush up any debris, tooth dust, necrotic tissue, and the like. When the sodium hypochlorite and the hydrogen peroxide combine, they cause an **effervescent** or bubbling action and should not be used interchangeably from one luer loc syringe to another. Each syringe should be color-coded and kept separate from the other. *Many dentists choose to use only the sodium hypoclorite solution because it not only rinses but also disinfects.

Broaches, files, and reamers are small endodontic instruments used to remove matter from the inside of the tooth and enlarge and smooth the canal. They are color-coded or marked to show size. They can be used in a slow-speed handpiece or operated by use in the fingers. More dentists use the hand-held fingertip reamers and files to remove debris and prepare the canal because of the sensitivity that can be felt with the fingertip touch. All reamer, files, broaches, and tips are sterilized before use in the tooth. A quick method to sterilize at the chair is accomplished by inserting the instrument into the hot glass beads (450°F) contained in the glass bead sterilizer for 10 seconds and then after the procedure. Each instrument is cleaned and either autoclaved or placed in a dry heat sterilizer between patients.

All debris and matter present is removed before the cleaning and smoothing of the canal walls. **Irrigation** from the two syringes is used to remove the dentin dust and debris. Paper points are used to absorb and dry the canal after the irrigating solutions have been used. (See Figure 7–10 for a typical tray setup for endodontic treatment.)

During the use of the small endodontic instruments, the dentist is careful not to probe too deeply into the canal. The final instrument and filling insertion is recommended to be approximately 1 to 2 mm from the apical foramen. To prevent penetration, the dentist requests the length to be marked from one instrument to another. This is accomplished by placing "stoppers" of small rubber band pieces to mark the depth (Figure 7–11).

Another method of measuring is to place a line for the desired length and then positioning the instruments and points into a pair of locking pliers set at the desired spacing. The dentist orders or exposes an x-ray of the tooth periodically to determine the correct length positions and gauge (thickness) of the instruments.

The assistant records the length of the last instrument used and the color-coded size (thickness) of the last reamer or file used. In this manner, no penetration occurs and the walls of the canal are cleaned thoroughly.

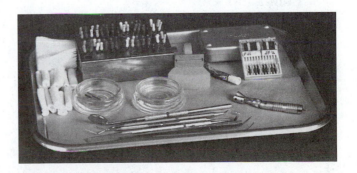

FIGURE 7-10 Examples of the root canal equipment needed for treatment.

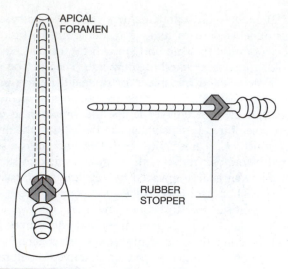

APICAL FORAMEN

RUBBER STOPPER

FIGURE 7-11 The stopper indicates the length of the canal. The following instrument must be marked with the present length to avoid penetrating the apical foramen.

8 Assist with Medication of the Canal

In cases of bacterial infection, such as decay, abscessing, or old fractures, the dentist may wish to chemically sterilize and treat the area. Antibiotic pastes or chemical sterilizers such as parachlorophenol or camphor may be placed into the pulp canal. This is accomplished by placing the desired medicine on a small cotton pellet and inserting into the pulp chamber. The **medicament** may be permitted to remain encased in the area until the next visit. To stop the medicament from oversaturating the canal and leaking into the bloodstream and nearby tissues, the assistant dips a pellet into the medicine and blots it to almost a dry state.

9 Assist with Temporary Filling of the Canal and Tooth

After the medicated pellet has been situated and is in position, the assistant passes another sterile cotton pellet in college pliers to the dentist. While the pellet is being placed in the crown area over the medicine, the assistant prepares the temporary filling material, which may be a mixture of two pastes, a powder and liquid mixture, or straight from a tube. The pliers are received and a double-ended PFI or condenser instrument with filling material on the PFI side is passed. The assistant holds the slab of material near the work site for refilling until the temporary restoration has been completed.

10 Clean up Patient, Area, and Instruments

The assistant passes the dental dam clamp holder to the dentist, who removes the clamp and returns the holder and clamp. The assistant receives the frame and napkin and passes the scissors for cut of ligatures and dam material. When the scissors are returned, the assistant holds a gauze square near the work site to receive the ligature pieces and then receives the dam material, which is checked for any missing pieces.

The mouth is rinsed and evacuated. If the temporary restoration has been placed on a biting surface, the assistant passes articulating paper for a check of the height of the restoration. If needed, the assistant passes the PFI, carver instrument, or finishing bur in a slow handpiece to the dentist to adjust the biting surface of the temporary restoration.

The patient is cleaned up, given postoperative instructions, and requested to call the office if any pain returns to the area. The patient is dismissed after another appointment is made for the next visit.

The area is cleaned up in the usual manner. The assistant checks to be sure that the last length, size, and number of the reaming and filing instruments were written on the records.

Visit 2

A second visit may be necessary if a large infection was present. The instruments and materials for visit 2 are the same as visit 1. The procedure is the same, with the exception of the anesthesia. Since the pulp tissue is removed, there may or may not be sensation. The dentist chooses if an injection is to be given.

The dentist opens the tooth, removes the dressings, and enlarges and smooths the root canal area. A medicated pellet and temporary restorative material are placed, and the patient returns for a third visit.

Visit 3

11 Assemble Equipment and Prepare the Patient

The setup for the last endodontic root canal therapy is the same as for visits 1 and 2, except for the addition of:

- ▶ gutta percha points, chloroform solvent
- ▶ root canal cement and equipment
- ▶ cement spreader
- ▶ root canal plugger
- ▶ alcohol torch or propane burner, match
- ▶ spoon excavator
- ▶ final restorative material or cover and equipment

The patient is seated and prepared for the last visit. The health history is reviewed, and the procedure is explained. PPE is donned.

12 Assist with Placement of Dental Dam

The dental dam is reapplied, and the tooth and material are disinfected by swabbing with an applicator of Metaphen or a suitable solution.

13 Assist with Removal of Temporary Restoration

The assistant aids in the removal of the temporary restoration by passing the handpiece and round bur. Next, an explorer is passed to remove the cotton pellets used to fill the pulp chamber and carry the medicament.

14 Assist with Cleaning the Canal

The dentist determines the amount of reaming, filing, and irrigation needed and requests the appropriate instruments or syringes. All instruments used are sterile and may be re-sterilized at the chair in the glass bead sterilizer. Small hand instruments are marked with stoppers at the recorded length. The assistant remains ready to pass what is desired and maintain visibility and a dry field. Radiographs of the tooth may be periodically taken to determine if the canal is fully opened and cleaned.

15 Assist with Fitting of Central Core for Canal

When the canal has been treated, cleaned, and properly smoothed, the dentist fills the area so no bacteria may accumulate to form other abscesses. The canal may be filled with a silver point, gutta percha point, or a combination of the two.

The dentist requests a silver or gutta percha point similar in size to the last largest instrument. The point may be inserted into the canal, positioned, then x-rayed for proper fit. This serves as the master cone. If any opening remains in the canal after the fitting of the master cone, slender gutta percha points are inserted to take up the void.

If the master cone correctly fits the canal, a pair of cotton pliers is passed for the dentist to mark the proper length on the point while it is in position. The master cone is withdrawn and returned to the assistant, who prepares the root canal cement according to the manufacturer's recommendation.

16 Prepare Root Canal Cement

The assistant wipes the slab with alcohol and prepares the cement to a thick, creamy state. A cement spreader is rubbed onto the cement and passed to the dentist, who fills the canal with cement. The assistant holds the slab near the site to recoat the cement spreader.

17 Assist with Cementation and Filling of Canal

The assistant receives the cement spreader, places the master cone in the cement paste, rolls it for coverage, and passes it to the dentist, who inserts it into the canal. The pliers are returned, and the assistant passes a plugger to the dentist to condense the gutta percha cone.

The assistant dips smaller gutta percha points into the mixed paste or sealer solvent and passes these to the dentist, alternating plugger with point with plugger. As the dentist plugs or condenses the canal with the plugger, the assistant dips and prepares to pass another point. While the point is being inserted, the assistant dips the plugger tip into solvent and wipes it clean to be passed again. The process is repeated until the canal is filled (Figure 7–12).

The dentist requests a final radiograph of the root canal, which the assistant assists with or exposes. Overgloves are donned again, and the film is processed. If the dentist is satisfied with the filling results, the assistant heats a spoon excavator and passes for the dentist to remove any gutta percha ends remaining in the crown area. The assistant holds gauze near the site to receive the cut off ends and wipe the instrument.

When the spoon excavator is returned, the assistant passes a disinfectant-moistened cotton pellet to the dentist to clean the crown area prior to the restoration. The assistant receives the pellet and pliers.

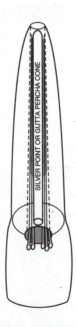

SILVER POINT OR GUTTA PERCHA CONE

FIGURE 7–12 After the canal is completely filled, the excess material in the crown is removed; a restoration is placed.

18 Assist with Final Restoration and Cover

The assistant prepares the restorative material of choice, passes it to the dentist, and gives the condensers and carvers as needed. The assistant maintains visibility and evacuates the area throughout the procedure.

19 Clean Up Patient and Dismiss

The dental dam is removed. The assistant holds articulating paper on the occlusal surface (if needed) to test the occlusal height of the restoration. If adjustment is necessary, the assistant passes a carver or handpiece with finishing bur. The mouth is rinsed and evacuated. The patient is cleaned up. Instructions are given, and the patient is released.

20 Clean Up Operatory and Equipment

The assistant gathers contaminated materials and equipment and takes it to the sterilizing room. Latex exam gloves are removed, and the hands are washed. The assistant gathers the records and films, updates the patient's chart, and returns the chart to the front desk.

The assistant returns, dons utility gloves and PPE, and disinfects or sterilizes all items. The area is cleaned up. The gloves are washed, disinfected, and removed; the hands are washed.▲

THEORY RECALL

Endodontic Root Canal Treatment

1. Why is the patient requested to wear protective eyeglasses during endodontic treatment?

2. Why is the tooth receiving treatment isolated during the procedures?

3. How can one determine the size of the reamers and files to be used?

4. What is used to sterilize the reamers and files at the chairside?

5. What is used to carry and hold medicine in the root canal during therapy?

6. What material is used to fill the root canal?

7. What material is used as a temporary filling during therapy?

8. Why are "stoppers" used during root canal therapy?

9. What material is used as a permanent filling in root canal therapy?

10. Where are the x-rays taken during therapy kept when treatment is over?

Now turn to the competency Evaluation Sheets for Procedures 36A and 36B, Assisting with Root Canal Therapy (Visits 1–3), located in Appendix C of this text.

REMOVABLE PROSTHODONTICS

Prosthodontics is the branch of dentistry that deals with the **reconstruction** or replacement of teeth with artificial appliances. Prosthodontics may be removable or fixed.

Preparing and constructing a prosthodontic appliance is a very complicated process that requires more than one appointment. Removable appliances may be an artificial tooth, a group of teeth, or an entire dentition replacement that may be placed and removed by the patient.

The procedure for the fabrication of a removable appliance is basically the same for a partial **denture** (a few teeth) as it is for a complete denture (all teeth in the arch) (Figure 7–13). Choice of impression materials and technique for fitting may differ the most, but the dentist determines the specific type and action.

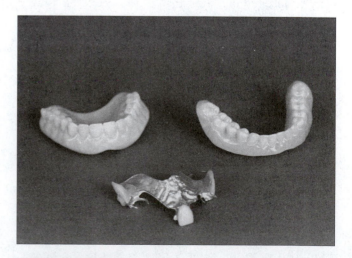

FIGURE 7-13 Example of a partial appliance and a complete denture.

Assisting with Prosthodontic Impressions

Active participation in procedures and moisture evacuation is not as demanding in prosthodontics as in some other types of operative dentistry; assistants may be of value in preparation, organization, cleanup, support, material preparation, and laboratory work.

Prosthodontic care involves more than one visit, as laboratory work must be performed between each step. Appointment scheduling must be staggered and made to accommodate lab work time between visits. Most removable appliances need three or more appointments, depending on the extent of treatment involved.

The patient's first appointment requires an impression to be taken of the mouth, which is poured up into a study cast. A custom tray is constructed on this cast so a second impression will be exact and form fitting.

The dentist may also require photographs, radiographs, and mouth preparations to be completed before the construction of the appliance. *Mouth preparation may require root canal therapy, abutment preparation, restorative procedures, or necessary dental treatment for a partial appliance. The patient may require an alveoplasty, tissue preparation, or surgery for root tip impaction of complete dentures.

During the patient's second visit, another impression is taken. This one is completed in a custom tray constructed between visits. Before the patient's next visit, a custom **acrylic** tray is formed and prepared on top of the study cast. This provides the prosthodontist with an impression tray conforming to the patient's individual shape and form.

A second impression is taken using the custom tray. The prosthodontist may choose any type of impression material, such as rubber or silicone base. This second impression, when completed, will be poured up and used as the working cast for the fabrication of the denture base (Figure 7–14).

The laboratory work of custom tray and denture construction may be performed in the lab section of the office or it may be sent to a commercial laboratory. All lab work to be completed must be accompanied by a work order filled out and signed by the prosthodontist or dentist. The prescription bears the patient's name and age, denture material of choice, tooth shade and mold shape, as well as any other particular modification or instructions desired.

The original impression to construct the study cast may be done in alginate material, poured and trimmed.

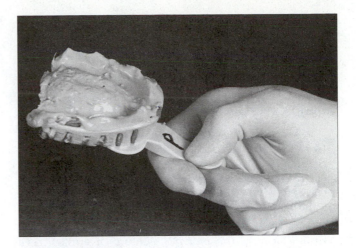

FIGURE 7–14 A light-bodied impression material or wash is placed in the patient's tray for an impression.

2	Prepare the Impression Tray
3	Prepare the Impression Material
4	Assist with the Removal of the Impression Tray
5	Repeat the Procedure for the Other Arch
6	Assist with the Bite Registration
7	Assist with Tooth Selection
8	Clean Up, Dismiss the Patient, and Sterilize

The patient has already had a preliminary impression taken, which was sent to the laboratory to be poured up and used as a master cast for a custom tray for a full denture or a base for appliance fabrication for a partial denture. Since taking alginate impression procedures are previously covered and fabrication of custom trays is covered in Unit 9, the second visit needed for removable prosthodontia is stressed in this procedure.

1 Complete the Preparations

The equipment and materials necessary for the second impression appointment follow:

- custom tray constructed from previous study model
- wax rope for edging trays, spatula, alcohol torch
- basic setup
- sundry setup, including denture cup (if applicable)
- adhesive liquid and brush
- impression materials and mixing equipment
- wax or bite registration material
- shade and mold guides

PROCEDURE 37

Assisting with Prosthodontic Impressions (Visit 2)

1 Complete the Preparations

▶ millimeter rule or boley gauge
▶ record card
▶ disinfectant and bag for impressions, bite registration

The assistant greets and seats the patient, who is draped and bibbed around the neck. The procedure is explained. The assistant dons PPE.

2 Prepare the Impression Tray

The custom tray constructed from the study model is prepared when the assistant paints the tray adhesive on the inside of the tray. The tray edges are lined with a wax roping material and adapted to the tray. The assistant accepts the patient's denture or appliance (if applicable) and places it in a denture cup filled with cool water. The tray is passed and received from the dentist, who has tested the tray for fit. If no adjustment is needed, the tray is painted or sprayed with an adhesive material to ensure the impression material adheres to the tray. The mixing of impression materials may begin. If the tray does not fit properly, more wax is adapted to or removed from the tray edge with a warm wax spatula.

3 Prepare the Impression Material

The assistant mixes the impression material according to the manufacturer's directions (Table 7–2). The choice of the material is made by the dentist. Many prefer an elastic type of two viscosities when working with undercuts and when teeth are present. The assis-

tant mixes equal amounts of the lighter flowing elastic material and **catalyst** to a **homogeneous** color, loads it into the syringe and passes the syringe to the dentist, who will dispense the material around the dried teeth. While the dentist is placing the syringe material, the assistant mixes the heavier elastic material in the same manner and loads the prepared custom tray, which is passed when the impression syringe is returned to the assistant. The filled tray is inserted over the syringe impression material already in place on the teeth. Both materials blend into one impression.

The dentist may prefer a syringe impression material, which is prepared and dispensed according to recommendations of the manufacturer. Some impression materials are now packed in an automatic mixing container that combines the impression material and catalyst through the mixing syringe tip (Figure 7–15). The double barreled container is placed into the pump syringe. When the pressure is applied, both materials descend the inner circular tube, which evenly combines the two materials and replaces the assistant's task of mixing. While this method may be more expensive, the mixture is regulated and the mixture is effortlessly and correctly done.

The dentist may prefer a zinc oxide impression material for the secondary impression of a denture patient. The assistant mixes the two pastes together to a creamy consistency, fills the tray, and passes it to the dentist for insertion. When working with this material, it is wise to have a piece of gauze and orange solvent to clean up the patient's face and the instruments used.

Another impression application that may be used is

TABLE 7-2

Prosthodontic Impression Materials

MATERIAL	PURPOSE	DISPENSE	MIX METHOD	MIX	WORK	SET TIME
wash	tissue detail	equal amount of pastes	spatulate to even color	30 sec. or more	5 min.	5 to 10 min.
syringe—light or heavy viscosity	fine form, some support	pastes, autopump	automix, self spatulate to even color	20 to 30 sec.	2 to 3 min.	4 to 5 min.
putty	form and shape	pump, scoop, activate with drops or paste	score, activate, knead to even color	45 sec.	2 to 2½ min.	4 to 5 min.
			GENERAL RULES			

1. Use overgloves to prevent cross contamination and latex reaction with some impression materials.

2. Read manufacturers' directions for dispensing amounts, methods for mixing, and setting times. (All companies differ.)

3. Do not mix materials from different companies since formulas are not the same.

4. Tray used for impression must be rigid and prepared with adhesive before placement of impression material.

5. Check manufacturers' directions for disinfection of finished impression; some may be immersed in disinfectant.

6. Become familiar with materials to be used; many are color-coded for easy identification.

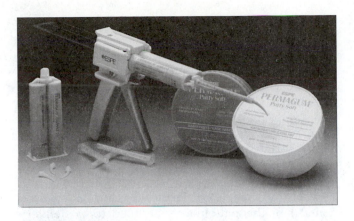

FIGURE 7-15 **Example of automatic mixing impression syringe. These devices save time and material and lessen cross contamination. (Courtesy of ESPE America.)**

a putty or dough consistency. The assistant scoops out the recommended amounts for the impression needed, adds the manufacturer's suggested amount of catalyst drops, and kneads the dough to a homogeneous color. When properly mixed, the dough is placed into the prepared tray and passed to the dentist for insertion. In approximately four minutes, the tray is removed, disinfected, and bagged for the laboratory. When teeth or severe undercuts are present, the dentist may request a lighter viscosity of putty material to be mixed, placed in a syringe and dispensed around the teeth before the tray insertion. These two materials unite during the impression into one mass.

4 Assist with the Removal of the Impression Tray

After the impression has been taken, the dentist hands the tray to the assistant who rinses the impression and then sprays with a disinfectant. The impression and tray are inserted into a plastic bag, without touching the outside of the bag. An applicator stick may be placed in the bag opening to keep it spread apart. After the patient is dismissed and the assistant returns to get the patient's notes, the assistant may touch the outside, close, and zip lock the bag with the impressions and bite registration inside.

5 Repeat the Procedure for the Other Arch

The procedure is repeated for the other arch using the same technique and method and appropriate tray.

6 Assist with the Bite Registration

The assistant warms a wax bite registration block or a piece of base plate wax and passes it to the dentist for a bite registration. After the patient bites on the wax, the assistant may pass or use the syringe to apply cool water to wax for a setup. The HVE is used to evacuate the mouth. The wax is removed; the assistant rinses it in cold water, disinfects it, and places it with the impression in the plastic bag. The dentist may prefer a syringe-dispensed silicone registration material, which is dispensed directly on the occlusal or facial surfaces and allowed to set. When firm, it is removed to be used as a registration of the patient's bite. The assistant collects the piece, spray disinfects it, and places it into the plastic bag. Edentulous patients may have bite registration completed while wearing wax denture prosthesis.

7 Assist with Tooth Selection

The assistant helps with the tooth shade selection by wetting the shade guide and passing it to the dentist. The light is turned off or directed into another area as the shade guide should be wet like the tooth and viewed in a natural light. When the correct shade is chosen, the assistant records the number on the record card.

The mold selection is completed in the same manner. The dentist may signal for a millimeter rule or a boley gauge to measure length. The patient may have been requested to bring an old photograph to show the smile and the shape of the original teeth, if none are present. When the dentist has chosen the desired shape, the assistant records the mold number on the card.

8 Clean Up, Dismiss the Patient, and Sterilize

When the shade and shape are chosen, the patient's mouth is rinsed and the assistant washes off the appliance or denture and returns it to the patient. Then the patient is dismissed.

The assistant gathers the contaminated materials and equipment and takes them to the sterilizing room. All shade and mold guides placed out on the tray are sterilized, even if they were not used in the mouth. The assistant removes the exam gloves, washes hands, and records the treatment.

The assistant dons utility gloves and disinfects and sterilizes in the usual manner. The gloves are washed, disinfected, and removed; the hands are washed.

The impressions and bite registration in the plastic bag are taken to the office laboratory or prepared for shipment to a commercial lab. The prescription or work orders are included in the box.▲

Removable Prosthodontics

1. What are removable appliances?

_____

2. In what way do the impression taking for a partial and complete denture differ?

_____

3. What is constructed on the study cast that will be used in later impressions?

_____

4. Besides the impression, what might the dentist require at the first appointment?

_____

5. What mouth preparation may be required of a patient receiving a partial appliance?

_____

6. Which material does the assistant prepare first in a two-viscosity mix?

_____

7. What type of impression material may a dentist prefer for a full denture impression?

_____

8. What does the assistant do to the impression and tray after the dentist removes it from the patient's mouth?

_____

9. Why does the assistant wet the shade guide and move the lamp during the shade selection?

_____

10. Why may the dentist request the patient to bring an old photo when selecting the mold for the dentures?

_____

Now turn to the Competency Evaluation Sheet for Procedure 37, Assisting with Prosthodontic Impressions (Visit 2), located in Appendix C of this text.

TRY IN AND DELIVERY APPOINTMENTS

The third appointment in the removable prosthodontic chain is the try in session. The dentist or commercial laboratory has completed the appliance in a waxed or partial formed shape. The dentist tries the appliance or denture in the patient's mouth and makes any adjustments before the final preparations are completed.

If the patient is receiving a complete denture, the denture base is fabricated of wax. The teeth set in the wax plate are the actual teeth of the future denture. The dentist checks the articulation and fit and makes adjustments in the wax before it is sent to the lab to be finalized.

If the patient is receiving a partial appliance, the framework with wax bite plates are placed in the mouth for adjustments and fit. The appliance is returned to the lab, which adds the final acrylic base material and teeth.

When the completed denture is returned from the dental lab, the patient is scheduled for a delivery appointment. After seating and positioning the patient, the temporary or old dentures are removed and placed in cool water in a denture cup. The disinfected, new dentures, which have been moistened, are inserted into the patient's mouth. The appearance, function, and comfort are tested; any adjustment is performed. Once the prosthodontist or dentist and patient are pleased with the results, the patient is reviewed in the use and care of artificial teeth and dismissed with a return appointment scheduled to reevaluate the fit.

Assisting with Try In and Delivery Appointments

Try in Appointment
1 Complete the Preparations
2 Assist with Placement of the Appliance
3 Assist with Adjustment of the Appliance
4 Instruct and Dismiss the Patient
5 Clean Up and Sterilize
6 Complete the Lab Work Order

Delivery Appointment
7 Complete the Preparations
8 Assist with Placement
9 Assist with Adjustment
10 Dismiss Patient, Disinfect and Sterilize

Try In Appointment
1 Complete the Preparations

The equipment and materials needed for the try in appointment follow:

▶ basic setup
▶ sundry setup
▶ appliance or denture from the laboratory, which is

disinfected and rinsed
▶ denture cup to hold patient's old appliance during treatment
▶ hand mirror for patient viewing
▶ articulating paper and holder
▶ adjusting instruments, including wax spatula, pliers, alcohol torch, match, and wax for addition
▶ slow handpiece with finishing burs for framework
▶ boley gauge for measuring
▶ patient prescription notes
▶ hand mirror

The patient is greeted and seated. A drape and bib are placed on the patient and the procedure is explained. The assistant dons PPE.

2 Assist with Placement of the Appliance

The assistant accepts the patient's old denture and appliance, rinses it, and places it in a denture cup filled with cool water. The assistant passes or uses the syringe to spray rinse the patient's mouth. The disinfected try in appliance is dampened and passed to the dentist for insertion. Articulating paper is either passed or held by the assistant while the patient tests the new bite.

3 Assist with Adjustment of the Appliance

If adjustment is necessary the assistant passes whatever is requested by the dentist. The assistant is prepared to pass a warm spatula to remove excess wax or to reset a tooth or to pass pliers for realignment of a rest or uncomfortable part of the metal appliance. (See Figure 7–16 for crimping of the framework.)

Wax may be heated and placed where the dentist desires. Articulating paper is passed and the bite retested. The dentist may request a millimeter rule or boley gauge to measure adjustments. All adjustments are recorded on the dental lab prescription. Any time the appliance is out of the mouth for alteration, it is rinsed and dampened before reinsertion.

When the adjustment is completed, the patient is handed a mirror for viewing and comments. The completed appliance or denture is passed to the assistant, who rinses it, disinfects it, and places it in a plastic bag.

4 Instruct and Dismiss the Patient

The patient is cleaned up and prepared for dismissal. The old appliance is washed, rinsed, and handed to the patient for insertion while wet. The patient is dismissed after an appointment is made for the final delivery session.

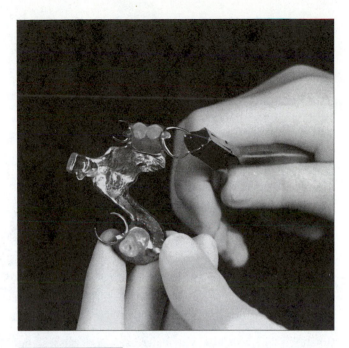

FIGURE 7–16 Pliers can be used to adjust the fit of the metal appliance during the try in appointment.

5 Clean Up and Sterilize

The assistant cleans up the operatory, removes gloves, washes hands, and records treatment on the patient's chart. Utility gloves are donned and the cleanup, disinfection, and sterilization are completed. The gloves are washed, disinfected, and removed. The hands are washed.

6 Complete the Lab Work Order

The assistant gathers the plastic bag with the try in appliance and prepares it for the dental laboratory. The prescription is checked, and the dentist is given the notes and prescription for final orders. The prescription and try in appliance are wrapped with directions and notes on disinfection processes and then sent to the lab.

Delivery Appointment

7 Complete the Preparations

The preparations are completed. The materials and equipment used in the previous appointment are assembled. The final appliance or denture is disinfected, rinsed, and placed in cool water until insertion.

The patient is greeted, seated, draped, and bibbed. The procedure is explained, and the assistant dons PPE.

8 Assist with Placement

The patient is requested to remove old appliances, which the assistant takes and places in a denture cup. The syringe is passed or used to spray rinse the patient's mouth. The new appliance is removed from the cool water and handed to the dentist for insertion. The patient is handed a mirror for viewing.

9 Assist with Adjustment

Articulating paper is passed or held for the patient to test the new bite. If any adjustment must be made, the assistant passes the slow handpiece with finishing or acrylic bur to reduce any high spots or areas (Figure 7–17). Any adjusting or trimming areas must be polished and smoothed before the patient is dismissed.

Pliers may be passed for metal readjustment for a partial appliance. The assistant passes the requested items of adjusting and refining. When adjustment is finished, the assistant washes, rinses and passes the dampened dentures or appliance to the dentist for insertion. The hand mirror may be re-passed also.

10 Dismiss Patient, Disinfect, and Sterilize

The patient is cleaned up. The old dentures are placed in a plastic bag and given to the patient. The patient is instructed in the care and reviewed on the insertion and removal process. The patient is cautioned to clean the appliance over a sink filled with water to lessen the chance of breaking in a fall. The appliances must be washed daily in tepid water as hot water may warp and water that is too cold may make the dentures brittle. The assistant may let the patient perform a cleaning process before leaving.

The assistant removes the contaminated materials and equipment to the sterilizing room, removes gloves, and washes hands. The treatment is recorded on the patient's chart. The utility gloves are donned; the cleanup, disinfection, and sterilization are completed. The gloves are washed, disinfected, and removed; the hands are washed.▲

◤ T H E O R Y   R E C A L L

Try In and Delivery Appointments

1. What is done on the third appointment for a denture or appliance?

2. What teeth are placed in the wax try in denture?

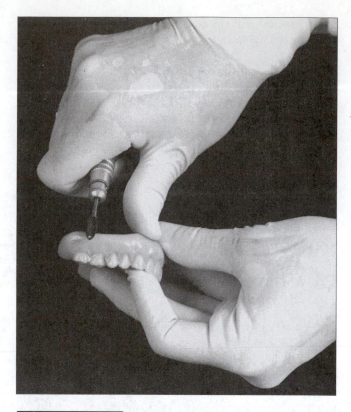

FIGURE 7–17 When the denture is relieved by an acrylic bur, a polishing or finishing bur must be used to smooth the correction.

3. What will be done with the try in appliances or dentures after the try in appointment?

4. Where does the assistant place the patient's dentures during the try in appointment?

5. What may the dentist request to record the length of adjustment to be made?

6. What does the assistant do with the appliance whenever it is taken out of the mouth and needs reinsertion?

7. What does the assistant do to try in denture before placing it in the bag to be sent to the laboratory?

8. What must the assistant be sure to have present before the delivery appointment?

9. What does the assistant pass or hold to test the articulation of the new appliance?

10. What instructions does the assistant give to the patient regarding appliance or denture care?

Now turn to the Competency Evaluation Sheet for Procedure 38, Assisting with Try In and Delivery Appointments, located in Appendix C of this text.

FIXED PROSTHODONTICS

Fixed prosthodontics deals with the placement of an artificial tooth or an appliance cemented in the mouth that cannot be removed by the patient. The most common fixed appliance is the **dental crown**, which fully or partially covers the tooth. When a tooth has extensive decay or breakdown, the dentist may suggest an artificial crown for the restorative work. A full crown covers the prepared tooth with an anatomically shaped and fitted cover made of a precious or semiprecious metal. A partial crown covers three-quarters of the tooth structure, leaving only the facial aspect (Figure 7–18).

The plain metal crown may be cemented onto a prepared tooth or the patient may choose to have a veneer covering applied to the structure to make the appliance more natural. Veneer facings are porcelain material placed and baked on the roughened surface of the crown. When fully fabricated, the artificial crown greatly resembles a natural tooth. Veneer facing may be placed on the total crown or only on the facial (front) aspect.

Dental crowns may be applied to a single prepared tooth or may be part of a multiple united structure called a bridge. When the patient has a missing tooth area to be restored, the dentist may suggest a bridge.

Crowns may be placed upon the teeth **adjacent** to the missing area to support the artificial tooth substituted or become part of the appliance, rendering support and stability. The substitute tooth part of the bridge is called a **pontic** and the prepared teeth, which serve as supports for the crown parts on each side of the pontic, are called abutments. Fixed bridgework is designated by the amount of units involved. Each tooth, present or being replaced, is considered one unit each (Figure 7–19).

Crowns prepared to be part of a bridge or being fabricated solely as a single tooth cover are constructed in the same manner. The initial visit is rather long and complicated since many procedures are completed. The impression is taken for a temporary crown; the tooth or teeth are prepared for a covering; the final impression is taken for the construction of the artificial appliance. The prepared teeth are covered with a temporary crown cover to protect, while the construction is completed on the permanent appliance.

P R O C E D U R E   3 9

Assisting with Fixed Crowns (Visit 1)

1 Complete the Preparations

2 Assist with the Impressions

3 Assist with the Anesthesia

4 Assist with Tooth Shade Selection

5 Assist with Crown Preparation

6 Assist with Final Impression Tray or Tube Fit

7 Assist with Gingival Retraction Cord

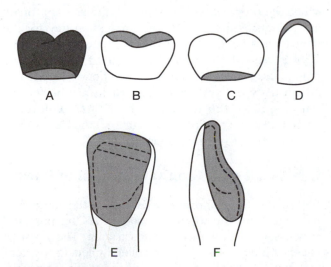

FIGURE 7–18 Examples of crowns: A, B, C, and D are full crowns; E and F are examples of three-quarter crowns.

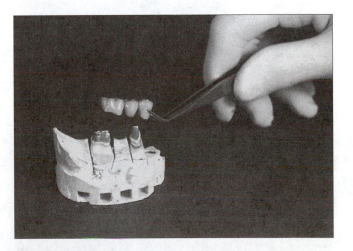

FIGURE 7–19 The three-unit bridge. Appliances are counted by the number of units used in the fabrication.

1 Complete the Preparations

The equipment and materials needed for the first visit follow:

- basic setup
- sundry setup, including floss, threader, and articulating paper
- anesthesia setup
- alginate impression materials, tray, adhesive, and setup
- high-speed handpiece with diamonds, disks, and burs
- hand instruments, spoon excavators, scalers
- tooth-shade guide
- gingival retraction cord and pusher or PFI
- final impression tray
- impression material and mixing equipment
- bite registration material
- compound, alcohol torch and tube (optional), or elastic-type impression material and tray
- crown and collar scissors
- acrylic cover material and dappen dish
- temporary cement and mixing materials
- slow handpiece with finishing burs
- varnish
- bite stick
- bag for impression
- wax for blocking space

The patient is greeted, seated, and prepared for the visit. The procedure is explained. The assistant dons PPE.

2 Assist with the Impressions

The assistant passes or uses the syringe to rinse the patient's mouth and passes an impression tray to the dentist for a fit. The recovered tray is painted with an adhesive material and alginate impression material is mixed. The tray is loaded and passed to the dentist, who takes an impression of the work site area. The procedure is repeated for the other arch. If the area involves a missing tooth, the blank area is blocked off with a wax insert, which the assistant passes to the dentist before the impression. The alginate impression is rinsed and wrapped in moist paper toweling until later use in the procedure.

3 Assist with the Anesthesia

The assistant aids with anesthesia by passing a piece of gauze to dry the injection site followed by an applicator with topical anesthesia. The anesthetic syringe is passed and received by the assistant, who caps the needle with a one-handed motion and monitors the patient's reactions.

4 Assist with Tooth Shade Selection

While waiting for the anesthesia to take effect, the assistant passes a dampened shade guide to the dentist to determine the correct tooth shade. The assistant either turns the lamp off or moves the beam so that natural light may be used for the judgment. The assistant receives the guide and records the choice.

5 Assist with Crown Preparation

The assistant aids in the crown preparation by passing the high-speed handpiece with a diamond rotary instrument or a fissure carbide bur. The assistant cools the area with a spray of water to the work site and increases visibility by evacuating and retracting. The assistant remains prepared to pass hand instruments on demand and to exchange burs and stones as requested.

6 Assist with Final Impression Tray or Tube Fit

When the preparation is completed, the assistant rinses and evacuates the mouth. The impression tray for the final impression is passed to the dentist for a fitting. Wax is passed for any adjustment. If it is a single crown, the dentist may prefer a compound material or an elastic-type impression material in a tube for the impression of the prepared tooth. An explorer is passed after the seating of the tube so the dentist may etch the correct seating position.

7 Assist with Gingival Retraction Cord

Before the final impression is taken, the gingiva is retracted from the tooth preparation so the prepared crown securely fits in the gingival area. The assistant passes a piece of cord in the college pliers to the dentist, who places the cord around the tooth. The assistant passes a hand instrument, a pusher or PFI, for the dentist to push the cord into the sulcus area beneath the gingival crest.

There are different kinds of gingival cords. Some are impregnated with chemicals, which help retract tissue. Some contain a vasoconstrictor, epinephrine, which is dangerous for a patient with a heart or blood pressure condition. The assistant must check with the dentist for the proper selection of cord. Cords also offer a selection in thickness. The dentist may prefer a thin-, or thick-gauged cord width.

8 Assist with Final Impression

The assistant dons overgloves to prevent cross contamination from touching materials and also to prevent chemical reaction of the latex exam gloves with some impression materials that may retard setting times. The college pliers are passed to the dentist, who retrieves the gingival cord and returns both. The assistant mixes the impression material according to the manufacturer's directions, fills the syringe, and gives it to the dentist for insertion around the prepared tooth. While this is being accomplished, the assistant mixes the thicker impression material, loads the tray, and passes it to the dentist for insertion. Mixing syringe materials, which are easily dispensed, may be used instead of the manually mixed ones.

When the impression material has set up (approximately four minutes), the tray with both materials is removed and returned to the assistant. The assistant rinses the impression, disinfects it, and places it in the plastic lab bag. Overgloves are removed.

9 Assist with Bite Registration

The assistant aids in the bite registration by preparing the bite tray and impression material. If the dentist wishes to use the dough ball technique, the assistant mixes a thicker ball of impression material and passes it to the dentist for insertion, bite, and setup. Silicone syringe impression material may be expressed onto the occlusal surfaces or pressed onto the facial surfaces, permitted to set up, and removed; or, a wax wafer can be warmed for the patient to bite and record. The dentist selects the material to use. In any case, the impression material is removed, rinsed, disinfected and placed in the plastic lab bag.

10 Assist with Temporary Cover Construction

The alginate impression that was taken and wrapped in moist toweling at the beginning of the appointment is retrieved. The assistant passes or uses the syringe to rinse the patient's mouth. The temporary acrylic material may be prepared directly in the impression by first expressing a few drops of monomer into the crown (Figure 7–20) and then shaking some shaded acrylic powder into the drops (Figure 7–21). The drip and

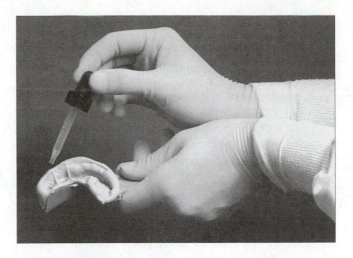

FIGURE 7–20 The drops of monomer are placed into the tooth indentations of the first alginate impression.

shake of the two products is repeated until the crown area is three-quarters full. When the sticky gloss appearance has left, the impression is reinserted onto the preparation site, which has been painted with varnish. The impression is permitted to remain until the form has taken.

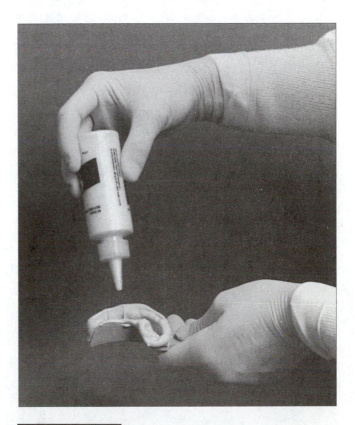

FIGURE 7–21 The shaded powder is shaken into the monomer liquid that was placed in the impression material.

An alternate method for preparation of a temporary cover is to complete a mixture of temporary acrylic in a paper cup and left to stand until the gloss is gone. During this time, a pellet moistened with varnish is passed to the dentist in college pliers. The dentist treats the prepared tooth. The acrylic mixture is spatulated into the preparation area of the first impression, passed to the dentist for seating, and allowed to set up. The tray is removed and returned to the assistant. The mouth is rinsed and evacuated again.

11 Assist with Finishing of the Cover

After setup and before total hardening, the impression is removed and the temporary cover is taken from the alginate. Any material that has oozed out of the site (flashing) is cut off (Figure 7–22), and the soft cover may be crimped for shape. When the material hardens, any rough edges are trimmed with a finishing bur or disk set in a slow handpiece (Figure 7–23). The finished cover is cemented onto the prepared tooth and worn until the finished crown is ready to be inserted.

12 Assist with Cementation of the Cover

The mouth is isolated with cotton rolls which have been passed from the assistant to the dentist. The assistant mixes the temporary cement at the dentist's signal and fills the cover. The dentist is handed a small PFI with cement, and the assistant holds the mixing tray near for refills. At the signal, the assistant passes

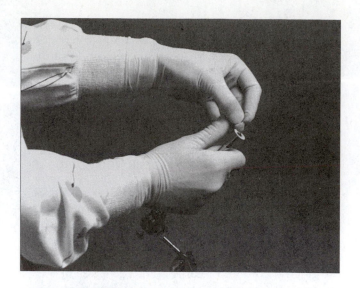

FIGURE 7–23 All rough edges must be smoothed and polished before the cover is cemented onto the tooth.

the cemented cover, and the dentist seats the crown cover. The assistant passes a bite stick for the patient to bite on. A sponge is passed to wipe off wet, excess cement.

The cement is allowed to dry. The assistant receives the bite stick and passes a scaler or explorer to the dentist to remove excess dry cement and check the fit. Dental floss is passed to check interproximal spaces. If the temporary cover involves a missing tooth area, the assistant passes a piece of dental floss in a floss threader to remove any loose cement under the bridge area.

The assistant holds articulating paper in the holder for the patient to bite on to test the bite. If adjustment is necessary, a slow handpiece with finishing bur is passed to adjust height. The mouth is rinsed and evacuated.

13 Dismiss Patient, Clean Up, Disinfect, and Sterilize

The patient's face is cleaned, and the drape and bib are removed. The patient is given postoperative instructions and a hygiene demonstration. The patient is dismissed.

The contaminated and used materials and equipment are taken to the sterilizing room. The latex gloves are removed, and the hands are washed. The treatment and color shade are written on the patient's chart. The plastic bag of impressions and bite registration is taken to the lab or prepared for shipment.

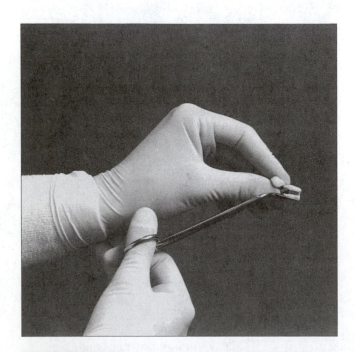

FIGURE 7–22 The excess material (flashing) is removed with scissors.

The utility gloves and PPE are donned. Cleanup, disinfection, and sterilization are completed. The gloves are washed, disinfected, and removed. The hands are washed.▲

T H E O R Y   R E C A L L

Fixed Prosthodontics

1. What does fixed prosthodontia involve?

   _____

2. Name four procedures that take place at the first prosthodontics appointment.

   a. _____

   b. _____

   c. _____

   d. _____

3. If the area for the impression involves a blank or missing space, what is placed in that area before the impression?

   _____

4. What is the assistant's duty during the preparation of the teeth for the prosthesis?

   _____

5. What is done to the gingiva before the final impression?

   _____

6. What does the assistant mix for the temporary crown cover?

   _____

7. After the cover is removed, what is done with it before cementation?

   _____

8. What is passed for isolation before the cementation of the cover?

   _____

9. What is used to remove cement from the interproximal spaces?

   _____

10. What is used to remove excess dry cement from under the temporary bridge?

   _____

Now turn to the Competency Evaluation Sheet for Procedure 39, Assisting with Fixed Crowns (Visit 1), located in Appendix C of this text.

FIXED CROWNS (FINAL VISIT)

The final visit for the dental crown is not as involved as the previous work. The completed crown is fitted and cemented onto the prepared tooth. Any needed adjustments are made, and the patient is dismissed. The crown should be a vital and useful addition to the patient's dentition that will last for a considerable amount of time if good oral hygiene practice is maintained.

When the crown is a part of bridgework, the patient is required to make an extra visit to try in and arrange the individual bridge units into position. The completed units (crowns and pontics) are placed into position, and an impression is taken to establish the proper alignment. Once this is finished, the temporary cover is replaced; the patient returns home until the units have been soldered together as bridgework.

The patient's final visit is basically the same for bridgework as for a single crown, except the appliance being placed is larger and more complicated.

P R O C E D U R E   4 0

Assisting with Fixed Crowns (Final Visit)

1 **Complete the Preparations**

2 **Assist with the Anesthesia**

3 **Assist with Temporary Cover Removal**

4 **Assist with Permanent Crown Try In**

5 **Assist with the Crown Adjustment**

6 **Assist with the Crown Cementation**

7 **Assist with the Final Crown Adjustment**

8 **Clean Up Patient, Disinfect, and Sterilize**

1 **Complete the Preparations**

The materials and equipment necessary for the final visit follow:

► basic setup
► sundry setup, including floss and articulating paper
► anesthetic setup
► slow handpiece with finishing burs, prophy handpiece, cups, brushes, and paste
► crown remover, crown seater, mallet
► bite stick
► hydrogen peroxide solution
► cement and mixing equipment
► PFI, scaler
► hand mirror

The patient is prepared and the procedure is explained. The assistant dons PPE.

2 Assist with the Anesthesia

The assistant rinses and evacuates the mouth. The injection site is dried with a piece of gauze. Topical anesthesia is applied to the site. The dentist is summoned and removes the applicator sticks. The anesthetic syringe is passed and received, and the needle is recapped with a one-handed motion. The patient's reaction to anesthesia is monitored.

3 Assist with Temporary Cover Removal

The assistant passes the crown remover to the dentist, which is returned with the temporary crown. The patient's mouth is rinsed and evacuated. The assistant passes a mirror and explorer to the dentist for an examination. Excess cement is removed by the explorer or with a scaler if requested. The mouth is rinsed and evacuated again.

4 Assist with Permanent Crown Try In

The assistant receives the mirror and explorer and passes the permanent crown, which is positioned on the preparation. The assistant passes the wood bite stick for the patient to bite on. If there is difficulty with the fit, the dentist may request a mallet and use the bite stick edge and mallet for force. When seated, the mallet and bite stick are returned; the assistant passes the mirror and explorer for examination of the fit.

5 Assist with the Crown Adjustment

Articulating paper is held on the occlusal surface, and the patient makes a test bite. The assistant may pass the slow handpiece with finishing bur to reduce any high areas. If the crown has a porcelain covering, special grinding wheels must be used; special polishing should be done to retain the glaze.

When the adjustment is finished, the assistant receives the handpiece and passes the crown remover. The crown is returned with the crown remover and checked for any dents or rough edges.

6 Assist with the Crown Cementation

The assistant uses the slow handpiece with a rubber disk or polishing wheel to polish the crown, which is cleaned out with hydrogen peroxide solution. Cotton rolls are passed to the dentist for isolation followed by college pliers with a varnish moistened to treat the prepared tooth. *If the crown area has received extensive removal, the dentist may choose to place retention pins into the tooth and build up the core before placing the crown onto the tooth.

The pick ups are returned. At the dentist's signal, the assistant mixes the permanent cement. The assistant places cement on the inside of the crown and passes a loaded PFI to the dentist to cement the preparation. Extra cement is held nearby for the dentist to refill.

The assistant receives the PFI and passes the crown, which is re-seated on the preparation. The bite stick is passed, and the patient bites down. If a mallet is necessary, the dentist signals. A piece of gauze to wipe off wet cement is passed when the stick and mallet are returned.

7 Assist with the Final Crown Adjustment

The assistant places a saliva ejector in the patient's mouth and lets the cement harden. When the cement has set, the assistant removes the saliva ejector and cotton rolls and hands the dentist a mirror and explorer for examination. Excess cement is removed. If a scaler is needed, the dentist signals.

When the cement is removed, the mouth is rinsed and evacuated. The assistant passes or holds articulating paper on the occlusal surface for a bite check. If adjustment is needed, the assistant passes the slow handpiece and a finishing bur or stone.

When adjustment is finished, the assistant receives the handpiece and prepares the prophy angle with brush and paste for polishing. The mouth is rinsed and evacuated. Dental floss is passed to check and clean the interproximal surfaces.

8 Clean Up Patient, Disinfect, and Sterilize

The patient's face is cleaned and the assistant passes a hand mirror to the patient for viewing the new crown. Instructions for care and hygiene are reviewed. The patient's bib and drape are removed. The patient is dismissed.

The assistant gathers contaminated materials and equipment and takes them to the sterilizing room. The gloves are removed and the hands are washed. The treatment is recorded on the patient's chart.

The assistant dons utility gloves and PPE, disinfects, cleans, and sterilizes in the usual manner. The gloves are washed, disinfected, and removed; the hands are washed.▲

THEORY RECALL

Fixed Crowns (Final Visit)

1. What procedures are accomplished on the final visit for a crown placement?

_____

2. When are the adjustments completed?

_____

3. What instrument is passed to the dentist to remove the temporary crown?

_____

4. What does the patient bite on to seat the crown?

_____

5. If the patient's bite is not sufficient to seat the crown, what instrument may the dentist call for to seat the crown?

_____

6. What is the crown checked for after removal from the test seating?

_____

7. What is used to clean out the permanent crown before cementation?

_____

8. What type of cement is used to cement the crown?

_____

9. What does the assistant place in the patient's mouth while the cement is setting?

_____

10. What does the assistant hand to the dentist when the cement has set?

_____

Now turn to the Competency Evaluation Sheet for Procedure 40, Assisting with Fixed Crowns (Final Visit), located in Appendix C of this text.

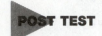

Total possible points = 100 points
80% needed for passing = 80 points

Total points this test _____ pass _____ fail _____

MULTIPLE CHOICE: Circle the correct answer. Each question is worth 3 points for a total of 60 points.

1. A dental crown is considered which type of dental appliance?
   a. orthodontic   b. fixed   c. removable   d. operative

2. How long is an endodontic instrument left in the glass bead sterilizer?
   a. 10 to 15 seconds   b. 10 to 15 minutes   c. 2 to 4 hours   d. overnight

3. The alginate impression taken of the tooth before crown preparation is used
   a. for legal proof.
   b. for study models.
   c. to serve as a model for the permanent crown.
   d. to serve as a model for the temporary crown.

4. A pulpotomy is a
   a. partial removal of pulp tissue.
   b. total removal of pulpal tissue.
   c. capping of pulp tissue.
   d. calcification of pulp tissue.

5. All laboratory work sent to a commercial lab must have
   a. a prescription.   b. the fee posted.   c. the assistant's comments.   d. a boxing permit.

6. A ten-year-old child is said to have what type of dentition?
   a. mixed   b. primary   c. secondary   d. partial

7. The purpose for the use of endodontic "stoppers" is
   a. to control bleeding.
   b. to regulate thickness.
   c. to regulate length.
   d. to stop bleeding.

8. A dental crown may be part of a larger appliance called
   a. orthodontic bond.   b. a mobile fixator.   c. a bridge.   d. an endo tracker.

9. Which of the following is *not* considered a preventive measure for pediatric treatment?
   a. sealants   b. fluorides   c. restorations   d. gold crowns

10. Dental dam isolation is used in endodontics to (1) control bleeding, (2) control tongue movement, (3) provide visibility, (4) keep the field sterile, or (5) protect from chemicals.
    a. 1 and 2   b. 1, 3 and 5   c. 3, 4 and 5   d. all of the above

11. The tooth shade is moistened before use to
    a. imitate natural conditions.
    b. make insertion easier.
    c. enhance denture color.
    d. prevent cracking.

12. A good material to use for pulp capping is
    a. zinc phosphate.   b. calcium hydroxide.   c. resin.   d. hydrogen peroxide.

13. In denture fabrication, a custom tray is made
    a. for study models.
    b. to give better impression detail.
    c. to test accuracy of alginate impression.
    d. for fluoridation.

14. Sealants placed on primary teeth must be used on teeth that have been
    a. rinsed and dried.   b. isolated.   c. precleaned.   d. all of these conditions

15. Which of the following materials is *not* suitable for crown fabrication?
    a. amalgam   b. gold   c. resin over metal   d. chrome

16. Endodontic files and reamers are used for which purposes? (1) to enlarge canals, (2) to smooth canals, (3) to measure canals, or (4) treat canals.
    a. 1 and 2   b. 1, 2, and 3   c. 1, 3, and 4   d. all of the above

17. Which of these endodontic tests is conducted using finger pressure? (1) percussion, (2) thermal, (3) vitality, (4) questioning, (5) examination, (6) x-ray, (7) mobility, (8) palpation, or (9) transillumination.
    a. 8   b. 7 and 8   c. 1, 7, and 8   d. all of the above

18. Fluoride ingested in food or drink is said to be which type?
    a. topical   b. systemic   c. aciduphosphate   d. liquid

19. Pulpotomy and pulpectomy treatments require
    a. sterile technique.   c. impression methods.
    b. permanent covering.   d. sealant covering.

20. For which purposes are paper points used in endodontic treatment? (1) to dry canals, (2) to moisten canals, (3) to irrigate pulp, (4) to maintain pressure, (5) to measure canals, or (6) to x-ray indicator of length.
    a. 1   b. 3 and 6   c. 4, 5, and 6   d. all of the above

MATCHING: Place the letter from Column B in the correct blank in column A. Each question is worth 2 points for a total of 40 points.

	Colulmn A		Column B
___ 1.	gutta percha	a.	permanent cement
___ 2.	alginate	b.	sedates pulp and stimulates secondary dentin growth
___ 3.	calcium hydroxide	c.	controls pulp bleeding
___ 4.	monomer/polymer acrylic	d.	fills pulp canal; used in thermal testing for endodontics
___ 5.	pumice	e.	used for impressions
___ 6.	cast gold	f.	used for isolation of teeth
___ 7.	sealant	g.	acrylic protection for newly erupted teeth
___ 8.	dental dam	h.	material for temporary crown cover
___ 9.	zinc phosphate	i.	polishing material
___ 10.	Formo-cresol	j.	permanent crowns

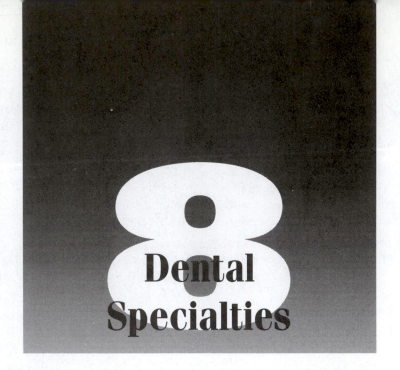

8

Dental Specialties

◤ OBJECTIVES

Upon completion of this unit, the student will achieve a score of 80% or better on the Post Test covering the following material.

1. Discuss the importance of the preliminary examination for the orthodontic patient, including the causes, treatments, and procedures used in this specialty.
2. Describe the duties and responsibilities of the dental assistant during the orthodontic banding appointment.
3. Describe the duties and responsibilities of the dental assistant during the orthodontic bonding appointment.
4. Demonstrate the techniques necessary for the placement and removal of the arch wires, including the tie in with ligatures.
5. Discuss the type of procedures performed by the oral surgeon and the types of patient and cases referred for specialist care.
6. Discuss the duties and responsibilities of the dental assistant during the multiple extraction, postoperative, and suture removal procedures.
7. List the various types of soft tissue surgical techniques performed by the oral surgeon and the role the dental assistant plays during these procedures.
8. Discuss the importance of the preliminary examination for periodontal services and list the various patient influences for the condition of the periosteum.
9. Describe the duties and responsibilities of the dental assistant during the gingivectomy and surgical packing treatment procedure.

◤ KEY TERMS

activator	curettage	malocclusion
alveolitis	debride	PFI
alveoplasty	dry socket	protrude
biopsy	exudate	retruded
brackets	festoon	spicules
buccal tube	frenum	supernumerary
cariogenic	I & D	supragingival
contouring		

ORTHODONTICS

Orthodontics is the branch of dentistry that deals with the alignment of teeth and jaw structure (Table 8–1). Treatment may be of a corrective, preventive, or interceptive nature. It normally is not an immediate process but involves growth and development occurring over a period of time.

Preventive or interceptive orthodontic treatment is designed to address various mouth conditions, which, when left untreated, may develop into orthodontic problems. Common conditions may be premature loss of teeth, which may call for space maintenance devices, or habit-control measures to deal with thumb sucking, tongue thrusting, fingernail biting, or other bad habits.

Corrective orthodontics, the treatment of existing **malocclusion** conditions, is usually completed with the use of removable or fixed intraoral and extraoral appliances.

The orthodontist must include a variety of diagnostic procedures, such as x-rays, photographs, impressions, clinical exams, health history interviews, and dental examinations to determine a special, individualized treatment plan for the patient.

At one time, orthodontics was considered for only the child patient, but today many adult patients are seeking and receiving orthodontic care. The procedure plan outlined is for the child patient but may be easily adapted for the adult.

The preliminary exam is the preparatory appointment and may be called the workup or pretreatment visit. The dentist obtains the information necessary to plan orthodontic care by completing a multitude of procedures. The assistant aids or performs some of these procedures, depending on the State Dental Practice Act of the state employed and the training and competence level of the individual.

When the procedures are completed, the patient and parents receive a consultation appointment in which the dentist presents and explains the orthodontic plan, gives a time estimate, and makes financial arrangements. Future appointments are centered around the information gathered by the preliminary exam and the orthodontist's study of the data.

P R O C E D U R E 4 1
Assisting with the Orthodontic Preliminary Examination

1 Assist with Interview and Preparation

2 Assist with or Expose Photographs

3 Prepare the Patient

4 Assist with Clinical Examination

5 Assist with or Expose Radiographs

6 Assist with or Take Full-Mouth Alginate Impressions

TABLE 8–1

Possible Causes and Treatments for Tooth Malocclusion

CAUSES

Genetic—large teeth for small bones, small teeth for large bones, inherited growth patterns and abnormalities, such as **supernumerary** teeth, cleft palate, improperly sized tongue, **frenum**, or lips.

Habits—tongue thrusting, finger and thumb sucking, nail biting, mouth breathing

Health—diseases, injuries, and physical conditions, such as TMJ trouble, cysts, growths, carious, and missing teeth

TREATMENT

Preventive	▶ restorative work to prevent loss of teeth
	▶ space maintainer to hold space of missing tooth
	▶ monitoring of growth and development of teeth and bones
	▶ alertness for abnormalities
	▶ correction of bad habits affecting oral health
Interceptive	▶ removal of teeth retained over functional time
	▶ placement of incline plane appliances to guide growth
	▶ regaining of lost space through space-seeking maintainers
	▶ tooth removal to prevent overcrowding of arch
Corrective	▶ use of bands, brackets, tubes, wires, and appliances to alter or correct and control growth to proper correct alignment

7 **Dismiss the Patient**

8 **Clean Up, Disinfect, and Sterilize**

1 Assist with Interview and Preparation

The setup for the preliminary exam follows:

Interview Needs

► patient information records
► health and medical history records
► business and financial records
► patient folder and pen
► camera and cheek retractors

Examination Needs

► basic setup
► sundry setup
► alginate impression and equipment setup
► radiographic films and machine

The exam begins in the consultation room where the orthodontist interviews the parent and child to determine the interest and need. The health and medical history, including habits and allergies, which may already have been previously gathered by the assistant, are noted. This information is important to help determine the cause or reason for the malocclusion and the course of treatment needed. Any data gathered regarding the patient is recorded on the history chart.

2 Assist with or Expose Photographs

The assistant may expose photographs of the patient. The child is asked to hold clear cheek retractors, which permit better exposure of the teeth and gingival areas. An identification plate with name and case number and date may be prepared ahead of time and placed around the child's neck. A full face view and each side view are taken. Photographs are important records that provide appearance and progress data for pretreatment assessment. Photographs are taken regularly throughout the treatment period.

3 Prepare the Patient

The operatory or dental chair area is prepared for the patient to be seated after the interview and photographs. The patient is draped and a bib is placed. The atmosphere remains casual but businesslike. Conversation regarding the patient's interest is started, establishing a rapport with the child. The assistant dons the PPE.

4 Assist with Clinical Examination

The assistant records the findings of the clinical examination. The orthodontist begins by appraising the facial structure, abnormalities, and occlusion classification.

Malocclusion conditions may be classified into one of three types—Class I, Class II, or Class III—according to a system devised by Dr. Edward Angle. In 1899, Dr. Angle based the classification on the relationship of the maxillary first permanent molar with the mandibular first permanent molar while in occlusion (Figure 8–1).

In Class I, the mesiobuccal cusp of the maxillary first permanent molar lies in the mesiobuccal groove of the mandibular first permanent molar. The maxillary permanent cuspid lies between the mandibular permanent cuspid and first bicuspid or premolar. While the jaws seem in good relationship, some occlusion problem exists, such as malpositioned, missing, or unerupted teeth; open, cross, or overbite, or excessive spacing within the teeth.

In Class II, the distobuccal cusp of the maxillary permanent first molar lies in the mesiobuccal groove of the mandibular first permanent molar, and the cuspid is mesial to the lower cuspid. The jaws have a bite appearance of a **retruded** lower jaw or overjetting upper jaw. Teeth may be tipped, crowded, or overlapping. The anterior teeth position also subdivide this classification into type 1 and type 2.

In type 1, the maxillary incisors are extremely tipped toward the lip (labiovertically); in type 2, the maxillary incisors are normal or tip slightly toward the tongue (linguovertically). The maxillary lateral teeth often overlap the central incisors by tipping labially and mesially.

In Class III, the mesiobuccal cusp of the maxillary permanent first molar is distal to the mandibular first permanent molar, and the upper cuspid lies distal to the lower cuspid. The jaws have an appearance of a **protruded** lower jaw and a retruded upper jaw.

The assistant may pass a mirror when the orthodontist examines the teeth and gingival tissues and remains ready with the syringe for air or water spray as signaled. All findings are neatly and accurately recorded.

5 Assist with or Expose Radiographs

Depending on the State Dental Practice Act, the assistant either exposes or assists with the exposure of the radiographs needed for the case study. X-rays determine the position of the exposed teeth and the unerupted teeth to follow. Bone density and growth prediction may be obtained through radiographs. The orthodontist requires a set of intraoral radiographs, an occlusal, and a panoramic view. A cephalometric (full-head) radiograph

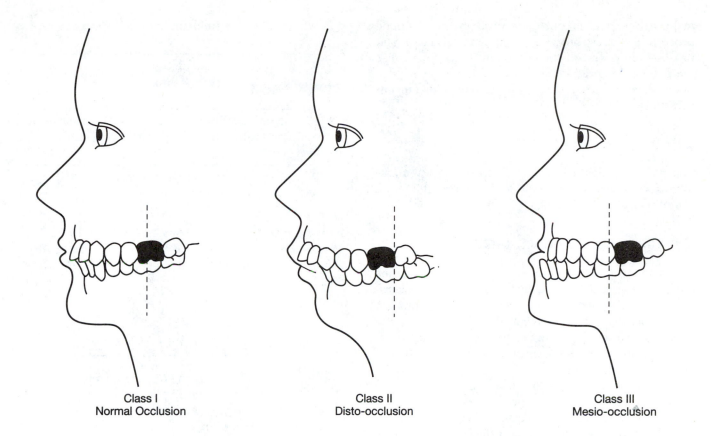

Class I
Normal Occlusion

Class II
Disto-occlusion

Class III
Mesio-occlusion

FIGURE 8–1 Each type of malocclusion exhibits specific characteristics.

also is taken to measure, trace, and predict future growth (Figure 8–2).

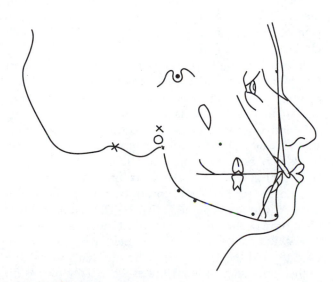

FIGURE 8–2 Cephalometric drawings can help determine future bone growth. (Photo courtesy of DENTSPLY International, Inc., GENDEX Corporation, Midwest Dental Products Corporation.)

6 Assist with or Take Full-Mouth Alginate Impressions

When the mouth exam and radiographs are completed, the assistant may help with or complete the alginate impressions for study casts. These are used for diagnosis and preparation. These casts show the best view of the lingual side of the tooth development and also provide a replica of the mouth for measurement and appliance fitting.

The assistant passes trays to determine a correctly sized tray fit. Any wax adaptation or padding needed to improve the mucobuccal fold involvement is performed at this time and retested for fit. The syringe is passed for the dentist to spray rinse the mouth, and the assistant mixes the alginate material to a smooth, creamy texture.

The tray is loaded and passed to the dentist, who seats and holds the alginate in the tray until the material sets. The tray is removed and examined for proper indentations. If acceptable, it is rinsed in water, disinfected, and wrapped in a wet disinfectant tissue. After a spray rinse and evacuation, the second arch is completed in the same manner.

The assistant softens base plate wax or a bite wafer in warm water and hands it to the orthodontist to make a bite registration to be used in the trimming process. The assistant receives the bite registration and passes the syringe to the orthodontist to spray rinse the patient's mouth. The bite registration is rinsed, disinfected, and placed in the plastic bag with the impressions.

7 Dismiss the Patient

The patient is cleaned up and dismissed. An appointment for a consultation meeting of parents, child, and orthodontist is arranged.

8 Clean up, Disinfect, and Sterilize

The operatory area is cleaned up. The impressions and bite registration are bagged and taken to the laboratory. The exposed radiographs are bagged and taken to be processed. The contaminated materials and equipment are gathered and taken to the sterilizing area. The assistant removes the exam gloves, washes hands, and records treatment.

The assistant dons utility gloves and performs the operatory and sterilizing room techniques. Utility gloves are washed and disinfected when work is completed. Gloves are removed, and the assistant washes hands.▲

THEORY RECALL

Orthodontics

1. Orthodontics is the branch of dentistry that is concerned with what?

_____

2. What does the orthodontist need to determine the special individualized treatment plan for a patient?

_____

3. What type of appointment is the preliminary examination?

_____

4. What determines the amount of help the assistant may give in a preliminary examination?

_____

5. What type of appointment is given to the parents and patient when the preliminary exam is completed?

_____

6. Around what are future orthodontic appointments centered?

_____

7. Where does the preliminary examination begin?

_____

8. What does the patient hold during the photographic session?

_____

9. What type of atmosphere does the assistant try to establish in the preliminary exam appointment?

_____

10. What types of radiographs does the orthodontist require in the preliminary exam?

_____

Now turn to the Competency Evaluation Sheet for Procedure 41, Assisting with the Orthodontic Preliminary Examination, located in Appendix C of this text.

PLACEMENT OF ORTHODONTIC BANDS

Orthodontic treatment to correct malocclusion and to improve facial contour is completed by the use of push and pull forces. Movement is accomplished by the application of tension and strain from springs, elastics, and wires. Pressure applied to the crown of a tooth transmits the length of the tooth and eventually pushes and compresses the tooth against the periodontal bone causing resorption of the tissue. This loss of resistance permits the tooth to move into the space.

When the tooth is pulled into a space, there is an opening or gap on the other side where the tooth was previously present. This stretch area is soon filled in with bony tissue and with time will calcify until tooth movement is complete.

In order to apply pressure to the tooth, there must be some way to attach the forceful appliances. This is accomplished by two methods—banding the crown of a tooth or bonding appliances to the tooth surfaces.

When banding teeth, the orthodontist attaches stainless steel circles around specific teeth. These bands may be custom-made in the office by sizing the strip around a tooth and then spot welding it into a circle or may be ordered constructed for each type of tooth in various generalized sizes. The bands may be plain or may already have attached brackets or tubes.

Brackets are placed on the anterior bands and are used to hold the U-shaped arch wire that gives shape to the entire arch. **Buccal tubes** are usually placed on the molar bands and are used for inserting the ends of the arch wire that encircles the surfaces of the teeth. Both the brackets and tubes are placed on the facial side for attaching devices, and lugs or buttons may be placed on the lingual side for assistance in seating the band. The gingival edge of the band is straight edged, while the incisal or occlusal end is beveled. The bands may be applied at one setting or may be progressively applied according to the individualized treatment plan (Figure 8–3).

Before the band application appointment, separators may be placed in the interproximal spaces of the teeth to provide space for the banding visit. These separators may be made of latex elastic circles, plastic wedges, or metal springs. The assistant may be permitted, in some states, to insert and remove these separators, which are placed during an appointment scheduled a few days before the banding visit. Elastic circles are "sawed" into the interproximal area much like dental floss, plastic dumbbell-shaped wedges are pressure forced into the area and the metal spring separators are clamped in.

The assistant advises the patient not to eat foods or chewy candies and to avoid chewing gum. The patient is also advised that some separators may drop out before the banding appointment. This is not a problem. It only indicates that the spacing has been accomplished.

At the banding appointment, which usually is the longest visit, the assistant prepares the patient and removes the remaining separators. Bands for fitting and adapting are passed until the proper ones have been chosen. The assistant organizes the bands and, upon their removal, takes them to the lab for the final preparation.

The cementation of the bands is accomplished with a team effort. The assistant mixes the cement, loads the band by evenly coating the insides and passes it to the orthodontist until all have been seated. When the cement has hardened, the assistant may be permitted to remove the excess or assists the operator in doing so.

Arch wires and ligatures may be applied at the banding appointment, or the patient may be scheduled for another appointment to receive these appliances. The orthodontist determines the exact treatment per visit.

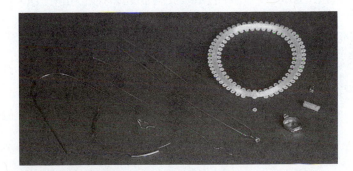

FIGURE 8–3 Examples of orthodontic appliances.

Before the patient is dismissed, the assistant instructs in the care of the appliances and the oral hygiene and nutrition attention that must be given the appliances.

P R O C E D U R E 4 2

Assisting with Placement of Orthodontic Bands

1 Prepare for Banding Appointment

2 Seat the Patient

3 Assist with Selection of Bands

4 Assist with Preparation of Bands

5 Assist with Crown Polish

6 Assist with Cementation of Bands

7 Clean Up Patient and Dismiss

8 Clean Up, Disinfect, and Sterilize

1 Prepare for Banding Appointment

The setup for the banding appointment follows:

► basic setup
► sundry materials, including cotton rolls and holders
► assorted presized bands with or without brackets and tubes
► band block receptacle
► band-applying instruments—pushers, adaptors, contouring pliers, band driver, band file or smoother, band seater, burnisher, and band remover
► cement and mixing equipment
► plastic filling instrument (PFI)
► handpiece with prophy cup and paste
► scalers

Lab setup includes:

► assorted brackets and tubes
► electric welder
► finishing bur
► wax and pins

2 Seat the Patient

The assistant greets and seats the patient, placing a bib around the neck. The assistant reviews the health history by inquiring into any illnesses or accidents since the last visit and then explains the procedure. PPE is donned and the orthodontist is summoned.

3 Assist with Selection of Bands

The assistant begins the appointment by handing the orthodontist an explorer to check the teeth. Any separators needing removal are taken out at this time. *In some states, the assistant is permitted to remove the separators and may do so before summoning the orthodontist. The syringe may be passed for a water spray and air dry. The assistant receives the syringe and passes a try in band for sizing.

Some orthodontic bands are numbered according to the Palmer method, where a bracket mark indicates the arch and the numbers 1–8 indicate each tooth in the arch. Color-coding is also useful in identifying the various sizes of the bands. Marked bands are passed, followed by the band pusher; adapting and **contouring** instruments are passed as signaled by the orthodontist.

When a properly sized band has been chosen, the assistant passes an explorer to the orthodontist to scratch a mark indicating the position of the band or to place a bracket. The explorer is received as the assistant passes a band remover to the orthodontist to remove the fitted band. The assistant receives the band remover and band and places the sized band on an arch block in the appropriate place designated for that tooth. The procedure is followed again for each tooth to be banded at this appointment.

4 Assist with Preparation of Bands

The patient is advised of the rest period, which occurs while the assistant takes the bands to the lab for final preparation. Overgloves are donned and the arch band block with the fitted bands is gathered. The waiting procedure is explained to the patient, who is given a book or game to occupy the time. Children and many adults enjoy the hand-held computer games, which help to pass time while band processing is going on. The assistant takes the bands to the lab area.

In the lab area the bands are prepared for cementation. The edges are checked for any roughness. Any dents or sharp areas are smoothed off with a handpiece and finishing bur. If the fitted bands have brackets, the bands are fitted with pins or wax in the openings to prevent cement from filling the bracket holes and making the brackets useless for retaining the arch wire.

If the bands do not have brackets, the assistant selects a bracket, places it on the scratched mark and spot welds the two metals together. The finished bracketed band is waxed and pinned also. All bands are lubricated on the outside for easy removal of cement after they have been placed in the mouth. The bands are rechecked for proper positioning and placed on designated areas on the band block for proper use.

5 Assist with Crown Polish

The assistant returns the prepared bands to the chairside, summons the orthodontist, and removes the overgloves. A slow handpiece with prophy cup and paste is passed to the orthodontist, and the excess is held near the work site. The assistant passes or uses the syringe to rinse and the HVE to evacuate as needed. If calculus or tartar buildup is present, the orthodontist may call for a scaler to remove the debris before cementation. Dental floss is also passed so the orthodontist may check the interproximal spaces. In states where permitted, the assistant may perform this procedure and then summon the dentist for cementation of the bands.

6 Assist with Cementation of Bands

The assistant passes cotton rolls or a loaded cotton roll holder to the orthodontist for isolation of the banding area. The assistant mixes the zinc phosphate cement according to the manufacturer's directions and loads the first band, making sure to load from the gingival edge and cover the entire inside of the band. The loaded band is placed on a small tab of masking tape that helps to hold the little appliance for passing to the orthodontist. The orthodontist places it on the tooth. The assistant passes the band driver and any other instrument the orthodontist may call for until the band is properly seated.

A wet piece of gauze is placed near the work site for the orthodontist to wipe off excess cement on instruments. The assistant also holds a wet gauze to wipe instrument tips. The HVE tip is used to maintain a dry field. The banding procedure is repeated again on another tooth until all scheduled bands have been cemented or until the cement has lost its gloss and requires a new mix to be prepared. In such a case, a new batch of cement is prepared and the appointment continues until all scheduled banding is completed.

7 Clean Up Patient and Dismiss

The patient is permitted to sit and wait until the cement has finished its final set. The assistant monitors the patient during this period, perhaps returning the book or hand game to amuse the patient. When the cement has set, the isolation is removed and the orthodontist is summoned. The assistant passes a scaler for removal of excess cement on the bands. The assistant passes or uses the syringe for a water spray rinse and the HVE to evacuate the area until all cement is removed and the bands are clean. Again, if permitted by the State Dental Practice Act, the assistant may perform this procedure.

The patient's face is cleaned and the parent is brought into the room. The assistant gives the patient a hand mirror to view the bands. While parent and patient are together, the assistant gives instructions in care, hygiene, and nutrition (Table 8–2). The patient is dismissed.

8 Clean Up, Disinfect, and Sterilize

The assistant gathers the contaminated materials and equipment, takes them to the sterilizing room, removes gloves, and washes hands. The treatment and band sizes are marked on the patient's chart, which is taken to the front desk.

The assistant returns, dons utility gloves and PPE, and disinfects the operatory area. The disposable articles are placed in the proper containers. The large items are disinfected, and the instruments are cleaned and prepared for sterilizing. All bands that have been tried or exposed at the chair are sterilized, regardless if they were used or not. The area is cleaned up; the gloves are washed, disinfected, and removed. The assistant washes hands.▲

THEORY RECALL

Placement of Orthodontic Bands

1. How is orthodontic treatment and facial recontouring completed?

   _____

2. Pressure to the tooth transmits the entire length and eventually compresses what tissue?

   _____

3. What two methods may be used to attach appliances to the teeth?

   _____

4. Tubes are usually placed on which bands, anterior or molar?

   _____

5. Are brackets and tubes placed on the facial or lingual side of the band?

   _____

6. What may be placed on the lingual side of the band?

   _____

7. In what three materials may separators be purchased?

   a. _____

   b. _____

   c. _____

8. What advice is given to the patient when separators are placed?

   _____

9. What are some of the duties the assistant may perform during a banding appointment?

   _____

10. What type of instructions does the assistant give the patient upon dismissal?

   _____

Now turn to the Competency Evaluation Sheet for Procedure 42, Assisting with Placement of Orthodontic Bands, located in Appendix C of this text.

TABLE 8–2

Postoperative Instructions for the Orthodontic Patient

1. Maintain good oral hygiene. It is very important to keep the teeth and appliances clean. Use a soft bristle brush to clean all areas after eating and at bedtime. It will do no good to align and correct the teeth if poor oral hygiene leads to caries and possible tooth loss.

2. Follow prescribed home care. Place appliances and elastics as directed for the specific time and method indicated. Orthodontic care is a team effort. The patient is responsible to maintain appliances as specified.

3. Avoid eating high **cariogenic** (sweet, sticky) and hard foods. Avoid or cut down on soda, substitute fruit drinks, if possible. Some foods tend to adhere to the teeth more than others, and carbonated drinks can cause some deterioration of the appliance cements.

4. If any of the appliances placed in the mouth become loose, call the office for an appointment. If left unattended, one loose piece will place strain on other pieces and destroy the effectiveness of the appliance.

5. Keep all appointments scheduled with the office. The treatment plan is made up with a time frame sequence that should be followed.

BONDING BRACKETS

The orthodontist may decide to place brackets or tubes directly onto the tooth surface when preparing for arch wire support. This process, called direct bonding of bands (DB), is effective in cases in which the crowding of teeth does not permit placement of stainless steel bands. Some orthodontists prefer the DB system because they are faster to apply, less traumatic to fit, and more attractive in appearance. Also, the patient may be able to maintain oral hygiene easier with less artificial structuring present in the mouth.

Direct bonding brackets are supplied in four materials—plastic, ceramic, composite, and metal. Plastic and composite brackets (clear and designer colors) need to be preconditioned before being placed in the bonding material. Ceramic brackets need a special bonding adhesive, and metal brackets and tubes have a thin mesh backing that helps to adhere to the surface.

The duties of the assistant in bonding are similar to the banding visit. The assistant helps prepare the brackets and tubes, assists with or performs the coronal polish, and then aids with the etching of the tooth enamel surface prior to the cementation of the appliances.

Direct bonding is completed by cementing the attachments onto the prepared tooth surfaces. There are two types of bonding cements—one is self-activated and the other is light cured. In the auto-cured cement, the two materials are mixed and placed on the tooth surface, bracket, or tube. The curing is completed in the manufacturer's set time. Fresh cement must be mixed to complete the entire mouth when the time period has expired for the first mixture. Cement that is too tacky due to curing limits will not adhere properly, and leakage can occur.

Light-activated cement permits more working and preparation time than other types of cement. The cement is applied to the surfaces, the attachment is placed, and then the tip of the light is held close for the manufacturer's recommended time period, usually a few seconds. Once these hooked attachments have been applied and cured, the assistant may help or perform the cleanup removal of any excess cement. The orthodontist may wish to proceed with the attachment of the arch wires with ligatures or make an appointment for this procedure at a future date.

PROCEDURE 43

Assisting with Cementation of Brackets

1 Assemble Equipment

2 Prepare the Patient

3 Assist with Bonding Preparation

4 Assist with Acid-Etch

5 Assist with Bracket and Tube Bonding

6 Clean Up Patient

7 Clean Up Operatory

8 Disinfect and Sterilize

1 Assemble Equipment

The setup for the bonding appointment follows:

- ▶ basic setup
- ▶ sundry material setup with cotton roll holders
- ▶ slow handpiece with prophy angle and paste
- ▶ etching material and equipment
- ▶ activator material and equipment
- ▶ bonding material and equipment
- ▶ curing lamp for light cured material (if used)

2 Prepare the Patient

The assistant greets and seats the patient inquiring into the patient's health history. The procedure is explained to the patient. PPE is donned, and the orthodontist is summoned. An illustration of the bonding process may be found in Figure 8–4.

3 Assist with Bonding Preparation

An explorer is passed to the orthodontist for checking the teeth and preparing for etching. To perform the crown polishing (Figure 8–4A), the slow handpiece with prophy angle, cup or brush, and paste are passed when the explorer is returned. The assistant holds the prophy paste at the work site and passes or uses the syringe for water spray rinsing. The HVE tip is used for evacuation of the mouth. *In some states, the trained assistant may perform the coronal polishing.

The assistant passes the syringe for drying of the tooth surfaces and receives the syringe while passing cotton rolls or a loaded cotton roll holder for isolation. In place of the cotton rolls, the orthodontist may prefer to isolate the teeth by placing a dental dam, particularly for the etching process.

4 Assist with Acid-Etch

The tooth surfaces must be acid-etched to soften a microscopic layer of the enamel tissue, which permits the better adhesion of the bonding cement for the tooth and bracket or tube (Figure 8–4B and C). To assist with the etching of the tooth, the assistant dons overgloves to work with the bonding material syringes to prevent contamination between patients. The syringes nevertheless are disinfected when the procedure is over.

The material is prepared, and a loaded applicator tip is passed to the orthodontist, who places a drop of the gel on the facial surface of the tooth or teeth. The assistant holds the gel syringe nearby for refills to the applicator tip. The assistant monitors the timing (approximately 60 seconds) and passes the syringe for a water spray rinse. The HVE tip is used to evacuate the mouth. The used cotton rolls are removed.

5 Assist with Bracket and Tube Bonding

When the etching is completed, the assistant passes fresh cotton rolls for re-isolation. The activator material is prepared and the applicator brush is passed to the orthodontist, who places the activator on the etched surface. The assistant places some activator on the bracket being held in the pliers (Figure 8–4D).

The assistant passes the pliers with bracket and **activator** to the orthodontist and receives the activator brush. The assistant prepares the bonding material, places a small amount on the bonding brush, and paints the back of the bracket or tube the orthodontist is holding. The orthodontist places the bracket on the activator paste with a twisting motion. Occasionally, the dentist may wish to adjust the angle placement of the bracket and request a straight hand instrument for slight movement of the hook (Figure 8–5). The assistant times the process (35–45 seconds) (Figure 8–4E).

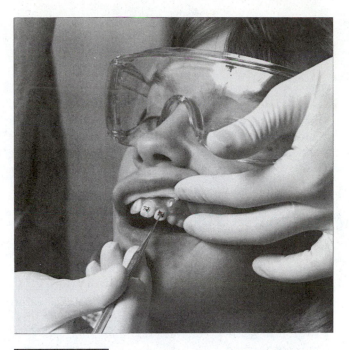

FIGURE 8–5 The brackets may be bonded directly to the tooth surface. They may be clear or in designers' colors.

When the cement has set, a scaler is used to remove any excess (Figure 8–4F). The blade edge of the scaler is moved in a direction away from the center of the bracket to avoid loosening the article from the tooth. The scaler instrument is used in short strokes from center to outer surface. A scaler is passed to remove the cement or the procedure is performed by the assistant in areas where permitted. The activating and bonding process is repeated for each tooth to be bracketed.

When all have been bracketed, the assistant removes the overgloves and the patient's isolation and passes the syringe for a spray rinse of the mouth. The HVE is used to evacuate the area.

If a light-cured bonding material is used, the assistant holds the light and shield near the area of the bracket bonding for the manufacturer's designated time. If the orthodontist is using plastic brackets, the brackets are preconditioned by placing the activator on the bracket two minutes prior to seating.

6 Clean Up Patient

When all the brackets are cemented on the teeth, the assistant passes a scaler to the orthodontist for removal of excess cement. The scaler is received and an explorer is passed for the orthodontist to check the adhesion and position of the brackets. If the orthodontist is satisfied with the seating, the placement of the arch wire may proceed after four minutes of final setting. The patient may be reassigned another appointment for the arch wire placement.

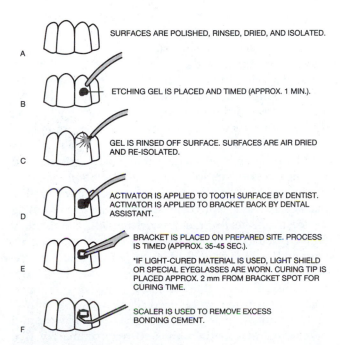

A — SURFACES ARE POLISHED, RINSED, DRIED, AND ISOLATED.

B — ETCHING GEL IS PLACED AND TIMED (APPROX. 1 MIN.).

C — GEL IS RINSED OFF SURFACE. SURFACES ARE AIR DRIED AND RE-ISOLATED.

D — ACTIVATOR IS APPLIED TO TOOTH SURFACE BY DENTIST. ACTIVATOR IS APPLIED TO BRACKET BACK BY DENTAL ASSISTANT.

E — BRACKET IS PLACED ON PREPARED SITE. PROCESS IS TIMED (APPROX. 35-45 SEC.).

*IF LIGHT-CURED MATERIAL IS USED, LIGHT SHIELD OR SPECIAL EYEGLASSES ARE WORN. CURING TIP IS PLACED APPROX. 2 mm FROM BRACKET SPOT FOR CURING TIME.

F — SCALER IS USED TO REMOVE EXCESS BONDING CEMENT.

FIGURE 8–4 The acid-etching process for direct bonding of brackets and tubes.

The patient is cleaned up and the parent summoned. The assistant gives instructions in care, hygiene, and nutrition. The patient is dismissed.

7 Clean Up Operatory

The assistant gathers the contaminated materials and equipment and takes them to the sterilizing room. The latex exam gloves are removed and hands are washed. The assistant records the treatment on the patient's chart and takes it to the front desk.

8 Disinfect and Sterilize

The assistant returns, dons utility gloves and PPE, and disinfects the operatory area. The disposable articles are placed in the proper containers. The instruments are cleaned and prepared for sterilization. The large items are disinfected. The area is cleaned up; the gloves are washed, disinfected, and removed. The hands are washed.▲

THEORY RECALL

Bonding Brackets

1. Why do some orthodontists prefer direct bonding over band placement?

_____

2. In what materials are direct bond brackets supplied?

_____

3. What must be done to plastic brackets before placement in bonding?

_____

4. What does the orthodontist do to the tooth surfaces before etching?

_____

5. Where is the etching gel placed for direct bonding?

_____

6. Where is the activator material placed in direct bonding?

_____

7. Why does the assistant don overgloves when working with the bonding material syringes?

_____

8. What is the approximate time the bonding material needs for setting?

_____

9. What does the assistant hand to the orthodontist to remove excess bonding?

_____

10. How soon can arch wires be placed after the bonding of the brackets?

_____

Now turn to the Competency Evaluation Sheet for Procedure 43, Assisting with Cementation of Brackets, located in Appendix C of this text.

ARCH WIRE AND LIGATURE PLACEMENT

Once the teeth have received the brackets and tubes necessary for the placement of the arch wire, this procedure is begun. An arch wire is a heavy or thick band of wire formed into a horseshoe or arch shape. Once in place, the teeth are pushed, pulled or tilted toward this shape for the formation of the arch line. The orthodontist may choose to "seat and tie" in the arch wire at the banding appointment or reschedule the patient for a separate arch wire appointment.

The arch wire is preformed on the study case poured up from the preliminary examination. The form and shape of the arch wire is prescribed by the orthodontist, who places pressure loops and strength bends in areas of particular need. In order for the arch wire to hold the prescribed shape, the arch wire is preheated and conditioned before the patient is scheduled for the placement visit.

In some states, the assistant may be permitted to place and tie in the arch wire. If not allowed, the assistant may aid in the treatment plan, which begins with the insertion of the distal ends of the wire into the molar buccal tubes. The wire is then placed into the brackets beginning with the anterior area and working toward the rear until all brackets enclose on the preformed wire. (See Figure 8–6 for an example of arch wire set into tubes and brackets.)

When the arch wire is set into place, it is secured by one of two methods or a combination of both. Very small elastics may be used to wrap around the bracket and arch wire and stabilize the arch-forming device to the teeth brackets, or the orthodontist may prefer placing a thinner ligature wire around the arch wire and bracket flanges. A 4- to 5-inch piece of ligature wire is bent in half and compressed to a 45 degree angle at the middle bend or a smaller preformed ligature bent wire may be used (Figure 8–7).

The tight loop is placed over the arch wire and bracket ends and then twisted approximately five times. The excess wire is cut off leaving only a three to five millimeter ending that is twisted up and under the bands so no irritation is caused by the sharp

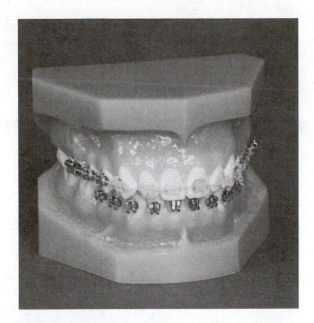

FIGURE 8–6 Typodont with arch wire and direct bonded brackets and tubes.

points. To prevent the arch wire from coming out of the tubes, the distal ends of the arch wire extending through the tubes are bent forward and tucked under.

After all brackets and tubes have been ligated, the patient is requested to feel with the tongue for any sharp areas or wire points, which are tucked into the recessed area. The assistant gives appliance care, oral hygiene, and nutrition instruction and makes a future appointment for about three to four weeks to determine the progress of the treatment.

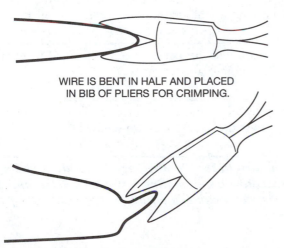

WIRE IS BENT IN HALF AND PLACED
IN BIB OF PLIERS FOR CRIMPING.

BEFORE RELEASING PLIERS, THE CRIMPED PART IS BENT
SIDEWAYS (SLIGHTLY) TO ACCOMMODATE THE BRACKETS.

FIGURE 8–7 The ligature wire is crimped and passed to the orthodontist, who loops it over the arch wire and twists it for tying in.

PROCEDURE 44

Assisting with Arch Wire and Ligature Placement

1	Assemble Equipment and Material
2	Prepare the Patient
3	Assist with Arch Wire Insertion
4	Assist with Ligature Placement
5	Assist with Ligature Cut and Tuck
6	Clean Up Patient
7	Clean Up Operatory, Disinfect, and Sterilize

1 Assemble Equipment and Material

The equipment necessary for this appointment follows:

- basic setup
- sundry setup
- preformed arch wire
- ligature wires, shapes
- ligature tying pliers
- Howe pliers
- ligature cutters
- ligature director or Schure instrument
- needleholder
- crimping pliers

2 Prepare the Patient

The assistant seats the patient, reviews the health history and explains the procedure. PPE is donned, and the orthodontist is summoned.

3 Assist with Arch Wire Insertion

The assistant passes and receives a mirror for examination. The previously preformed arch wire is passed in Howe pliers and visibility with regulation of moisture control is completed by using the HVE tip and positioning the light. The end tips of the arch wire are inserted into the buccal tube situated on the last molar on each side of the arch. The wire body is inserted into the bracket spaces, beginning at the anterior and working toward the back. The distal ends of the arch wire extending through the buccal tubes are bent mesially and tucked under.

4 Assist with Ligature Placement

The assistant receives the Howe pliers and passes a ligature wire that has been crimped into a 45 degree angle at the middle of the halfway bend. The small

226

loop eye is placed over the arch wire and bracket edges. The ligature tying pliers are passed, and the free ends are twisted approximately five times to tighten over the arch wire. The orthodontist may prefer to stabilize the arch wires by using elastics to hold the brackets and wires together. The assistant must remain prepared to pass either or both elastics and ligature wires.

5 Assist with Ligature Cut and Tuck

The ligature cutting pliers are passed to the orthodontist who snips the ligature wires to approximately three to four millimeters closeness. The assistant holds a hand nearby to retrieve the cutoff ends of ligature wire.

When all ends have been cut, the assistant receives the ligature cutters and passes a ligature direction instrument, which the orthodontist uses to push the ends to tuck under the wires. When they have been tucked, the assistant receives the tucking instrument and passes crimping pliers for pressing edges together. The patient is instructed to run the tongue over the edges to point out any sharpnesses. If any areas are found, the assistant passes the ligature tucking or Schure instrument to the orthodontist for tucking.

6 Clean Up Patient

The patient's mouth is rinsed and dried. The face is cleaned off and the drape and bib are removed. The assistant gives instructions in hygiene, care, and nutrition. The patient is dismissed but rescheduled for approximately three to four weeks later. If the patient is using elastics, the assistant may provide them with a "take home" extra supply to place when needed. Sometimes a small piece of wax rope will be given for the patient to apply to any sharp area until care can be rendered. The patient is instructed in the method of applying the elastics and wax roping when not in the office.

7 Clean Up Operatory, Disinfect, and Sterilize

The assistant gathers the contaminated materials and equipment and removes them to the sterilizing room. The exam gloves are removed, and the hands are washed. Since the orthodontist must make observations and notes more frequently and more extensively than general dentistry, notetaking may be completed on paper and then copied onto the patient's chart after exam gloves are removed. The original contaminated notes are then disposed of with the swipes, gauze, and other disposables. The assistant must copy the notes exactly and neatly. *Some offices dictate notes to a recorder which is foot-lever activated. These recordings are transcribed to the patient's records at a later date.

The assistant returns, dons utility gloves and PPE, and disinfects the operatory area. The disposables are removed and placed in correct containers, the large items are disinfected, and the instruments are cleaned and prepared for sterilization. The area is cleaned up; the gloves are washed, disinfected, and removed. The hands are washed.▲

THEORY RECALL
Arch Wire and Ligature Placement

1. What procedure must be finished before the placement of the arch wire and ligatures?

2. What is used to preform the arch wire before the placement appointment?

3. What does the assistant pass to the orthodontist to tie off the arch wire?

4. What is passed to the orthodontist to cut the ligature wire ends?

5. How close to the gingival area does the orthodontist cut the ligatures?

6. When all the ligatures are cut, what instrument does the assistant pass?

7. What does the orthodontist use to tuck in the ligature edges?

8. Why is the patient requested to run a tongue around the mouth after the tie in?

9. When will the patient be rescheduled to come in for another appointment?

10. Why does the assistant copy the orthodontist's notes after the gloves are removed?

Now turn to the Competency Evaluation Sheet for Procedure 44, Assisting with Arch Wire and Ligature Placement, located in Appendix C of this text.

ARCH WIRE, BAND, AND BRACKET REMOVAL

nce the patient's alignment has reached the desired position, the orthodontist schedules the patient for band removal. In this appointment, the patient has all intraoral appliances removed. The teeth are cleaned of cement and polished with a fluoride paste.

An impression is taken of the new bite. The impression is poured up into new study casts that are used to prepare a retainer for the patient. Retainers may be constructed as a clear acrylic bite tray or a framework appliance with an acrylic palate area (Figure 8–8).

Since the bones are not yet fully calcified in their new position, a retainer will be worn for support for a period of time, perhaps one to two years. The new study casts are used not only as a pattern for a retainer but serve as records of the after- or post-orthodontic treatment condition as compared with the study casts of the initial preliminary appointment.

Photographs may be taken at this time to show the difference in the appearance of the patient at the end of the corrective treatment and the beginning of care.

P R O C E D U R E 45

Assisting with Arch Wire, Band, and Bracket Removal

1 Assemble Equipment and Materials, Prepare the Patient

2 Assist with Ligature Wire Removal

3 Assist with Arch Wire Removal

4 Assist with Band and Bracket Removal

5 Assist with Cement Removal

6 Assist with Impression

7 Assist with Photographs

8 Clean Up and Dismiss Patient

9 Clean Up, Disinfect, and Sterilize

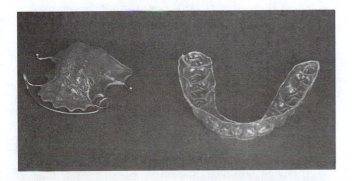

FIGURE 8–8 Retainers are worn until the new mouth position becomes calcified and strong.

1 Assemble Equipment and Materials, Prepare the Patient

The equipment needed for the removal appointment follows:

▶ basic setup
▶ sundry setup
▶ scalers, hand and ultrasonic
▶ Schure instrument
▶ ligature cutters
▶ needleholder
▶ Howe pliers
▶ band removing pliers
▶ slow handpiece with prophy angle and fluoride paste
▶ safety glasses for patient

The patient is seated, draped, and bibbed. The patient is requested to don a pair of safety eyeglasses, and the procedure is explained. The assistant dons PPE and summons the orthodontist.

2 Assist with Ligature Wire Removal

The assistant passes a scaler or Schure instrument to the orthodontist to retrieve and release the cut ends of the ligature wires. When all ends are obvious, the assistant receives the scaler or Schure and passes the needleholder and ligature wire cutters. The assistant holds a piece of gauze near the work site to receive the ligature pieces. After all ligatures are removed, the assistant receives the needleholder and ligature cutter.

3 Assist with Arch Wire Removal

The assistant passes the scaler or Schure instrument to the orthodontist to release the crimped ends of the arch wire situated in the buccal tubes. The instrument is returned and the assistant passes the Howe pliers for arch wire removal. The arch wire is pulled straight out of the tubes, bracket slots, and the mouth. When it has been removed, the assistant receives the Howe pliers and the arch wire.

4 Assist with Band and Bracket Removal

Depending on what type of appliance has been holding the arch wire, the assistant passes the correct removal instrument. For brackets, a pair of ligature cutters is passed to cut and twist the bracket from the tooth surface. The assistant holds gauze near the site to receive the removed brackets.

When removing bands, the assistant passes band-removing pliers and holds gauze near the site to receive the removed bands. The assistant is prepared

228

to pass the blunt end instrument or scaler to aid in band removal.

5 Assist with Cement Removal

After all appliances have been removed, the assistant removes the retained cement, if permitted, or passes the mirror and scaler to the orthodontist for cement removal. The orthodontist may request the ultrasonic scaler for removal of gross amounts of cement. The assistant should have the ultrasonic scaler "tuned" and ready for use.

The slow handpiece with prophy cup and fluoridated paste is passed for the crown polish after the assistant receives the mirror and scaler. During the polishing of the teeth, the assistant maintains a dry field and operates the syringe water rinse as needed.

6 Assist with Impression

When the teeth are cleaned and polished, the assistant aids with the alginate impression of the new bite. The assistant passes trays to the orthodontist for fit, adapting with wax when and if needed. Once the trays are chosen, the assistant mixes the alginate according to manufacturer's directions, fills a tray from the lingual side, and passes the tray to the orthodontist for seating.

When the impression has set, the orthodontist gives the tray to the assistant, who passes the syringe for a water spray rinse. The assistant evacuates the mouth and washes the impression under running water. The impression is disinfected and placed in a plastic bag.

The assistant prepares the other tray and repeats the steps for the impression of the other arch. Base plate wax is softened in hot water and passed to the orthodontist for a bite registration, which is rinsed, disinfected, and placed in the plastic bag with the two completed impression trays.

7 Assist with Photographs

To record the difference between the appearance and position of the teeth from the beginning visit to the removal session, the orthodontist may request photographs to be taken. These serve as records of the before and after presentation. The assistant follows the same procedure as in the beginning, requesting the patient to hold or wear cheek retractors and then exposing a full face view and one of each side. The patient wears an identification tag with name and date preprinted.

8 Clean Up and Dismiss Patient

The patient is cleaned up and given a hand mirror to see the new smile. Do not be too surprised that the

patient feels a bit "odd" without the appliances. The orthodontic patient has been wearing these devices for some time and now looks at a different view. The patient adapts to the clear mouth very rapidly. The assistant reviews the appliance care, oral hygiene and nutrition instructions, and dismisses the patient.

9 Clean Up, Disinfect and Sterilize

The assistant gathers the contaminated materials and equipment and takes them to the sterilizing room. The gloves are removed and the hands washed. The assistant copies notes and treatment on the patient's chart, which is taken to the front desk.

The assistant dons utility gloves and PPE, disinfects the operatory area, places disposables in the proper container, disinfects large items, cleans, and prepares instruments for sterilization. The area is cleaned up. The gloves are washed, disinfected, and removed; the hands are washed.▲

THEORY RECALL

Arch Wire, Band, and Bracket Removal

1. When the desired alignment has been obtained, what type of orthodontic appointment is scheduled?

2. What happens in a band removal appointment?

3. How long may a patient wear a retainer after band removal?

4. What use are the study casts taken at the band removal appointment?

5. What is the patient requested to wear during the band removal appointment?

6. What does the assistant pass to the orthodontist to expose the tucked in ends of the ligatures?

7. What does the assistant pass to the orthodontist to remove the ligatures?

8. Once the bands and brackets are removed, what does the orthodontist do next?

9. What instrument does the orthodontist use to remove the cement?

10. When the cement is removed, what does the orthodontist do next?

Now turn to the Competency Evaluation Sheet for Procedure 45, Assisting with Arch Wire, Band, and Bracket Removal, located in Appendix C of this text.

ORAL SURGERY PROCEDURES

The specialty of oral surgery is the part of dental practice that deals with the diagnosis, surgical, and adjunctive treatment of the diseases, injuries, and defects of the human jaw and associated structures. Although oral surgical procedures are taught and practiced in general dentistry, complicated tooth extraction, jaw fractures, bone reduction and reconstruction, implantation and other procedures are referred to the oral surgeon, a specialist in this type of dentistry.

Patients with compromising health conditions which may turn a simple surgical procedure into a delicate situation are also sent to the oral surgeon for treatment in the office or hospital in- or out-patient setting. A dentist referring a patient to the oral surgeon sends a copy of the patient's dental record, current x-rays, and a prescription or recommendation for surgical treatment to the surgeon for the examination visit.

Since many of the procedures are complicated, the surgeon may prefer to premedicate or supplement anesthesia with a nitrous oxide analgesia; therefore, investigation into the health and medical history of the patient is stressed. Vital signs may be taken and recorded. The surgeon may consult with the patient's physician or order laboratory testing prior to surgery.

Pre-surgical planning is extremely important in oral surgical procedures. Radiographs supplied by the referring dentist and any taken related to the surgery are examined closely before the surgeon outlines the procedure. During the examination, the patient is advised of the treatment plan, financial cost, and recuperative period before treatment is scheduled.

The oral surgical assistant must be well prepared before treatment. All materials and equipment must be present in the surgical area, and asepsis must be maintained throughout the process. Instrument setups are prepared using sterile techniques prior to surgery and arranged in the order of use. Pre-set surgical trays are wrapped or covered by a sterile towel until time of use. Standby trays for emergencies or complications are placed nearby for retrieval if needed.

One of the more common procedures completed in the oral surgeon's office is that of the multiple extraction. Not only are the teeth extracted or removed from the mouth but the alveolar ridge must be prepared to receive a partial or complete denture. Therefore, when scheduling for a multiple extraction, the assistant must also prepare for a total or partial alveoplasty (smoothing of the alveolar bone).

The assistant should become familiar with the oral surgery instruments and equipment, particularly the forceps. Each forceps is designed and manufactured for a specific tooth or area of the mouth. The nibs or beaks of the forceps are curved to wrap around and grasp the tooth giving the best leverage available. Forceps may be for designated upper or lower teeth, anterior or posterior teeth, groups or universal, meaning usable for more than one tooth or area.

Oral surgery procedures definitely call for assistant care and participation. The assistant must anticipate the surgeon's needs in order to pass and receive instruments, maintain visibility by suction, place the light, retract the tissue and tongue, monitor patient reaction, review postoperative instructions, and render general aid.

The assistant may also (in some states) be trained to remove the patient's sutures in four to six days following surgery (Figure 8–9A). Once the patient has been seated, the assistant, who is wearing PPE, examines the mouth and then rinses with a spray bath. The sutures are located and then disinfected by dabbing with wet disinfectant applicator (Figure 8–9B).

The assistant gently lifts the suture and inserts the small end of the suture scissors under the loop of the material. The scissors are moved to the side of the loop furthest from the knot and then snipped (Figure 8–9C). With the college pliers, the assistant lifts the knot gently and removes the suture material (Figure 8–9D). The removed suture is placed on a piece of gauze and counted to see if the number matches the patient's surgical record count.

Once the sutures are counted and removed, the mouth is rinsed again and the dentist may check the area to evaluate the healing process. In areas where the assistant is not permitted to perform the procedure, the assistant may aid the surgeon by passing and helping with the removal.

PROCEDURE 46

Assisting with Multiple Extractions and Suture Removal

Multiple Extractions

1 Assemble Equipment and Materials

2 Prepare the Patient

3 Assist with Anesthesia

4 Assist with Extraction of Teeth

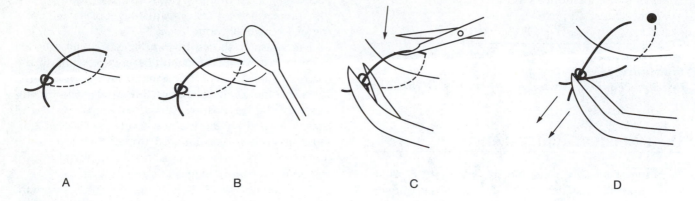

A   B   C   D

FIGURE 8–9 Suture removal technique: (A) suture placement, (B) disinfection of suture, (C) snip of suture (away from knot), and (D) gentle lift and removal of suture.

5   **Assist with Alveoplasty**

6   **Assist with Artificial Clot Material (If Needed)**

7   **Assist with Suturing**

8   **Clean Up and Dismiss Patient**

9   **Clean Up, Disinfect, and Sterilize**

Removal of Sutures

10   **Assemble Materials and Equipment, Prepare the Patient**

11   **Remove Sutures**

12   **Clean Up the Patient, Area, Equipment, and Materials**

Multiple Extractions

1 Assemble Equipment and Materials

To assist in the most common oral surgical procedure, removal of teeth, the assistant must prepare the following equipment and materials:

▶ patient chart, x-rays, and treatment plan
▶ surgical tray of basic setup
▶ sundry setup, including sterile gauze and artificial clotting material
▶ anesthesia setup
▶ prep and removal instruments—elevators, specific forceps
▶ bone and tissue instruments—scalpel, periosteal elevator, rongeurs, bone file
▶ hemostats, tissue pick ups
▶ elevators, root tip picks

▶ handpiece with surgical burs
▶ suture instruments—needleholder, prepared sutures, suture scissors
▶ suction tip—extra tips with small, medium, and large openings
▶ wire for clogged tips

Once the assistant has reviewed the surgical plan, prepared the trays, placed the x-rays on the viewer and checked that operatory equipment is working properly, the patient may be brought into the surgical area.

2 Prepare the Patient

The patient is seated and positioned for the surgery. Some patients may need to receive premedication, which is given after reviewing the health history. The assistant checks to see if all permission and consent forms are signed and in order. Oxygen outlets are checked to determine if the valves are open and operating, and the emergency tray is kept within reach.

The patient is prepared with a drape. The face is washed with a disinfected soap, rinsed, and patted dry with sterile gauze; a sterile towel is placed around the neck. The procedure is explained.

The assistant dons the PPE. A surgical coat or dress is placed over the clothes. Some operators prefer to don a disposable cap to cover hair during the procedure. The mask and eyewear are placed, and the hands are scrubbed with microbial soap and dried on a sterile towel. Surgical latex gloves are drawn on with aseptic technique.

3 Assist with Anesthesia

The assistant may assist with anesthesia by rinsing the patient's mouth and applying a topical anesthetic to the injection site or sites. Some patients may have received a premedication or are given a general or partial anesthesia, called analgesia.

When the surgeon arrives, the assistant receives the used applicators and passes the prepared syringe, guards against sudden movements, and receives the syringe, which is capped in a one-hand motion. The assistant monitors the patient for anesthetic reaction.

4 Assist with Extraction of Teeth

At the surgeon's signal, the assistant passes an explorer for the surgeon to test the effect of the anesthesia. The explorer is returned and the assistant passes an elevator for loosening of the tissue and ligaments around the tooth or series of teeth. The assistant holds a gauze square nearby to wipe the tip free of debris and is prepared to aspirate the area with the surgical suction tip, which is thinner than the HVE tip.

The dentist returns the elevator, and the assistant passes the correct forceps for the tooth being extracted. Each forceps is designed and shaped for a specific tooth. The assistant should check with the surgeon first if not familiar with the exact forceps required.

The assistant receives the forceps and tooth, which the surgeon checked to see if all pieces were attached. If a root tip is missing, the assistant suctions the socket and passes an elevator or root tip pick to the surgeon for root removal. The assistant maintains visibility and a dry field at all times.

5 Assist with Alveoplasty

After multiple extractions, the ridge of alveolar bone points must be evened off so the patient will be able to be fitted for dentures. The surgeon performs an **alveoplasty** (smoothing or contouring of the alveolar bone) to prepare the bone for denture wear.

The assistant passes a scalpel to incise the tissue. After receiving the scalpel, the assistant passes a periosteal elevator for relieving the gingiva and exposing the alveolar bone beneath.

When the bone points are exposed, the assistant receives the elevator and passes the rongeurs for snipping off the points or crests. The assistant may pick up the bone **spicules** or slivers with a hemostat or with the suction tip and place them on a piece of sterile gauze.

The surgeon returns the rongeurs and is handed a bone file to smooth off the edges. Some surgeons prefer a surgical bur in a straight handpiece that causes less trauma to the bone. Visibility and a dry field are maintained.

6 Assist with Artificial Clot Material (If Needed)

If the surgeon desires to place artificial clotting material in the socket areas, the assistant passes small pieces of medicated sponge or gauze to the surgeon in a pair of college pliers. The medicine glass holding other slivers of clotting material is held nearby for refill. The assistant may use sterile gauze to dab the area clean as suction may aspirate the clotting material away.

7 Assist with Suturing

The assistant passes tissue pick ups and a needleholder loaded with a prepared suture and holds the trailing ends high off the patient's chin to avoid contamination. The assistant uses suture scissors to cut the suture when and where indicated by the surgeon.

8 Clean Up and Dismiss Patient

The patient is cleaned up. The mouth is wiped out and sterile gauze pads are placed in the mouth for the patient to bite on. The face is wiped off and the drape and bib removed. The bib is placed over the dirty instruments and materials.

The patient's companion or friend is brought into the room and the assistant reviews the postoperative instructions. Most offices have a printed instruction sheet the assistant may read with the people (Table 8–3). The patient is dismissed after changing the sterile pads for new ones on which to bite. A patient is never released and permitted to leave the office with dirty, bloody gauze protruding from the mouth.

9 Clean Up, Disinfect, and Sterilize

The assistant gathers all equipment and materials for the sterilizing room. Surgical gloves are removed and the hands are washed. The assistant records the surgical procedure on the chart listing all teeth and areas affected, type and amount of anesthesia, amount of sutures, and prescriptions given. The chart is taken to the front desk.

The assistant dons utility gloves and PPE, disinfects, sterilizes, and cleans up the areas. The gloves are washed, disinfected, and removed, and the hands are washed.

Removal of Sutures

10 Assemble Materials and Equipment, Prepare the Patient

Approximately five to seven days after surgery, the patient returns to have the sutures removed. The assis-

TABLE 8-3

Postoperative Instructions for the Oral Surgery Patient

1. Bite on gauze pack that has been placed in mouth. If necessary, change in 30 minutes. If bleeding persists for over 30 minutes, wrap cooled, used tea bag in sterile gauze, place on operative site and bite down. Call office if bleeding does not stop within one hour.

2. Avoid rinsing mouth on day of surgery. Cool sips of water may be taken after bleeding has stopped. Do not use straw for sipping, as suction may disturb clot.

3. Place cool packs on face tissue over operative site. Remove pack for 15 minutes after each half hour application. Apply as soon as possible.

4. Eat only soft food on day of surgery and later as needed. Drink ample fluids.

5. On day after surgery, cleanse mouth by gently brushing remaining teeth with a soft brush. Use a mouthwash or warm salt water, $1/2$ to 1 teaspoon of salt to 8 ounces of water, after meals and at bedtime. Avoid excessive swishing, use gentle movements.

6. Take medications as prescribed by the dentist or oral surgeon.

7. On day of surgery, avoid excessive exercise; sleep with head elevated.

8. Do not place tongue or fingers into operative site as this will cause irritation and possible infection.

9. Notify office of any excessive bleeding, pain, or condition that concerns.

Surgeon's Name

Surgeon's Phone Number

---

tant trained to perform this task assembles a mirror, college pliers, and suture scissors. An applicator, bottle of disinfectant, and piece of gauze are also placed on the tray. The assistant reviews the patient's chart, listing the area involved and the amount of sutures to be removed.

The patient is seated and positioned in the chair. The assistant inquires about the patient's condition and experiences since last in surgery. A mirror is used to view the mouth area and sutures in particular. If no unusual or inflammatory conditions are present, the assistant rinses and evacuates the mouth. An applicator tip is moistened and swabbed on the sutures.

11 Remove Sutures

The assistant or operator picks up the tail of the suture with the college pliers and identifies the knot. The suture scissors are inserted under the suture loop and placed close to the gingiva but away from the knot. A cut is made and the college pliers are used to gently pull the knot which brings the suture out of the gingiva.

The sutures are placed on the gauze and counted. When all are removed, the mouth is inspected and rinsed again. The assistant passes the mirror to the surgeon who examines the area and dismisses the patient.

12 Clean Up the Patient, Area, Equipment, and Materials

The assistant cleans up the room, removes the latex gloves, washes hands, and records treatment on the patient's chart. The assistant dons utility gloves and

PPE, disinfects, and sterilizes. Utility gloves are washed, disinfected, and removed; the hands are washed.▲

THEORY RECALL

Oral Surgery Procedures

1. What type of oral surgery procedures does the oral surgeon perform?

2. Besides complicated cases, what type of patients may a dentist refer to an oral surgeon?

3. What does the referring dentist send with the patient to the oral surgeon?

4. During the initial exam, what subjects do the oral surgeon and the patient discuss?

5. What preoperative duties does the assistant have?

6. How is the patient prepared for an oral surgery procedure?

7. What is the term applied to the smoothing and contouring of the bony alveolar ridges?

8. After placement of artificial clots, why does the assistant dab the area instead of aspirating the blood at the site of the extraction?

9. To whom does the assistant give postoperative instructions?

10. How long after surgery does the patient return for suture removal?

Now turn to the Competency Evaluation Sheet for Procedure 46, Assisting with Multiple Extractions and Suture Removal, located in Appendix C of this text.

MINOR TISSUE SURGERY

Dry Socket

Occasionally, a few days after surgery a patient experiences severe and lasting pain in the operative site. The assistant, suspecting a **dry socket**, infection, or both requests the patient to return for emergency treatment.

A dry socket occurs when the clot in a surgical wound has not properly formed or has prematurely dissolved or washed away. The operative site is retaining food and mouth debris. Intense pain occurs from lack of covering on the alveolar bone.

The patient is seated and may receive local anesthesia. After examination, the socket is irrigated and cleaned of all debris and foreign matter. Depending on the condition of the opening, the oral surgeon may elect to either **curettage** the area and add artificial clot material to the new blood to form another clot or just place some iodoform clotting gauze into the socket site.

Once the medication is in place, sutures may be placed to prevent the loss of the new clot or the collection of foreign matter in the wound site. The patient is dismissed but should return in a few days for reevaluation.

The procedural steps for a dry socket (**alveolitis**) are:

1. Complete Preparations
2. Assist with Anesthesia
3. Assist with Curettage
4. Assist with Suturing
5. Dismiss and Cleanup

Incision and Drainage

Another emergency patient may be one in pain from an abscess or infection causing a large infected area.

Accumulation of pus, lymph, dead cells, and matter causes swelling, heat, tenderness, and intense pain. The patient is referred because of the potential septic problem and the difficulty in providing anesthesia to the congested area.

Antibiotic therapy is usually recommended for patients with acute abscesses. A review of the patient's health history and allergy reactions is very important before the writing of a prescription.

Once the patient is seated and the exam determines incision and drainage (I & D) treatment, the area may be anesthetized. An incision is made into the swollen area and the opening is enlarged by placing a hemostat in and stretching the incision for the drainage of the **exudate** and matter. A small piece of dental dam material may be placed into the opening to prevent the natural closing and healing over in this area and to aid in the draining of the pus. Suturing may be required to keep the material in place.

The patient, who may feel almost immediate relief as the pressure is relieved when the drainage occurs, is rescheduled for treatment in a few days after the antibiotics and drainage have cleared the area of sepsis.

The procedural steps are:

1. Complete Preparations
2. Assist with Anesthesia
3. Assist with Incision and Drainage (**I & D**)
4. Assist with Suturing (If Needed)
5. Assist with Cleanup, Dismissal, Disinfection, and Sterilization

Biopsy

A **biopsy** is the surgical removal of a piece of tissue that is sent to the laboratory for microscopic examination to help determine the diagnosis and future treatment. This type of patient may be scheduled or may occur as an emergency if a troublesome or suspicious area is found during an examination. The patient is seated and after examination of the area, the oral surgeon determines which type of biopsy is to be made. There are three ways to perform a biopsy in the oral surgeon's office:

1. Exfoliative cytology—scraping of area
2. Incisional biopsy—cut into lesion
3. Excisional biopsy—removal of lesion

When completing the exfoliative cytology style, the surgeon scrapes the area or suspect tissue several times in the same direction with a tongue blade or other flat object. The collected matter is smeared on two glass slides starting at the center and spreading evenly out to the ends. The slides are flooded with a 70 percent alcohol fixative, which is allowed to remain for 20 minutes and then removed by gently tipping the slides. They are permitted to air dry in a clean area and when completely dry are packed in a vial and sent to the laboratory for analysis. *Spray fixants are also available. This procedure is very much like the Pap smear that women undergo for testing for cancer.

In the excisional biopsy, the surgeon removes the entire lesion plus a small amount of normal adjacent tissue for comparison and sends all to the laboratory for analysis. This type of testing is done only when the lesion is very small or not in an area where removal may cause trouble with function or appearance.

The incisional biopsy is the most popular method used in the oral surgery office. The surgeon removes a wedge of the lesion and a small amount of normal tissue. The specimen is placed into a bottle of solution labeled with the patient's name, date, and area of excision and sent to the laboratory for analysis. Occasionally, the surgeon includes a drawing of the area to be sent with the specimen. Future treatment depends on the results gained.

P R O C E D U R E 4 7
Assisting with Minor Tissue Surgery

Dry Socket (Alveolitis)

1 Complete Preparations

2 Assist with Local Anesthesia

3 Assist with Curettage

4 Assist with Suturing

5 Clean Up the Patient, Area, and Equipment

Incision and Drainage (I & D)

6 Complete Preparations

7 Assist with Anesthesia

8 Assist with Incision and Drainage

9 Assist with Suturing

10 Clean Up the Patient, Area, and Equipment

Biopsy

11 Complete Preparations

12 Assist with Anesthesia

13 Assist with Biopsy

14 Clean Up the Patient, Area, and Equipment

15 Prepare Biopsy for Laboratory

Dry Socket (Alveolitis)

1 Complete Preparations

The patient arrives in the office as an emergency patient. The assistant prepares for a dry socket setup,

---

TABLE 8–4

Examples of Tissue Surgery

A. DRY SOCKET

A clot washed away or did not form.

Treatment:
► clean out socket
► encourage bleeding (place artificial clot)
► possible suture

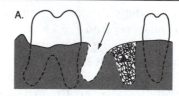
A.

B. INCISION & DRAINAGE (I & D)

Infection causes swelling and pain.

Treatment:
► incision into swollen area
► opening of wound to permit drain
► possible insertion of dental dam material into incision

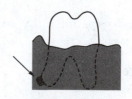
B.

C. BIOPSY

Tissue color or growth is questionable.

Treatment:
► excision and removal with biopsy
► specimen sent to laboratory for staining and microscopic study

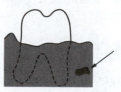
C.

prior to the patient's arrival. The equipment necessary for treatment follows:

- basic setup
- sundry setup
- anesthesia setup and equipment
- curette and scalpel to debride and incise
- artificial clotting material and college pliers
- sutures, needleholder, and tissue pick ups
- x-ray, if requested
- indelible pencil

The patient is prepared for surgery in the usual manner, except for premedication. Since the expected treatment is not complicated, premedication may not be required. Anesthesia may or may not be needed. An x-ray may be taken if the surgeon requests one. The face is prepared with a scrub and the assistant uses aseptic technique to set up the surgical tray. The hands are surgically scrubbed and PPE gear is donned.

2 Assist with Local Anesthesia

The assistant helps with local anesthesia if needed. Sometimes the small amount of curettage needed to **debride** (clean out) and stimulate bleeding does not warrant local anesthetic injection pain. The surgeon determines the use of anesthesia. The assistant is prepared for the procedure.

3 Assist with Curettage

The assistant helps with curettage by passing a mirror and curette or large spoon excavator to the surgeon for debridement of the socket. The assistant passes a syringe of warm water or hydrogen peroxide to irrigate and wash the site. A surgical tip aspirator is used to aspirate the area. If curettage is not enough to stimulate new blood to form a clot, the surgeon may request a scalpel for incision. The assistant is prepared for both.

When the socket is clean and filled with fresh blood, the surgeon may request artificial clotting material, which the assistant passes in sterile college pliers.

4 Assist with Suturing

The area may be sutured to ensure the new clot will remain. The assistant aids by passing the needleholder with suture and holding the tail of the suture material off the face. When the suture has been knotted, the assistant clips the ends of the material in the area indicated by the surgeon.

5 Clean Up the Patient, Area, and Equipment

The patient is cleaned up, and postoperative instructions are reviewed. Sterile gauze is placed on the wound and the patient is instructed to bite. The pa-

tient is dismissed, and the assistant performs the cleanup chores.

Incision and Drainage (I & D)

6 Complete Preparations

The assistant prepares for an emergency surgical treatment, prepares the patient for surgery, and dons PPE. The patient may be premedicated, depending on the severity of the infection, or the surgeon may prefer to administer nitrous oxide analgesia during surgery. The assistant is prepared for both.

7 Assist with Anesthesia

Local anesthesia is difficult in infection sites. The swelling and accumulation of exudate may prevent the absorption of the anesthetic solution. The assistant may ask the surgeon which area to apply topical anesthesia. The assistant aids in local anesthesia in the usual manner. In some cases, no anesthesia is attempted as incision offers some type of relief immediately.

8 Assist with Incision and Drainage

The assistant passes the mirror to the surgeon for an examination of the site. Upon receiving the mirror, the assistant passes the scalpel for incision. After the cut, the assistant aspirates the wound to collect infectious matter. A hemostat may be passed to penetrate and enlarge the opening.

The assistant receives the scalpel and passes a piece of dental dam material in sterile college pliers. The surgeon inserts the dam into the wound to prohibit closing of the wound and permit drainage. The assistant receives the college pliers.

9 Assist with Suturing

If the surgeon desires to suture the dam material into the wound site to ensure the material is not washed away, sutures are placed. The assistant is prepared to assist with suture placement.

10 Clean Up the Patient, Area, and Equipment

The patient's mouth is rinsed and aspirated. The assistant avoids aspirating in the wound site so the dam drain is not disturbed. The patient is cleaned up, given postoperative instructions, and dismissed. Clean up is done in the usual manner.

Biopsy

11 Complete Preparations

The assistant prepares for the tissue surgery in the usual manner, except that a specimen bottle containing a preservative solution is placed with the surgical instruments. The bottle may be labeled with the date and patient's name before the treatment.

12 Assist with Anesthesia

The assistant helps with the topical and local anesthesia. Premedication is rarely given in this minor surgery. While the anesthesia is taking effect, the oral surgeon may mark off the incisional area with an indelible pencil or marker.

13 Assist with Biopsy

The assistant passes the mirror to the surgeon for the examination of the site. The mouth may be rinsed and evacuated. The assistant may pass the scalpel and tissue pick ups to the surgeon, who incises and removes a small amount of tissue. The assistant accepts the tissue into the waiting specimen bottle and caps the bottle. If bleeding is profuse, the surgeon may request suture placement, which the assistant is prepared to assist with. If bleeding is minor, the assistant may pass a sterile gauze for the surgeon to pack the wound site.

14 Clean Up the Patient, Area, and Equipment

The patient is cleaned up. Postoperative instructions and assurances of notification are given to the patient; the patient is dismissed. The assistant cleans up in the usual manner.

15 Prepare Biopsy for Laboratory

After cleanup is accomplished, the assistant finishes the biopsy instructions. The assistant checks the laboratory orders and includes them with the specimen bottle. The form includes the patient's name and address; the dentist's name and address; and a detailed description of the lesion, including the size, location, color, consistency, and shape. The vial or box is prepared for mailing or sent to the laboratory for examination. The biopsy treatment is marked on the patient's chart, and the patient's name is placed on the outgoing lab sheet.▲

THEORY RECALL
Minor Tissue Surgery

1. What are symptoms of a dry socket?

_____

2. When does a dry socket occur?

_____

3. Why does the surgeon use a curette in the wound site of a dry socket?

_____

4. Why must the assistant be sure *not* to aspirate the wound site after the placement of the artificial clot?

_____

5. What causes the pain, heat, and swelling in a mouth infection?

_____

6. If the patient is undergoing intense pain, what type of pain control may the surgeon use in conjunction with local anesthesia?

_____

7. Why is local anesthesia difficult at the swollen infection site?

_____

8. Why is the dental dam material permitted to remain in the I & D wound?

_____

9. What is a biopsy?

_____

10. After the surgery, what does the assistant do with the biopsy specimen bottle?

_____

Now turn to the Competency Evaluation Sheet for Procedure 47, Assisting with Minor Tissue Surgery, located in Appendix C of this text.

PERIODONTICS

Periodontics is the branch of dentistry that deals with the cause and treatment of diseased tissues surrounding the teeth. Although many periodontal problems are routinely handled by the general dentist, difficult cases may be referred to the specialist for treatment.

One of the most important procedures for the periodontist is the preliminary examination, a thorough and comprehensive accumulation of data that dictates future treatment. This initial visit includes not only the clinical data of the exam, radiographs, probes, and measurements but considers lifestyle, habits, and personal interviews. The physical and mental fitness of the patient must be evaluated to determine if stress, endocrine imbalance, allergies, or some other problem is reflected in the health of the gingival tissues. The periodontist is involved with the holistic view of the patient, who not only needs treatment but actively seeks to work for a cure.

The assistant can be of value to the periodontist by making preparations before and after the examination and treatment. The recording of data and maintaining of charts plays a very important part in the treatment plan. The assistant also offers help during the procedures and works to maintain visibility. Periodontal procedures may often have a copious amount of blood present, and the elimination of fluids during the exacting treatment is very necessary. Patient education and postoperative instruction, along with monitoring of the patient during treatment can be delegated to the assistant.

PROCEDURE 48

Assisting with Periodontal Exam and Prophylaxis

Examination

1 **Complete Preparations**

2 **Assist with Interview**

3 **Assist with Clinical Examination**

4 **Assist with Radiographs**

5 **Assist with Periodontal Probing**

6 **Assist with Mobility Testing**

Prophylaxis

7 **Assist with Anesthesia**

8 **Assist with Scaling**

9 **Assist with Curettage**

10 **Assist with Root Planing**

11 **Assist with Polish of Teeth**

12 **Clean Up and Dismiss Patient**

13 **Clean Up Area, Disinfect, and Sterilize**

Examination

1 **Complete Preparations**

The assistant aids the periodontist by setting up for the initial appointment. The equipment and materials required follow:

- basic setup
- sundry setup, including articulating paper
- radiographs and equipment
- periodontal probes and charts
- photographic equipment, intra- and extraoral
- charts and records

The patient is seated in the operatory, draped, and bibbed. The assistant reviews the procedure while establishing a rapport with the patient.

2 **Assist with Interview**

The first part of the appointment requires mainly note-taking. The periodontist interviews the patient regarding the patient's medical and health status, trying to determine if an underlying disease or present medication could affect the vitality of the gingiva.

The patient's diet and nutrition level will have an effect on the healing process. The types of food and the frequency of meals may hinder proper tissue regeneration. The patient may be directed to keep a food diary for a few days for later analysis.

Lifestyles and habits may have a direct effect on the periodontal tissues. Unusual biting or chewing habits may cause pressure points or tooth movement. Articulating paper may be used to determine proper occlusion. A person's lifestyle may not encourage frequent and thorough mouth cleansing or cooperation with a home care program.

Throughout the interview, the assistant takes notes using the patient's own words as close as possible. The patient's own words may indicate the intensity or desire for good dental health. The periodontist may include orders or findings to be recorded also.

The assistant may don plastic gloves and expose photographs, both intra- and extraoral. These can be used in the diagnosis and case plan as well as a record of pre-existing conditions.

3 **Assist with Clinical Examination**

When the periodontist has finished the interview, the assistant dons PPE for the clinical examination. The syringe may be passed for a spray rinse and evacuation before the assistant passes a mirror to be used in the mouth scan.

The periodontist surveys the mouth, investigating the tissues of the cheek, tongue, and throat as well as the periosteum. A generalized reading of the plaque and calculus formation as well as a classification of the gingival involvement are recorded.

Classification of gingival involvement may be:

Class I Gingivitis—inflammation of tissues, redness, puffiness, may bleed

Class II Slight periodontitis—redness, swelling of tissue, bone compression

Class III Moderate periodontitis—increased redness and swelling, bone loss

Class IV Advanced periodontitis—deep pocket formation, bone loss, mobility

Class V Refractory progressive periodontitis—tissues deeply affected, necrotic, severe bone loss and tooth mobility

4 Assist with Radiographs

The assistant may help with or expose radiographs, which may include a full mouth series to show individual areas and a panoramic view to show the overall alveolar crest. The assistant dons overgloves while processing the films.

5 Assist with Periodontal Probing

In the periodontal probing procedure, the assistant passes the periodontal probe to the periodontist, who inserts the tip of the probe into three areas on the facial and lingual side of the tooth (mesial, distal, and midtooth) (Figure 8–10).

The assistant uses the HVE tip to maintain visibility, records three numbers for each side, and places these numbers on the chart under or over the specific tooth. When the periodontal probing depth is recorded, the assistant may draw a connecting line showing the gingival crest, giving a visual plot line.

6 Assist with Mobility Testing

The periodontist may test the mobility of the teeth next. This procedure is accomplished by placing an instrument (mirror and probe) on each side of the tooth and pressing for movement. Fingers cannot be used as reference points because of the "give" of the skin tissues.

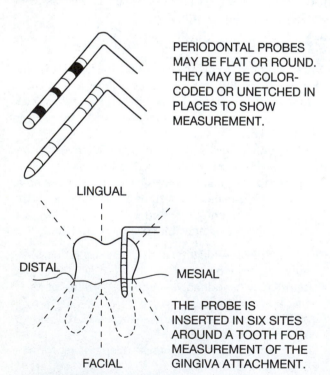

PERIODONTAL PROBES MAY BE FLAT OR ROUND. THEY MAY BE COLOR-CODED OR UNETCHED IN PLACES TO SHOW MEASUREMENT.

LINGUAL

DISTAL

MESIAL

FACIAL

THE PROBE IS INSERTED IN SIX SITES AROUND A TOOTH FOR MEASUREMENT OF THE GINGIVA ATTACHMENT.

FIGURE 8–10 The periodontal probe measures the depth of the pocket involvement.

Mobility is classified as 0 for normal, +1 for facial-lingual movement, +2 for mesial-distal movement, +3 for both 1 and 2, and +4 for depression and rotation in the socket. The assistant records the periodontist's findings in the block around the specific tooth.

Prophylaxis

When the examination is completed, the periodontist and patient have a consultation. The periodontist shows the clinical data and explains the treatment plan, both office and home care, financial cost, and proposed outcome (prognosis).

The first step of the treatment is the prophylaxis. Some cases are so severe and involved that only one quadrant may be scheduled at a time. Each case is managed individually, according to the needs of the patient. The periodontist may employ a dental hygienist for the prophylaxis treatment. The dental assistant may be of great use to the hygienist in this procedure.

The equipment and materials needed for the prophylaxis follow:

- ▶ basic setup
- ▶ sundry setup, including dental floss and tape
- ▶ prophylaxis handpiece and brush, cups, and paste
- ▶ ultrasonic unit and tips
- ▶ hand scalers, curettes, hoes
- ▶ HVE tip
- ▶ periodontal aids
- ▶ dappen dish with disinfecting solution

The patient is seated, draped, and prepared. The assistant dons PPE.

7 Assist with Anesthesia

Because the gingival tissues are inflamed and irritated, the patient may be given some topical or local anesthetic. The amount and kind are determined by the periodontist. The assistant prepares to give a disinfecting, analgesic mouthwash, paints the gingiva with a topical anesthetic, or passes the anesthetic syringe for local anesthesia.

8 Assist with Scaling

The assistant aids in the scaling of the **supragingival** calculus and plaque by passing a hand scaler or the ultrasonic handpiece and tip. The assistant will learn the operator's choice of instruments after a few sessions. The assistant may dip the tip of the instrument into a dappen dish of hydrogen peroxide solution or a commercial disinfecting solution before passing or exchanging instruments with the operator.

Throughout the scaling procedure, the assistant maintains visibility by rinsing and evacuating the mouth as needed. The operator may request the air syringe to dry the pockets for better viewing and access.

9 Assist with Curettage

The assistant aids in the curettage by passing the curettes and ultrasonic tips as requested. Visibility and a dry field are maintained by the assistant. A gauze square should be held near the work site to clean the instrument.

10 Assist with Root Planing

Root planing is carried out in the same manner as the scaling and curettage. The instruments are passed at the operator's request. The assistant dips the tips of the instruments into the disinfecting solution, passes, and exchanges as needed. Visibility is maintained by the air or water syringe and the HVE. All instruments used must be sterile for the procedure, and an aseptic technique should be used throughout the visit.

11 Assist with Polish of Teeth

The assistant aids in the polishing of the teeth by passing the handpiece with prophy cup and paste or the air polisher handpiece. The assistant holds the excess paste near the work site for refill and rinses and evacuates the mouth as needed.

Dental floss or tape is passed to polish the interproximal areas after the polishing of the crowns. If the operator desires to use any periodontal aids such as a stimulator or bridge cleaner, the assistant passes them as requested.

12 Clean Up and Dismiss Patient

The patient is cleaned up after the prophylaxis. Home care instructions are given and rehearsed with the patient. Diet and nutrition talks may also be stressed at this appointment (Table 8–5). If there is great tenderness in the area, the patient may be requested to maintain home care in all other areas, but to rinse thoroughly in the operative site. The patient is rescheduled and dismissed.

13 Clean Up Area, Disinfect, and Sterilize

The assistant gathers instruments and materials to take to the sterilizing room, removes gloves, and washes hands. The treatment is recorded on the patient's chart.

The assistant dons utility gloves, disinfects, sterilizes, and cleans up in the usual manner. The gloves are washed, disinfected, and removed; the hands are washed.▲

TABLE 8–5

Postoperative Instruction for the Periodontal Patient

Because of the delicate surgery performed, some bleeding, discomfort, and swelling may be expected. The surgical area has been packed with a periodontal dressing to protect and treat the tissues. Some pieces of this dressing may flake off. If discomfort or pain is present, please notify the office.

On the day of surgery, cold packs may be placed on the facial tissues in the operative area. Remove the pack for 15 minutes after each half hour of use.

Do not eat spicy, hard, or sour foods. Drink ample amounts of liquids. Try to avoid chewing in the area covered with the periodontal dressing.

Gently brush and floss the remaining teeth not covered by the packing material. After the first 24 hours, a mouthwash or warm salt water ($1/2$ to 1 teaspoon of salt per 8 ounces of water) may be used to gently rinse the mouth.

Take the medication prescribed for you. Avoid excessive exercise on the day of surgery and if any excessive bleeding, discomfort, or problems occur, notify the office at once.

Doctor's name

Doctor's phone number

THEORY RECALL
Periodontics

1. Periodontics is the branch of dentistry that deals with what?

2. What is one of the most important procedures for the periodontist?

3. What are the assistant's main duties in the interview section of the preliminary exam?

4. What effect does the patient's diet and nutritional level have on periodontal therapy?

5. What problems could habits have on the patient's dental health?

6. What would recording notes in the patient's own words show about the patient?

_____

7. What do radiographs show in the periodontal exam?

_____

8. How many readings with the periodontal probe does the periodontist make?

_____

9. What is the classification number for moderate periodontitis?

_____

10. How may the assistant aid the operator during the scaling, curettage, and root planing of the prophylaxis?

_____

Now turn to the Competency Evaluation Sheet for Procedure 48, Assisting with Periodontal Exam and Prophylaxis, located in Appendix C of this text.

GINGIVECTOMY AND REMOVAL OF PERIODONTAL PACKING

A gingivectomy is the surgical removal of the diseased tissues surrounding the tooth. The need for this surgery is indicated when the response to therapy has not occurred or when the tissues have deteriorated beyond repair.

The procedure for a gingivectomy is to remove the unattached, inflamed, necrotic tissue, removing irritating calculus and deposits, and packing the area with a soothing palliative dressing to permit regrowth of new, healthy tissue.

A gingivectomy may be performed in a localized area or completed as a full mouth therapy. When extensive tissue removal is needed, the patient is scheduled for multiple visits, usually receiving a quadrant at a time with one week intervals between visits.

The assistant may aid the periodontist by making pre- and postoperative preparations and cleanup. Helping to maintain visibility through suction, dabbing, light movement, and tongue control is important during the surgical procedures. The assistant also helps during the procedure with the mixing of materials, the handling and cleaning of instruments, monitoring the patient's reaction, and giving postoperative instructions to patients after surgery. During the removal of periodontal packing, the assistant aids in the periodontal procedure by preparation, patient care and cleanup, instruction, and visibility control, if not permitted by the State Dental Practice Act to remove the packing material.

PROCEDURE 49

Assisting with Gingivectomy and Removal of Periodontal Packing

Packing Placement

1 Complete Preparations

2 Assist with Anesthesia

3 Assist with Gingivectomy Procedure

4 Prepare Periodontal Packing Material

5 Assist with Placement of Packing Material

6 Clean Up and Instruct Patient

7 Clean Up Area, Disinfect, and Sterilize

Packing Removal

8 Complete Preparations

9 Assist with Removal of Packing

10 Clean Up Patient, Disinfect, and Sterilize

Packing Placement

1 Complete Preparations

The setup for the gingivectomy procedure follows:

► basic setup
► sundry setup
► anesthetic setup
► periodontal pocket markers, indelible pencil
► gingival knives and scalpel
► periosteal elevator
► scalers, curettes, assortment
► periodontal packing, pad, stiff spatula, and alcohol
► PFI instrument
► aspirating handle, extra tips, wire
► suture needle, sutures, suture scissors
► tissue scissors, pick ups, nippers

The patient is greeted and seated. The patient may need premedication if the tenderness and severity of inflammation is excessive. The assistant checks the orders and washes the patient's face with an antimicrobial soap. A drape and sterile bib are placed around the neck. The procedure is explained to the patient.

The assistant makes sure everything is ready. The tray may have been pre-set and wrapped with a sterile towel. The machines and equipment are checked. The assistant dons the gown, mask, and eyewear, scrubs hands, and dons surgical sterile gloves.

2 Assist with Anesthesia

The assistant may offer a disinfectant mouthwash to the patient. Topical anesthesia is placed on the injection site, and the periodontist is summoned. The assistant passes and receives the anesthetic syringe, recapping the needle in a one-handed motion. If analgesia (nitrous oxide and oxygen) are to be used, the mask is set and adjusted.

3 Assist with Gingivectomy Procedure

To assist with the surgical removal of tissue, the assistant passes a mouth mirror to the periodontist for a mouth exam. An explorer is passed to test the anesthetic level. The assistant passes periodontal pocket markers to the periodontist, who inserts the blunt end into the sulcus area and squeezes the tips together. The pointed end stabs the loose tissue and leaves a mark. The markers are inserted in all pocket areas. The periodontist may use the indelible pencil to mark a line from one point to another to set the path for the incision (Figure 8-11).

Cotton rolls or a gauze pack are placed in the area, and the assistant passes a scalpel or periodontal knife to the periodontist to incise the tissue. When the incision line has been made, the assistant receives the scalpel or knife and passes the periosteal elevator to lift the tissue away. The periosteal elevator is received, and the assistant passes tissue pick ups and tissue scissors or nippers. The loose tissues are clipped off, and the assistant holds gauze near the work site to receive the tissue pieces. Throughout the entire procedure, the assistant maintains visibility and a dry field by aspirating, retracting, and evacuating the mouth.

With the necrotic tissue removed, the periodontist may view and remove deposits. The assistant passes scalers or curettes as requested while holding gauze near the site to clean instruments and gather deposit debris.

4 Prepare Periodontal Packing Material

When the surgical procedure is finished, the assistant may make a periodontal pack out of eugenol and zinc oxide or a commercial mixture. This may be made up ahead of time to save time during the surgery.

The assistant dons overgloves and places a spot of eugenol approximately the size of a nickel on a glass slab or treated pad that has been wiped with alcohol. A heap of zinc oxide powder (approximately one or two large tablespoons) is placed nearby. Using a sterile, stiff stainless steel spatula, the powder is drawn into the liquid and mixed to a stiff doughy consistency. The dough is rolled in zinc oxide powder until it takes its limit. The roll is approximately two inches long and slightly thinner than a pencil. The overgloves are removed. If prepared ahead of surgery, the rolls may be wrapped in clear plastic wrap, placed in an airtight container, and kept in a cool place until needed.

A commercial periodontal packing material may be purchased. This product is supplied in a two-paste system. Equal lengths of paste are extruded from the two tubes onto a treated paper mixing pad (Figure 8-12). The materials are mixed to a homogeneous color and texture (Figure 8-13) and then are pressed into a roll to be placed on the surgical site (Figure 8-14).

If profuse bleeding occurs, the periodontist may wish to apply a suture or two before the packing. The assistant must be prepared for the event.

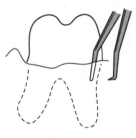

THE BLUNT END OF MARKER IS INSERTED INTO POCKET. TIPS ARE SQUEEZED TOGETHER. THE SHARP END PUNCTURES THE GINGIVA.

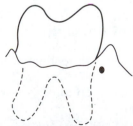

PUNCTURE MARKS INDICATE DEPTH OF POCKET AND GIVE INCISION PATTERN FOR THE GINGIVECTOMY.

FIGURE 8–11 Pocket markers are used to indicate the depth for tissue removal.

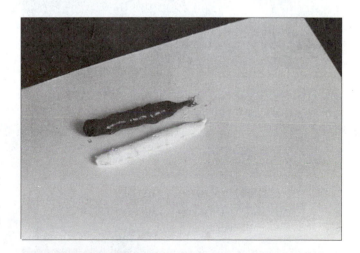

FIGURE 8–12 Equal lengths of the two mixtures are placed on a treated paper pad.

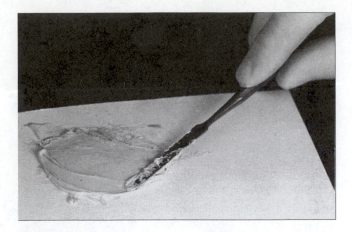

FIGURE 8-13 The materials are mixed until they form a homogeneous mixture.

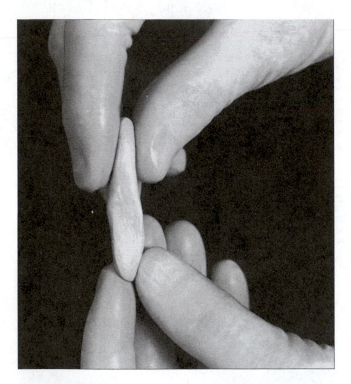

FIGURE 8-14 The mass is kneaded and fingered into a thin roll for placement.

5 Assist with Placement of Packing Material

The assistant aspirates or blots the area dry with sterile gauze then passes the periodontist a roll of packing and a **PFI** (plastic filling instrument) instrument for compressing the roll into the interproximal areas. When the facial side has been compressed, the lingual side may be packed. The assistant passes a damp, sterile gauze for the periodontist to compress the packing.

When the packing has been compressed and **festooned** (fitted) into the interproximal areas, the assistant passes a scaler to cut and smooth off the gingival edge of the packing. The assistant receives the scaler and the packing and passes the syringe for a gentle rinse of the mouth.

Small strips of foil or plastic wrap may be placed over the packing until it is dry. The patient is warned that this covering may work off and not to worry about it.

6 Clean Up and Instruct Patient

The patient is cleaned up and the assistant gives postoperative instructions to drink cool drinks at first, avoid rough, spicy, and hot foods, avoid smoking, and maintain hygiene on other teeth. The patient should rinse the operative area and expect a small amount of bleeding and pieces of packing to fall off. If there is any pain, the patient should call the office. The patient will return in a week for pack removal and a checkup (Table 8–5). The patient is dismissed.

7 Clean Up Area, Disinfect, and Sterilize

The assistant cleans up, records treatment on the patient's chart, and dons utility gloves for disinfection and sterilization. The gloves are washed, disinfected, and removed; hands are washed.

Packing Removal

8 Complete Preparations

The patient returns in one week and is seated in the chair, draped, and bibbed. The assistant dons PPE. The necessary equipment follows:

▶ basic setup
▶ sundry setup
▶ scaler or PFI instrument
▶ dental floss or tape
▶ suture removal equipment (if needed)

9 Assist with Removal of Packing

*In some states the trained assistant is permitted to remove surgical packing. If the State Dental Practice Act does not allow the assistant to perform this task, the assistant should aid the dentist.

The assistant passes the mirror for the exam. The syringe is passed for a spray rinse and evacuation is done. The scaler or PFI is passed. The periodontist pries the packing loose and removes it in pieces, placing the packing in the gauze that the assistant is holding at the work site. The assistant also holds the HVE tip to aspirate the area.

When the packing has been removed from the mouth, the assistant passes dental floss or tape for cleaning of the interproximal areas and passes or uses the syringe for a rinse. If sutures were previously placed, they are now removed.

10 Clean Up Patient, Disinfect, and Sterilize

The patient is cleaned up, given a review of oral hygiene practices, and dismissed. The assistant gathers contaminated materials and takes them to the sterilizing room. The gloves are removed, and the treatment is recorded on the patient's chart. The utility gloves are donned and the cleanup, disinfection, and sterilization are completed. The gloves are washed, disinfected, and removed; the hands are washed.▲

THEORY RECALL

Gingivectomy and Removal of Periodontal Packing

1. When is the need for a gingivectomy indicated?

2. What is the procedure for a gingivectomy?

3. Where is the blunt end of the periodontal pocket marker placed?

4. What does the assistant pass to the periodontist to remove the exposed calculus deposits after the gingiva is removed?

5. What does the assistant don before the mixing of the periodontal pack?

6. To what consistency does the assistant wish to mix the periodontal pack?

7. Which side of the teeth's surfaces receive the periodontal packing first?

8. What may the periodontist place over the packing material to preserve it until it is dry?

9. What postoperative instructions may be given the gingivectomy patient?

10. What instrument is used to loosen the packing material?

Now turn to the Competency Evaluation Sheet for Procedure 49, Assisting with Gingivectomy and Removal of Periodontal Packing, located in Appendix C of this text.

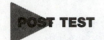
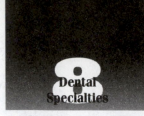

Total possible points = 100 points
80% needed for passing = 80 points

Total points this test _____ pass _____ fail _____

MATCHING: Place the letter from column B in the correct blank in column A. Each question is worth 2 points for a total of 20 points.

Column A	Column B
_____ 1. periodontist	a. total removal of questionable lesion
_____ 2. Class II malocclusion	b. protruding lower jaw feature
_____ 3. I & D	c. alveolitis
_____ 4. orthodontist	d. specialist in surgical procedures of mouth and jaw
_____ 5. exfoliative biopsy	e. scraping method for biopsy use
_____ 6. dry socket	f. partial removal of lesion for biopsy
_____ 7. Class III malocclusion	g. specialist in gingival care
_____ 8. oral surgeon	h. specialist in tooth alignment
_____ 9. incisive biopsy	i. incision and drainage of abscess
_____ 10. excisive biopsy	j. protruding upper jaw feature

Multiple Choice: Circle the correct answer. Each question is worth 4 points for a total of 80 points.

1. Removal of the entire questionable lesion is considered which type of biopsy?
   a. excisional   b. incisional   c. enfoliative   d. operative

2. The consistency of periodontal packing material should be
   a. stiff and tacky.   b. soft and sticky.   c. hard.   d. doughy.

3. A dry socket after extraction is caused by
   a. too much ice application.   c. lack of or loss of clot.
   b. too little anesthesia.   d. lack of anesthesia.

4. The purpose of an arch wire used in orthodontics is to
   a. determine the length of the arch.   c. provide stability in appliance.
   b. hold the brackets in place.   d. set a pattern for alignment.

5. Which of the following is *not* considered part of periodontal treatment?
   a. scaling   b. curettage   c. root planing   d. sealant

6. In suture removal, the suture scissors are placed to snip
   a. near the knot.   b. away from the knot.   c. through the knot.   d. midway.

7. If a perio-involved tooth exhibits facial-lingual movement, the mobility is classified as
   a. 0.   b. +1.   c. +2.   d. +3.

8. Orthodontic brackets and tubes are attached to which side of the band?
   a. facial   b. occlusal   c. mesial   d. distal

9. The smoothing and contouring of the bony ridges left after multiple extractions is called
   a. osteographics.   b. gingivectomy.   c. frenectomy.   d. alveoplasty.

10. Teeth to get orthodontic bonded appliances must first receive
    a. restoration.   b. etching.   c. band sizing.   d. crowning.

11. A forceps designed to remove teeth in either arch is called
    a. anterior.   b. posterior.   c. clinical.   d. universal.

12. Orthodontic separators are placed prior to bands to
    a. prepare for the feel of bands.   c. provide relationship measurement.
    b. prepare and strengthen enamel.   d. provide space for bands.

13. A periodontal pack is placed after a gingivectomy surgery to (1) prevent bleeding, (2) prevent infection, (3) protect the area, (4) provide better esthetics, (5) soothe the wound, or (6) prevent irritation.
    a. 1, 2, 3, 5, and 6   b. 2, 4, and 6   c. 1, 3, and 6   d. all

14. Which of the following patients is most likely *not* to be referred to an oral surgeon?
    a. a patient needing single extraction   c. a patient in compromising health condition
    b. a patient needing multiple extraction   d. a patient with a complicated impacted tooth

15. A patient is exhibiting the following symptoms: deep periodontal pockets, supportive bone loss, tooth mobility, swelling of tissues, profuse redness and bleeding. In which gingival stage will the patient be classified?
    a. Class I—gingivitis   c. Class III—moderate periodontitis
    b. Class II—slight periodontitis   d. Class IV—advanced periodontitis

16. When orthodontic brackets and tubes are cemented on the tooth enamel, the procedure is called
    a. direct bonding.   b. bracket banding.   c. auto-banding.   d. workup ortho.

17. Orthodontic treatment may be completed by using which type of appliance?
    a. fixed   b. removable   c. Hawley   d. a, b, and c

18. A cephlometric radiograph is taken during the preliminary orthodontic exam to
    a. detect carious lesions.   c. detect broken teeth.
    b. determine bone growth.   d. detect rotated teeth.

19. Orthodontic treatment, which deals with correction of the effects of bad habits such as thumb sucking, is said to be which type of treatment?
    a. corrective   b. preventive   c. interpretative   d. behavioral

20. Which classification of malocclusion is exhibited by a condition in which the mesiobuccal cusp of the first permanent maxillary molar is mesial to the mesiobuccal groove of the mandibular first permanent molar, and the upper cuspid is anterior to the lower cuspid giving a retruded lower jaw appearance:
    a. Class I   b. Class II   c. Class III   d. Class IV

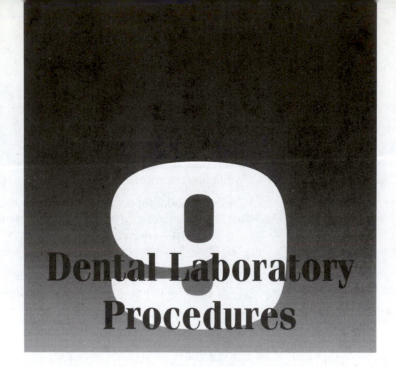

9 Dental Laboratory Procedures

▶ **OBJECTIVES**

Upon completion of this unit, the student will achieve a score of 80% or better on the Post Test covering the following material.

1. Discuss the properties, uses, and preparation procedures for gypsum products.
2. Demonstrate techniques for the pouring of alginate impressions with gypsum products to form study models.
3. Demonstrate the method for the separation of alginate impressions and poured gypsum study models.
4. Discuss and demonstrate the procedures for the trimming of study models constructed from gypsum products.
5. Demonstrate the technique to articulate gypsum study models into patient occlusion.
6. Demonstrate the procedure for the construction of wax occlusal rims and base plates prepared for construction of dentures.
7. Discuss the need and demonstrate the method to construct custom trays.
8. Identify the steps necessary for assisting with the fabrication of temporary crowns in a preparation appointment.
9. Discuss and demonstrate the method for the preparation of lab cases for shipment to commercial dental laboratories.

▶ **KEY TERMS**

acrylic	esthetic	polymer
alginate	fabrication	polymerization
alignment	functional	preliminary
anatomic	gypsum	pulverized
articulator	indentations	replica
base form	inverted	spatula
bite registration	luting	study models
consistency	monomer	tuberosity
custom tray	occlusion	vibrator
deteriorate	parallel	void
edentulous	peripheral	

FABRICATION OF STUDY MODELS

There are two types of **gypsum** products used in the dental office—laboratory plaster and dental stone. Both come from stone quarries. The processing makes them different. The gypsum rock is **pulverized** and heated to drive off the moisture. This produces a finished product called plaster of Paris or dental laboratory plaster. Gypsum stone, which is pulverized and then autoclaved, produces another kind of powder called dental stone. When joined with water, both powders form a bond and become hard. The amount of water each powder takes differs. Laboratory plaster requires 60 milliliters (ml) of water to 100 grams of plaster powder, while dental stone needs 30 ml per 100 grams of stone powder, unless stated differently by the manufacturer.

Laboratory plaster is not as strong as dental stone; therefore, it is used in the dental office for study models, impressions, or utility purposes. Dental stone is strong and dense; it can withstand more pressure, abrasion, and use than laboratory plaster. Stone is used in the dental office for orthodontic study models, dies, and projects that require extensive work or resistance.

Since both laboratory plaster and dental stone come from the same source, they are the same color in the natural state. Many manufacturers add color, usually a buff or yellow shade, to the dental stone to designate a difference on sight. Gypsum, which has been super heated, is even more dense and more resistant; it may be colored different shades, such as pink or green.

Gypsum products can be purchased in many weight quantities from premeasured envelopes of a few grams up to 50-pound barrels or drums. Gypsum must be stored in a cool, dry place. It should not be ordered too far in advance of anticipated use or the gypsum powder will take moisture out of the air and eventually **deteriorate** to the point where it will not get hard. One can tell when gypsum products are deteriorating by how fast it sets up. As gypsum ages and picks up moisture, it takes longer to get hard properly.

Gypsum also has another amazing quality in setting up. It will get hard under water. That quality is why a dental assistant must be careful with excess soft gypsum mixtures. Leftover gypsum products should be scraped out of the bowl and placed in a waste receptacle. They should *never* be washed down the sink because soft gypsum will set up; if not flushed out of the drains, it will harden in the pipes and clog them. All mixing bowls should be scraped clean, wiped with paper toweling, and then washed.

To get a proper mixture of a gypsum product, the assistant must combine a correct amount of water to the powder. The manufacturer will suggest the amount; usually, to 100 grams of powder, it is recommended to add 60 ml plaster and 30 ml water to dental stone. A graduated measuring cup can be used for the water measure and a dietary scale can be used to weigh the powder. Some professionals who have been preparing gypsum mixtures for some time will guesstimate the proportions; for a strong and proper finished product, it is best to measure.

One of the most popular dental uses for gypsum material is in making a **study model**, which is a **replica** of a patient's mouth. While the patient is in the office, an impression of the teeth and a **bite registration** are made. An impression material, usually **alginate**, is placed in an impression tray and inserted into the mouth. The impression tray loaded with soft alginate is pressed onto the teeth and surrounding structure and held for a short time until it stiffens or sets up. It is then removed, giving the dentist an impression of that arch. The process is repeated for the other arch and then a bite registration is taken. To record a patient's normal bite, the dentist uses a piece of soft material, perhaps a doubled up piece of base plate wax or a commercial bite wafer, and places it into the mouth. The patient is instructed to bite down on this material until indents are made. It is withdrawn, cooled, disinfected, and saved until the models are poured up in gypsum and are to be trimmed.

After the impressions and bite registration have been made, they are taken to the dental laboratory to be poured and trimmed. This is a process in which the assistant fills up the impression material with a gypsum product adding extra on the bottom to make the model more **functional** and appealing. This extra part is called the base. Together the impression and the base make an exact replica of the patient's mouth, which the dentist may use for planning and measuring in the patient's absence (Figure 9-1).

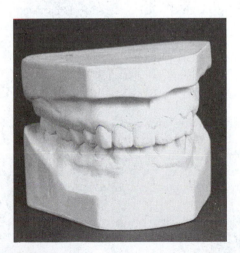

FIGURE 9-1 Study models can be used as patterns for construction, legal records, examples of before-and-after treatment, as well as planning and preparation.

PROCEDURE 50

Fabrication of Study Models

1 Assemble Equipment and Materials

2 Don PPE

3 Disinfect Impressions and Bite Registration

4 Mix Gypsum Product

5 Pour Gypsum into Impression

6 Make Art Base Form

7 Repeat Process for Other Arch

8 Identify Study Models

9 Clean Up Work Site and Equipment

1 Assemble Equipment and Materials

To prepare a mixture of gypsum, the following materials are needed:

- two rubber mixing bowls (flexibowls), one for each arch
- two semiflexible, broad-bladed spatulas
- dietary scale for weighing powder
- bottle of room-temperature water with dispenser
- graduated measuring cup
- scoop to carry powder
- paper cup to hold powder
- mechanical mixer used to mix materials (optional)
- electrical vibrator (optional)

To complete the pouring procedure, the following materials and equipment are needed:

- impressions and bite registration (disinfected)
- base formers or boxing wax (if desired)
- glass slabs or flat smooth surface to set poured impressions

2 Don PPE

Before the mixing and pouring of the impression can begin, disinfecting must be done. The dental assistant must don utility gloves and PPE, including eyeglasses or a face shield. Spraying or splashing of the mixture may carry pathogens into unprotected areas.

3 Disinfect Impressions and Bite Registration

The assistant sprays the trays with impression material and the bite registration with disinfecting solution or immerses them into a disinfectant solution for less than 30 minutes, since alginate has a tendency to ab-

sorb moisture and distort the impression shape. All traces of blood, saliva, or debris must be removed, not only for sanitation practice, but also so that the setting process of the gypsum material is not affected. If there is a large amount of foreign material in the impression or if saliva strings are attached, the dental assistant may make up a runny plaster mixture and run this mixture through the impression material to pick up this debris. The impression is then rinsed clear of the runny plaster mixture and most debris is removed.

When the impression is cleaned and disinfected, the dental assistant removes the moisture drops from the impression. If these droplets are permitted to remain during pouring, they will cause a hole or **void** effect in the model. To remove excess moisture, a small piece of absorbent cloth toweling can gently dab up and absorb the drops. A light spray of compressed air may be used, but care must be given not to dry out the alginate impression material. If the dental assistant is using a spray of compressed air to dry the impression, a mask should be worn to prevent contamination to the operator.

4 Mix Gypsum Product

After assembling the materials and equipment, the dental assistant should:

a. Place a paper cup on the dietary scale and adjust the scale to zero.

b. Scoop enough powder to weigh 100 grams and place it in the cup on the scale.

c. Dispense enough room-temperature water to make the correct powder-water ratio for desired powder—60 ml for plaster, 30 ml for dental stone. *Note:* Room-temperature water is used because hot or warm water makes the mixture set up sooner and cold water retards the setting. As a further protection against infection, some offices are mixing sodium hypochlorite solution up to one-quarter volume in the mixing water.

d. Rinse out the rubber bowl and empty the contents to ensure no measured water will be used to moisten the bowl.

e. Sift powder into the water and let it be absorbed (Figure 9-2).

f. Gently cut through the mixture in a figure-eight pattern to moisten the powder particles (Figure 9-3).

g. When mixture is moist, spatulate evenly, trying not to trap in air. *Note:* If using a mechanical mixer, cover and rotate the knob until the mixture is smooth and creamy (Figure 9-4).

h. When the mixture is smooth (Figure 9-5), place the bowl on the **vibrator** or bounce the bowl on a table top to bring trapped air to the surface (Figure 9-6).

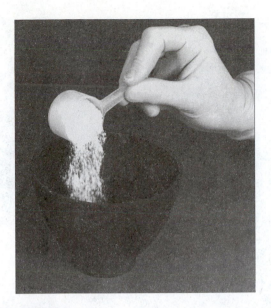

FIGURE 9-2 Mixing gypsum material. Powder is gently shaken into the water to prevent clumping of material.

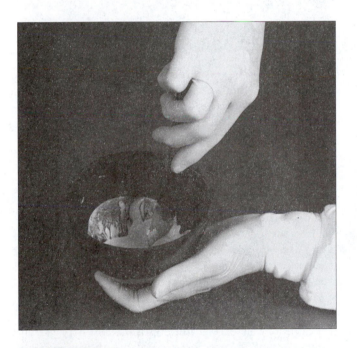

FIGURE 9-3 A figure-eight motion is used to unite the water and powder materials.

As noted, water temperature can help determine how fast gypsum products get hard. The setting time can be hastened also by adding a little table salt to the mixture, or the setting time can be slowed or retarded by putting in a pinch of borax to the mixture. Usually, the room-temperature water and powder mixture works in a proper and comfortable manner.

The choice of plaster or stone is determined by the dentist or the policy of the office for that procedure.

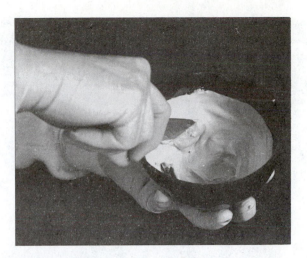

FIGURE 9-4 When materials are moistened, the mixture is stirred to a smooth condition.

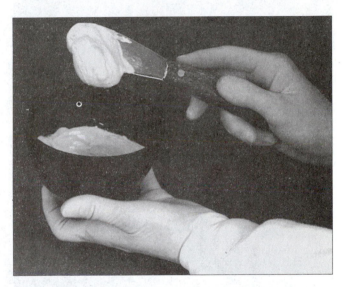

FIGURE 9-5 The mixture must be smooth and have no lumps.

The dental assistant must make the correct water-powder ratio for the gypsum material of choice. When it is mixed smoothly with air bubbles removed, it is placed in the impression.

5 Pour Gypsum into Impression

The alginate impression in the tray is held on an angle on the vibrator (or tapped gently on the table top). A small amount of gypsum is carried by the spatula to the rear of the molar area (Figure 9-7). Here, it is gently flowed into the molar **indentations**. Another small amount of gypsum is placed in the same area and the material is flowed onward through the molars toward the anterior region, taking care to push the air out ahead of the gypsum and avoid trapping any air under

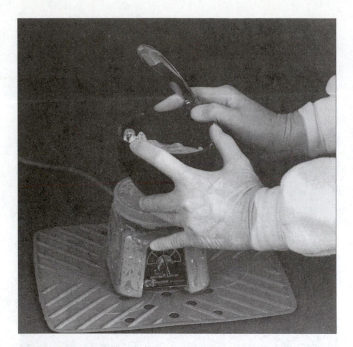

FIGURE 9–6 The bowl of gypsum mixture is placed on a vibrator to eliminate air bubbles.

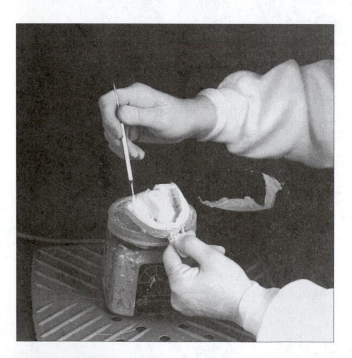

FIGURE 9–7 Pouring tray series. Small amounts of gypsum are vibrated into the posterior tooth indentations and vibrated forward.

the mixture. More and more small amounts are added until the mixture has flowed into all the tooth impressions. When these indent areas have been filled, the rest of the impression is filled (Figure 9–8).

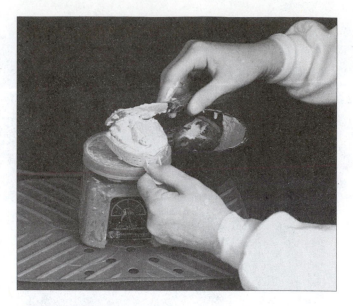

FIGURE 9–8 The gypsum material is flowed along the tooth indentations pushing out the air and filling the depressions. The tray is completely filled.

6 Make Art Base Form

There are different ways to make the base of the study models. The dental assistant can place some boxing wax around the impression tray carefully **luting** (melting) the meeting edges together to form a box. Gypsum material is then vibrated into this "box" to form a base. This method is called boxing an impression.

Some offices, particularly the orthodontists', use a preformed base or base former filled with gypsum to make the base. The base form is filled with the soft gypsum material and then the poured impression is set into the center of the wet gypsum in the former with the teeth side up. This method is called setting an impression.

A more common method to complete the **base form** is to do the **inverted** pour method. The dental assistant increases the initial proportion of gypsum mixture by a half portion. This excess amount of mixture is placed in a pile on a glass or smooth slab after the impression has been filled. The impression filled with the gypsum is then inverted over the excess pile (Figure 9–9). A **spatula** is used to smooth the two parts together. Care is taken not to spread the mixture on the tray. Keep the tray **parallel** to the floor (Figure 9–10). When uniting the mandibular impression with the base, the tongue area must be smoothed out or a piece of alginate or wet paper towel can be used to stuff the tongue area to keep it open. Any excess left in the tongue area is cut and smoothed out when trimmed.

If one chooses to do so, the inverted pour method may be completed in two steps called a double pour.

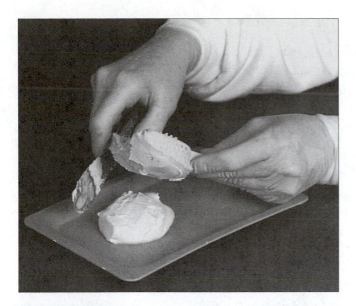

FIGURE 9-9 The filled tray is inverted over a pile of thick gypsum material.

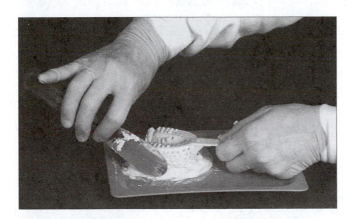

FIGURE 9-10 The sides are smoothed into a union. Care is taken to avoid smearing onto the tray.

After the teeth impression part has been filled in, the top surface is left rough. A second mixture is made up, and the base is formed to which the teeth impression is added. In all methods of making the base, enough gypsum should be placed to provide a base large enough to be one-third the size of the models when finished.

7 Repeat Process for Other Arch

The mandibular impression needs attention in the tongue area before pouring the impression with gypsum. This space needs to be filled in to avoid the harder task of carving out the gypsum after setting. The tongue area may be stuffed with alginate, a piece of softened base plate wax, wet toweling rolled into a wad, or a pile of dough.

When both arches have been filled and completed, they are set aside to permit the mixture to set up and get hard. This process usually takes about an hour. Gypsum material gives off heat before the setting is final.

8 Identify Study Models

Some form of identification is made and placed near the poured impressions. It may be a piece of paper with the patient's name written on it or the name in crayon on the glass slab when the impressions are setting up. Once the models have cooled, the impression and gypsum parts can be separated and trimming can begin.

9 Clean Up Work Site and Equipment

Cleanup work can be completed whenever there is a lull or a wait for a process to finish. All disposable items, such as masks, overgloves, and towels, may be placed in the plastic bag that held the impressions and bite registration, closed, and placed into the trash receptacle. A clean and tidy laboratory is easier and more pleasant to work in than one where nothing is put away or cleaned up.▲

THEORY RECALL
Fabrication of Study Models

1. The two types of gypsum products found in the dental office are

   a. _____

   b. _____.

2. The formula for preparation of plaster of Paris or laboratory plaster is _____ml of water to _____ grams of plaster.

3. The formula for preparation of dental stone is _____ ml of water to _____ grams of dental stone.

4. How is gypsum stored?

   _____

5. Why must gypsum products never be flushed down the drain?

   _____

6. Why is room-temperature water used for mixing gypsum products?

   _____

7. Before the process of the pouring of the impressions can begin, what must be done to the impressions?

   _____

8. If moisture drops are permitted to remain on and in the impression when pouring, what will be evident in the finished product?

_____

9. The gypsum mixture is flowed into the teeth impression beginning at what part of the impression?

_____

10. Why does the dentist request study models be taken of a patient's mouth?

_____

Now turn to the Competency Evaluation Sheet for Procedure 50, Fabrication of Study Models, located in Appendix C of this text.

SEPARATION OF MODELS AND IMPRESSION

After the gypsum models have dried and are cool to touch, the assistant may separate them and prepare to trim the models. This procedure may be completed about an hour after the pouring or they may be left until the next day or so when there may be more time to complete the separation and trimming tasks. The urgency of the separation and trim depends on the work that must be planned and the scheduling of the patient's next visit.

PROCEDURE 51

Separation of Models and Impression

1 Assemble Materials and Equipment

2 Don PPE

3 Examine Models

4 Release Gypsum and Impression Materials

5 Remove Impression Material

6 Identify Models

7 Cleanup Procedures

1 Assemble Materials and Equipment

To complete the separation procedure, the assistant gathers the following:

► poured models in impression trays
► laboratory knife
► marking pen
► safety glasses
► overgloves and utility gloves

2 Don PPE

Before beginning the separation procedure, the assistant dons safety glasses to protect the eyes from chips and flying pieces of gypsum. Utility or overgloves are worn to protect against infection.

3 Examine Models

The assistant tests to see if the model is hard and cool. Cooling is an indication that the chemical process of setting up has been completed. The assistant may attempt a knife puncture to test the firmness.

4 Release Gypsum and Impression Materials

To separate the impression from the gypsum, the assistant takes a knife and cuts away all overhanging and excess impression material, thus exposing the impression tray. The point of the knife is inserted between the tray and the hard model and gently twisted causing a small separation of the two and letting air enter between them. The knife tip is rotated and gently twisted at various spaces around the tray until the tray and the material are loosened.

5 Remove Impression Material

Avoiding any sharp angles, the impression is then lifted up and off the model. The assistant is careful to lift the material straight up and off as twisting may snap off any small incisor teeth of the model.

6 Identify Models

The models' identification is checked and rewritten if not present. The assistant inspects the models and places them and the bite registration near the model trimmer.

7 Cleanup Procedures

The impression trays are cleaned, washed, rinsed, and prepared for sterilization. All litter and gypsum flakes are picked and cleaned up. PPE is disinfected and removed. The hands are washed. The gypsum models are ready to trim.▲

THEORY RECALL

Separation of Models and Impression

1. What procedure must be performed to the models and impression before trimming?

_____

2. What determines the urgency of the separation of the models and the impression?

_____

3. Why does the assistant wear safety glasses during the separation procedure?

_____

4. Before the separation, what does the assistant cut away from the impression and models?

_____

5. Why is the knife tip inserted and twisted between the impression material and the models at the start of the separation?

_____

6. In what motion is the model removed from the impression material?

_____

7. What harm can occur from twisting the material during the separation procedure?

_____

8. Which teeth are the most susceptible to snapping off during the separation procedure?

_____

9. How are the models identified after separation?

_____

10. What is the next procedure to occur after the models are separated from the impression material?

_____

Now turn to the Competency Evaluation Sheet for Procedure 51, Separation of Models and Impression, located in Appendix C of this text.

TRIMMING GYPSUM MODELS

When the poured impressions have set and the gypsum is removed from the alginate impression material, a positive reproduction of the patient's mouth is present in the gypsum casts. These reproductions are used by the dentist to help with diagnosis and future treatment planning; therefore, they are called study models. They may also serve as permanent records of oral conditions prior to treatment and later may be compared with a posttreatment cast. In some cases, these models are used as patterns for appliances or measurement of dental restorations.

The assistant prepares these models to be more appealing and functional by trimming them to a standard pattern and finishing them to improve their **esthetic** nature. An electric grinding machine, called a model trimmer, is used to eliminate gross amounts of gypsum, while a rasp and sandpaper smooth and prepare the models' surfaces.

The study models are trimmed in a conventional, standard method. A bite registration will be used in the cutting procedure to ensure that the models will be in the patient's normal occlusal pattern. The casts are composed of two parts—an **anatomic** area, which includes the teeth and the surrounding periodontal tissues, and an art base, which is added to improve the looks and to make the set more stable and functional. The anatomic part of the model comprises two-thirds of the entire height with the art base holding only a third.

When finished with the trimming, the models are approximately three inches tall and are seated in occlusion with the maxillary anterior region in a point to include the labial frenum. The mandibular anterior area is rounded. The sides are parallel to the occlusal surfaces of the premolars and heel cuts are made perpendicular opposite the cuspids. The surfaces contain no voids; they should be smooth and glossy. The edges are beveled. The study models bear the name of the patient and the date of preparation.

PROCEDURE 52

Trimming Gypsum Models

1 Assemble Materials and Equipment
_____

2 Don PPE
_____

3 Prepare Model Trimmer
_____

4 Trim Maxillary Base Cut
_____

5 Trim Maxillary Posterior Cut
_____

6 Trim Maxillary Lateral Cuts
_____

7 Trim Maxillary Heel Cuts
_____

8 Trim Maxillary Anterior Cut
_____

9 Trim Mandibular Posterior Cut
_____

10 Trim Mandibular Base Cut
_____

11 Trim Mandibular Lateral Cuts
_____

12 Trim Mandibular Heel Cuts
_____

13 Trim Mandibular Anterior Cut
_____

14 Finish Models
_____

15 Identify Models
_____

16 Cleanup Procedures
_____

1 Assemble Materials and Equipment

The equipment needed follows:

- model trimmer
- safety glasses, gloves
- pencil and compass
- ruler
- models with bite registration
- lab knife
- rasp, wet and dry sandpaper
- soap solution, polishing cloth

If some time has elapsed between the trimming and pouring and the models have dried out, they should be soaked in cool water for five minutes to permit easier reductions with the model trimmer. Damp models do not drag or chip off as readily as dry ones.

2 Don PPE

A model trimmer could be a dangerous piece of equipment if used improperly. Eye protection must be worn. Hair should be tied back. No jewelry or hanging ties on clothes should be evident. Attention should be concentrated on the job at hand, which is grinding plaster and stone to proper proportions.

3 Prepare Model Trimmer

The model trimmer must have a steady stream of water circulating over the grinding wheel so the surface does not become clogged and the model trims smoothly. The water is turned on, and the model trimmer is started. Once the water is moving over the grinding wheel properly, the trimming may begin. The operator must always remember to hold the models to be trimmed steady and flat on the trimming table, gently feeding the gypsum with steady pressure into the grinding wheel. This leaves a flat and smooth trimmed surface.

4 Trim Maxillary Base Cut

In many cases, the maxillary dentition is wider but may be shorter than the mandibular dentition; therefore, trimming begins on the maxillary model or whichever is larger. The model is set on the table top with the teeth down. Take a compass's plain point and run along the table edge. The other edge of the compass should mark a line on the base parallel to the table (Figure 9–11). Circulate the pencil line around the entire model, then trim off excess hard gypsum above the line. This forms the base cut, which gives the height to the model. The base should be approximately 1½ times the length of the maxillary canines or one-third of the study model height.

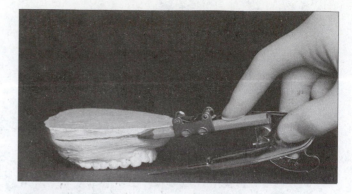

FIGURE 9–11 Trimming model series. The base cut line is parallel to the table top.

5 Trim Maxillary Posterior Cut

The maxillary posterior cut is next. The model is set on the table with the teeth up. The plain compass point is inserted between the mesial interproximals of the centrals on the palate side. With the pencil end extended to ¼ inch longer than the last molar, make a slight mark on the **tuberosity** area. Draw a line down the central occlusal area of the last molar extending to cross the first mark, making an *X* on the tuberosity area (Figure 9-12). Complete this process on the other side, which leaves two *X*s. Hold a ruler to the two *X*s and draw a straight line. The marked area should be measured and checked against the length of the mandibular model, being careful to include enough in the posterior to cover the mandibular teeth. Trim off the excess hard gypsum to this line, which leaves the posterior smooth and even.

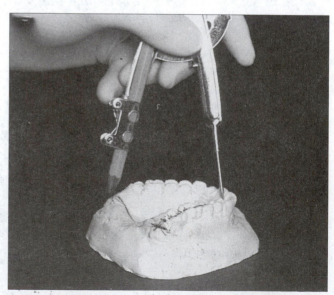

FIGURE 9–12 The compass is used to make an even line for the back cut. The tips must extend as much as possible on the maxillary because the lower jaw is usually longer.

2. What instrument is used to trim gypsum models?

_____

3. Why is it important to wear overgloves when trimming gypsum models?

_____

4. Why is water flow critical in model trimming?

_____

5. Why should safety glasses be worn when working with the model trimmer?

_____

6. The anterior portion of the maxillary model is trimmed in what shape?

_____

7. The anterior of the mandibular model is trimmed in what shape?

_____

8. Rough scratch marks may be removed by using _____ or a _____ to finish up a model.

9. What two purposes do soap solutions serve?

a. _____

b. _____

10. Finished models are marked with what information when completed?

_____

Now turn to the Competency Evaluation Sheet for Procedure 52, Trimming Gypsum Models, located in Appendix C of this text.

ARTICULATING GYPSUM MODELS

Study models may or may not be mounted on **articulators**. The future use of the models determines if such a procedure will be undertaken. Articulators are hinged metal devices that imitate the movement of the jaw.

When impressions have been poured up, trimmed, prepared, and mounted on the articulator, the dentist may observe the maxillary and mandibular jaws and the teeth in occlusion.

Articulators vary from simple disposable styles to a complicated type of device using facebows and other attachments. A complex method of preparing this type is performed by the dentist or prosthodontist; the methods vary according to the designs of the operator.

The simple type of articulator is mounted by using a clean articulator, study models, and laboratory plaster. The bite registration wax plate is used to determine the patient's normal bite pattern. Each arch is attached with wet laboratory plaster to a ring or flange

of the articulator. When dry and set, the models are fixed on the articulator, functioning and working as the patient's own dentition.

PROCEDURE 53
Articulation of Study Models

1 Assemble Equipment and Materials
2 Soap Model Bases
3 Stabilize Models
4 Assemble Articulator
5 Prepare Gypsum Material
6 Place Models on the Articulator
7 Test Articulation
8 Cleanup Procedures

1 Assemble Equipment and Materials

The equipment needed for this procedure follows:

► prepared models
► bite registration wafer or form
► articulator
► elastic band and stabilizing material
► gypsum mixing materials and equipment
► soap solution
► pencil for marking

2 Soap Model Bases

To prepare the study models for easy removal from the articulator when the case is finished, the assistant soaps the top and bottom of each model with a soap solution. This may be accomplished by painting a thin film of detergent on the bases' top or bottom or they may be dipped in soap solution with the teeth facing up. The soap on the bases is permitted to dry while the preparations for the articulation are being made.

3 Stabilize Models

The patient's bite registration is placed between the models establishing the occlusal bite, then the models are stabilized by securing some melted, sticky wax in scattered areas around the teeth or by placing a thick rubber band around the two arches while in occlusion (Figure 9–17).

4 Assemble Articulator

A clean articulator is obtained and checked for function and use. It is adjusted for sizing to contain the set of models or poured impressions.

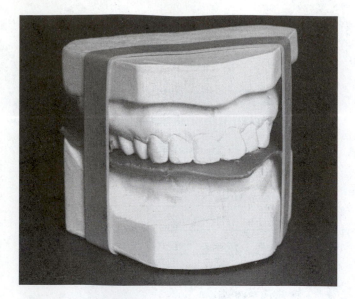

FIGURE 9–17 The study models are placed in occlusion and stabilized by an elastic band or sticky wax.

5 Prepare Gypsum Material

A half mixture (50 grams plaster to 30 ml water) of laboratory plaster is mixed to a smooth **consistency**, slightly thicker than for study models.

6 Place Models on the Articulator

Half the plaster mix is placed on the mandibular ring or bar in a pile. The base of the mandibular model, which has been painted with a soap solution to permit easy separation, is placed on the wet pile in an even and parallel manner (Figure 9–18). The remainder of

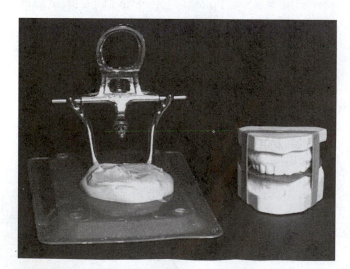

FIGURE 9–18 Plaster is placed on the greased lower articulator ring. The model will be seated in this area.

the laboratory plaster is placed on the maxillary ring or bar and the top part of the base of the maxillary model, which has also been painted with soap solution. The plaster is smoothed over after the models have been seated (Figure 9–19).

7 Test Articulation

The assistant checks to see if the models are parallel to the floor and evenly set. A quick check is made to see that all areas are clear and able to function properly. Care is taken to avoid smearing a lot of wet plaster around the articulator. Clean up of hard plaster is difficult and not needed.

When the plaster holding the models has dried, the elastic band may be cut and trimmed off close to the plaster piles; the bite registration is removed. The articulator should open and close in a manner resembling the patient's mouth movements.

8 Cleanup Procedures

All materials and equipment are cleaned up and put away. *When the articulator has been cleaned and before it is put into storage, a light coat of petroleum jelly on the metal makes the next cleanup easier. The assistant washes hands when finished.▲

THEORY RECALL
Articulating Gypsum Models

1. Study models are mounted on which laboratory instrument?

   _____

2. What is the purpose of mounting the gypsum study models?

   _____

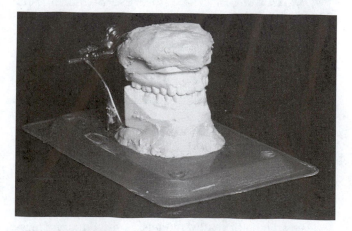

FIGURE 9–19 Models that have been articulated will imitate the movements of the patient's bite and function.

3. The bite registration form serves what purpose when mounting gypsum models?

_____

4. What material is used to attach the study models to the articulator?

_____

5. What material is used to prepare the study models for easy removal from the articulator when the case is finished?

_____

6. What can the assistant use to hold and stabilize the models together while mounting the gypsum set?

_____

7. What materials can be used to maintain the finished condition of the articulators between use?

_____

Now turn to the Competency Evaluation Sheet for Procedure 53, Articulation of Study Models, located in Appendix C of this text.

CONSTRUCTION OF BASE PLATES AND OCCLUSAL RIMS

Base plates and occlusal rims are used by the dentist in construction of dentures. The base plate represents the body of the denture, and the occlusal rim is a wax block on which the dentist or dental technician places the actual denture teeth.

When the teeth have been placed and tested on the articulator and in the patient's mouth and all final fittings have been completed, the last step in construction begins. The base plates and occlusal wax with the denture teeth are invested in or covered with material (alginate or investment). After this material hardens or sets into place, the wax is heated or melted out and then replaced by an **acrylic** material mixture forming the denture base. Since the wax is the pattern for the denture base and tooth placement, it is important that the base plate with rims is exact, comfortable, and esthetic in nature.

Base plates can be made of two materials—base plate wax and a gutta percha material, which, like wax, softens with heat (hot water) and hardens when cooled. Once in a softened state, the two are prepared in the same manner.

Base plate wax can be purchased in one- or five-pound boxes. It comes in colored sheets, either red, pink, or yellow and in various consistencies of soft, medium, tough, or extra tough.

Occlusal rims are blocks of the same type of wax. They are shaped like a horseshoe and are approximately 4½ inches long and ½ inch square shape.

They are pink and come packed 100 in a box. Occlusal rims need not be commercially made. Base plate wax sheets can be tightly folded over and over until they meet the same dimensions. Commercial rims are easier to use, save time, and are more likely not to have any void areas.

PROCEDURE 54

Construction of Base Plates and Occlusal Rims

1 Assemble Equipment and Materials

2 Prepare the Edentulous Models

3 Adapt the Base Plate to the Edentulous Model

4 Trim Excessive Wax

5 Contour Wax Sheet into Mucobuccal Fold

6 Place Occlusal Rim on the Plate

7 Fill Space Between the Rim and Plate

8 Cut Heel Slant

9 Level Occlusal Surface

10 Finish Plate and Occlusal Rims

11 Prepare Opposite Arch in Similar Manner

12 Cleanup Procedures

1 Assemble Equipment and Materials

To construct base plates with occlusal rims, the following equipment and materials will be needed:

► edentulous model
► indelible pencil
► talc or baby powder
► Bunsen burner or alcohol torch, match
► base plate wax
► commercial bite rims (optional)
► spatula
► glass slab or large putty knife
► pencil eraser end
► soft cloth
► lab knife and scissors

Hair is tied or pulled back when working with the open flame of the Bunsen burner or alcohol torch. All tubing is kept to a minimum and placed to the back of the table out of reach and accident area.

2 Prepare the Edentulous Models

The edentulous model is checked for smoothness and irregularities. An indelible pencil or marker is used to mark around the area where the denture is to fit. Baby powder or talc may be sprinkled onto the model and rubbed in to help prevent the base plate wax from sticking to the form. After the model is prepared, long hair is pulled back and sleeves turned up to prevent a fire mishap with the lit Bunsen burner.

3 Adapt the Base Plate to the Edentulous Model

A sheet of base plate wax is softened over the flame in a gentle moving motion. When the sheet is soft and draping, it is placed over the **edentulous** model and finger pressed onto the form (Figure 9–20).

4 Trim Excessive Wax

Excess wax is cut off with a lab knife, scalpel or scissors ⅙ to ¼ inch around the mucobuccal fold area. Trimmed wax may be saved for later use (Figure 9–21).

5 Contour Wax Sheet into Mucobuccal Fold

Now that there is less weight and bulk hanging over the model edge, a closer fit can be made by gently pressing the material closer to the model in the mucobuccal fold. The tip of a pencil eraser is a handy object to use; it will not puncture or tear as easily as an instrument. The wax edge is tilted back and then

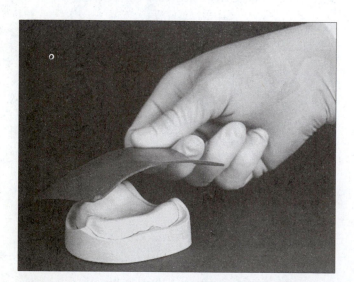

FIGURE 9–20 The softened base plate wax is draped over the edentulous model.

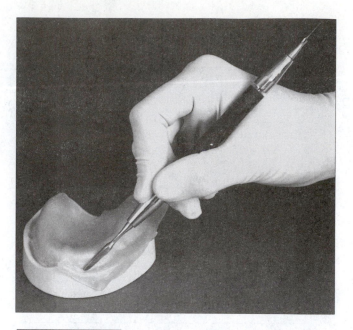

FIGURE 9–21 The excess wax is cut off and saved for uniting and filling in gaps in the rim and plate union.

pressed against the plate conforming to the premarked indelible pencil line. The wax is reheated throughout the procedure as necessary for movement and conformity. An alcohol torch with a forced flame director is handy in this procedure.

Occasionally, the inside of the base plate must be checked to determine if any pinches, ridges, voids, or irregularities have occurred. The base plate should be even in thickness.

6 Place Occlusal Rim on the Plate

After the base plate is constructed, the occlusal rims are added. Commercial rims or those made with base plate wax may be used. The thick blocks are softened in warm water and bent to conform to the shape of the arch. The rims are centered over the plate and pressed over the occlusal ridge (Figure 9–22).

7 Fill Space Between the Rim and Plate

These two pieces are then united to look and act as one. Excess wax trimmed from the base plate is melted and dripped or spooned into the voids and gaps between the two. A warm spatula can smooth the edges for an even surface (Figure 9–23).

8 Cut Heel Slant

To permit an opening and closing of the rims while in articulation, a small cut is taken at the heel of each plate. The lab knife is placed on the surface of the rim

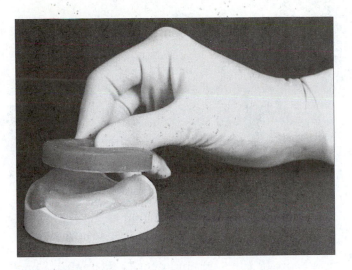

FIGURE 9-22 The softened rim is contoured and placed over the occlusal ridge of the base plate.

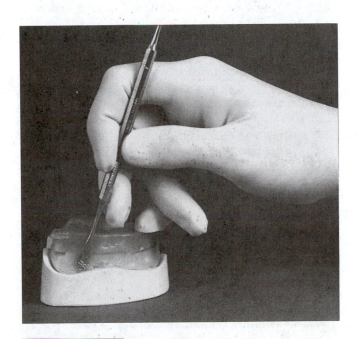

FIGURE 9-23 The union of the plate and rim is smoothed and filled in.

and sliced on an angle toward the posterior. This is called a heel cut (Figure 9-24).

9 Level Occlusal Surface

A large glass slab or large putty knife is heated and placed on the occlusal surface of the rims. This heated object is placed parallel to the floor and ensures a flat, even, occlusal plane (Figure 9-25).

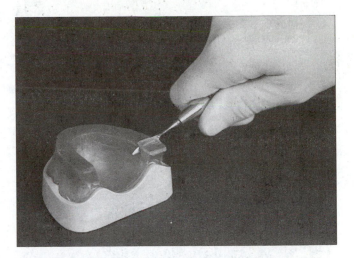

FIGURE 9-24 A diagonal cut is made at the end of the rim over the heel cut. This permits the opening and closing motion of the jaw to occur.

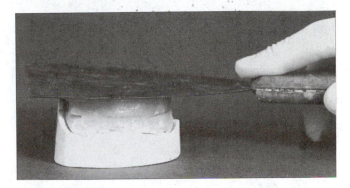

FIGURE 9-25 A large heated spatula or glass slab is used to level the rims.

10 Finish Plate and Occlusal Rims

After all cuts, heatings, and filling in are completed, the inside of the plate is rechecked for irregularities. The inside of the base plate must be smooth as this is the part of the finished denture that touches the mucous membranes. The wax plate and rims are buffed with a soft cloth and made smooth and shiny (Figure 9-26).

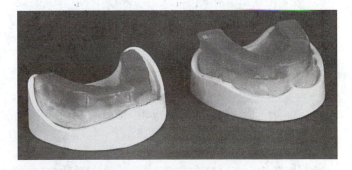

FIGURE 9-26 An example of finished base plates and occlusal rims.

11 Prepare Opposite Arch in Similar Manner

The opposite arch is completed in the same manner.

12 Cleanup Procedures

The work area is cleaned up and the materials and equipment are put away, leaving the lab in proper order. The assistant washes hands.▲

THEORY RECALL

Construction of Base Plates and Occlusal Rims

1. Base plates and occlusal rims are used by the dentist for what purpose?

   _____

2. The base plate represents which part of the denture?

   _____

3. What is the purpose of the occlusal rims?

   _____

4. What two materials are used in the manufacture of base plates?

   a. _____

   b. _____

5. To facilitate easy removal of wax from the model, with what is the model dusted?

   _____

6. How is the base plate wax prepared for placement onto the model?

   _____

7. How close is the excess base plate wax trimmed from the model edge?

   _____

8. Where is the occlusal rim placed on the base plate?

   _____

9. What is used to unite the occlusal rim and the base plate?

   _____

10. Why is the corner removed on the heel of the base plate and occlusal rim?

    _____

Now turn to the Competency Evaluation Sheet for Procedure 54, Construction of Base Plates and Occlusal Rims, located in Appendix C of this text.

CONSTRUCTION OF CUSTOM TRAYS

Occasionally, a patient, because of an abnormal size or shape of mouth or an anatomic deformity, requires a special impression for final models in the construction of dentures. There are also some dentists and prosthodontists who routinely desire a final impression to obtain a closer and more defined edentulous model to be used in the **fabrication** of dentures. This final impression is completed by constructing a custom tray. This specially made tray will fit the contours of the patient's mouth better than any used to take an exacting, fitting impression, which is poured up to be the mold for a base plate and rims.

Construction of a **custom tray** is done in the dental laboratory or lab room in a dental office. After a preliminary impression has been completed and poured into a gypsum form, a custom tray can be completed. The materials used for custom tray construction are an acrylic mixture of **monomer** (liquid) and **polymer** (powder). This material is stiff enough, when completed, to hold impression mixtures and maintain its custom shape and contours.

Acrylic resin can be purchased in two forms. A pelletized resin dough mixture can be softened into a moldable state when it is placed in hot water (145° to 180°F) for a short period of time. This dough is formed over the patient's preliminary model and hardens in a few minutes, or more quickly if placed in cold water. The second type of acrylic resin is a mixture of liquid and powder that is formed, shaped, and adapted over the preliminary model. This tray mixture can be purchased in colors of pink, blue, or white and can be obtained in one-, three-, or five-pound bulk, while the liquid is sold in 8-, 16- or 32-ounce bottles. The quantity ordered is determined by the amount of use and need in the office. Because the liquid is pungent in odor and irritating to mucous membranes, ventilation is needed when in use.

PROCEDURE 55

Construction of Custom Trays

1 **Assemble Materials and Equipment**

2 **Prepare Model**

3 **Place Spacer on Model**

4 **Prepare Tray Material**

5 **Contour Acrylic Wafer**

6 **Attach Handle**

7 **Remove Tray from Model**

8 **Smooth Tray Edges**

9 Identify Trays

10 Cleanup Procedures

1 Assemble Materials and Equipment

The equipment and materials necessary for construction of custom trays follow:

▶ edentulous model
▶ indelible pencil or marker
▶ base plate wax
▶ lab knife
▶ paper cup
▶ acrylic resin material
▶ petroleum jelly
▶ tongue blade
▶ sandpaper and dental lathe and trimming wheels
▶ talc or baby powder
▶ Bunsen burner, a match

*Safety glasses may be worn as protection from splashing liquid. A face mask may be donned to protect from inhalation or powder mist or pungent fumes.

2 Prepare Model

After the material and equipment have been gathered, the preliminary edentulous model is prepared. The model is marked with an indelible pencil or marker line indicating the **peripheral** edge for denture fit. Any abnormalities or special considerations are marked off or filled in with wax if needed. The model is lightly dusted with talc or baby powder for easy wax removal.

3 Place Spacer on Model

A sheet of base plate wax is warmed, draped over, and contoured to the edentulous pattern model. This wax is trimmed to the marked denture line and will serve to leave space for a final impression material in the last impression for dentures; therefore, this wax form is called a spacer (Figure 9–27).

Some dentists may require a double layer of base plate wax to permit more space or may wish to have "stop" indicators for how deep to set the tray. The assistant may make a small "stop" hole on each side, on the occlusal ridge, being careful not to place the holes over a prep area.

4 Prepare Tray Material

Once the spacer is formed and closely contours the model, it may be painted with a liquid foil separating medium that will permit the easy removal of the spacer from the finished custom tray (Figure 9–28).

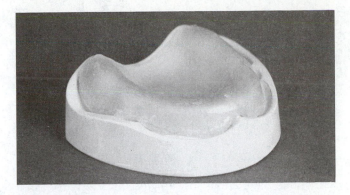

FIGURE 9–27 Custom tray series. A spacer is placed on the model. When the custom tray has been made, the wax is removed to make room for impression material.

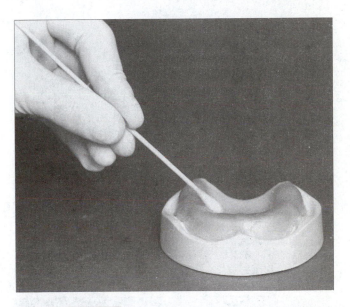

FIGURE 9–28 The wax spacer is painted with a separating liquid for easy removal.

An acrylic resin or dough tray is constructed. When using the mixture of resin, care must be taken to keep good ventilation and protect the skin of the hands from acrylic resin setting up on them. Petroleum jelly rubbed over the gloves or fingers prevents the mixture from sticking. *To avoid wearing gloves, the edentulous stone model may be soaked in a disinfectant solution prior to the custom tray procedure.

Acrylic resin can be a messy material and will stick to utensils, so it is wise to use disposable items when possible. Resin liquid and powder should be mixed in a paper cup, which can be pulled apart to lay flat, and should be stirred with a tongue blade snapped in half lengthwise. Both items may be discarded after use.

Manufacturer's recommendations are followed to obtain correct measurements for powder and liquid ratios. The powder is placed in the paper cup, and the liquid is added to the powder. A piece of tongue blade stick or applicator stick is used to stir the mixture, which only needs to mix the two materials together and moisten each other. The chemical action causes the bonding. The mixture is quite sticky at first but when allowed to sit for a minute or so, it loses the stickiness and becomes tacky (Figure 9–29).

5 Contour Acrylic Wafer

Once the material has lost its gloss and is massed in a tacky condition, fingers lightly greased with petroleum jelly can roll and pat the material into a wafer shape to be placed over the surface of the **preliminary** edentulous model. A commercial wooden board and rolling pin can be purchased to roll the dough into a wafer (Figure 9–30).

This thin $1/16$ to $1/8$ inch pliable wafer is pressed closely to the model covering the base plate wax spacer (Figure 9–31). If one is using the resin dough material, the process is the same, except the dough pellets are warmed in hot water, shaped into a wafer, and contoured onto the preliminary model. Both materials are kept smooth and close fitting. Excess material is cut off with a lab knife, taking care to avoid causing a tearing rough edge (Figure 9–32).

6 Attach Handle

The excess material that was removed is compressed and formed into a small handle, which is attached

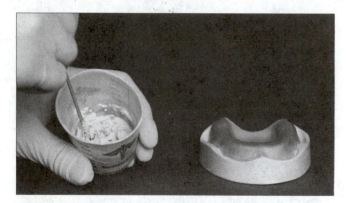

FIGURE 9–29 The materials are mixed to moisten all particles. Chemical bonding finishes the combining.

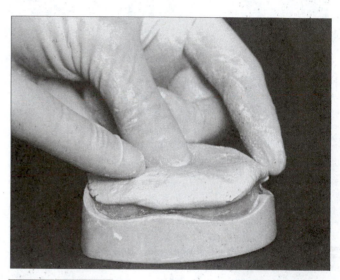

FIGURE 9–31 The wafer is placed over the wax spacer and finger pressed outward. Avoid pushing too far and too fast. Excessive pushing and movement wrinkle the finished product.

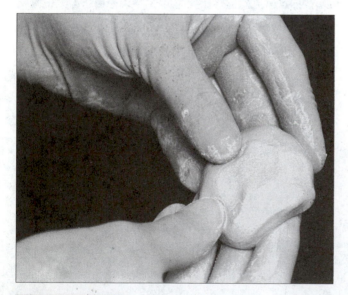

FIGURE 9–30 After the gloss has left and the material is not sticky, the mass is formed into a wafer.

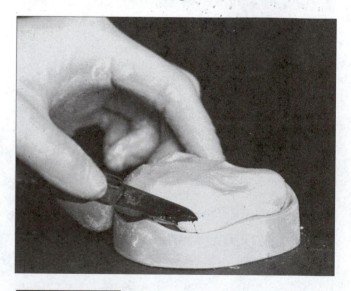

FIGURE 9–32 The excess material is cut off with a sharp knife.

onto the anterior of the newly constructed impression tray. This small handle will aid in the removal of the tray at the impression appointment. When applying the handle to the tray, keep it parallel to the floor. At the attachment end of the handle, bend the handle slightly up and then out. This leaves room for the lips to close down over the tray in the impression-taking process. The handle is attached by pressing onto the soft tray material and is completed before setting up has occurred. If the acrylic plate seems too dry to accept the small handle, a brush of a little resin liquid may help it to adhere better (Figure 9–33).

7   Remove Tray from Model

After the impression tray has set up and become hard, it is removed from the model. Unless indicated by the dentist, the wax spacer is removed, and the tray is tested for any sharp edges or overhangs that will cut or irritate the tissues during the impression appointment.

8   Smooth Tray Edges

Rough edges may be trimmed by sandpaper, emery disks, or acrylic trimming wheels or burs. These burs and disks may be used in a lab bench slow handpiece or the tray may be smoothed on finishing wheels in the dental lathe. The amount of trimming and finishing to be completed is determined mainly by the care taken in the construction of the trays.

9   Identify Trays

Once the trays have been smoothed, they are marked with the patient's name in permanent marker and cleaned and stored for future use (Figure 9–34).

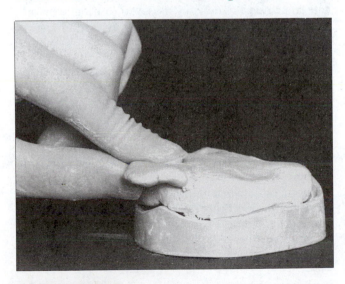

FIGURE 9–33 The excess material is used to make a handle for the tray.

10   Cleanup Procedures

The area is cleaned up and the equipment and materials are returned to their proper places. The assistant washes hands.▲

THEORY RECALL

Construction of Custom Trays

1. Name two reasons for the construction of a custom tray.

   a. _____

   b. _____

2. Where is the construction of a custom tray completed in the dental office?

   _____

3. What two materials are used for custom tray construction?

   a. _____

   b. _____

4. Acrylic resin is a mixture of a _____ and a _____ and is combined in a _____ .

5. What is the sheet of wax placed between the model and the tray material called? What is its use?

   _____

6. What is placed on the fingers to prevent resin from sticking to the skin?

   _____

7. How thick should the dough or resin mixture be when placed over the model?

   _____

8. For what is the excess trimmed tray material used?

   _____

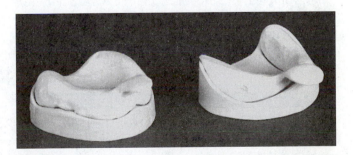

FIGURE 9–34 An example of finished custom trays.

9. What is used to smooth edges of the tray after the material has hardened?

_____

10. What is the best prevention to use to avoid excessive trimming of the finished tray?

_____

Now turn to the Competency Evaluation Sheet for Procedure 55, Construction of Custom Trays, located in Appendix C of this text.

FABRICATION OF TEMPORARY CROWNS

Another use for acrylic resins is in the fabrication of a temporary crown. It takes more than one appointment to complete a crown for a patient, because laboratory work time must be included in the procedure. When a person receives a crown, it is understood that a large percentage of tooth surface will be lost, either to the previous decay or to the tooth preparation needed. After the dentist has prepared the tooth for a crown, he or she will provide protection for this preparation because the remaining tooth surfaces will be sensitive and very susceptible to new decay.

A standard practice is to make a temporary crown for the prepared tooth, which the patient will wear until the final crown has been completed and is ready to be placed. Many dentists prefer acrylic resin as the material for fabrication of temporary crowns.

Acrylic resin comes in a liquid (monomer) and a powder (polymer). Unlike the acrylic resin used in the custom trays, the powder is obtained in a variety of tooth shades. Since the patient will be wearing this temporary crown, it will be made with esthetic consideration as well as function in mind. Acrylic resins used in the temporary coverage are supplied in small amounts because a much smaller dose is used in this procedure than in custom trays. These materials usually come in a set or kit, with an assortment of shades and one main bottle of liquid. Occasionally, there will be some powder or liquid left over when starting a new kit but it is advisable not to interchange these materials, especially if a new kit is from a different manufacturer. Although the process is the same, manufacturers differ in the preparations, and brands should not be interchanged. When using a new product, it is always advisable to read the manufacturer's directions before proceeding.

PROCEDURE 56

Assisting with Fabrication of Temporary Crowns

1 Complete the Preparations

2 Assist with Alginate Impression

3 Assist with Crown Preparation and Impression

4 Prepare Acrylic Crown

5 Pass Tray and Mix to Dentist

6 Clean Acrylic Crown Cover Prep

7 Finish Acrylic Crown Cover

8 Return Finished Crown Cover to Dentist

9 Prepare Crown Prep Impression for Lab

10 Cleanup Procedures

1 Complete the Preparations

The equipment needed for assisting with the fabrication of a temporary crown follows:

▶ monomer and polymer kit
▶ alginate impression
▶ crown and collar scissors (curved)
▶ slow handpiece with trimming burs, disks, and stones
▶ contouring pliers
▶ dropper
  *It may be noted that the fabrication of this temporary crown may or may not be completed at chairside, in the laboratory, or in a combination of the two.

2 Assist with Alginate Impression

The procedure for making a temporary cover begins at the crown appointment. An alginate impression is taken in a quadrant tray. Due to the nature of the alginate impression material, it is saved in a tight jar or a humidor, or it is wrapped in moist towels after a spray or disinfection until future need.

3 Assist with Crown Preparation and Impression

Crown preparation requires gross removal of tooth tissue; therefore, the assistant helps with the local anesthetic procedure. Once the loss of sensation is accomplished, the dentist begins the crown preparation, followed by gingival retraction and impression of the preparation (see Procedure 39). The original alginate impression is retrieved for temporary crown fabrication.

4 Prepare Acrylic Crown

A dropper of liquid monomer is used to place a few small drops of liquid into the alginate indentation of

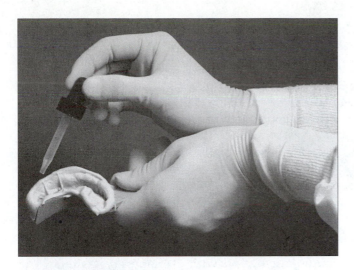

FIGURE 9-35 Drops of monomer are placed into the indentation of the prepared tooth.

the tooth that is to receive the cover (Figure 9–35). Then a small amount of the shaded powder, one which closely resembles the patient's natural color, is shaken into the liquid (Figure 9–36). This step is repeated as many times as necessary until the indentation is about three-fourths filled. Since the basis of uniting these materials is chemical (**polymerization**), the chemicals do the work. There is no need for mixing or stirring. When the powder and liquid are moistened together, they will set up; therefore, care should be taken to ensure the powder is getting evenly distributed and dampened in the indentation.

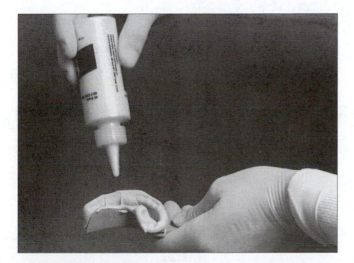

FIGURE 9-36 Powder is shaken into the liquid and absorbed. The process is repeated until three-quarters full.

5 Pass Tray and Mix to Dentist

A few moments are allowed for the mixture to start the polymerization and to lose its stickiness. When the mixture is doughy, the alginate impression is seated over the work site quadrant. The prepared tooth, which has been protected with a painting of liquid tinfoil substitute or cavity liner, is inside this mixture making its own shape. The tray is kept on the quadrant for approximately three to five minutes and then removed from the mouth. The mixture completes the final hardening out of the mouth. If the dentist is satisfied that the impression in the mixture was successful, the trimming may begin.

6 Clean Acrylic Crown Cover Prep

The trimming of the temporary cover may or may not be done at chairside. If it is taken to the laboratory to be finished, some sanitation procedures must be taken. To go to the laboratory section, the impression tray and material must be cleaned and spray disinfected. The assistant, who has been working at chairside, must don new gloves or overgloves to work in the laboratory. To avoid contamination to the laboratory and to other cases present, the impression and temporary cover must be considered an outside case and be treated in the customary manner.

If the preparation for the cover has been completed neatly, it may be finished at chairside. In either condition, the trimming procedure is the same, once the sanitation has been completed.

7 Finish Acrylic Crown Cover

Once the acrylic mixture has been taken out of the mouth and is holding shape, it is removed from the alginate impression. Any flashing (a thin layer of mixture extending out beyond the gingival line) is carefully cut off with the curved crown and collar scissors. The scissors are positioned in harmony with the curve to avoid any tears or rough areas (Figure 9–37). All rough edges are smoothed with sandpaper disks or small round burs placed in a slow handpiece (Figure 9–38). The margins of the cover can be gently crimped inward to provide a closer marginal adhesion. Care must be taken not to crimp too hard or before polymerization has been completed. After the cover is smooth and there is no roughness, it is cleaned out. All loose shavings and grinding dust must be removed. A swabbing of the cover with a wet applicator of hydrogen peroxide can be used to give a final cleansing and freshening before the cover is placed back into the mouth.

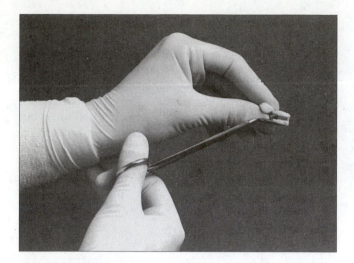

FIGURE 9-37 The flashing is cut off the newly formed, temporary crown.

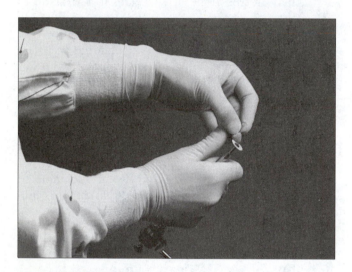

FIGURE 9-38 All rough edges are smoothed and trimmed.

8 Return Finished Crown Cover to Dentist

When the temporary crown has been placed in the mouth and the dentist is satisfied with the fit, a temporary cement is mixed and the crown is cemented with a temporary ZOE-type cement over the prepared tooth. The patient will wear this crown cover until rescheduled to return to receive a permanent crown.

9 Prepare Crown Prep Impression for Lab

The impression of the prepared tooth is disinfected, bagged, and sent to the laboratory for construction of the permanent crown. The patient is dismissed, and the procedure is recorded on the patient's chart.

Some dentists prefer to use a preformed crown cover as protection for a prepared tooth. Instead of constructing a cover from the acrylic mixture, they will purchase an assortment of preformed resin covers. The chairside appointment is the same for the preformed cover as the custom mixed, except there is no need to take an impression for a pattern. After the tooth preparation is completed, the empty crown surface area is measured mesially-distally for size; a suitable preformed crown cover is selected. In most cases, there will be additional trimming, adapting, and smoothing for the individual. The same trimming and finishing process is applied to the preformed crown cover as the acrylic resin mixed one. Either crown cover when properly prepared and fitted is then cemented on the tooth preparation with a temporary cement. The patient is scheduled for another appointment.

10 Cleanup Procedures

All equipment used is washed, rinsed, and prepared for disinfection or sterilization. The area is wiped clean and disinfected. All disposable items are placed in the proper receptacle. The PPE is washed, dried, and disinfected. The assistant washes hands at the end of the procedure.▲

THEORY RECALL
Fabrication of Temporary Crowns

1. What is the purpose of a temporary crown cover?

2. Is it wise to combine acrylic resin powders of one manufacturer with a liquid of another manufacturer? Why or why not?

3. What is the first procedure completed before the tooth preparation in a resin mix coverage type of temporary crown?

4. Where is the monomer and the polymer mixed for fabrication?

5. By what process do the monomer and polymer unite?

6. What is flashing?

7. What instruments are used to trim and smooth the temporary cover?

8. What precautions must be taken if the temporary cover is taken into the office laboratory section?

_____

9. If a dentist chooses to do so, what may be used to cover a prepared tooth, other than a resin mixed cover?

_____

10. How is the preformed crown cover trimmed and smoothed?

_____

Now turn to the Competency Evaluation Sheet for Procedure 56, Assisting with Fabrication of Temporary Crowns, located in Appendix C of this text.

PREPARING LABORATORY CASES FOR SHIPPING

Not all laboratory procedures are completed on site. Even if a practice is equipped with a full dental laboratory setup, there can be some items that may be sent to a commercial laboratory to be fabricated or repaired. How much and how often the services of a dental laboratory are required depends greatly on the amount of time and expertise a dentist may have available.

Commercial laboratories may be located in the same building, down the block, across town, or even many miles away from the office. Usually, the dentist will have a good working relationship with two or more laboratories and make use of their services. No matter which lab is used or where it is located, all dental laboratories have one thing in common. They are required to have orders to perform their procedures. A written note, much like a medical prescription, is prepared and placed with the item sent to the lab for work. Whether the case is picked up, delivered, or sent by mail, a written prescription or work authorization must accompany it.

If the article being sent to the commercial dental laboratory has been contaminated with blood or any other potentially infectious material, it is disinfected as well as possible and a note indicating what procedures were followed is included. In this way, the laboratory personnel will be aware of what procedures and cautions to take upon its arrival.

Since the written prescription is the major line of communication between the dentist and the laboratory, it must be exact and clearly understood by both parties. The dentist writes the order for the work, but the assistant may help lighten the task of preparing the prescription. The assistant may fill in the patient's name, age, sex, shade number, and any other notations that have been recorded. The date of the next appoint-

ment is written so the lab will be aware of the time frame for the work. The writing must be legible and written hard enough to pressure into the duplicate copies. All orders must be exact and neat; poor communication may result in a costly error. A copy of the prescription is kept in the patient's file, and the record is noted when the shipment has occurred.

Most laboratories have corrugated boxes, shipping labels, and methods of packing, such as bubble paper wrappers, that they prefer. The assistant should follow the instructions from the lab. Basically, note the following items:

1. All orders and necessary information on the prescription should be completed and legible.
2. All case materials relative to the procedure are present and packed in the designated manner.
3. All disinfection procedures have been indicated and noted with the case.
4. The patient's records are updated, and the transaction is recorded.
5. The shipment is made correctly and immediate.

Doing these things correctly can make the difference between an efficiently run office or one of confusion and interruptions.

PROCEDURE 57
Preparing Laboratory Cases for Shipping

1. **Assemble Materials and Equipment**
2. **Don Utility PPE**
3. **Gather Impression or Item to be Sent to the Commercial Lab**
4. **Disinfect the Item**
5. **Bag the Item**
6. **Clean PPE and Wash Hands**
7. **Fill Case Carton**
8. **Prepare Case Carton**
9. **Record Transaction on Patient's Chart**

1 Assemble Materials and Equipment

To prepare laboratory cases for shipping, the assistant will need:

► the item to be shipped
► a carton for shipment
► bubble paper or pellets for shipping
► a plastic sealing bag
► the patient's chart

- an office lab work authorization form
- sealing tape
- mailing label

2 Don Utility PPE

If the item to be shipped has not been disinfected previously and must be handled, the assistant should don utility gloves or a pair of overgloves for protection from infection or contamination. After the item has been sealed in a plastic bag, the gloves may be removed.

3 Gather Impression or Item to be Sent to the Commercial Lab

When the gloves are in place, the assistant gathers the item being sent to the commercial laboratory. Care must be taken to ensure that all pieces and parts of the impression or item are present and in good shape.

4 Disinfect the Item

If the item has not yet been disinfected, it now receives this treatment. After rinsing to remove gross debris and air drying to avoid diluting the germicide, the item may be immersed in disinfecting solution or may be sprayed with a disinfectant. Whatever method is employed, the name or type of disinfectant and time are noted on a piece of paper to be included with the item being sent.

5 Bag the Item

All components of the item being sent to the laboratory are encased in a plastic bag for shipment. If the office has a sealing device, the ends are closed and sealed. If no device is present, the assistant may use the common plastic lock top bags, making sure that the closure seal or contact is properly made.

6 Clean PPE and Wash Hands

Once the item has been disinfected and sealed in a plastic bag, the assistant may disinfect, wash, rinse, and remove the utility gloves and wash hands. If the overgloves were used, they may now be properly disposed of and the hands are washed before continuing the procedure.

7 Fill Case Carton

The plastic bag containing the items may be wrapped in bubble paper to protect during shipment. If bubble paper is not available, the assistant may use the foam shipping pellets to isolate the bag in the corrugated carton. Many labs provide the cartons and labels for shipping.

The work authorization form, which has been checked to see if it is fully and properly made out, and the disinfection procedures taken during handling are included in the carton (Figure 9–39).

8 Prepare Case Carton

When the items and papers are set into the carton, it is closed and sealed with tape. The shipping label, which was prepared previously, is applied to the carton.

The prepared carton is sent to the laboratory by various means. The assistant may call the lab for a pick up or may take the box to the post office or shipping service to be sent to the laboratory.

9 Record Transaction on Patient's Chart

The laboratory transaction is recorded on the patient's chart. The laboratory, work order, time designated, day, and means of departure are recorded on the patient's chart. The duplicate copy of the work authorization form is placed in the patient's file.

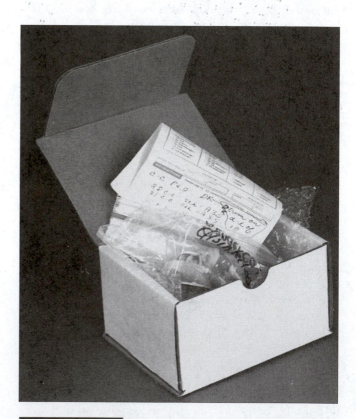

FIGURE 9–39 The lab carton must contain the item to be used for fabrication or repair, the completed and signed work authorization form, the disinfection notice, and enough protective wrapping to prevent damage in shipping.

Most offices have a laboratory work sheet near the desk that specifies the day of departure and recommended work time. The lab case is entered on the master chart, which will be consulted when nearing the completion and return date. When the item is returned, the master chart is marked with the date. In this way, the assistant knows the whereabouts of each lab case.▲

THEORY RECALL

Preparing Laboratory Cases for Shipping

1. How much and how often a dentist uses the services of a commercial dental laboratory may depend on what two factors?

   a. _____

   b. _____

2. Where is the commercial dental laboratory located?

   _____

3. What is required from a dentist before the commercial dental lab may begin work?

   _____

4. List four items an assistant may write on a prescription to help facilitate its preparation.

   a. _____

   b. _____

   c. _____

   d. _____

5. How does the office keep track of lab cases that have been sent to the commercial dental laboratory?

   _____

6. Who supplies the case boxes and shipping labels to the office in many instances?

   _____

7. List five tasks the assistant must be sure to complete when preparing laboratory cases for shipping?

   a. _____

   b. _____

   c. _____

   d. _____

   e. _____

Now turn to the Competency Evaluation Sheet for Procedure 57, Preparing Laboratory Cases for Shipping, located in Appendix C of this text.

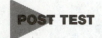
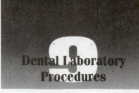
Total possible points = 100 points
80% needed for passing = 80 points

Total points this test _____ pass _____ fail _____

MATCHING: Place the letter from column B in the correct blank in column A. Each question is worth 2 points for a total of 20 points.

Column A

_____ 1. custom tray
_____ 2. study model
_____ 3. model trimmer
_____ 4. base plate and rim
_____ 5. lab order
_____ 6. dental lathe
_____ 7. articulator
_____ 8. vibrator
_____ 9. lab work schedule
_____ 10. acrylic

Column B

a. required for commercial dental lab procedure
b. record of status of lab cases
c. used for final impression for dentures
d. machine used to grind or adapt gypsum products
e. machine used to imitate jaw movements
f. machine used to smooth, shape, and finish trays
g. machine used to elevate air bubbles
h. used to set teeth and shape for dentures
i. positive reproduction of mouth
j. material used for temporary crowns

MULTIPLE CHOICE: Circle the correct answer. Each question is worth 4 points for a total of 80 points.

1. The water ratio for the mixing of 100 grams of dental stone is
   a. 25 ml.   b. 30 ml.   c. 50 ml.   d. 60 ml.

2. What is the name of the part of the study model that does not contain the anatomy of the mouth?
   a. art base   b. fulcrum   c. anatomic base   d. articulation end

3. What is placed on the fingers to prevent the warmed custom tray material from sticking to the skin?
   a. baby powder   b. wax   c. rubber or overgloves   d. petroleum jelly

4. What material is used to unite the base plate and the occlusal rims?
   a. plaster   b. cement   c. wax   d. auto-cured resin

5. What is used to smooth the edges of the custom tray after the material has hardened?
   a. knife   b. model trimmer   c. dental lathe   d. polishing cloth

6. The anterior portion of the maxillary gypsum study models are trimmed to what shape?
   a. pointed   b. round   c. zigzag   d. left alone

7. The posterior end of the heel of the occlusal rim situated on top of the base plate is cut off to
   a. facilitate contour of the plate.   c. facilitate teeth.
   b. allow for opening and closing.   d. facilitate movement.

8. To accelerate the gypsum setting time, what is added to the mixture?
   a. borax   b. sand   c. baby powder   d. salt

9. When trimming study models, what is used to permit the operator to trim the maxillary and mandibular models in the patient's normal occlusion?
   a. an articulator b. a bite registration   c. a boley gauge   d. photographs

10. What is the name applied to the piece of base plate wax that is placed between the gypsum model and the custom tray material?
    a. spacer   b. connector   c. insulator   d. bite registration

11. In the base plate and occlusal rim setup, what part of the denture does the wax base plate represent?
    a. anatomic   b. functional   c. teeth position d. palate and tissue

12. Which one of the following is *not* the purpose of the temporary crown?
    a. to maintain space   b. protection   c. to guide occlusion   d. to restore function

13. What must accompany the laboratory case to the commercial lab?
    a. payment   b. a picture of the patient   c. work authorization   d. materials

14. An electric appliance used to bring air pocket bubbles to the surface of the freshly mixed gypsum material is called
    a. a trimmer.   b. a lathe.   c. a vibrator.   d. a handpiece.

15. How close is the base plate wax being prepared for occlusal rims trimmed to the peripheral edge of the stone edentulous model?
    a. 0.4 ml   b. 1/4 inch   c. 10 ml   d. 1 inch

16. Before the process of pouring gypsum in the impression, what is done to the impression first?
    a. It is dried.   b. It is disinfected.   c. It is autoclaved.   d. Nothing.

17. Where is the impression for the fabrication of a temporary crown taken?
    a. in the mouth   b. from study models   c. from the denture   d. none used

18. In the preparation of a temporary crown, what is flashing?
    a. excess expressed material   c. moving of light for color selection
    b. blending of the monomer and polymer   d. time used to trim material

19. Which of the following information is *not* included on the work sheet sent to the dental laboratory?
    a. the patient's name   b. the patient's address   c. the patient's age   d. the patient's tooth size

20. What is the first procedure completed before the tooth preparation in a resin mix coverage type of temporary crown?
    a. periodontal probe   b. x-ray   c. cementation   d. impression

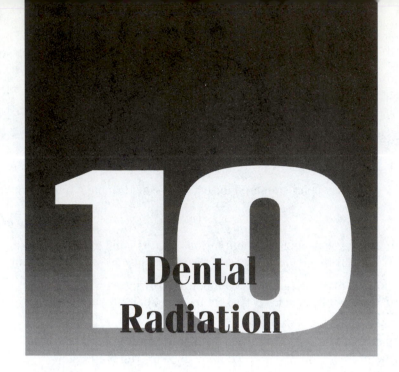

10 Dental Radiation

Upon completion of this unit, the student will achieve a score of 80% or better on the Post Test covering the following material.

1. Discuss the restrictions and dangers concerned with the exposing of dental radiographs. Describe methods of safety protection for the patient as well as the operator and office staff.
2. Identify various types, sizes, uses, and numbering systems of dental radiographic film. Discuss the procedures for the purchase, storage, and handling care of dental radiographic film.
3. List general and specific rules for x-ray exposure for full-mouth series and bitewing views using both parallel and bisecting techniques.
4. Discuss and demonstrate methods and techniques for the manual and automatic processing of dental radiographs.
5. Demonstrate procedures for mounting, marking, storing, and using processed dental radiographs.
6. Describe the common errors and resulting radiographs that may occur during the exposure and processing of dental radiographs.

▶ **KEY TERMS**

ALARA	edentulous	panoramic
automatic	exposure	parallel
bisecting angle	extraoral	penetrate
technique	fixer	periapical
cassette	intensifying	PID
cephalometric	intraoral	radiograph
cumulative	ionize	replenishing
effect	kilovoltage	safelight
developer	manual	technique
dosimeter	milliamperage	

RADIATION SAFETY KNOWLEDGE

Dental **radiographs** are of great benefit in the diagnosis and treatment of hidden problems in the oral cavity. These invisible rays can expose decay, infection, foreign bodies, growth irregularities, cysts, retained roots, and many other conditions requiring professional attention.

While these radiographs can be very helpful, they can also be quite harmful. X-rays have the ability to **penetrate** tissues but they also possess the ability to **ionize** change, or alter these tissues. Growing or immature cell tissue is the most sensitive to the ionizing effect but any tissue may be permanently damaged by improper radiation exposure. Sensitivity to radiation occurs in the following most sensitive to least sensitive order: embryonic (in pregnant women), blood and bone marrow, skin, connective tissue, nerve, brain, muscle cells, bone, and enamel tissue.

Radiation has a **cumulative effect** upon tissue; that is, **exposure** effects are long lasting. As x-rays penetrate the body and proceed to the film and lead backing for absorption, some weaker rays may remain in the cells. These few affected bodies will be sloughed off in a short period of time, usually less than 24 to 48 hours. However, repeated radiation, exposure upon exposure may cause a situation in which the body does not have enough time to slough off, and permanent tissue damage can occur.

Excessive dosages of radiation, such as nuclear explosion or exposure, can be too powerful and affecting to be cast off by cells and cause damage and death to cells and tissues. Therefore, knowing the dangers of radiation exposure should dictate that radiation exposure be exact and infrequent in use.

When working with dental x-rays the assistant must be careful to protect not only the patient but the operator as well. There are safety precautions that must be observed for everyone's benefit. The best protection that can be offered is knowledge of radiation and safety habits (Table 10–1).

The federal government established the Consumer-Patient Radiation Health and Safety Law in 1981, which decrees each state must monitor and regulate the dental practice law, specifying the requirements of those permitted to expose radiographs in its borders. Each state decides the amount of training and testing necessary to ensure competent exposure practices. Some states permit only the dentist and dental hygienist, while others allow trained auxiliaries who have been tested and certified to take x-rays. Each dental assistant must check the requirements for the state in which he or she is employed.

Although the dental assistant is not responsible for the purchase and performance of the dental x-ray machine, the regular scheduling of testing or complet-

---

TABLE 10–1

Dental Radiation

Types

Primary—radiation given off by tubehead, desired x-ray exposure

Secondary—radiation coming from bounce or deflection

Scattered—radiation escaping from faulty tubehead or source, undesirable x-ray

SAFETY PRECAUTIONS

General Safety Practices

- ▶ Use of fast-speed films
- ▶ Properly functioning machine, quality testing
- ▶ Good processing techniques and facilities
- ▶ Proper handling and storage of films
- ▶ Good exposure techniques
- ▶ Understanding of machine functions and use

Patient

- ▶ Questioning about last exposure
- ▶ Lead apron, collar

Operator

- ▶ Use of dosimeter
- ▶ Barrier or shield used during exposure
- ▶ Never hold film for patient

---

ing of testing exposures may be the duties of the assistant. Most states offer or require periodic quality control test checks of radiation machines to determine if the filtration and safety features are working properly. The dental assistant may have the responsibility to obtain a testing kit or tool and make regulated exposures and processing exercises. The radiographs are compared to the kit's test strip to determine if skin exposure is acceptable. Such routine tests may be cataloged and saved for legal purposes and offer assurance of compliance with state regulations (Figure 10–1).

Some effective safety practices for radiation use follow.

Machine Operation Knowledge

The trained assistant must be knowledgeable in the operation of the dental x-ray machine. The assistant must know the location of the on/off control and how to adjust the machine controls for **milliamperage** (mA), **kilovoltage** (kVp), and exposure time. The assistant, if permitted to expose radiographs, must know the effects that increasing and decreasing the amounts of mA, kVp, and time will have upon the x-ray film. The assistant must be able to regulate each and be able to

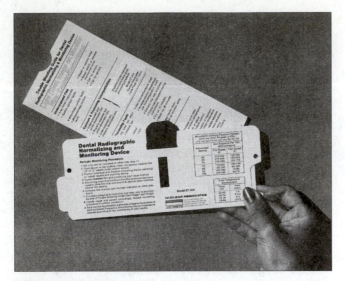

FIGURE 10–1 The assistant follows the direction of the manufacturer to complete the quality assessment of the x-ray machine. Results are recorded in the OSHA safety procedure book. (Courtesy of Nuclear Associates, 100 Voice Road, Carie Place, NY.)

follow the manufacturer's exposure chart specifying each requirement necessary for the maximum efficiency of the film.

Milliamperage increases or decreases will affect the amount of possible x-ray electrons, which, in turn, affects the density of the ray. An increased milliamperage will increase density and darkness of the film.

Kilovoltage increases will increase the speed or penetrating power of the x-ray electrons. Denser objects may require an increase in the amount of kVp power.

Exposure time is the amount of regulated exposure or production of the radiation. Once the mA, kVp, film-focal distance, and type of film to be used have been selected for the exposure purpose, the assistant may check the exposure guidelines chart for the suggested exposure impulse time. The assistant may use the conversion chart (Figure 10–2) to compute seconds or decimals if the machine in use works on a system other than impulse exposure. Regulated exposure time is also affected by the target (patient) size. Children are exposed for shorter periods. Most offices determine the best setting for their particular machine and operate on a standard pattern.

Knowledge of Positioning Devices

The assistant must be able to exchange position indicating devices (PID) as needed or as requested by the

Exposure Guidelines for KODAK EKTASPEED Dental Film

Region	Vertical Angle	70 kV 7 mA Adult* 8"	70 kV 7 mA Adult* 12"	65 kV 10 mA Adult* 8"	70 kV 10 mA Adult* 8"	70 kV 10 mA Adult* 16"	80 kV 10 mA Adult* 8"	80 kV 10 mA Adult* 16"	90 kV 10 mA Adult* 8"	90 kV 10 mA Adult* 16"	65 kV 15 mA Adult* 8"	70 kV 15 mA Adult* 8"	70 kV 15 mA Adult* 12"	80 kV 15 mA Adult* 8"	80 kV 15 mA Adult* 16"	90 kV 15 mA Adult* 8"	90 kV 15 mA Adult* 12"	90 kV 15 mA Adult* 16"	Office kV	Office mA Adult	Office mA Child
Maxillary Incisor	+40°	7	16	8	5	20	4	14	3	13	5	3	7	2	10	2	5	8			
Cuspid	+45°	7	16	8	5	20	4	14	3	13	5	3	7	2	10	2	5	8			
Bicuspid	+30°	9	20	10	6	25	4	18	4	16	7	4	9	3	12	3	6	10			
Molar	+20°	10	22	11	7	27	5	20	4	17	7	5	10	3	13	3	6	12			
Mandibular Incisor	−15°	5	12	6	4	15	3	11	2	9	4	2	6	2	7	2	4	6			
Cuspid	−20°	5	12	6	4	15	3	11	2	9	4	2	6	2	7	2	4	6			
Bicuspid	−10°	6	14	7	4	17	3	12	3	11	3	3	6	2	8	2	4	7			
Molar	−5°	7	16	8	5	20	4	14	3	13	5	3	7	2	10	2	5	8			
Anterior Bite-Wing Size 1 Adult	+8°	5	12	6	4	15	3	11	2	9	4	2	6	2	7	2	4	6			
Size 1 Child	+8°	4	8	4	2	10	2	7	2	6	3	2	4	2	5	1	2	4			
Posterior Bite-Wing Size 2 or 3 Adult	+8°	7	16	8	5	20	4	14	3	13	5	3	7	3	10	2	5	8			
Size 0 Child	+8°	4	10	5	3	12	2	9	2	8	3	2	5	2	6	1	3	5			

*Children: Reduce adult exposure time about one-third.   Edentulous areas: Reduce exposure time about one-quarter.

To avoid fractional impulses, some 8" exposure times have been rounded off to whole numbers. Mathematically, these 8" times will not comply with the inverse square law in relation to the 16" exposure times.

The above guidelines were developed following recommended time-temperature processing with Kodak chemicals. Method to compute mAs or mAi: mAs is the product of milliamperage times seconds of exposure; mAi is the product of milliamperage times the impulses of energy. If the product is the same in either case, the quantity of radiation produced is essentially the same.

Examples:
mA x sec = mAs; mA x imp = mAi
10 x 1/2 = 5 ; 10 x 30 = 300
15 x 1/3 = 5 ; 15 x 20 = 300

Health Sciences Division
EASTMAN KODAK COMPANY
Rochester, New York 14650

Kodak, Ektaspeed, and Ultra-Speed are trademarks.

FIGURE 10–2 The exposure guideline serves as a quick reference for the proper settings when taking a dental radiograph. (Reprinted with permission of Eastman Kodak Company.)

dentist. **PID**s (Figure 10–3) may be round or rectangular and are supplied in 8-, 12-, or 16-inch lengths. The shorter length is used for a bisecting exposure technique, and the longer PID is employed in the paralleling exposure technique. The rectangular PID permits less scattered radiation at the film site, but both types of PIDs are lead lined or glassed to prevent radiation loss.

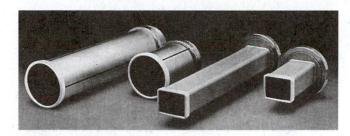

FIGURE 10–3 The Position Indicating Devices (PIDs) are lead lined to provide a concentrated beam of radiation and to lessen secondary radiation. (Courtesy of Rinn Corporation.)

In an exchange of PIDs, aluminum filtration disks, which may have been placed between the device and tube window are repositioned to maintain the filtration safety against weak x-ray waves.

Adjustment of the machine's timing exposure control must be made with each exchange of positioning devices, because the length of the PID will affect the time needed for exposure. The ability to position each PID should be demonstrated by the assistant.

Film Handling and Storage

Proper film storage and handling is important in radiation safety. The assistant must rotate the stock and take the oldest box of film from the cool, dark storage area, which is not located around chemicals. The refrigerator may be used for film storage, but the film is taken out a few hours before use to allow the film chemicals to return to room temperature.

After checking the expiration date, the packets are placed into a lead-lined dispenser. Some offices now purchase films packed in barrier coverings, or the assistant places the dental films into barrier packets before exposure so at developing time the barriers can be removed for germ-free processing.

The assistant dispenses a film, noting the type and film amount. Most offices use fast films (speed D and E) to reduce patient exposure time. Sometimes the dentist is aware that radiographs may need to be sent to insurance companies or to another dentist for referral, so a film packet with two films inside is requested. The color code and printing on the back of the film packet indicates the speed of the film and the amount of film inside the packet. Available film sizes and types are discussed later.

Once the film has been inserted into the mouth and exposed, the assistant places the film aside in a protected space until developing time. If barrier shields or a barrier film has been exposed, the assistant may open the pack and drop the film into the lead-lined box. The untouched films may be taken into the darkroom and processed in the usual manner. No gloving or sterilizing technique is required after barrier use. The protective barrier covers are placed on a paper towel until the procedure is completed and then disposed of in the contaminated waste container.

Proper Exposure Techniques

There are a few specific **techniques** to use for patient safety. The dental office must use the **ALARA** principle, which is *a*s *l*ow *a*s *r*easonably *a*chievable exposure. The patient must be questioned as to the last time of exposure and the reason. If exposure has occurred recently, or if the patient is pregnant, dental x-ray surveys should be postponed for another time. The dentist specifies which and how many radiographs to take and makes the recommendations only when the exposures are necessary.

If a patient is to be exposed to radiation, the assistant covers the subject with a lead drape and perhaps a lead collar or possibly a combination drape-collar apron. These devices are placed over the front of the patient to cover the sex glands and the throat to cover the thyroid and parathyroid glands. When the lead protective devices are not in use, they are carefully hung over a towel bar or other device to avoid twisting or crumbling the shields.

Proper exposing technique ensures less radiation for the patient because retakes will not be necessary. Any dental personnel who is delegated the responsibility of radiation exposure must know the proper positioning of patient, film, and tubehead. Film positioners hold film in position in the patient's mouth and are used instead of the patient inserting and holding a film with a finger, which increases body exposure.

Operator Safety Techniques

Operators must be careful in x-ray exposure. The assistant who exposes films should never hold a film in the patient's mouth. If the patient is unable to maintain the film, the person who brought the patient to the office is requested to assist.

Operators should wear radiation **dosimeters** (Figure 10–4). Dosimeters, whether a badge, pen, or ring, do not protect from radiation but only indicate the amount of radiation received. Any person receiv-

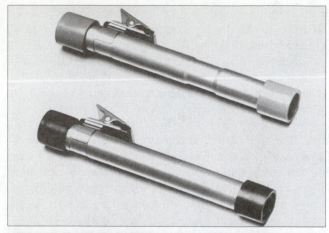

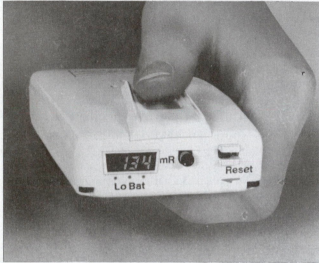

FIGURE 10–4 Dosimeters do not protect the assistant from radiation. A dosimeter only records the amount of radiation received during the use period. (Courtesy of Nuclear Associates, 100 Voice Road, Carie Place, NY.)

ing a high dosage reading from the monitoring firm should check procedures or equipment before exposing again.

Operators should not stand in the direct line of radiation exposure. If a lead shield is available, the operator should stand behind the shield during the activation time. If no shield is present, the operator should stand to the side of the tube head, at least six feet away from the source.

Proper Processing Techniques

The last method to apply as a general safety rule for radiation is in the developing of the films, called processing. If mistakes are made in this procedure, more exposure to the patient must be made in retakes. The assistant must make sure that the darkroom is clean and light free. The safety light must be the strength designed to work with the film being processed, and

the assistant should employ good techniques in the processing of films. Any errors in light or processing will make the film useless.

Proper application of safety habits ensures the best results for the patient at the least amount of risk.▲

THEORY RECALL
Radiation Safety Knowledge

1. List four oral problems a dental x-ray may expose.

   a. _____

   b. _____

   c. _____

   d. _____

2. Besides the ability to penetrate tissues, what other property does a dental x-ray possess?

   _____

3. Which tissues are the most sensitive to dental x-rays?

   _____

4. What is the cumulative effect in dental radiation?

   _____

5. What does the Consumer-Patient Radiation Health and Safety Law require?

   _____

6. Who has the responsibility of checking state dental laws for the permission to expose dental radiographs?

   _____

7. What responsibility may an assistant have toward monitoring the safety of the dental radiation machine?

   _____

8. List the four controls on the x-ray machine that the assistant must know how to operate.

   a. _____

   b. _____

   c. _____

   d. _____

9. What controls may need adjusting when a change of a PID has occurred?

   _____

10. What does ALARA mean?

   _____

For additional activities related to this lesson, turn to Assignment Sheet 10.1, Radiation Safety Knowledge, located in Appendix B of this text.

RADIATION FILM KNOWLEDGE

Dental radiographs are supplied in different sizes and shapes (Figure 10–5). Each film is designed for a specific area of placement for optimal use. Some are used in the mouth (oral), and some are placed outside the mouth (**extraoral**) for larger area views. Some films are prewrapped and oth-

Bitewing Films

Periapical film may be placed in a positioning device or a paper loop with the tab positioned on the outside of the front of the film. The loop tab is centered so the patient's bite is evenly distributed between the maxillary and mandibular jaws.

Another way to modify a periapical film into a bitewing film is to place a sticky tab on the center front of the film; when the patient bites on the tab, the film's face is centered behind the teeth evenly.

When using a positioning device for exposing bitewing radiographs, the films are placed into the bite

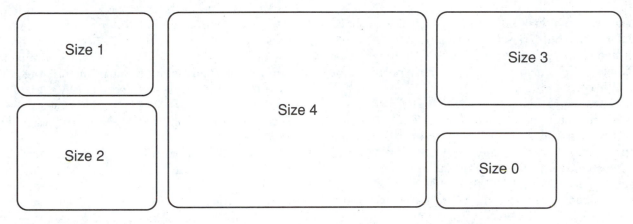

FIGURE 10–5 Dental radiation films are supplied in a variety of sizes and shapes. Each film is selected for use in a specific exposure. (Reprinted with permission of Eastman Kodak Company.)

ers come in a box of film and are singularly placed in a **cassette**. Each film has its own speed, which is determined by the type of chemical emulsions placed on the film when it is manufactured. The assistant must take time to learn the various types and kinds of dental radiographs.

Intraoral

Intraoral films are exposed within the mouth. The most common film is the **periapical** film, size 2. It is $1\frac{1}{4}$ inch by $1\frac{5}{8}$ inches in size and may be used in the anterior or posterior area of the mouth. When used in the anterior portion of the mouth, the film is placed in a vertical position. When used in the posterior part of the mouth, the film is placed horizontally.

An adult patient with a smaller or more angulated mouth or a child aged six to eight may be more comfortable with the smaller, size 1 periapical, which is $1\frac{5}{16}$ inch by $1\frac{9}{16}$ inches. For the younger child's mouth (3 to 5 years), there is a smaller periapical film, size 0. This film is $\frac{7}{8}$ inch by $1\frac{3}{8}$ inches and is positioned anteriorly and posteriorly as the larger periapical film.

block in the same position as periapical shots. The anterior bitewing's exposures are vertical films and the posterior exposures are horizontal.

Two film views are usually necessary when using the periapical film in a bitewing position. One is placed more in the bicuspid region, and the other is moved into the molar region. Sometimes the operator may adjust the film slightly by sliding the film in the loop toward the view to be taken. When exposing a molar bitewing, the film is moved in the loop more to the molar side.

There are two commercial bitewing films—a posterior film, size 3, and an anterior bitewing film, size 1. The posterior film is $\frac{11}{16}$ inch by $2\frac{1}{8}$ inch and placed horizontally in the posterior part of the mouth for views of the maxillary and mandibular tooth crowns and alveolar crest.

The anterior bitewing film is $\frac{15}{16}$ inch by $1\frac{9}{16}$ inches. The film is placed vertically while the patient bites on the tab with the teeth edge to edge. Both the maxillary and mandibular crowns and alveolar crests are viewed in this film.

All intraoral films have a protruding bump, sometimes called a pimple, on the front of the film packet and a concave area, called the dimple, on the back. The bump faces the tubehead and is used in mounting the finished radiographs. When holding the radiograph with the bump toward the operator, the operator faces the patient, the same as the tubehead. The back of the film packet is marked to show the speed, film amounts, as well as the rear of the film.

The occlusal film, size 4, may be used in or out of the mouth. This film, which is $2^{1}/_{4}$ by 3 inches, is used to view larger areas of the mouth. It may be placed for maxillary or mandibular views of the arches. It too has a dimple-pimple arrangement.

Extraoral Films

The occlusal film may be used in extraoral exposures. The film may be exposed to examine the TMJ area, impacted teeth, or cystic bone losses of the maxilla or mandible. The dentist will request the type of exposure needed.

A **panoramic** film is a special film that offers a view of the entire mouth area (Figure 10–6). This film must be placed in a special cassette in a panoramic exposure machine. The patient either sits or stands in a designated spot while the tubehead and film cassette rotate around the head. When completed and developed, the dentist can view the entire lower part of the face.

Cephalometric x-rays are larger, extraoral films taken to view the head. The orthodontist usually requires such a radiograph to determine future growth plotting. The film is loaded into a cassette and placed in a special holder. The patient is positioned, using the ear as a focal point; the exposure is made. When finished and processed, the dentist or orthodontist has a view of the entire head.

Other extraoral films may be taken in the dental office. These films are larger 5 × 7 or 8 × 10 films that are placed in cassettes. When loaded, the cassettes are positioned on the outside of the head, and the radiation exposure is done extraorally. Special training usually is necessary to position these films. When completed, the dentist can view the TMJ area, jaw fractures, or large disorders of the mouth.

Cassettes

Extraoral films, with the exception of the occlusal film, must be loaded into a cassette for use. These film cassettes may be made of metal, vinyl, or paper. The metal extraoral cassettes are the more popular and both the metal and vinyl have an intensifying screen inside the cassette to reflect and intensify the radiation exposure to the film. This intensification of the ray lowers the amount of time necessary for patient exposure to radiation.

Intensifying screens must be kept clean and smear proof. Fingerprints on the screen will show up on the finished x-ray and may obscure the view. The assistant may use a commercial solution to provide static control and wipe clean the inside of the cassette or alcohol on a gauze pad to clean the surface.

All loading and unloading of film in the cassette is done in the darkroom or daylight loader. The film is handled by the corners only. When loading, the film is taken out of the box still wrapped in its yellow paper.

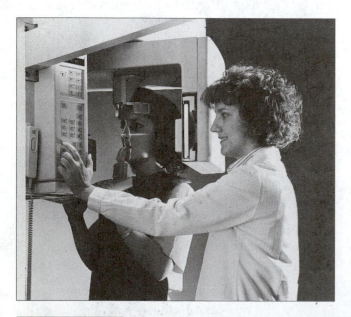
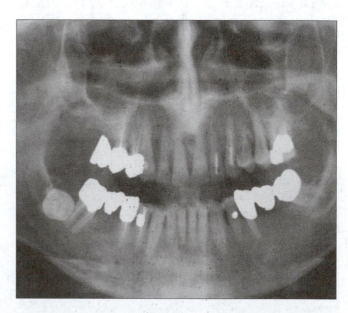

FIGURE 10–6 An example of a panoramic radiographic exposure. The entire mouth area may be viewed with this type of film. (Courtesy of DENTSPLY International Inc., GENDEX Corporation, Midwest Dental Products Corporation.)

The lid of the film box is immediately replaced. The assistant picks the film by the corner and places it into the cassette. A gentle finger probe into the four corners ensures the film is in proper position. The lid is closed and the metal spring is engaged. The yellow wrapper paper is placed in the trash.

Vinyl cassettes are used in some panoramic cassettes that are curved around a target area. These are flexible but work on the same principle as the metal cassettes. Loading is done in the dark and all is sealed before exposure to the light.

Paper cassettes do not have intensifying screens and are merely covers that keep out light rays. When using a paper cassette, the assistant unwraps it in the darkroom, places the film inside, closes the paper cassette, and seals it shut. Exposure times may need to be adjusted for paper cassettes.

Film Coding

Dental films are marked to show their content. The markings are on the back of the film packet and indicate the speed and the amount of films inside the packet. Companies color code these packets on the back side for easy and quick identification of the product.

Storage

Dental x-ray films are stored in a cool (50 to 70°F), dry (40 to 60 percent humidity) area away from chemical storage spots. When storing for a period of time, these films are wrapped in aluminum foil to protect from moisture. They may be placed in a refrigerator but must be allowed to warm to room temperature before use.

Film stock is rotated. The first in is the first out. The assistant checks the expiration date marked on each box. If the time has expired on the film, it is destroyed and not used.

Exposure Chart

Film manufacturers provide film exposure and developing charts (refer back to Figure 10–2) that condense the information into a small area. The assistant must be able to interpret the various lines for exposure of the different types and speeds of films. Practiced use of these charts will make the assistant more proficient at following manufacturer's directions.

By taking care of film and using it properly, the assistant will ensure better and more constant good results in dental radiation.▲

THEORY RECALL

Radiation Film Knowledge

1. What is the term for dental radiographs used in the mouth? out of the mouth?

2. What is the most common intraoral film? What is its size number?

3. In what position is the periapical film placed for an anterior shot?

4. How does the patient bite on an anterior bitewing film?

5. What is the size number of the child-sized periapical film?

6. Where can the occlusal film be used?

7. How is the periapical film position modified in a bitewing film exposure?

8. How many views are necessary for bitewing exposures when using the modified periapical films?

9. What are some uses for the occlusal film extraorally?

10. What does the panoramic film show in an x-ray exposure?

For additional activities related to this lesson, turn to Assignment Sheet 10.2, Radiation Film Knowledge, located in Appendix B of this text.

EXPOSURE OF DENTAL RADIOGRAPHS

Exposure of dental radiographs should be completed by competent, trained personnel. Each state has requirements for the licensing or permission of qualified persons to perform radiographic exposures. It is the duty of the dental assistant to inquire into the particular state requirements of the state where employed. If dental auxiliaries are permitted to expose x-rays, the auxiliary should perfect the practice procedure. If the auxiliary is not permitted, the assistant should still have a good working knowledge of the procedure to be of better assistance in the process.

There are two methods for dental x-rays exposure—the **bisecting angle technique** and the paralleling technique. In the bisecting angle method, the film is positioned to be placed against the long axis of the tooth being exposed. In the paralleling method, the film is put into a holder that keeps the film **parallel** to the long axis of the tooth being exposed (Figure 10–7). Both procedures are accepted methods of exposure and are used in dental offices.

When using either technique, there are a few general exposure rules that apply to both methods. Exposure to radiation must be ALARA (as low as reasonably achievable); therefore, the film placed in the patient's mouth must be maintained by a holding device instead of by digital or finger stabilization. There are commercial holders. Rinn's BAI (bisecting angle) and XCP (paralleling) holders are quite popular. The indicator rods and aiming rings of this set can be used for either technique if the proper holding blocks are employed.

In the bisecting technique, smaller blocks (Figure 10–7, part A) hold the film against the tooth. In the parallel method, the longer blocks (Figure 10–7, part B) hold the film away from the long axis of the tooth. Holding devices can be made from a hemostat or the patient may use a simple commercial plastic clamp device.

Another method for obtaining radiographic intraoral views of teeth and supporting tissues is called video imaging x-ray application. This method requires a specific radiographic system including a sensor wand for placement in the mouth and computer screen for immediate imaging and analysis. Being computer generated, the image can be enhanced, enlarged, reduced, lightened, darkened, or sharpened. Image printouts can be activated onto a printer or the image may be recalled from the archive at any time (Figure 10–8).

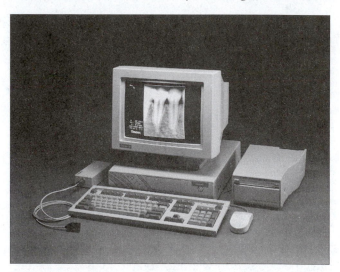

FIGURE 10–8 The VIXA video imaging x-ray system. (Courtesy of DENTSPLY International Inc., GENDEX Corporation, Midwest Dental Products Corporation.)

All patients to be exposed to radiation are questioned regarding the last time and type of exposure. Patients are positioned in the dental chair with the occlusal plane of the teeth parallel to the floor. When the mouth is closed or lower jaw is dropped open for maxillary exposure, the patient's head is placed with the chin down. For exposures of the mandibular arch, the patient is positioned with the head back. If the operator can imagine a pencil positioned on the biting surface (occlusal plane) and keep this pencil parallel to the floor, the patient's head will be well placed. The head must also be centered and level. This is accomplished by placing the imaginary facial midline perpendicular to the floor (Figure 10–9).

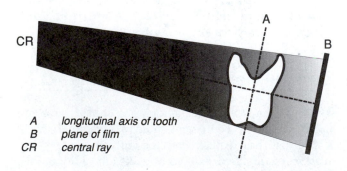

A	longitudinal axis of tooth
B	imaginary bisecting line
C	plane of film
CR	central ray

A	longitudinal axis of tooth
B	plane of film
CR	central ray

FIGURE 10–7 The two common, recommended methods of dental radiographic exposure are (A) the bisecting angle technique and (B) the paralleling technique. (Courtesy of Rinn Corporation.)

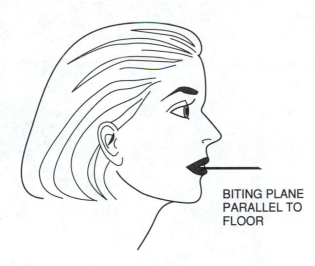

BITING PLANE
PARALLEL TO
FLOOR

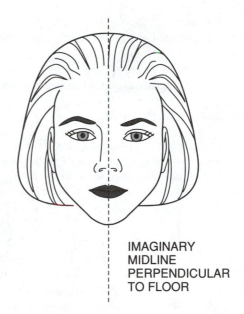

IMAGINARY
MIDLINE
PERPENDICULAR
TO FLOOR

FIGURE 10-9 The assistant uses the imaginary lines on the patient's face to ensure a level and even placement for the dental films.

Seven views are necessary to complete a series of exposures for an arch: one central and two, right and left each, for the canines or cuspids, premolars or bicuspids, and molars. Anterior teeth views must have the film placed in vertical position and posterior teeth films must be placed horizontally. All biting edges of the teeth should be approximately ⅛ inch from the edge of the film when placed by the tooth.

The dental radiograph must have the smooth or plain side of the film touching the tooth, which requires the back side of the film to touch the plate of the holding device. To assist with the mounting of films, it is suggested that the assistant or operator place the "pimple" or raised dot toward the mesial and the biting surface.

When not using film-holding devices with indicator rods and aiming rings, the assistant should be extremely concerned with the vertical angles of the PIDs. For proper exposure, PID placement should be positioned in approximated angle markings found on the tubehead. The suggested vertical angle degrees follow.

	MAXILLARY	MANDIBULAR	BITEWING
Central incisor	+40 degrees	-15 degrees	+8 degrees
Canine or cuspid	+45 degrees	-20 degrees	
Bicuspid or premolar	+30 degrees	-10 degrees	
Molar	+20 degrees	-5 degrees	

P R O C E D U R E   5 8

Exposure of Intraoral Radiographs—Bisecting and Paralleling Techniques

1 Assemble Materials and Equipment

2 Prepare the Patient

3 Prepare for Procedure

4 Practice Operator Safety Precautions

5 Bitewing Exposure

6 Expose Maxillary Radiographs

7 Expose Mandibular Radiographs

8 Dismiss the Patient

1 **Assemble Materials and Equipment**

To expose a full-mouth survey, including bitewings, the assistant must prepare the operatory and assemble:

▶ unexposed films
▶ barrier envelopes (if used), gloves
▶ holding cup or lead-lined container
▶ radiographic machine
▶ positioning device set with holding blocks
▶ BIA short blocks for bisecting angle technique
▶ XCP longer blocks for paralleling technique
▶ radiographic dosimeter, shield
▶ cotton rolls, may be placed to help hold blocks in mouth

▶ exposure chart
▶ patient radiation protection devices (drape and collar)

The assistant reviews the orders for the radiographic exposure, dons overgloves, and wears a dosimeter.

2 Prepare the Patient

The patient is greeted and seated in the operatory. The assistant questions the patient regarding the last x-ray exposure occurrence and the possibility of pregnancy. If radiation has been experienced lately or the patient is pregnant, the assistant advises the dentist and awaits orders.

Once seated, the patient is protected from secondary radiation by the placing of the lead apron and thyroid collar. The patient is positioned for the x-ray film position. Maxillary and bitewing exposures require the chin to be down; mandibular exposures need the chin to be positioned up, so that the occlusal plane of the teeth being exposed is parallel to the ground.

3 Prepare for Procedure

The assistant dons the dosimeter if not already worn and prepares the film for exposure. If barrier envelopes are being used, they are placed on the film and put aside out of exposure range. The waiting cup is marked with the patient's name.

The assistant washes hands and dons latex exam gloves or overgloves. The patient's mouth is spray rinsed or the patient is offered a mouth rinse. The mouth is examined for any disturbances or irregularities and the assistant begins the survey.

4 Practice Operator Safety Precautions

Throughout the entire procedure, the assistant practices good radiation safety habits, such as standing behind a shield or six feet away from and behind the tubehead, cautioning the patient to close the eyes and not to move during exposure. All films exposed and unexposed are kept out of radiation range, and the exposure timer is set before film placement to quicken exposure and lessen time for film in the mouth.

5 Bitewing Exposure

If commercial films size 3 are not being used, molar bitewing films are prepared from horizontally spaced periapical film using loops or sticky tabs. The biting tab is on the plain side of the film. The film is placed in the mouth covering the three-molar area. The tab is held on the occlusal plane and the patient is instructed to gently bite on the tab. The assistant makes sure the tab (center of film) is midway between the maxillary and mandibular arches. The head is positioned for the

occlusal plane to be parallel with the floor and the imaginary midline perpendicular to the floor (Figure 10–10). The PID, set at a positive vertical angle of

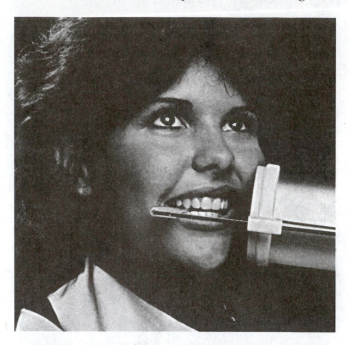

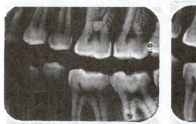

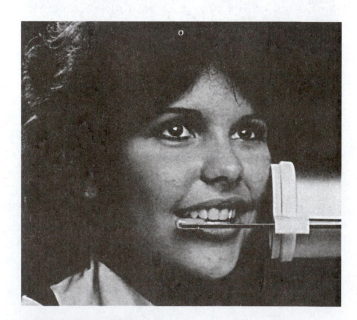

FIGURE 10–10 Positions for bitewing (interproximal) exposures. (Courtesy of Rinn Corporation.)

eight degrees, is brought next to the cheek positioning it so the central ray is aimed to the center of the film in the middle. The assistant stands behind the shield, cautions the patient, and activates the machine. The film is removed and placed in the waiting cup.

If a film-holding device is used, the device is prepared by inserting the indicator rod pins into the two forward holes of the plastic, disposable bite block. The aiming ring is slid onto the indicator rod, and the film packet is placed into the slot at the rear of the bite block. The assistant tests to make sure the film is securely placed and the plain side of the film is aimed toward the PID. All anterior exposures are performed with an anterior vertical bite block. The posterior exposures require the posterior horizontal bite block.

Once the film device and film are ready, the film block with film is placed into the patient's mouth. The film is centered behind the premolar area with the arm of the block over the occlusal surface of the mandibular teeth. The patient is advised to slowly close down and bite on the block. The aiming ring is slid down the rod until it touches the cheek surface. The open circle of the PID is aligned with the circle of the ring. Once these two rings are sandwiched together and the indicator rod and PID are parallel, the assistant steps behind the barrier and activates the preset timer for exposure of the film. Once exposed, the film is removed from the mouth and placed aside for processing. These bitewing exposures are considered to be the easiest to complete. The patient is complimented on the good performance, and the process is repeated for the molar view and the two views on the other side of the mouth.

6   Expose Maxillary Radiographs

When exposing the maxillary central area, the film is placed vertically in the holding block and both are placed directly behind the central and lateral incisors with the plain side of the film facing the tubehead. A cotton roll may be placed between the teeth of the opposing arch and the holding block to help retain the bite block. Cotton rolls can also be used to help balance the blocks in **edentulous** areas where teeth are missing.

In the bisecting technique, the base of the block is shorter, and the film leans against the incisors. A shorter PID (8 inches) is used (Figure 10–11, part A). In the paralleling technique, the block base is longer and the film sets into the mouth deeper, paralleling the teeth image onto the film. A longer PID (16 inches) is recommended but a short one may be used (Figure 10–11, part B).

The indicator rod protrudes from the center of the mouth and the aiming ring is drawn down the rod to the lips or cheek. The PID is lined up parallel to the indicator rod and is centered against the ring. The

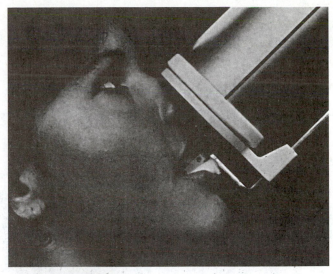

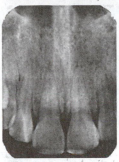

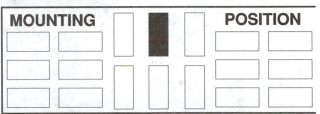

MOUNTING   POSITION

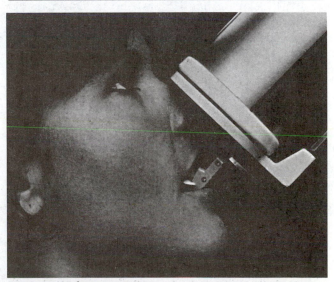

FIGURE 10–11 Positions for maxillary incisor exposure. (A) Paralleling technique and (B) Bisecting +40° technique. (Courtesy of Rinn Corporation.)

assistant moves behind the shield and activates the preset timer.

The maxillary canine or cuspid exposure is completed in the same manner and positioned the same way as the central exposure except that the cuspid and the first premolar are centered on the film in the block. The indicator rod protrudes out straight. The aiming ring is drawn down the rod to touch the cheek. The PID is centered against the ring and parallel to the rod (Figure 10–12). The assistant stands behind the shield and activates the preset timer. The procedure is completed in the same manner on the other side of the mouth but the assistant may wait until the bicuspid and molar exposures are completed on alternate sides.

The maxillary premolar or bicuspid exposure requires the film to be placed horizontally into the holding block. The indicator rod must be positioned into the block so the angle is facing the operator (coming out of the mouth). The back of the film touches the bite plate of the block and the film and block are centered behind the premolars or bicuspids (the shorter block for BAI and the longer block for XCP). The aiming ring is drawn up the protruding indicator rod to the cheek, and the PID is placed parallel to the rod and against the ring (Figure 10–13). The assistant stands behind the shield and activates the preset timer. The same method is used on the other side of the mouth for the maxillary premolar or bicuspid exposure.

The maxillary molars exposure is completed in the same manner, but the film and block are centered behind the three-molar area. The patient is instructed to bite on the block and cotton roll; when all is secure, the aiming ring is drawn up the indicator rod until it is next to the cheek. The end of the PID is placed against the ring and aligned with the indicator rod. The assistant stands behind the shield and activates the preset timer (Figure 10–14). When finished with the molar exposure on one side of the mouth, the assistant may move to the other side and complete the canine, premolar, and molar exposures in sequence.

7 Expose Mandibular Radiographs

When exposing the mandibular teeth, the patient is positioned with the chin up so when the mouth is opened, the occlusal plane is parallel to the floor. The anterior exposures require the film to be placed in the anterior holding block in a vertical position, and the film is centered behind the incisors. A cotton roll may be added for comfort and assistance in holding. When the block and film are securely placed in the mouth, the assistant moves the aiming ring up the indicator rod to the cheek and positions the PID parallel to the

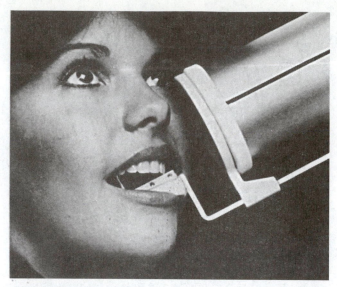

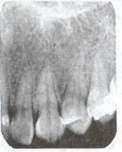

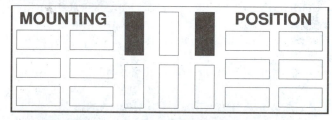

MOUNTING   POSITION

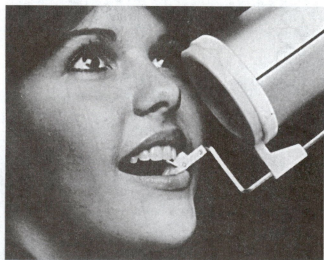

FIGURE 10–12 Positions for maxillary canine or cuspid exposure. (A) Paralleling exposure and (B) Bisecting exposure +45°. (Courtesy of Rinn Corporation.)

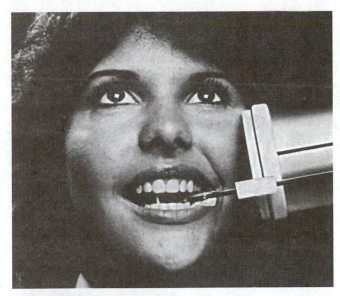

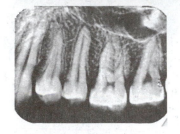

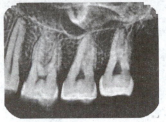

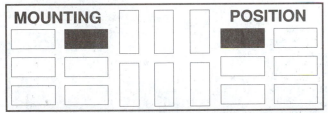

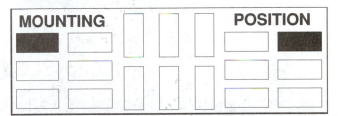

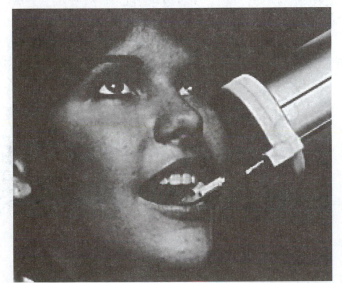

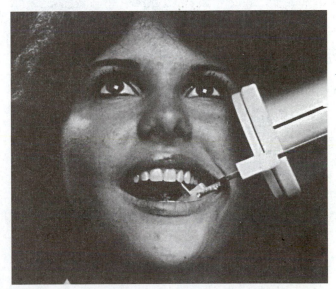

FIGURE 10–13 Positions for maxillary premolar or bicuspid exposure. (A) Paralleling exposure and (B) Bisecting exposure +30°. (Courtesy of Rinn Corporation.)

FIGURE 10–14 Positions for maxillary molar exposure. (A) Paralleling exposure and (B) Bisecting exposure +20°. (Courtesy of Rinn Corporation.)

rod sandwiched next to the ring (Figure 10–15). Standing behind the shield, the assistant activates the preset timer exposure button.

The mandibular canine or cuspid exposure is completed in the same manner as the lower incisors, but the film and biting block are moved to the side so the cuspid and some of the first premolars are centered on the film. After the patient bites on the block and cotton roll to secure the film in the mouth, the aiming ring is drawn up the indicator rod until it touches the cheek. The PID is sandwiched against the ring and aligned with the indicator rod (Figure 10–16). The assistant activates the preset timer after moving behind the shield or six feet away from the tubehead. The procedure is completed in the same manner on the other side of the mouth.

The mandibular premolars or bicuspids require the film to be placed in a horizontal position in the holding block, and the posterior indicator rod is placed into the block so the angle faces the operator when it comes out of the mouth. The securely placed film is centered behind the premolars or bicuspids. The patient bites on the biting block and cotton roll, and the aiming ring is drawn up the indicator rod until it touches the cheek. The PID is placed parallel to the rod and against the ring (Figure 10–17). The timer is activated after the assistant stands behind the shield and cautions the patient to close eyes and hold still. Both sides of the mouth are exposed using the same technique.

The mandibular molar exposure is completed in the same manner as the premolar or bicuspid exposure except the film and biting block are placed distally to include the three-molar area. After the patient carefully bites on the bite block and cotton roll, the aiming ring is drawn up the indicator rod. The PID is placed parallel to the rod and against the ring (Figure 10–18). The timer is activated after the assistant stands behind the shield.

8 Dismiss the Patient

When the series of film exposures is completed, the patient is repositioned into a comfortable sitting position. The drape and collar are removed and the patient is dismissed. The latex exam gloves are removed, and the hands are washed. The treatment is marked on the patient's chart and the cup with the exposed films is taken to be processed.

The assistant dons utility gloves, disinfects, sterilizes, and cleans up in the usual manner. The lead safety apron and collar are draped over the chair. The surface of the items receive the spray-wipe-spray disinfecting treatment and then are placed on the towel bar or hooks to dry. Folding of the lead apron is avoided because the lead padding inside the apron

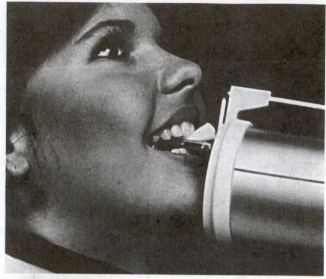

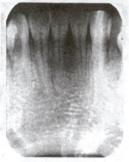

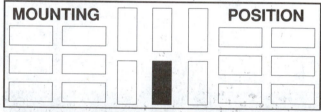

MOUNTING   POSITION

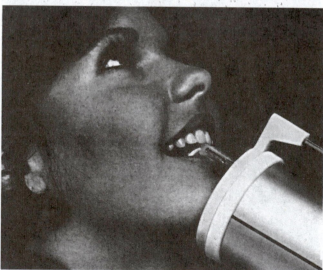

FIGURE 10–15 Positions for mandibular incisors exposure. (A) Paralleling exposure and (B) Bisecting exposure –15°. (Courtesy of Rinn Corporation.)

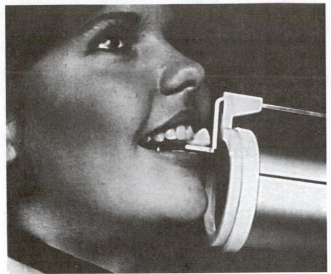

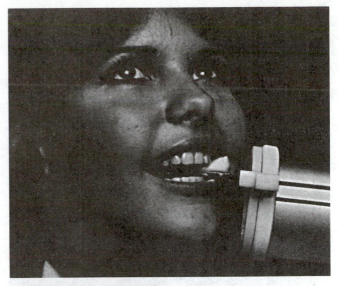

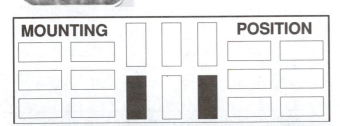

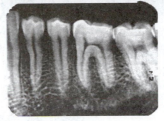

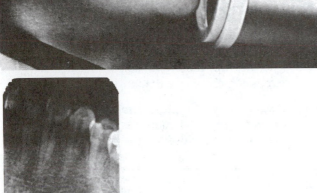

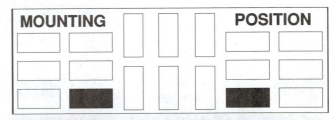

MOUNTING						POSITION	

MOUNTING						POSITION	

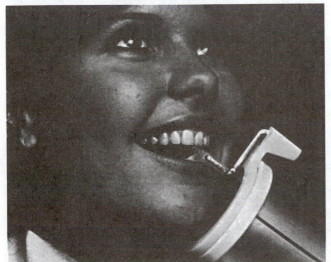

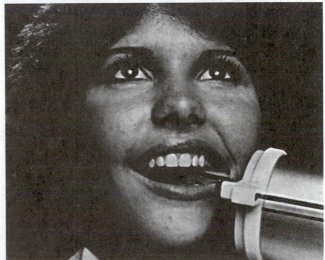

FIGURE 10–16 Positions for mandibular cuspid or canine exposure. (A) Paralleling exposure and (B) Bisecting exposure –20°. (Courtesy of Rinn Corporation.)

FIGURE 10–17 Positions for mandibular premolar or bicuspid exposure. (A) Paralleling exposure and (B) Bisecting exposure –10°. (Courtesy of Rinn Corporation.)

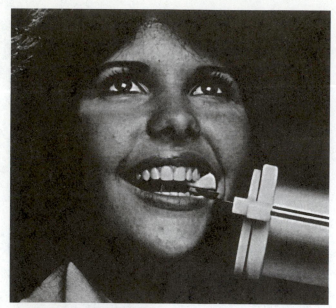

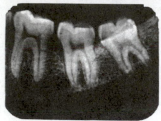

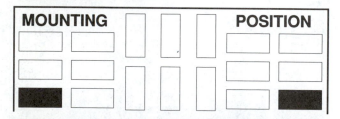

MOUNTING **POSITION**

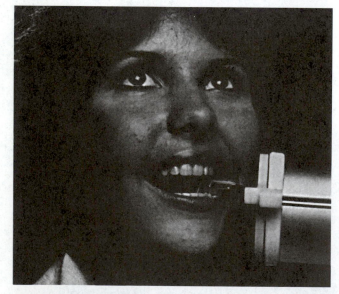

FIGURE 10-18 Positions for mandibular molar exposure. (A) Paralleling exposure and (B) Bisecting exposure −5°. (Courtesy of Rinn Corporation.)

may crack and crumble, leaving an ash of lead in the hem of the apron and little coverage where needed.

In the sterilizing area, the disposable blocks are placed in the contaminated trash receptacle. The indicator rods and aiming ring may be treated in the same manner as an instrument. They may be placed in the ultrasonic cleaner and then autoclaved or sterilized in a chemical bath. After all materials are cleaned, disinfected, and sterilized, the area is cleaned up. The gloves are washed, disinfected, and removed; the assistant washes hands.▲

THEORY RECALL
Exposure of Dental Radiographs

1. Who sets the requirements for the licensing and permission to expose dental x-rays?

   _____

2. What are the two methods of exposing dental x-rays commonly used in the dental facility?

   a. _____

   b. _____

3. Why does the assistant draw an imaginary line down the patient's face and place it perpendicular to the floor?

   _____

4. How close are all biting edges placed to the edge of the dental film?

   _____

5. Which side of the dental film faces the tubehead?

   _____

6. Are the films placed horizontally or vertically for a posterior view?

   _____

7. Where are exposed and unexposed films kept during exposure?

   _____

8. Why is the timer preset before the film placement?

   _____

9. Where is the PID placed?

   _____

10. Where does the assistant stand when activating the timer button?

   _____

Now turn to the Competency Evaluation Sheet for Procedure 58, Exposure of Intraoral Radiographs—Bisecting and Paralleling Techniques, located in Appendix C of this text.

PROCESSING DENTAL RADIOGRAPHS

Once dental radiographs have been exposed with radiation, they need to be chemically processed to display the results of the exposure. This processing is called film developing. There are two chemical baths that must be used to bring out the radiation image. One is **developer** and the other is **fixer**. The third bath used on the films is water, which is used to remove or wash away the other chemicals.

There are two ways to develop dental radiographs—manually and in an automatic film processor. The processing is the same, only the technique is different. In the **manual** method, the assistant manually transfers the films from the developing solution to the water, to the fixer, and back into the water bath. In the **automatic** processor (Figure 10–19), the film is placed on rollers which causes it to travel through the three baths.

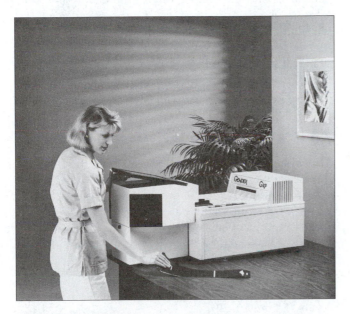

FIGURE 10–19 The assistant uses a daylight loader apparatus that permits processing radiographs without a darkroom. The same automatic processor may be used in the darkroom, without the loader attachment. (Courtesy of DENTSPLY International Inc., GENDEX Corporation, Midwest Dental Products Corporation.)

When working with the processing of films, it is very important to maintain an area of cleanliness. Spills or spots of solution can cause chemicals to neutralize or films to predevelop. Fixer solution, when spilled or carried into developing solution, can alter the developer's action. When working with the solutions, the assistant always should fill, stir, or work with the fixer first to avoid splashing some fixer solution into the developer solution.

If drops of developing solution are spilled or splashed onto unprocessed film, that spot will begin processing and become darker than the rest of the film. Spilling fixer on the unprocessed film will destroy that area for processing and viewing. The assistant must clean up all spills and messes before beginning the developing process.

The chemical solutions used in the developing process must be monitored daily for temperature, amount, cleanliness, and use. Temperature plays an important part in the chemical processing. The hotter the temperature, the faster the chemicals work, and developing time should be shortened. The assistant checks the temperature of the solution and the manufacturer's chart before setting the timer for developing in the manual method. The automatic processors are automatically set for temperature levels, and the assistant should read the manufacturer's directions before any adjusting.

The chemical solutions must fill the bath area where the films are to be placed. The assistant should check the levels of the solutions before beginning developing. **Replenishing** liquid should be added to the developing solution tank each working day. Automatic machines need 12 ounces daily and many automatic processors complete this function automatically while the assistant must do this chore each day for the manual system. It is suggested that 8 ounces of replenisher be added per gallon of developer per workday. Automatic machine requirements should follow manufacturer's demands. Although both methods of developing the radiographs are similar, the processing chemicals for the manual and automated uses are different types and composition and should be noted when ordering new supplies.

When not in use, lids should be left on the manual developing tank to avoid oxidation, but the cover should be removed at night from the automatic processor (unless otherwise noted by the manufacturer) to avoid condensation collection. Solutions should be changed every three or four weeks or more often if used excessively or if their appearance is dirty, or if it is suggested by the manufacturer of the processor.

PROCEDURE 59

Processing Dental Radiographs

1 **Prepare Films for Processing**

2 **Assemble Equipment and Material**

3 **Prepare the Chemicals**

1 Prepare Films for Processing

When preparing to develop films, the assistant should take precautions to avoid contaminating the darkroom equipment and materials. The chain of asepsis should be maintained in the developing process also. Films that have been exposed in the patient's mouth must be carefully handled to avoid contamination of the darkroom.

Some offices have a barrier shield on the dental x-ray films. These shields are placed over the film before placement in the patient's mouth. Some films may be purchased already wrapped in a barrier shield. When the film is exposed and removed from the patient's mouth, the shield is pulled open, the film is expressed or dropped into a lead-lined box or paper cup and taken to the darkroom for processing.

If no barrier shields are used, the assistant should don overgloves, take the paper cup of films into the darkroom, remove the lid on the lightproof container, and lay out a paper towel on the counter. Using only the **safelight**, the assistant opens the waterproof packet, grasps the black paper wrapper tab and pulls up the film and wrapper paper. The untouched films should then be dropped into a lightproof container. When all exposed films have been emptied into the lightproof container the lid is replaced. All contaminated papers should be placed on the waiting paper towel and later bundled up and disposed of in the contaminated trash container. The assistant can then remove the overgloves, which are placed into the contaminated trash container. Now the processing procedure beings. *A hemostat may be used to remove the film from the black paper wrapper and place the film into the lightproof container for storage if desired. The hemostat is kept in a dry container and is used only to pick up the untouched film. Some concern has been shown about powder residue on hands after removal from latex gloves in the darkroom. Powder may adhere to the films and interfere with the developing process. It is suggested that the assistant remove the latex gloves, wash hands, don overgloves, and enter the darkroom to remove the contami-

nated film wrappers. After the overgloves are removed and disposed of, the clean films may be taken out of the safelight container or off the towel and processed.

2 Assemble Equipment and Materials

With the exposed films in a lightproof container, the white light may be turned on for processing preparation. The assistant assembles the equipment needed for processing—stir rods, timer, thermometer, developing rack, pen or marker, and processing chart. All areas should be checked for cleanliness. No spills or spots should be present.

3 Prepare the Chemicals

The chemical solutions are checked for amount, cleanliness and temperature. Each solution is stirred with a separate marked stir rod to ensure even distribution of the chemicals. The developer rod is used to stir the developer, and the fixer rod is used in the fixer solution. Any replenishment is completed; water is changed or circulated, and the temperature of the developing solutions is noted. The assistant, if processing manually, checks the temperature with the manufacturer's chart for the proper time needed for processing and sets the timer for the appropriate time span length. If the automatic processor requires replenishing or temperature adjustment, which are not automatically controlled, the assistant completes the needed preparations.

4 Place Films on the Developing Rack

The white light is turned off. Using only the safelight, the assistant opens the lightproof container of exposed, unprocessed film. Each film is separately placed on the rollers of the automatic processor or on a developing rack, which has been marked with the patient's name. The assistant loads the first film on the lowest clip and alternates the loading from one side of the rack to the other while raising up the rack. The films are given a slight tug to determine if they have been placed securely (Figure 10–20).

5 Place Films in the Developer

The rack with films is placed in the developing solution. The assistant agitates them a few times and checks to see if the level of solution is covering all the films and that no films are touching each other or the sides of the tank. The lid is placed on the tank and the timer is activated. The rack stays in the solution until the time expires. In the automatic machine, the moving belt carries the films through the processing solutions.

6 Rinse Films in Water

When the timer goes off, the assistant lifts the rack and films up out of the developer and into the water

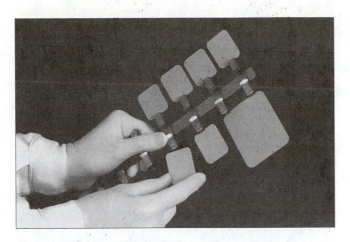

FIGURE 10-20 Films are placed on the rack in alternate order. When starting at the bottom, the assistant is assured that the film will be covered by the solutions when inserted into the tank.

bath where it is agitated for 30 seconds and then raised up over the water bath. The drip is allowed to fall into the water bath.

7 Place Films in the Fixer

The rack and films are placed into the fixer bath, where they are raised and lowered five times to remove the surface bubbles. The rack is hooked on the side and the lid is replaced after the assistant checks that the solution covers all the film surfaces and that none are stuck to the side of the tank or another film. The timer is set for manufacturer's recommended time (2 to 4 minutes). At the end of the fixing cycle, the rack is raised and moved to the water bath where the solution is permitted to drip off.

8 Place Films in the Water Bath

The rack and films are placed into the water bath and permitted to remain in the running water for ten minutes.

9 Dry Films

After ten minutes, the assistant may obtain the rack and films and place them under a running water stream. This process removes the chemicals and helps to clean the racks of solutions. The rack (with films) is placed in a clean area with circulating air to dry. When dry, the films are removed from the rack and mounted.

Automatic Processing

10 Prepare Films

When using an automatic processor, the procedure is the same. The films are prepared by removing the bar-

riers or the waterproof coverings and placed into a lightsafe container until processing. The overgloves are removed and the equipment is prepared.

11 Prepare Equipment

The automatic equipment is checked and prepared according to the manufacturer's directions. Each machine has its own processing method. Temperature and condition of the solutions are important factors to be checked.

12 Process Films

Using the safelight, the films are removed from the lightproof container and placed into the automatic processor rollers for the developing procedure. The films are placed at a regular interlude so as not to touch each other and permit solution coverage of all parts of the films.

13 Prepare Films for Display

When the procedure is done, the assistant retrieves the finished films and places them into a mount or on a marked rack until mounting time. All drips or water spots are wiped up, and the area is left in a clean and polished state.▲

THEORY RECALL

Processing Dental Radiographs

1. What are the two methods used to process dental radiographs?

   a. _____

   b. _____

2. Why is it important to maintain a clean area when processing films?

   _____

3. Why should lids be left on the developing tank of a manual processing unit?

   _____

4. How can the assistant prevent contamination of the processing procedure when working with dental x-rays?

   _____

5. Where are the contaminated waterproof coverings of dental x-rays placed after they have been removed?

   _____

6. Are the films removed from the waterproof coverings in a safelight or in a white light?

_____

7. Why are separate stir rods used on different solutions?

_____

8. In what pattern does the assistant place the films to be developed on the rack?

_____

9. Why are the films and rack rinsed under running water after processing?

_____

10. Where are the films placed for drying?

_____

Now turn to the Competency Evaluation Sheet for Procedure 59, Processing Dental Radiographs, located in Appendix C of this text.

MOUNTING DENTAL RADIOGRAPHS

Mounting dental radiographs is a systematic placement of a series of small films. When properly arranged this series offers a total view of the entire mouth area. X-ray mounts are made of dark, light, or clear cardboard, plastic or vinyl sheeting composition, and have horizontal and vertical windows to hold processed radiographs (Figure 10–21).

Since the exposure of dental radiographs is completed following a specific pattern, the placement of these finished films is completed to match this standard pattern. Anterior exposures require the film to be placed in the mouth in a vertical position; therefore, when the film is to be mounted, it is mounted with the film in a vertical position. Posterior films are placed in a horizontal position during exposure and are mounted in the same position.

Fourteen dental films are needed to complete a series of exposures for the entire mouth. If the dentist also wishes to include bitewing exposures in the series, two to four more films are included. If the commercial bitewing film (size 3) is used, the mount necessary to house this series will have six vertical windows for the anterior views, and eight horizontal views for the posterior teeth. In the center of the posterior areas, there could be another window made to accommodate the size 3 bitewings. If the office prefers two modified periapical bitewing exposures per side, the mount needed will have six vertical and twelve horizontal. Each office orders the style and composition type mount that accommodates the office exposure procedure.

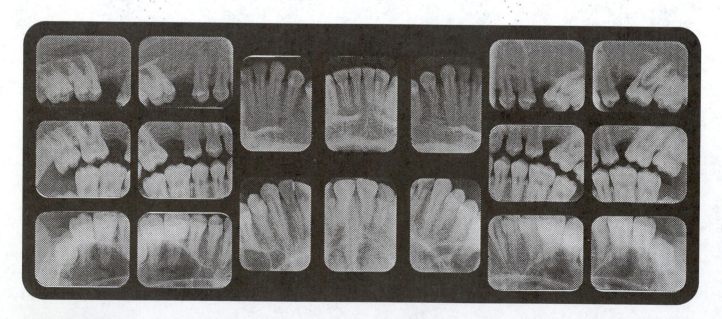

FIGURE 10–21 An example of a mounted set of dental radiographs.

PROCEDURE 60
Mounting Dental Radiographs

1 Assemble Equipment and Materials

2 Prepare Films for Mounting

3 Locate Pimple (Bump) and Dimple (Concave)

4 Arrange Films

5 Mount Molar Bitewings

6 Mount Premolar or Bicuspid Bitewings

7 Mount Maxillary Incisors

8 Mount Maxillary Canines or Cuspids

9 Mount Maxillary Premolars or Bicuspids

10 Mount Maxillary Molars

11 Mount Mandibular Incisors

12 Mount Mandibular Cuspid or Canines

13 Mount Mandibular Premolars or Bicuspids

14 Mount Mandibular Molars

15 Clean Up the Area

1 Assemble Equipment and Materials

When preparing to mount dental radiographs, the assistant washes and dries hands and assembles the necessary materials and equipment in a clean, dry area. Items needed follow:

▶ thoroughly dry, processed dental radiographs
▶ dental radiograph mount
▶ view box
▶ marker or pen
▶ gloves or finger stoles
▶ sheet of paper

2 Prepare Films for Mounting

The radiographs are assembled and removed from the rack (if manually processed) and placed on the clean sheet of paper. The assistant wears gloves or handles the films by only touching and using the film edges. The films are identified and the mount is marked with the patient's name and date. If the office uses a patient numbering system for radiographs, the patient's number is marked on the mount and recorded in the cross-reference file book.

3 Locate Pimple (Bump) and Dimple (Concave)

Touching only the sides of the film, the assistant picks up and examines a dental radiograph. By locating the dimple or pimple, the assistant rotates the film to be viewed from the pimple or the dimple aspect. If the dentist wishes to view the series from outside the mouth, the assistant places all radiographs with the bump (pimple) toward the operator. If the dentist wishes to view the series from the inside of the mouth, the assistant places all films with the concave area (dimple) toward the operator. Most offices prefer the protruding bump-style mounting.

4 Arrange Films

Using the knowledge of specific landmarks, the film is identified. The assistant has the choice of placing the film into the specific mount window for the film or placing it on the clean sheet of paper arranged in its proper area and mounted later. Some assistants prefer to mount directly, while others arrange the films on paper until all films are identified and situated in order.

*All films are mounted with either the pimple (bump) or the dimple (concave) facing the operator.

The landmarks for the mounting of the dental radiographs are as follows.

5 Mount Molar Bitewings

Identifying landmarks:

▶ bitewings (molar)
▶ coronal view of both arches
▶ three-molar area visible
▶ occlusal plane in center of film
▶ distal of second premolar or bicuspid
▶ ascending ramus to distal edge
▶ thicker teeth toward distal
▶ bifurcation of mandibular molar on bottom of film

6 Mount Premolar or Bicuspid Bitewings

Identifying landmarks:

▶ bitewings (bicuspid and premolar)
▶ coronal view of both arches
▶ occlusal plane in center of film
▶ both bicuspids or premolars, first molar
▶ distal of cuspid or canine
▶ bifurcation of mandibular molars on bottom of film
▶ maxillary sinus on top of film

7 Mount Maxillary Incisors

Identifying landmarks:

▶ film in vertical position
▶ two large central incisors, mesial portion of laterals

▶ incisal edge toward middle of mount
▶ crowns and roots fully shown
▶ nasal septum and fossae may be visible
▶ incisive foramen

8 Mount Maxillary Canines or Cuspids

Identifying landmarks:

▶ film in vertical position
▶ crown and root fully shown
▶ cuspid or canine in center of film
▶ distal of lateral
▶ mesial of first premolar, large lingual cusp
▶ possible view of maxillary sinus
▶ incisal edge toward center of mount

9 Mount Maxillary Premolars or Bicuspids

Identifying landmarks:

▶ film in horizontal position
▶ crowns and roots of both premolars and bicuspids
▶ maxillary sinus visible
▶ large lingual cusps
▶ mesial view of first molar
▶ distal of cuspid
▶ thicker, heavier teeth toward distal
▶ occlusal plane toward center of mount

10 Mount Maxillary Molars

Identifying landmarks:

▶ film in horizontal position
▶ crowns and roots visible for three-molar area
▶ maxillary sinus visible
▶ maxillary tuberosity
▶ crowded root area (three)
▶ full lingual cusps on premolars or bicuspids
▶ distal of second premolar or bicuspid
▶ thicker, heavier teeth toward distal
▶ occlusal plane toward center of mount

11 Mount Mandibular Incisors

Identifying landmarks:

▶ film in vertical position
▶ crowns and roots of centrals and laterals
▶ laterals slightly larger and wider than centrals
▶ distal view of cuspids or canines
▶ dense mandibular bone
▶ lingual foramen
▶ incisal edge toward middle of mount

12 Mount Mandibular Cuspid or Canines

Identifying landmarks:

▶ film in vertical position
▶ crown and root of cuspid or canine
▶ first premolar, distal of second premolar or bicuspid
▶ small lingual cusps on bicuspids or premolars
▶ dense mandibular bone, no maxillary sinus
▶ thicker, heavier teeth toward distal
▶ incisal edge toward middle of mount

13 Mount Mandibular Premolars or Bicuspids

Identifying landmarks:

▶ film in horizontal position
▶ crown and root of both premolars or bicuspids
▶ small lingual cusps of premolars or bicuspids
▶ mesial of first molar, distal or cuspid
▶ dense mandibular bone
▶ thicker, heavier teeth toward distal
▶ occlusal plane toward center of mount

14 Mount Mandibular Molars

Identifying landmarks:

▶ film in horizontal position
▶ crown and roots of three-molar area
▶ ascending ramus visible
▶ thicker, heavier teeth toward distal
▶ distal of premolar, small lingual cusp
▶ bifurcation of mandibular molar roots (two roots)
▶ mandibular canal
▶ occlusal plane toward center of mount

15 Clean Up the Area

Once the film is identified, the mounting is completed. All films are placed in order. The assistant reviews the entire series to make sure the films are related and in the proper sequence. The mounted series is then placed with the patient's records. The area is cleaned up, and the materials and equipment are returned to their proper places.▲

THEORY RECALL

Mounting Dental Radiographs

1. What is done in the process of mounting dental radiographs?

_____

2. What are dental radiograph mounts?

_____

3. In what color may dental radiograph mounts be purchased?

_____

4. Are anterior dental radiographs placed in a horizontal or vertical position for mounting?

_____

5. How many films are necessary to complete a mouth series if bitewings are not taken?

_____

6. What is the size of commercial bitewing film?

_____

7. What will the assistant wear to avoid smears and fingerprints when mounting radiographs?

_____

8. If the dentist wishes to review the series from the outside of the mouth, are the films viewed from the pimple or dimple side?

_____

9. If the assistant does not wear gloves, where are the films touched and handled?

_____

10. What is written on the mount before the films are placed in the mount?

_____

Now turn to the Competency Evaluation Sheet for Procedure 60, Mounting Dental Radiographs, located in Appendix C of this text.

ANALYZING THE QUALITY OF DENTAL RADIOGRAPHS

It is very important to be able to expose and produce an acceptable diagnostic tool when taking dental radiographs. Knowledge and practice of good exposure, storage, handling, and processing techniques help to provide a dental radiograph that can be used to detect hidden troubles and diseases. Occasionally, an error does occur. If the assistant is aware of what error has been made and the proper way to correct the mistake, the likelihood of this error occurring again is lessened.

Faulty radiographs can occur as a result of errors in any of the dental x-ray care or technique steps. These steps follow.

Purchase, Handling, and Storage

PROBLEM: FILMS ARE LIGHT; NO CONTRAST; FOGGY APPEARANCE. If films are expired and out of date, the emul-

sions may be weak and produce a light, undistinguishable radiograph. The assistant always checks the dates and rotates new and old stock when receiving a new supply. Never order more than can be used in six months. If there is a bargain discount available for multiple package purchases and the facility cannot use the minimum order amount, check with the manufacturer or supply house to see if the order can be made and paid for the larger amount but have arrangements for a back order delivery of part of the order at a later date when it will be needed. Films that have been heated or exposed to radiation or chemical vapors will also have poor contrast or look foggy.

Films that have been bent or twisted from too intense a softening of corners may show a dark line from a crack in the surface emulsion or a dark blur where the film was bent. Long fingernails or rough edges on racks may scrape the emulsion on the film and show a scratch mark on the finished product (Figure 10–22).

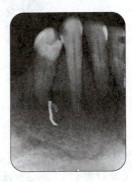

FIGURE 10–22 An example of a fingernail scratch.

Machine Settings

PROBLEM: FILMS TOO DARK OR TOO LIGHT; NO CONTRAST. When the x-ray machine settings are not placed in the proper position for the exposure and patient type, the results may give a film that is either too dark or too light to be of effective use (Figure 10–23). Milliamperage, kilovolt-

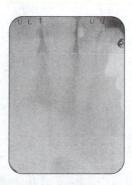

FIGURE 10–23 An example of improper machine settings. Poor exposure.

age, and exposure time must be set and regulated to fit the facility's machine potential. Once the desired settings are determined, they should be written somewhere near the control panel of the machine.

Film Placement Technique

PROBLEM: FILMS ELONGATED, FORESHORTENED, OVERLAPPED, HERRINGBONE EFFECT, CONECUT, OR IMPROPER PLACEMENT OF POSITION. When films are incorrectly placed and exposed, the resulting radiograph will be affected. Elongation errors happen if the vertical angle of the central ray coming out of the tubehead does not penetrate the film at the proper position. When the vertical angle is too low, the image of the tooth shown on the film will be longer than the actual tooth. Increasing the vertical angle will improve this condition (Figure 10–24).

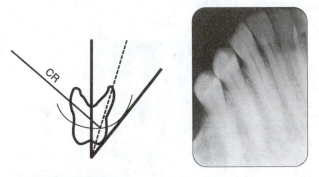

FIGURE 10–24 An example of elongation exposure. When the central ray does not perpendicularly intersect the bisecting plane between the tooth and film, an error occurs.

The opposite effect happens when the vertical angle of the central ray is too high. The resulting effect on the film will show an image of a tooth shorter than the actual tooth size. This error is called foreshortening (Figure 10–25). A reduction of vertical angulation improves this condition.

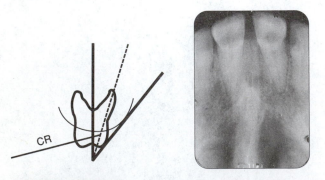

FIGURE 10–25 Example of foreshortening exposure. Central ray does not perpendicularly intersect bisecting plane.

When the central ray is placed in an incorrect horizontal angle, the radiation will cause an overlapping effect upon the waiting film. The shadow of the teeth will project over the adjacent teeth and make the film unreadable. This condition is called overlapping (Figure 10–26). To improve this condition, the tubehead must be aligned parallel to the head so the central ray may penetrate to the film in a perpendicular manner.

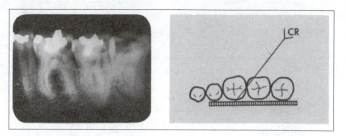

FIGURE 10–26 Example of overlapping exposure. Horizontal angle does not intersect perpendicularly to the center of the film.

If the central ray from the tubehead misses the film because it was placed too far horizontally mesial or distal from the center, the resulting error will show a picture with a white unexposed arch in the corner (Figure 10–27). This error is called conecutting, because the cone misplacement cut part of the image off. Centering the PID over the film area will correct this problem.

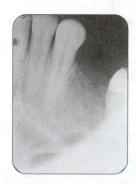

FIGURE 10–27 Example of conecutting exposure. Circle of radiation misses part of film. The central ray is too far mesial or distal to the center.

If films are not placed in the proper position behind the teeth to be exposed, the result will show either lacking crowns, roots, or adjacent teeth. Anterior teeth must be exposed with the films in vertical position while posterior teeth must be in horizontal position. Films also must be placed with the plain side facing the tubehead. If the x-ray film is placed with the back to the radiation source, the results will be a light film with a herringbone effect (Figure 10–28). This is caused by the exposure and image of the lead backing, which is placed inside the film packet. Correct placement of the film will eliminate the view of the herringbone effect.

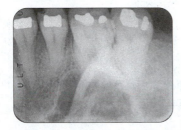

FIGURE 10–28 Example of herringbone-effect exposure. The film is light and the lead backing shows.

Exposure and Processing Time

PROBLEMS: BLURRY; DOUBLE EXPOSURE; SPOTTED FILM; STAINED FILM. Other errors can happen during the exposure time. Movement by the patient, machine, or film in the mouth can cause a blurred radiograph. Using films twice, an error caused when films are laid next to unexposed films, can cause a useless double exposure effect.

Processing of the film must be accomplished with care. All the proper handling and techniques during exposure will be lost if the films are damaged in the developing procedure. Some errors that can occur at this time follow:

▸ blank or clear film—wrong sequence of solutions, use developer, water, fixer
▸ dark spots—developer drips on film before processing
▸ white or blank spots—fixer drips on film before processing
▸ black or dark film—improper safelight, too warm solution temperature
▸ partial image—processing solutions low, film not covered by solution, films touched sides of tanks or each other on belt
▸ stained glass effect (reticulation)—large temperature difference of solution baths (manual method)
▸ yellow-brownish stains—improper water bath
▸ iridescent stains—old solutions, particularly the developer

The assistant must be careful in all parts of the radiation procedure. Improper techniques in any of the areas involving dental radiographs can and will cause flaws and errors that require retakes and more radiation exposure to the patient.▲

THEORY RECALL
Analyzing Dental Radiographs

1. List three ways a dental radiograph may be spoiled from improper or faulty purchasing, handling, or storing.

   a. _____

   b. _____

   c. _____

2. List two faults in dental radiographs that may result in improper machine settings.

   a. _____

   b. _____

3. What type of dental radiographic error may occur when film, machine, or patient movement happens during exposure?

   _____

4. List the two types of dental radiographic errors that may occur if the vertical angle of the central ray is not perpendicular with the bisecting plane of the tooth and film angle?

   a. _____

   b. _____

5. What effect will occur to a dental radiograph if the horizontal angle of the central ray is not perpendicular to the center of the film?

   _____

6. What effect will occur to a dental radiograph if the central ray is not aimed at the center of the film and misses the end?

   _____

7. What would happen to a dental radiograph if a drip of developer fell on the film prior to processing.

   _____

8. A partial dental radiograph image may be caused by what error?

   _____

9. If a film is opened in a white light and then processed, what effect will the processed dental radiograph show?

   _____

10. Films which have or develop a yellowish-brown cast indicate what has happened during processing?

For additional activities related to this lesson, turn to Assignment Sheet 10.3, Analyzing Dental Radiographs, located in Appendix B of this text.

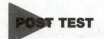

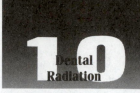

Total possible points = 100 points
80% needed for passing = 80 points

Total points this test _____ pass _____ fail _____

MATCHING: Write the letter from column B that best describes or matches the word in column A. Each question is worth 2 points for a total of 20 points.

Column A	Column B
_____ 1. elongation	a. improper horizontal central ray angle
_____ 2. paralleling block	b. bitewing film
_____ 3. iridescent stain	c. radiograph of head
_____ 4. conecutting	d. longer block to keep film away from site
_____ 5. interproximal	e. improper safelight
_____ 6. cephalogram	f. improper central ray vertical angle
_____ 7. bisecting block	g. old developing solution
_____ 8. periapical	h. shorter block to hold film against site
_____ 9. blurred image	i. intraoral film
_____10. black or dark film	j. movement during exposure

MULTIPLE CHOICE: Circle the correct answer. Each question is worth 4 points for a total of 80 points.

1. Which of the following cells is the least sensitive to radiation?
   a. skin   b. blood   c. muscle   d. bone

2. Which of the following dental radiographs is the most common one used in intraoral views?
   a. panoramic   b. occlusal   c. cephalometric   d. periapical

3. The protruding bump (pimple) on the dental x-ray film is located on which area of the film?
   a. the face of the film   b. the back of the film   c. the side of the film   d. anywhere

4. Which of the following would *not* be expected to be seen in a radiograph of a mandibular left premolar or bicuspid periapical shot?
   a. the root tip of both premolars and some of canine and possible first molar
   b. a view of crown and root sections of all premolars or bicuspids
   c. the film placed in horizontal position
   d. a view of the sinus

5. Which of the following safety items is considered useful for the patient? (1) collar, (2) drape, (3) dosimeter, (4) good techniques, or (5) shield
   a. 1 and 2   b. 1, 3, and 5   c. 1, 2, and 4   d. all

6. Intensifying screens are placed in metal cassettes to
   a. increase rays.   b. reflect rays.   c. decrease rays.   d. alter rays.

7. Which of the following radiographic films is *not* considered intraoral?
   a. panoramic   b. periapical   c. bitewing   d. occlusal

8. How many radiograph views are necessary to expose the maxillary arch?
   a. 6   b. 7   c. 14   d. 18

9. What is added to the developing solution when the quantity level drops?
   a. water   b. fixer   c. ice   d. replenisher

10. The bitewing views are usually mounted in which section of the mouth?
    a. the anterior section   b. the posterior section   c. it does not matter where

11. Which is the correct sequence of bath solution when processing films?
    a. water, developer, water, fixer   c. developer, fixer, water
    b. fixer, water, developer, water   d. developer, water, fixer, water

12. Which of the following would *not* be viewed on a maxillary molar shot?
    a. crowns and roots of the first, second, and third molars
    b. partial view of maxillary sinus
    c. partial view of second premolar or bicuspid
    d. clear view of two rooted (distal and mesial) molars

13. When mounting films, the posterior films will be placed in which position?
    a. vertical   b. horizontal   c. it does not matter

14. Barrier shields are placed on radiographic dental films to:
    a. stop cross contamination.   c. stop moisture leaks.
    b. stop stray radiation.   d. stop aging of film.

15. If drops of developing solution splash onto unprocessed film and the film is developed, how will the splash areas show up on the film?
    a. light spots   b. dark spots   c. clear spots   d. no effect

16. A radiographic cassette is used to
    a. hold pictures of dental procedures.   c. store processed films.
    b. hold radiographic film.   d. process films for viewing.

17. Which of the following are considered safety precautions for the operator? (1) collar, (2) drape, (3) dosimeter, (4) good exposure techniques, or (5) shield
    a. 1 and 2   b. 3, 4, and 5   c. 2, 3, 4, and 5   d. all

18. Radiation exposure devices, such as rings, pens, and badges, are used to
    a. absorb stray radiation.   c. measure exposure received.
    b. intensify radiation.   d. protect from radiographic penetration.

19. When viewing radiographs that have been mounted with the pimple or bump facing the operator, which way was the film placed in the mouth during exposure?
    a. toward the tubehead   b. away from the tubehead   c. it does not matter

20. Which of the following would *not* be expected to be present on a radiograph of a maxillary canine or cuspid?
    a. maxillary lateral view   c. possible start of sinus marks
    b. crown and root view of canine or cuspid   d. nasal septa

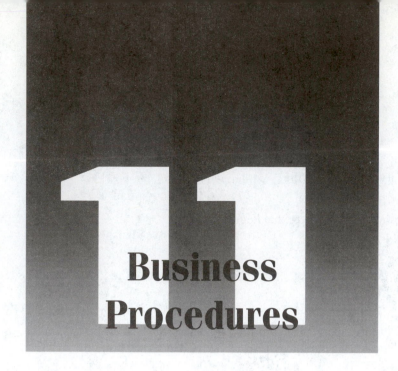

Business Procedures

► OBJECTIVES

Upon completion of this unit, the student will achieve a score of 80% or better on the Post Test covering the following material.

1. List and discuss the responsibilities of the receptionist and chairside dental assistant in relation to the opening and closing of a dental office.
2. Demonstrate dental office telephone techniques for general telephone use and specific tasks of appointment, professional, emergency, inquiry, collection, ordering, and followup calls.
3. Demonstrate techniques for efficient appointment making and control of office scheduling.
4. Discuss the techniques for collecting and recording data for the dental office.
5. List the steps and processes for the numeric, alphabetic, and chronologic methods of filing and processing dental records.
6. Demonstrate the method of recording daily dental office bookkeeping and record taking using the one write system.
7. Demonstrate the method for completion of dental insurance forms.
8. Discuss and demonstrate the techniques used to write checks and reconcile checking accounts.

► KEY TERMS

accommodate	cross-reference	placing
alphabetic	deductible	posting
buffer	dependents	pre-authorized
cancelled checks	deposit	reconciliation
chronologic	indexing	schedule of
confidentiality	inquiry	benefits
confirmation calls	ledger card	sorting
coordination	maximum	subscriber
of benefits	numeric	transaction
correspondence	outstanding	UCR
courtesy	payee	

OPENING AND CLOSING THE DENTAL OFFICE

The daily opening and closing of the dental office is a series of routine procedures that permit an efficient business to operate. The more thorough the preparation, the better and smoother the schedule will perform.

There is a multitude of minor procedures that should be completed before the workday begins. Preparation must take place in all the areas of the office to function properly. Many offices employ a dental assistant to complete the secretarial and business duties and one or more auxiliaries to work at chairside and in the laboratory. Working together, these auxiliaries can share preparation procedures; but in offices where only one assistant is employed, the duties are performed by that person.

PROCEDURE 61
Opening and Closing the Dental Business Office

1. **Open the Office**
2. **Perform Desk Duties**
3. **Prepare Reception Room**
4. **Sort Mail**
5. **Clean Reception Room and Desk Area**
6. **Complete Desk Work**
7. **Freshen Reception Room**
8. **Complete Mail Transactions**
9. **Close Area**

1 Open the Office

The secretarial assistant opens the office to prepare for the workday. If working strictly at the reception desk and area, the secretarial or business assistant is not required to don PPE but must put on a lab coat covering upon entering the operatory area. The secretarial assistant may wear street clothing to and from work but may choose to don the PPE outfits matching the other workers in the office.

Upon arriving at the office, the secretarial assistant turns on the lights and activates the thermal controls for patient comfort.

2 Perform Desk Duties

The desk duty to be addressed first is to check the phone answering machine or call the answering service for messages and act on the calls as soon as possible. A quick look into the fax machine may provide some **correspondence** replies or additional data to be added to patient's records.

The daily schedule for the day's activities is checked and posted in the designated areas. All patient's charts, records, and lab cases needed are assembled and prepared for use. If the office uses a computer for practice control, the assistant activates the machine and prepares for the day's business (Figure 11–1). If a daily log book or master sheet is used, the assistant prepares a new sheet for the day.

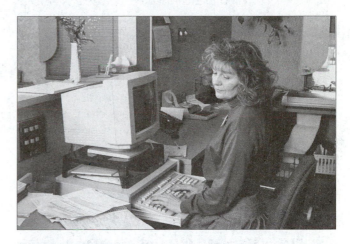

FIGURE 11–1 The receptionist prepares for the day by activating the computer. Many business procedures may be completed on the computer.

3 Prepare Reception Room

When the desk work is prepared, the assistant enters the reception room, dusts the furniture, rearranges the magazines (checking the timeliness and condition), and generally organizes the area. If flowers are present, dead leaves are picked off and the plant is watered on schedule. If the office supplies apples or coffee and tea treats, the supplies are replenished and fresh water is placed into the machine. The children's corner (Figure 11–2) is picked up. A periodic glance at

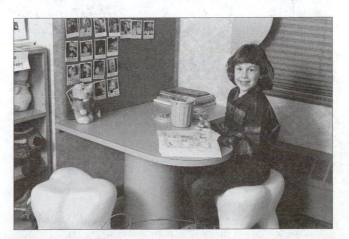

FIGURE 11–2 A children's corner can help to make a visit to the dentist a pleasant affair.

coloring book materials may suggest purchasing some new books; children rapidly use up pages when coloring. Sticky fingerprints are wiped off.

4 Sort Mail

If the mail has arrived, the assistant sorts and places the incoming materials in the proper place. All employer's correspondence marked personal is placed unopened on the doctor's desk along with journals and ads of interest. Some employers like to glance at the new magazines before their placement into the reception area.

Any lab cases or work boxes returned to the office are taken to the laboratory, and the arrival is marked on the lab work sheet and the patient's chart. Any bills are placed in a file with their matching inventory slip or packing list to await the payment procedure.

Patient payment and insurance checks are placed together until the assistant can complete the logging and receipt process. Junk mail is treated according to office policy.

5 Clean Reception Room and Desk Area

The thorough cleaning and disinfection of the front desk and reception room is done on a routine schedule, which may appear in an office manual and in the OSHA workbook. This cleaning involves the moving of chairs for sweeping and dusting and the disinfection of surfaces and items, including children's toys. This procedure may be completed by a cleaning service in the evening or done on a special morning when the doctor is scheduled for hospital surgery or some other routine event.

6 Complete Desk Work

To close the office at the end of the workday, the assistant completes the desk work. **Confirmation calls** have been made and the next day's schedule is printed up and copied so that each room has a print out of the scheduled appointments and upcoming planned dental procedures.

All charts and records for the following day are pulled and placed in an area for the next morning. Any needed materials that are not present are checked into. The financial **postings** are completed, and a deposit slip and bag are prepared for banking.

7 Freshen Reception Room

The reception room is freshened. All magazines are picked up, chairs may be put back into position, and trash baskets are tie bundled and removed, with new liners placed into the containers. Children's toys are

put back. If the dentist permits smoking in the reception area, the ashtrays are emptied and washed so that no lingering tobacco odor remains during the night.

8 Complete Mail Transactions

All outgoing mail transactions are prepared. Statements, records, lab cases, and correspondence are wrapped or enveloped, weighed, and postage stamped or metered for the correct amount. The assistant dispatches them on the way home or places the items in an area for pick up. Any faxing of correspondence may be completed at any time during the workday.

9 Close Area

When preparing to close for the day, the secretarial or business assistant engages the answering service or turns on the phone answering machine. All trash is gathered and taken to the pick up area. The air conditioner or heater may be turned up or down for the night. The office machines should be turned off. A hard copy of the day's business transactions must be made before the shut down of the computer.

Upon completing these procedures, the assistant may activate the security system employed by the office, secure the door, and leave.

PROCEDURE 62

Opening and Closing the Dental Operatory

Opening the Operatory

1 **Prepare for Work**
2 **Prepare Operatory**
3 **Prepare Sterilizing Area**
4 **Prepare Darkroom**
5 **Prepare Laboratory Area**

Closing the Operatory

6 **Clean Operatory Area**
7 **Clean Sterilizing Area**
8 **Clean Laboratory Area**
9 **Clean Darkroom Area**
10 **Change Clothing**

1 Prepare for Work

The duties of the chairside assistant are centered in the operatory, laboratory, and darkroom areas. The chairside assistant arrives 30 minutes before the first scheduled patient and prepares for the day by changing from street clothes into the PPE supplied by the dental office.

2 Prepare Operatory

The operatory is prepared first. The assistant checks the posted schedule of the day's appointments and begins preparation. The operatory is dusted, cleaned, and swept. Supplies are checked to make sure nothing will be needed in the middle of a dental procedure.

Any barrier shields employed by the office are applied, and the water lines are flushed to ensure fresh water. All barrier techniques are checked, and a quick scan of the room (including the ceiling) is made for acceptability and freshness before going into the sterilizing area. When the area is disinfected and prepared, the assistant sets out the items needed for the first appointment (Figure 11–3).

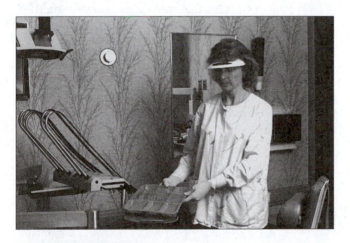

FIGURE 11–3 **The chairside assistant readies the operatory for the first appointment.**

3 Prepare Sterilizing Area

The assistant activates the dry heat sterilizer and prepares trays for the upcoming appointments. Any x-rays, records, charts, or lab materials needed for the appointment are gathered and placed with the tray.

The assistant checks the level of distilled water in the autoclave and the condition of the ultrasonic solutions. All supplies are replenished as needed. New sterilizing solutions are made up for the day, and spray bottles are filled for service.

4 Prepare Darkroom

The darkroom is prepared by checking for cleanliness. All solutions and temperatures are checked. The lid of the automatic processor is replaced after replenishing solution has been added if the machine does not complete this action automatically. Any dry x-rays are taken out of the darkroom, mounted, and placed with the patient's records. If processing is done with manual tanks, the solutions are replenished and stirred; temperatures are taken and adjusted as needed.

5 Prepare Laboratory Area

The laboratory area is prepared by activating the machines, such as hydrocolloid conditioners, the wax heater, and solutions. Many offices store their air compressor and nitrous oxide and oxygen tanks in the laboratory area. These tanks are turned on in preparation for the workday.

A quick review of the lab schedule confirms if all materials are ready for use. The supplies are checked and replenished, if needed, and the area is cleaned up. All completed cases are filed and placed in their proper positions.

Closing the Operatory

6 Clean Operatory Area

When closing up for the day, the assistant cleans the operatory area by donning utility gloves and PPE. All surfaces, areas, and hoses are disinfected. Traps for the saliva ejector and the HVE are cleaned out or replaced if using disposable ones. Contaminated barrier shields are removed and placed in the contaminated trash container bag, which is tie bundled and removed; a new liner is placed into the containers.

7 Clean Sterilizing Area

The sterilizing area is cleaned. All instruments and equipment present are cleaned, disinfected, sterilized, and replaced into the proper area for use on the next day.

Ultrasonic solutions are examined and replaced if needed. The tank is drained, washed out, rinsed, and filled with new solution. The condition of the autoclave water is examined; the machine is drained, cleaned out, and replaced with fresh, distilled water, if needed. Even if these solutions do not appear to need changing, they are purposely cleaned according to an office schedule. All trash is gathered, tie bundled, and removed; new liners are placed into the containers. Drips, smears, and fingerprints are polished off the counter tops and fronts. A quick check of the floors is made and any drips are quickly wiped up.

8 Clean Laboratory Area

The laboratory area is cleaned up in the evening. All machines are turned off and supplies are replaced. If condensation has collected in the air compressor, it is drained off; the gas machines are turned off and then drained to remove any gas in the lines. Lab orders for the next day are laid out; all trash is tie bundled and removed. New liners are placed in the containers.

9 Clean Darkroom Area

All spills and messes in the darkroom are cleaned up. Any racks used are cleaned and dried and placed back on the line. The automatic processor machine is turned off, and the assistant removes the cover to prevent condensation in the machine. If processing manually, the lid is placed on the solutions to prevent oxidation of the solutions. The trash is tie bundled and removed; new liners are placed in the containers. The door to the darkroom may be left open in the evening to permit an airing out of the chemical odors, particularly if the area is small and compact.

10 Change Clothing

To prepare to go home, the assistant washes and disinfects the utility gloves and removes them. The PPE gear is removed, and the assistant dons the personal articles worn to work. Dirty, contaminated laundry is placed into the laundry container, which is taken to the laundry room or pick up area. The trash is placed in the pick up area. The hands are washed, and the assistant prepares to leave for home.▲

THEORY RECALL

Opening and Closing the Dental Office

1. What do the opening and closing procedures in the dental office provide?

   _____

2. What are the first duties the receptionist performs in the morning?

   _____

3. Name four types of incoming mail and where it may be placed.

   a. _____

   b. _____

   c. _____

   d. _____

4. Before closing for the day, what kind of telephone calls does the receptionist make regarding the next day's schedule?

   _____

5. Name three examples of outgoing mail.

   a. _____

   b. _____

   c. _____

6. What must be done on the computer before closing down for the day?

   _____

7. Where are the duties of the chairside assistant centered?

   _____

8. What does the chairside assistant check before preparing for the day?

   _____

9. When closing for the day, what does the assistant do in the operatory?

   _____

10. What is done with the contaminated trash bundles and contaminated laundry at the end of the day?

   _____

Now turn to the Competency Evaluation Sheets for Procedure 61, Opening and Closing the Dental Business Office, and Procedure 62, Opening and Closing the Dental Operatory, located in Appendix C of this text.

TELEPHONE TECHNIQUES

One of the most important instruments in the dental office is the telephone. Telephone technique can make or break an office. The patient's first contact with the dental office is usually through the telephone, and business relations are maintained most frequently by phone conversations.

By using good telephone techniques, the assistant may make the office a more profitable and enjoyable place to work.

PROCEDURE 63
Telephone Techniques

1 **Assemble Equipment and Materials**

2 **Emergency Call Technique**

3 **Appointment Call Technique**

4 **Incoming Inquiry Call Technique**

5 **Personal and Professional Call Technique**

6 **Appointment Confirmation and Recall Technique**

1 Assemble Equipment and Materials

To efficiently work with the telephone, the dental assistant must be prepared. A pen or pencil and note pad should be beside each phone in every office area. The assistant must take notes when answering the phone because it is very easy to forget the call when times are busy or stressful. By making notes, the assistant is able to recall the conversation. Important facts, such as time of call, caller, reason, and message should be clearly and legibly written. The person taking the message should also sign the paper in the event there may be a question regarding the call.

Having an uncluttered area helps in the management of the telephone as an assistant may function better if not required to work around messy or cluttered materials.

The assistant answers the phone as soon as possible, speaking in a cheerful, plain, and distinct voice (Figure 11–4). Pencils, gum, or food in the mouth mumbles the speech, and the caller may not understand what the assistant is saying.

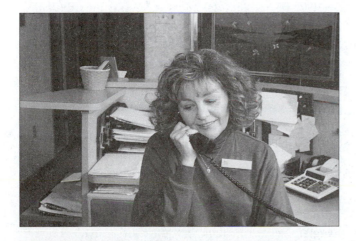

FIGURE 11–4 Telephone manners are very important as the phone is the lifeline of the dental facility.

When answering the phone, the office is identified. The speaker gives a name so that the party on the other side knows with whom the connection is made. The assistant identifies who is calling and uses the person's name frequently in the conversation.

2 Emergency Call Technique

When faced with an emergency call, the assistant must remain calm, identifying the caller and the problem as soon as possible. It is important to know how long the emergency has been occurring as some people may call with a "terrible" toothache that has been going on for two or three weeks.

An appointment may be given for immediate care, a referral may be offered, or the assistant may speak to the dentist to get advice on how to handle the emergency. Some offer of assistance is made for the patient's care.

3 Appointment Call Technique

When patients call for an appointment, the assistant screens the call by identifying the caller. If it is a regular patient, less information is needed. A new patient must be asked his or her name, address, and phone number so the office may be able to reach him or her in the event of an emergency or cancellation. These patients are also requested to bring in their card and benefit booklet if covered by insurance.

After determining the type of appointment needed, the assistant inquires about an acceptable time for the caller and offers that time or a selection of times close to the preferred period. Before hanging up, the caller is reminded of the date and time of the appointment. An appointment card may be sent to the caller if enough time permits between the call and the newly scheduled appointment.

4 Incoming Inquiry Call Technique

Many people call the office to make an **inquiry** into business or professional matters. The assistant identifies the caller and the problem, whether it be a question of insurance payment, statement, a "funny feeling" where the filling was placed, or whatever. If the problem needs research, such as looking up the insurance payments, the assistant asks the caller if he or she would prefer to be placed on "hold" or to be called back. If placing on "hold," the assistant never leaves for over 30 seconds without responding. When returning, always identify the caller before giving the information. The assistant makes sure the problem is settled and permits the caller to hang up first.

Care must be taken to maintain patient **confidentiality** and not to give out private information on the phone. When in doubt about the caller or the caller's intentions, inform them that the information needs to be looked up and offer to phone the caller at home with the answer. Look up the number on the record files and return the call personally.

5 Personal and Professional Call Technique

Personal and professional calls are always brought to the immediate attention of the dentist. Professional people offer the common **courtesy** of accepting calls as soon as possible. If the dentist is unable to come to the phone at that time, the assistant notifies the caller and suggests when the doctor will be free. The assistant offers to return the call at that time or lets the caller offer to call back. In either event, the dentist is notified that the call was received and the caller will return or expect a call at the earliest possible time.

If the call coming in is about a patient, the assistant obtains the records and takes them to the dentist so the information needed is at hand.

6 Appointment Confirmation and Recall Technique

The assistant places as well as receives calls. The most frequent type of calls made are appointment confirmation calls and recalls. The assistant calls the patient, identifies the office and caller, and confirms, not "reminds," the person of the upcoming appointment. Many broken or open appointment times are avoided by confirming the day before.

Recall appointments are made for patients previously scheduled to return to the office. When the dentist requests to see a patient in six months, the assistant writes the name and number on the recall page for six months ahead or enters it into the recall menu of the computer. On the first day of that month, the assistant calls the patient to schedule a recall appointment or runs off the computer's monthly recall list of printed postcards for scheduling time. Some patients schedule a recall appointment for future months and need only a reminder postcard sent. A few offices let the patient address the postcard and then hold it until a few days prior to the appointment. Repeat visits are handled in an assortment of ways.

If an appointment time suddenly becomes available, the assistant goes to the "on-call" list. Many people prefer to be called when there is some open time. These people may work in the same area or have irregular schedules that make appointment keeping difficult. When time becomes available, the assistant phones a patient on call, notifies him or her that a change in appointments has made a time available, and inquires if the patient wishes to take that time to come in.

7 Ordering Supplies Call Technique

The assistant uses the phone to make orders for supplies and materials. When calling a company to place an order, the assistant prepares before the call. A list of amounts, kinds, and stock numbers is made so all information is at hand when phoning. The assistant places the call, identifies the office and speaker, and places the order. A notation of the date ordered may be made if so desired.

8 Outgoing Inquiries Call Technique

The assistant also makes calls of inquiry, whether it be for prices, statements, laboratory case work, or lab results. When placing the calls, the assistant identifies the office and speaker and relates the problem. When satisfied with the reply, the results are noted and may be recorded on the patient's chart or invoice. It is best to prepare for outgoing calls. Knowing what is needed and required information makes the call more efficient and easy.

9 Collection Call Technique

Occasionally, the assistant makes a collection call. This is not a pleasant matter but must be done to maintain office expenditures. Before calling a patient, the assistant reviews the case with the dentist and gets permission to place the call. All phoning must be done at a reasonable hour so the patient is not inconvenienced. The assistant places the call, using a pleasant but matter-of-fact voice, stating the conditions of the account. Many people are just bad payers and need to be reminded, others have run into difficulty and need to rearrange their payment plan. The assistant listens to the patient and tries to establish some sort of payment. The results of the phone call and the arrangements made are recorded on the patient's card.

10 Followup Call Technique

The assistant places followup calls to patients who have had a difficult time or serious treatment. The assistant identifies the office and caller and inquires about the condition of the patient. Most patients enjoy the attention and relate their progress readily. The assistant listens to the conversation and lets the patient hang up when through. A quick jot is made on the patient's card to record the outcome.▲

THEORY RECALL

Telephone Techniques

1. When faced with an emergency call, how should the assistant act?

_____

2. Why is it important to get the name, address, and phone number of a new patient calling for an appointment?

_____

3. After making an appointment, what does the assistant do before hanging up?

_____

4. What does the assistant do before placing a caller on "hold?"

_____

5. If a professional is calling the dentist about a patient, what does the assistant do when putting the call through to the dentist?

_____

6. What is an "on-call" list?

_____

7. When placing a call to order supplies or make inquiries, what does the assistant do first?

_____

8. What does the assistant do before placing a collection call?

_____

9. Where are the results of the collection call conversation noted?

_____

10. What is a followup call?

_____

Now turn to the Competency Evaluation Sheet for Procedure 63, Telephone Techniques, located in Appendix C of this text.

APPOINTMENT SCHEDULING

The appointment book is the control center of the office. Bad scheduling may cause dull, unproductive days or times when patients are overcrowded and procedures are hectic and rushed. By choosing and placing patients into the right time slot, the dental assistant can organize the day and improve the work atmosphere.

To control the flow of patients correctly, the assistant must know how to operate the appointment book. A dentist may design an appointment book to **accommodate** the special office needs, use loose-leaf pages, or may purchase a standard one from the supply house. Most scheduling books are arranged so that when opened and flat on a surface the assistant may see a whole week at a glance. Some orthodontic practice appointment books provide views of monthly schedules.

Hours are divided into sections. The most popular divisions are the ten- and fifteen-minute sections or units. The day is divided into two or three columns, which can be used for scheduling patients for two chairs or for two or three operators. The dental hygienist may operate the hygiene patients from the central appointment book or may run one independently but coordinated with the doctor's scheduling.

The first thing an assistant does with a new appointment book is block or mark off any times the dentist will not be in the office. Hours before and after regular times are crossed out and special events or regularly scheduled meeting times are marked off as soon as planned.

Because changes in plans occur, appointments written into the scheduling book are done in pencil, preferably by one person. If the normal scheduling person is absent and another makes an appointment for a patient, the procedure is brought to the attention of the scheduler as soon as possible.

When penciling in an appointment, the assistant records the patient's name and phone number and the reason for the visit. New patients' names are circled or starred so the assistant can prepare the forms and necessary paper work before the patient arrives.

Each patient is allotted a specific amount of time by the manner in which the time periods are marked. When placing the patient's name in the book, the assistant assigns that time slot (10 or 15 minutes) to that person. If more time is needed to complete the procedure, the assistant draws an arrow down from the name line until enough time is reserved for the patient. Therefore, in a 15-minute unit block system, a one-hour appointment will take the original name line and three more lines reserved by an arrow (four units).

Just how much time to mark off for a patient may be difficult to judge, especially for a new assistant who does not know office procedures very well. Some offices keep office manuals specifying procedure needs and timing. If there is no manual, the assistant needs to write down and make a personal time frame to be prepared for scheduling. Many times the dentist writes on the patient's charge slip the time needed for the next appointment by putting down how many units to reserve, such as "3U."

It is also helpful to know or mark down how much lab time is needed between some appointments. The assistant must be careful not to schedule a patient's return before the lab work can be completed.

When scheduling for the day, the assistant tries to keep the day full but not rushed or crowded. Variety is also welcomed by the staff. No one wants to do the same procedure all day. More difficult patients are scheduled for the mornings or after lunch when everyone is fresher. Young children are scheduled in the morning before nap time and school children are scheduled after school for routine exams and minor work. If a school child requires a serious or complicated procedure, it may be scheduled for a school holiday or when the child may be excused from school. Usually the parent is quite helpful in the scheduling.

Patients are usually consulted about when they prefer to come to the dental office, and the assistant must work within their time frames. Some people go to the dentist before work, others want to come in after work, and still others may have transportation or babysitting problems and require more exacting times. Whatever the reason, the assistant should try to accommodate the patient's preference as much as possible. The assistant can write on the patient's chart the "best time" for future reference in scheduling.

Emergency patients call with problems and wish immediate attention. Many offices run a **buffer** time of one unit before lunch where emergencies can be placed. If no emergencies occur, the time may be used for catching up or preparing for the afternoon load. The dentist makes the decision whether or not to place a buffer unit in the schedule.

One word of caution: when scheduling the emergency patient, do not promise that the dentist will cure or fix the problem. The needed treatment may require a longer time period. Tell the patient that the dentist will look at the trouble and try to help. In this manner,

the assistant has not made a promise that the office cannot fulfill.

Everyone wears down during the day and the assistant should keep this in mind when scheduling. Minor visits, recall exams, and consultations may be scheduled for the late afternoon, if possible.

After reserving time for a patient in the appointment book, the assistant makes out an appointment card. This card serves as a reminder for the patient of the next visit. There are many different styles of attractive and eye-catching appointment cards; each card contains a space for the patient's name, date and day of appointment, and the time scheduled. The dentist's name, address, and phone number also should be on the card in the event the patient needs an appointment change.

Many offices use computers when scheduling dental appointments. While the practice may be different than writing into a book, the theory and background are the same. Instead of pencilling in an appointment time, the appointment page is called on the screen, and the patient's name is keyed into the computer. The same considerations for variety, blocks of time, and so forth are observed in both the computer and book scheduling processes (Figure 11–5).

```
                Appointments for 04-08-94 — Rooms 1 to 3

Time    :     Room #1       :     Room # 2        :     Room #3
────────────────────────────────────────────────────────────────
7:30am  :                   :                     :
7:45am  :                   :                     :
8:00am  : HOHMAN, MARY C.    : GILSON, FRANCIS      : KLINE, VIVIAN
8:15am  : Prov: #4           : Prov: #1             : Prov: #3
8:30am  : 18, 19 O -p+BASE   : 3,4 cc PREP & IMP    : Notes: EXM, P, CMX
8:45am  :    *     *         :       *     *        :     *      *
9:00am  :                    : MILLAR, JAMES P.     :     *      *
9:15am  :                    :       *     *        : Prov: #3
9:30am  :                    :       *     *        : Notes: EXM, P, FLU T
9:45am  :                    :       *     *        :     *      *
10:00am : KINGSTON, AUSTIN   : MANION, THOMAS A.    :     *      *
10:15am : Prov: #1           : Prov: #1             :     *      *
10:30am : Notes:  11 APICO   : Notes: A+18 MOD      : GILLIGAN, KRISTIN
10:45am :    *     *         :       *     *        : Prov: #3
11:00am :    *     *         :                      : Notes: EXM, P, BW
11:15am : SIEGAL, CATHERINE  : RODASH, OLGA--3 set  : GILLIGAN, KIMBERLY
11:30am : Prov: #2           : Prov: #2             : Prov: #4
11:45am : Notes: O BLEACH #2 :                      : Notes: EXM, P, BW
12:00pm :                    :                      :
12:15pm :                    :                      :
12:30pm :                    :                      :
12:45pm :                    :                      :
1:00pm  : SHOOTEST, KATHLEEN : BUSEMAN, MICHAEL     : BONFIDI, ROSA--PC-2
1:15pm  : Prov: #1           : Prov: #1             : Prov: #2
1:30pm  : Notes: 30 ROOT CANAL: Notes:6-10 C-C SPLINT: CABASH, JEFFREY
1:45pm  :    *     *         :       *     *        : Prov: #4
2:00pm  :    *     *         :       *     *        : NOTES: P,6X6 SEALANTS
2:15pm  :    *     *         :       *     *        :     *      *
2:30pm  : BEST, KERRI--8 MI R:       *     *        : DIEZ, CARLOS
2:45pm  : Prov: #2           :       *     *        : Prov: #1
3:00pm  :                    :                      : Notes: EXM, P, PROBE
3:15pm  :                    : ROCHARD, ASHEEM      :     *      *
3:30pm  : YOUNG, HARRY--SUT REM: Prov: #1           : BONNETT, ANNA
3:45pm  : BELL, MICHELE      : Notes: 3,4,5 BR #2   : Prov: #2
4:00pm  : Prov: #1           :       *     *        : Notes: CURETTAGE-L
4:15pm  : Notes: DENT ADJ    :       *     *        :     *      *
4:30pm  :    *     *         :       *     *        : CHIN, OKARI--PC#3
4:45pm  :    *     *         :       *     *        : Prov: #3
5:00pm  :                    :                      :
5:15pm  :                    :                      :
5:30pm  :                    :                      :
6:00pm  :                    :                      :
```

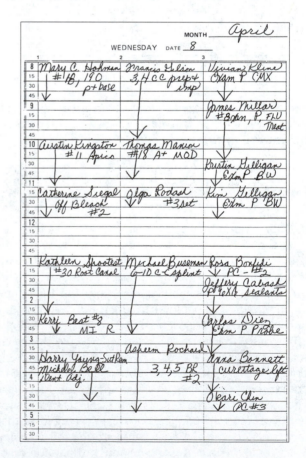

FIGURE 11–5 Whether the appointment control is (A) computer generated or (B) done in a book, the rules and considerations for scheduling patients are the same.

Making appointments seems like a difficult job at first, but it becomes very routine and relaxed once the assistant gets to know the office and the patients who visit. Everyone should feel comfortable about coming to the dentist and good appointment control starts the greeting process.▲

THEORY RECALL
Appointment Scheduling

1. What problems can bad scheduling cause to happen in the office?

_____

2. What are the time sections called?

_____

3. What is the first thing a dental assistant does with a new appointment book?

_____

4. What is written in the appointment book when making an appointment?

_____

5. Why is it important to list the phone number of a new patient in the appointment book?

_____

6. How does the assistant indicate the amount of time reserved for the patient after writing in the patient's name?

_____

7. What may a new assistant use to help determine the amount of time to reserve for a procedure?

_____

8. When are young children scheduled for dental office appointments?

_____

9. What is buffer time?

_____

10. What information is placed on an appointment card?

_____

For additional activities related to this lesson, turn to Assignment Sheet 11.1, Appointment Scheduling, located in Appendix B of this text.

PATIENT DENTAL RECORDS

New patients to the dental office receive special treatment starting with the making of an appointment. When the new patient's name is placed into the book it is starred or circled so that the assistant knows to schedule that person 15 to 30 minutes earlier than chair time. The new patient is given extra time to complete all the registration work necessary to complete the dental records of the office.

Exactly what preliminary information is needed for the office records is decided by the dentist, who should have questionnaires or blank fill-in forms to be completed by the patient. Most papers request statistical data, such as name, address, and phone numbers of patient, spouse, and work, plus insurance information. Health questionnaires may be short and minor or involved, depending on the nature of the dental office. The new dental assistant should become familiar with all forms before giving any to a patient. If the assistant does not understand the importance or relativity of a question, ask the dentist so that it can be explained if a patient makes inquiries.

Some offices hand a registration form and medical-dental health history inquiry to a patient to fill out and than review the answers with the patient using the information to make out the clinical file (Figure 11–6). Other offices interview the patient on a one-to-one basis to collect the information, perhaps keying the data into the computer, which prints out clinical records. No matter which method is used to obtain the data, both must be done in a quiet, private atmosphere. No one wishes to yell across a room what medication they are taking or any other personal information.

When interviewing or reviewing a patient's personal data, the assistant must act in a professional manner. Never show shock at an answer the patient gives and do not lose patience when the patient does not understand the questions. Take each question one at a time, and professionally write down the reply in the patient's own words or as near as possible to their words.

After the data has been collected, the receptionist may return the new patient to the reception room and offer a tour of the area, pointing out features, such as the location of the restroom, the lending library, the children's corner, or the beverage dispenser. Comments about other patients, whose pictures may be on a bulletin board, may help the patient feel as if he or she is being welcomed into a family or group. The new patient is introduced to the chairside assistant, who ushers the patient to the operatory area for the exam appointment.

Patient records involve more than registration data and medical-dental health history inquiries. Also included in the patient's file are the dentist's clinical examination, charting, and x-ray findings and any other items related to the care of the patient. Some offices include photographs or slide pictures and many offices, particularly the orthodontist, have case study models of each patient. All papers, mounted x-rays, pictures, and slides are kept in the patient's file. Case study models are stored in an arranged manner in a particular storage area.

DENTAL HEALTH HISTORY
(Confidential)

Today's Date_____

Patient Name_____ Birthdate_____
          Last   First   Initial

DENTAL HISTORY

Reason for Today's Visit_____

Former Dentist_____

Address_____

Date of last dental care_____ Date of last dental X-rays_____

Check (✓) if you have had problems with any of the following

☐ Bad breath   ☐ Grinding teeth   ☐ Sensitivity to hot
☐ Bleeding gums   ☐ Loose teeth or broken fillings ☐ Sensitivity to sweets
☐ Clicking or popping jaw   ☐ Periodontal treatment   ☐ Sensitivity when biting
☐ Food collection between teeth ☐ Sensitivity to cold   ☐ Sores or growths in your mouth

How often do you floss?_____ How often do you brush?_____

MEDICAL HISTORY

Physician's Name_____ Date of Last Visit_____

Have you had any serious illnesses or operations?_____ If yes, describe_____

Have you ever had a blood transfusion? ☐ Yes ☐ No   If yes, give approximate dates_____

(Women) Are you pregnant? ☐ Yes ☐ No   Nursing? ☐ Yes ☐ No   Taking birth control pills? ☐ Yes ☐ No

Check (✓) if you have or have had any of the following:

☐ AIDS   ☐ Cortisone Treatments   ☐ Hepatitis   ☐ Rheumatic Fever
☐ Anemia   ☐ Cough, Persistent   ☐ High Blood Pressure   ☐ Scarlet Fever
☐ Arthritis, Rheumatism   ☐ Cough up Blood   ☐ HIV Positive   ☐ Shortness of Breath
☐ Artificial Heart Valves ☐ Diabetes   ☐ Jaw Pain   ☐ Skin Rash
☐ Artificial Joints   ☐ Epilepsy   ☐ Kidney Disease   ☐ Stroke
☐ Asthma   ☐ Fainting   ☐ Liver Disease   ☐ Swelling of Feet or Ankles
☐ Back Problems   ☐ Glaucoma   ☐ Mitral Valve Prolapse   ☐ Thyroid Problems
☐ Blood Disease   ☐ Headaches   ☐ Nervous Problems   ☐ Tobacco Habit
☐ Cancer   ☐ Heart Murmur   ☐ Pacemaker   ☐ Tonsillitis
☐ Chemical Dependency   ☐ Heart Problems   ☐ Psychiatric Care   ☐ Tuberculosis
☐ Chemotherapy   Describe_____   ☐ Radiation Treatment   ☐ Ulcer
☐ Circulatory Problems   ☐ Hemophilia   ☐ Respiratory Disease   ☐ Venereal Disease

MEDICATIONS	ALLERGIES
List medications you are currently taking: _____ _____ Pharmacy Name_____ Phone_____	☐ Aspirin ☐ Penicillin ☐ Barbiturates (Sleeping pills) ☐ Sulfa ☐ Codeine ☐ Other_____ ☐ Local Anesthetic _____

SIGNATURE

The above information is accurate and complete to the best of my knowledge. I will not hold my dentist or any member of his/her staff responsible for any errors or omissions that I may have made in the completion of this form.

Date_ _____ Signature_____

FIGURE 11-6 A typical dental health history form. (Courtesy of Medical Arts Press, 1-800-328-2179.)

Throughout the active life of the new patient in the dental office, items will be added to the file. Copies of insurance billings, laboratory reports, updated films and exam findings, reference letters, and inquiries of any sort are kept together for quick reference.

All information included in the file is private and is the property of the dentist. The dental assistant is required by professional duty to maintain the confidentiality of all data.▲

THEORY RECALL

Patient Dental Records

1. How is a new patient designated in the appointment book?

   _____

2. Why does the receptionist request the new patient to arrive 15 to 30 minutes before chair time?

   _____

3. Who determines what information is needed for the dental office records?

   _____

4. What two methods are used to collect personal information from the new patient?

   a. _____

   b. _____

5. What two things should a dental assistant never do with a patient when collecting data?

   _____

6. What may the assistant do with the patient once the data has been collected?

   _____

7. What other records besides the registration information may be part of the patient's file?

   _____

8. What is added to the patient's file during the life of the account?

   _____

9. Whose property is the information in the patient's file?

   _____

10. What does "maintain confidentiality of the patient records" mean to the dental assistant?

   _____

For additional activities related to this lesson, turn to Assignment Sheet 11.2, Patient Dental Records located in Appendix B of this text.

RECORDS MANAGEMENT

Managing records is an important duty of the dental assistant. To run an office efficiently, the assistant must be able to locate data fast and often. Having a knowledge of filing can help the assistant locate items when needed and manage the flow of these records. There are four ways of filing items in the dental facility, **alphabetic**, **numeric**, **chronologic**, and by subject matter.

The most popular and common method is alphabetic. Papers, files, and items are placed according to the letter arrangement of their title. Most correspondence, patient files, and business papers fall into this sort of classification.

Patient's x-rays, study models, or photos may be assigned a number and be filed numerically. When a new patient is entered into the office computer, the machine accepts the data and assigns a patient number to the individual. In this manner, the file materials may be pulled up by using the patient's name or number. In the event that numbers are used to file or arrange items, a **cross-reference** book must be maintained. In cross-referencing, the name and number are given so the assistant may be able to locate the material by the patient's number or by the patient's name.

Names of recall patient's, future treatment plans, and some accounts that are on a payment plan are placed in a chronologic file arrangement. The patient's name may be placed in a file of a particular month and then filed numerically according to the due date.

Subject matter is used to place a collection of reports, items, or data relative to one particular subject. The assistant may use a subject matter file to place all invoices for utilities, another subject file for supplies to be ordered, another file for correspondence to be answered, or a file for insurance problems.

When an item falls into more than one category, the assistant places a cross-reference card in the file to help locate items. For example, if an insurance report concerning three family members has been received, the assistant may place the report in the insurance subject file and bright cross-reference cards in each patient's file to remind the assistant where to locate the paper.

Color plays an important part in the filing process. Many files have color-coded labels attached to aid in quick placement and retrieval. *As* may be colored bright orange, *Bs* may be pale blue, and so on. Color may be used to subdivide units also. *Aa* to *Am* may be yellow and *An* to *Az* may be black. By using this method, it is easy to spot a file that has been misplaced because it will bear a different color from the area in which it was placed. Color may also be added to indicate orthodontic cases, surgical, budget payment patients, difficult patients, or any other notation desired.

When working with either a vertical or horizontal file cabinet (Figure 11–7), the assistant must be careful to obey the safety rules. Never leave a file drawer open. Many people have bruised legs and fallen over drawers left open. Never pull out more than one drawer at a time. An entire filing cabinet could fall on the operator if too many drawers are pulled open and the weight is incorrectly distributed. Return all rotating horizontal files to their particular setting to avoid protruding file records.

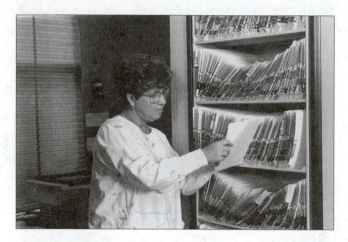

FIGURE 11-7 **A well-organized and managed filing system provides easy access to records.**

When it is necessary to remove a file, the assistant should insert an out file marker (a larger, bright-colored file sheet) in its place, close the drawer, and do the work required. When the job is completed, the drawer is reopened or the file is rotated into place, the out file marker is removed and placed in the back of the file contents for another time, and the patient's file is replaced in the proper slot. Never remove a file and loan it to another office without discussing it with the dentist and getting permission.

Preparation Procedure for Filing

The procedure for correct filing is **Indexing**, **Sorting**, and **Placing**.

INDEXING.   Indexing is the process of dividing the title of the item into divisions, called units. The title of the patient's file is the name of the patient. Names are separated into four units:

Unit 1 is the surname (last name of the patient).
Unit 2 is the given name (first name of the patient).
Unit 3 is the middle name or initial of the patient.
Unit 4 is the title or degree of the patient.

Other guidelines follow:
The most important rule of filing is that *nothing* is filed before *something*.

► When indexing a title, the assistant treats all hyphenated names as one.
► In all numbered names, such as 5th Avenue, the number is spelled out (Fifth Avenue).
► All possessive apostrophes, such as Coleman's Fish Market, are dropped (Coleman Fish Market).
► Abbreviations, such as St. Louis, are spelled out (Saint Louis).
► Compound names of towns, such as Las Vegas, are treated as one name. Businesses and firm names are treated in the same manner.

Some examples of indexing follow:

Title	1	2	3	4
Mrs. Richard Young (Mary Ellen)	Young	Mary	Ellen	Mrs. Richard
Rab. Max. Byestein	Byestein	Max		Rabbi
Miss Margaret Ann Brown	Brown	Margaret	Ann	Miss
George Fuller, Sr.	Fuller	George		Sr.
H. H. Harris	Harris	H.	H.	
Mr. Thomas Lyn-Smyth	Lyn-Smyth	Thomas		Mr.
19th Street Refuse Co.	Nineteenth	Street	Refuse	Co.
Gloria's Cleaners	Gloria	Cleaners		
St. Andrew's Golf Club	Saint	Andrew	Golf	Club
A-1 Auto Repair	A	one	Auto	Repair

SORTING.   Sorting is the process of arranging the indexed items in the sequential alphabetic order from A to Z, using the first letter of the first unit. If there is to be a choice in arrangement, the sorting continues through unit 1 and then into unit 2 and so on. That is why nothing is before something.

PLACING.   Placing is the process of putting the arrangement in properly and in order. All items are neatly placed. Any addition to the file is placed in the front of the file. Any items "borrowed" are noted with an out paper until returned.▲

Records Management

1. List the four methods of filing materials.

   a. _____

   b. _____

   c. _____

   d. _____

2. What item in the dental office may be filed numerically?

   _____

3. What is important to maintain when filing numerically?

   _____

4. Names of what kind of patients may be placed in a chronologic file?

   _____

5. List three subject matter files an assistant might maintain.

   a. _____

   b. _____

   c. _____

6. When an item falls into more than one category, what must an assistant do?

   _____

7. How does color help in the filing process?

   _____

8. What are the three procedures used for filing preparation?

   a. _____

   b. _____

   c. _____

9. How are hyphenated names treated in filing?

   _____

10. What is the most important rule of filing?

    _____

For additional activities related to this lesson, turn to Assignment Sheet 11.3, Records Management, located in Appendix B of this text.

BOOKKEEPING PROCEDURES

Bookkeeping procedures in the dental office can be completed on the office computer by entering files and following prompts or manually by inserting figures into papers with specific columns and adding and balancing totals at the end of the day, or monthly as for some recaps.

Pegboard or one write bookkeeping is a manual method of recording the business transactions of the day with a minimum of effort. Forms are strategically placed on a stiff-backed, pegged board so that a figure needs only to be written once. This system saves time by eliminating duplication of entries and lessens the chance of transposition errors (Figure 11–8).

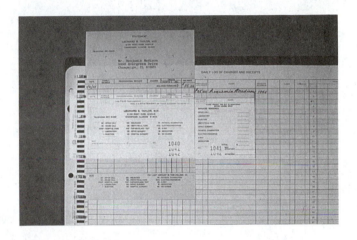

FIGURE 11-8 An example of a one write bookkeeping system. (Courtesy of Colwell Systems [Deluxe Forms].)

One Write Bookkeeping System

1 Assemble Equipment and Material

2 Register the Patient

3 Record Procedure and Charges

4 Record Payment

5 Make Future Appointments

6 Record Mail and Walk-in Payments

7 Assemble Insurance Superbill

8 Fill Out Deposit Slips

9 Reconcile Receipts

10 Clean Up Area

1 Assemble Equipment and Material

Before the first patient of the day arrives at the office, the assistant should get a new paper master sheet for the day's business and place it on a large board with pegs on the side (Figure 11–9). Even if the paper from yesterday still has room for entries, the assistant should place a new sheet for each day, and mark the date, and number as sheet 1 of 1. One sheet is usually enough for the typical office, but in a multiple practice, the assistant may need to place another sheet later in the day. This sheet will be labeled with the same date, but will be sheet 2 of 2, while sheet 1 becomes 1 of 2, and so on.

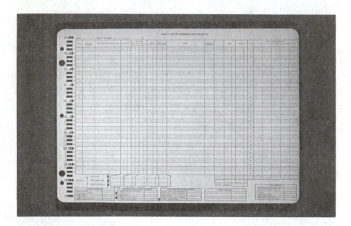

FIGURE 11–9 A new master sheet is placed on the pegboard each business day. (Courtesy of Colwell Systems [Deluxe Forms].)

After the master sheet is marked and in place, the assistant places a sheet of shingled charge slips and receipt papers on top of the master sheet (Figure 11–10). The first shingle fits on the first working line of the master sheet. These shingled papers are numbered, and the assistant starts today's shingle papers with the next number from yesterday's last receipt or charge number slip. For example, if the last entry yesterday was on #2478, today's entries start with the receipt or charge slip #2479.

The assistant should gather the **ledger cards** of the day's scheduled patients. Ledger cards are maintained on each account. They look exactly like a statement and show charges and payments made on the account. The ledger cards show the current balance of each account (Figure 11–11). When statement time nears, the assistant may make a copy of the ledger card and send it to the patient for payment. Since the ledger card file shows the financial charges and balances due the office, it is very important. Many offices place the file in the office safe at night or make sure the file is in a fireproof container and closed at the end of the office day.

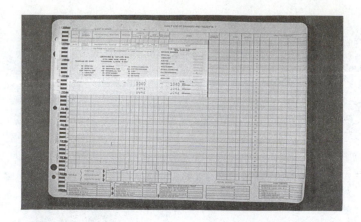

FIGURE 11–10 The charge and receipt slips are placed on the master sheet. Receipt numbers on the slips are kept in sequential order. (Courtesy of Colwell Systems [Deluxe Forms].)

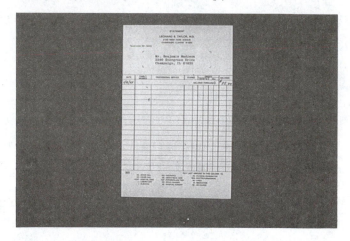

FIGURE 11–11 Each patient has a ledger card, which is used to record procedures and payments. (Courtesy of Colwell Systems [Deluxe Forms].)

To aid in the closing of the books and the depositing of the day's income, the assistant may use the **deposit** column on the master sheet by placing a preprinted deposit slip over the column and entering the figures throughout the day. At the end of the day, the column is totaled and the matched amount is placed in the bag with the slip, ready for deposit.

2 Register the Patient

When the patient enters, the pegboard system is activated by placing the patient's name on the charge slip and recording the receipt number on the master sheet. The assistant looks up the balance due by the patient and places that amount on the charge slip, which is then ripped off and clipped to the patient's file (Figure 11–12). The patient and the file are taken to the operatory for treatment and the dentist writes in the proce-

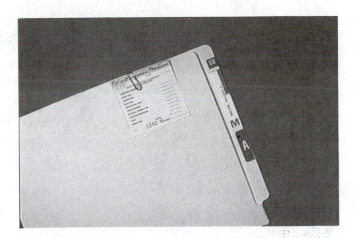

FIGURE 11-12 A charge slip is used to record services rendered, fees charged, and the need for future appointments. (Courtesy of Colwell Systems [Deluxe Forms].)

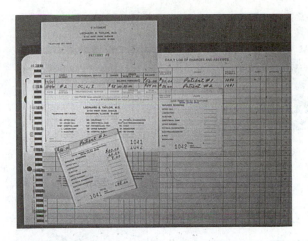

FIGURE 11-13 A completed master sheet. Each section of the sheet completes an individual bookkeeping service: (A) ledger card filled in, (B) charge and receipt data recorded, (C) deposit slip area, and (D) appointment card. (Courtesy of Colwell Systems [Deluxe Forms].)

dure completed and the charges to be made, if the office is not using a standard fee schedule. The dentist also notes how long before and how many appointments will be needed.

3 Record Procedure and Charges

The patient returns to the desk with the filled in charge slip. The assistant inserts the patient's ledger card under the receipt card and writes what was done in the procedure area and the charges made in the charge column and mentally calculates the new balance.

4 Record Payment

The assistant then asks how much the patient would like to pay on the account. This is a more positive statement than "Would you like to pay today?" When the patient gives an amount, the assistant writes that amount on the payment received area and computes and enters the new balance. The receipt card is removed from the pegboard. The ledger card is set aside and replaced later in the ledger file. Any cash or check payment made is marked in the appropriate column of the deposit section. In offices with more than one professional providing care, service fees may also be recorded in the appropriate column for the particular provider.

5 Make Future Appointments

If the dentist has requested a future appointment, as noted on the bottom of the charge slip, the assistant sets the time and date with the patient. The agreed on time is marked in the appointment book and on the bottom of the receipt or appointment card and given to the patient. The patient is dismissed, and the charge slip is placed in the patient's file (Figure 11–13).

6 Record Mail and Walk-in Payments

Occasionally, a patient will walk in to make payment on a bill. Each day the mail carrier delivers payments from patients and third parties (insurances). The assistant pulls the ledger card of the patient account receiving payment and places it on the first available line. No charge or receipt slip is used. In the receipt number column, the word "mail" is posted and in the professional services column the term ROA (received on account), is penned in. Payment is posted on the deposit slip area just as any other transaction.

If there is to be an adjustment, the dentist determines when to make an adjustment to the bill. The assistant places the amount of the payment in the payment column and the amount of the adjustment in the adjustment column, totals the two, and calculates the new balance for the patient.

7 Assemble Insurance Superbill

If the patient wishes to file for insurance coverage using the preprinted superbill, the assistant may remove the shingled receipt or charge slips and insert the superbill sheet (Figure 11–14). The processing is the same procedure, except the entire superbill is removed from the pegboard and sent to the operatory with the patient's file so the dentist may fill out the procedure, charge, and diagnosis.

When the superbill is returned from the operatory area, it is reinserted onto the pegboard and processed as the other slips. When processing is completed, the assistant removes the triple-layered superbill, has the patient sign the release of information and assignment

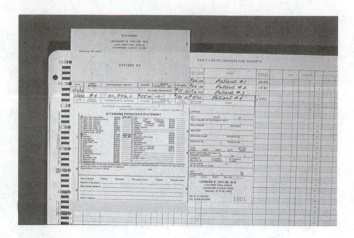

FIGURE 11–14 Many insurance companies accept the superbill which provides faster service and saves the assistant time in preparing the claim form, in lieu of the long form. (Courtesy of Colwell Systems [Deluxe Forms].)

of charges (if the payment is to come to the office), and gives two layers to the patient. One slip remains in the patient's file, the patient keeps one and mails the other to his or her insurance company for payment. The shingled receipt or charge slips are replaced on the pegboard. *Offices that use computer bookkeeping usually have a built in superbilling procedure that may be activated to print out a completed form.

8 Fill Out Deposit Slip

At the end of the day, the assistant totals the deposit cash and checks columns, the amount of cash on hand, and the checks, which were stamped "for deposit only," immediately upon receipt. The total figure for the cash and charge columns should match the amount of cash and checks on hand. The deposit slip is removed and placed in the bag with the cash and checks to be taken to the bank on the way home.

9 Reconcile Receipts

The books must be balanced at the end of the day. This is called proof of posting. Each column on the master sheet is added up, and the totals are placed in the designated lines at the bottom of the page. If the column totals match, the books balance and the processing is over (Figure 11–15). If they do not match, the assistant must review the entries until the error is found.

10 Clean Up Area

When proof of posting is completed, the bookkeeping duties for the day are done. The assistant checks the

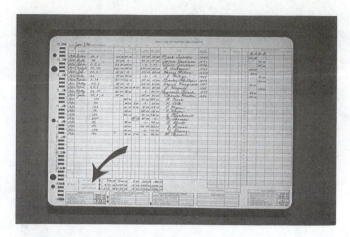

FIGURE 11–15 At the end of the day, a proof of posting ensures the bookkeeping practices are correct. (Courtesy of Colwell Systems [Deluxe Forms].)

patient's treatment cards to make sure the treatment and charges are entered correctly. The files are then replaced. The ledger cards are reviewed and replaced. If they are to be put in the safe, they are packed tightly together to prevent fire damage and put away for safekeeping.

The master sheet is removed from the pegboard and placed into a loose-leaf binder on top of yesterday's master sheet. The unused shingles are kept for tomorrow's use and the area is cleaned up for the day.▲

THEORY RECALL

Bookkeeping Procedures

1. What two methods may be used to complete bookkeeping procedures in the dental office?

    a. _____

    b. _____

2. What two benefits does the pegboard system of bookkeeping offer?

    a. _____

    b. _____

3. Where does the first shingle of the receipt or charge slip get placed?

    _____

4. What number should the first shingle slip contain?

    _____

5. Where does the assistant find the patient's balance due the office?

    _____

6. Where is the charge slip placed when it has been filled out?

_____

7. Where does the assistant insert the ledger card to receive charge and payment figures?

_____

8. If the patient requests a superbill for insurance purposes, where does the assistant place it?

_____

9. What does the total of the deposit slip match?

_____

10. Where is the master day sheet placed when the bookkeeping duties of the day are over?

_____

Now turn to the Competency Evaluation Sheet for Procedure 64, One Write Bookkeeping System, located in Appendix C of this text.

DENTAL INSURANCE

Part of the duties of the dental assistant involve working with dental insurance. Good management of dental insurance increases financial payments to the office and simplifies collection of accounts.

Although the procedure for filing claims is the same for most companies, each plan may be different. The assistant must be aware of the differences that can occur from policy to policy, even within the same company.

When a patient is making an appointment for the first visit, the assistant should inquire if there is dental insurance coverage. If so, the patient is requested to bring along his or her identification card and benefit booklet. The identification card shows the patient's policy numbers, which must be used on a claim form, and the benefit booklet explains just what type of coverage the patient may expect under this plan.

After reviewing the benefit booklet, the assistant may write down the type of coverage and requirements set by the insurance company (carrier). These items may be written into notes for the patient's file; if the office uses a computer, the information may be placed in the patient's data bank. When it is time to process a claim, the information will be at hand.

The assistant must know certain facts before processing a claim, such as if the carrier requires the dentist's services to be **pre-authorized** before work is started. Many companies require a claim form stating all proposed treatment to be submitted before work is to start, particularly if the total charge exceeds a specific amount. The assistant completes a claim, marks it pre-authorization in the upper left corner and submits it for approval (Figure 11–16). When the company sends approval, the work is completed. The claim is resubmitted, and payment is made.

One reason an insurance company may deny payment for services, is that the particular treatment desired is excluded, such as cosmetic dentistry or in some cases, orthodontic treatment. Another reason may be that the total for the treatment is too high. The policy may have a lifetime **maximum** or a yearly maximum, which limits the amount an insurance company may pay. If the limit is a yearly one, the policy book states if the limit is a calender year (January to December) or a policy year (one year from start date of policy).

If extensive and expensive treatment planning exceeds the policy limits, it is possible that one part of the desired services may be completed one year and another part of the treatment may be completed the following year.

Another reason for denying of payment may be that the patient is not covered by the policy. If the coverage is for individual membership, only the policyholder (**subscriber**) is covered. If it is for family coverage, the member (subscriber) and member's **dependents** (spouse and children) are covered, until the children reach a certain age, usually 18. If the child is still attending school after that age, the company may extend coverage until age 24 or 25. The policy book will state the rules of coverage for dependents.

Just how much payment the carrier will pay to the dentist or subscriber is determined by the type of coverage stated in the benefits booklet. The carrier pays

Dental Claim Form

Check one:	Carrier name and address
☐ Dentist's pre-treatment estimate	
☐ Dentist's statement of actual services	

P A T I	1. Patient name first m.i. last	2. Relationship to employee ☐ self ☐ child	3. Sex m f	4. Patient birthdate MM DD YYYY	5. If full time student school

FIGURE 11–16 The claim form may be sent in as a pre-authorization request or as a claim for services. The appropriate box is checked. (Courtesy of Colwell Systems [Deluxe Forms].)

by two methods—a **schedule of benefits** and **UCR** (usual, customary, and reasonable).

A schedule of benefits is basically just that, a table stating how much is allotted for each treatment service. The amount may or may not be the fee set by the dental office. The patient receives the scheduled payment; if the fee is higher, the patient is responsible for the remainder of the bill. Some government plans offer a set schedule that the dentist, if accepting this patient, agrees to accept as full payment.

UCR is the usual, customary, and reasonable fee for that type of treatment in that particular area. The carrier companies research these factors and set their UCR payment fees and pay accordingly. After averaging the survey the carriers arrive at a figure that is usual (U) for that area, a customary (C) charge by the dentists in that specified area, and a reasonable (R) fee for that particular service. Most companies pay percentages of the UCR after a deductible has been paid by the subscriber.

Deductibles are certain amounts that must be paid by the patient before the carrier considers payment. A deductible may be per individual or per family. The specific amount for each policy is written in the benefit booklet. Some preventive treatments, such as prophylaxis and examination do not require a deductible payment.

The percentage amount of UCR payment is also written out in the policy's benefit booklet. Most carriers pay 100 percent of UCR fees for preventive dentistry, such as exams, prophylaxis, and x-rays. Restorative dentistry services may receive only 60 to 80 percent of the UCR or whatever is in the booklet.

When a patient has coverage under more than one policy, a **coordination of benefits** principle determines which carrier pays what amount. The claim is sent first to a primary carrier. After that company pays its fees, the claim is resubmitted to the secondary company so it may pay its amount of payment. The employee's (subscriber) policy is the primary carrier and the spouse's company is the secondary company. When children in a family with double coverage need a claim filed, it is sent first to the carrier of the parent with the first birthday of the year and then to the carrier company of the other parent whose birthday is later in the year.

A claim must be submitted to the carrier for payment. There are different ways this processing may be completed. Offices using computer management of patient records, may key in procedures completed. The computer has already been programmed to process the codes and office fees per procedure. Since the assistant has programmed the patient information and insurance benefits from the booklet, the computer may print out a completed insurance claim to be sent to the company.

The assistant may be using a manual pegboard system of patient management. When registering the patient for treatment, the assistant places a superbill shingle on the pegboard and then clips it to the patient's file for the dentist to complete in the operatory. When the patient returns from the treatment, the assistant fills in the new charges and balances, gives the patient two copies, and keeps the third. The patient may then mail a copy of the superbill to the carrier for payment. The third method is to fill out a standard dental insurance claim form (Figure 11–17).

PROCEDURE 65

Processing a Dental Insurance Claim

1 Assemble Equipment and Materials

2 Complete Patient Section

3 Complete Attending Dentist Section

4 Complete Examination and Treatment Section

5 Obtain Signatures

6 Prepare Envelope

7 Clean Up Area

1 Assemble Equipment and Materials

To complete the procedure, the assistant needs:

▶ a dental insurance claim form
▶ patient information
▶ patient treatment record
▶ a booklet of procedures codes handy for listings

The assistant specifies if the claim is for payment or for pre-authorization and types in the carrier's name and address.

2 Complete Patient Section

The first section of the claim needs patient information (Figure 11–17A). The assistant types in the patient's information, which may be obtained from the patient records. If the patient is a child, the parents' names are used in the employee section. When both parents are employed, the father is usually placed as employee and the mother is placed in the spouse area.

3 Complete Attending Dentist Section

The second section requests the dentist's statistical information and inquires into the type and place of treatment (Figure 11–17B). The assistant can fill this data in from the treatment records.

Attending Dentist's Statement

Check one:
- ☐ Dentist's pre-treatment estimate
- ☒ Dentist's statement of actual services

Carrier name and address
Dental Care Insurance Company
1500 Western Avenue
Middleton, CA 98765

A — PATIENT SECTION

1. Patient name			2. Relationship to employee	3. Sex	4. Patient birthdate	5. If full time student
first	m.i.	last	☒ self ☐ child	m / f	MM DD YYYY	school city
Jason	P.	Rangers	☐ spouse ☐ other____	x	11 24 1950	--

6. Employee/subscriber name and mailing address
Self
2356 Harmony Avenue
Prospect, CA 98766

7. Employee/subscriber soc. sec. number
111-22-3333

8. Employee/subscriber birthdate
MM 11 DD 24 YYYY 1950

9. Employer (company) name and address
Sanders Refuse
14th&Main Sts.
Prospect, CA

10. Group number
4590

11. Is patient covered by another plan of benefits?
Dental none
Medical health

12-a. Name and address of carrier(s)
Maxima Health Ins.

12-b. Group no.(s)
2847B

13. Name and address of employer
none

14-a. Employee/subscriber name (if different than patient's)

14-b. Employee/subscriber soc. sec. number
same

14-c. Employee/subscriber birthdate
MM DD YYYY
----

15. Relationship to patient
☒ self ☐ parent
☐ spouse ☐ other____

I have reviewed the following treatment plan. I authorize release of any information relating to this claim. I understand that I am responsible for all costs of dental treatment.

► *Jasin P. Rangers* 8-15-xx
Signed (Patient, or parent if minor)   Date

I hereby authorize payment directly to the below named dentist of the group insurance benefits otherwise payable to me.

► *Jason P. Rangers* 8/15/xx
Signed (Insured person)   Date

B — DENTIST SECTION

16. Dentist name
Jay V. School

17. Mailing address
5600 Professional Building SuiteD
City, State, Zip
Prospect, CA 98766

18. Dentist Soc. Sec. or T.I.N.
999-88-7777

19. Dentist license no.
CA8476

20. Dentist phone no.
302-555-1111

21. First visit date current series
8/1/xx

22. Place of treatment
Office x Hosp. ECF Other

23. Radiographs or models enclosed?
No Yes x How many?

	No	Yes	If yes, enter brief description and dates.
24. Is treatment result of occupational illness or injury?	x		
25. Is treatment result of auto accident?	x		
26. Other accident?	x		
27. Are any services covered by another plan?	x		
28. If prosthesis, is this initial placement?			(If no, reason for replacement)
30. Is treatment for orthodontics?	x		

29. Date of prior placement

If services already commenced enter:
Date appliances placed
Mos. treatment remaining

C

Identify missing teeth with "x"

FACIAL
RIGHT UPPER PERMANENT PRIMARY LEFT
LOWER
FACIAL

32. Remarks for unusual services

31. Examination and treatment plan - List in order from tooth no. 1 through tooth no. 32 - Use charting system shown.

Tooth # or letter	Surface	Description of service (including x-rays, prophylaxis, materials used, etc.) Line No.	Date service performed Mo. Day Year	Procedure number	Fee	For administrative use only
		1 oral examination	08 01 xx	0 0120	24 00	
		2 Bite wing radiographs(2)	08 01 xx	0 2720	16 00	
		3 Prophylaxis	08 01 xx	0 1110	32 00	
8	M	4 Composite restoration 1 sur	08 15 xx	0 2330	44 00	
18	MO	5 Amalgam restoration 2 sur	08 15 xx	0 2150	48 00	
		6				
		7				
		8				
		9				
		10				
		11				
		12				
		13				
		14				
		15				

I hereby certify that the procedures as indicated by date have been completed and that the fees submitted are the actual fees I have charged and intend to collect for those procedures.

► _____ Date 8/16/xx
Signed (Dentist)

Total Fee Charged	164 00
Max. Allowable	
Deductible	
Carrier %	
Carrier pays	
Patient pays	

Form approved by the
American Dental Association
(ADS 85)
#29375 - Medical Arts Press 1 800 328 2179

FIGURE 11-17 A typical dental insurance claim form. (Courtesy of Medical Arts Press 1-800-328-2179.)

4 Complete Examination and Treatment Section

The treatment exam and plan section is the third section (Figure 11–17C). Here, the assistant types in tooth number, treatment, date of treatment, and procedure number, and then states the office fee. All services completed are placed on one claim and any services being planned in pre-authorization are included on another statement.

Procedure codes are numbers determined by the American Dental Association (ADA) to indicate certain services. Each treatment service has a particular five-digit number and may be found grouped into specialties or like services. For example, a prophylaxis group number is 011xx. An adult prophylaxis would have the number 01110 and a child's prophylaxis would have the number 01120. The payment rendered is based on these code numbers, so the assistant must be careful to use the correct code for the correct service. Keeping a list of the most frequent numbers and a code book of all code numbers handy will make the processing easy.

The mouth diagram on the chart is used to indicate position and placement of appliances. The dentist may or may not outline on this diagram. If the treatment is too complicated or a procedure number does not fit the exact service, the dentist may send a letter or drawing to help explain the treatment.

5 Obtain Signatures

There are three signature lines on the claim form: (a) The patient signs the release of information line, giving permission for the insurance company to make inquiries of the care. If the patient is a minor, the parent may sign. (b) The insured, which may or may not be the patient, assigns the carrier to pay the dentist for the services. Some offices require the patient to pay fully for the services and then submit claims without assigning the payment to the dentist. The patient is paid the benefits if the assignment line is not signed. (c) The dentist's signature line is in the dental section and is filled in and dated when the form is completed. The finished claim form is photocopied.

6 Prepare Envelope

An envelope addressed to the carrier is completed, and the claim is sent for processing. Any radiographs, slides, or other materials are included with the claim. The proper postage is placed on the envelope, and it is stamped and mailed.

7 Clean Up Area

The patient's chart is marked and dated, stating the insurance claim was sent. A copy of the claim is placed in the patient's file. The dental insurance log is filled in, noting the claim has been sent. An insurance log is a sheet of paper divided into columns. It indicates the progress of a claim. The patient's name, claim, carrier, and date are marked. When something occurs with the claim, it is noted on the log; the assistant knows the exact state of processing for the claim. When the claim has been paid, the name is erased or washed off the log sheet.▲

THEORY RECALL
Dental Insurance

1. What is the new patient requested to bring to the office if there is dental insurance coverage?

2. What is the difference between a pre-authorization and a claim form?

3. What is the difference between family and individual coverage?

4. What are the two payment methods used by insurance companies?

   a.

   b.

5. In coordination of benefits, which company pays benefits first?

6. The first section of a standard claim requests information about whom?

7. What are procedure codes?

8. Who signs the release of information line on the claim form?

9. Who signs the assignment of benefits line?

10. How may an assistant keep track of the progress of an insurance claim?

Now turn to the Competency Evaluation Sheet for Procedure 65, Processing a Dental Insurance Claim, located in Appendix C of this text.

CHECKING ACCOUNTS

Writing Checks

A check is a written order to the bank to pay a specific amount of money to a designated person. In most dental offices, it is the responsibility of the dental assistant to prepare the checks, but the authority to sign them rests with the dentist. Checks are usually written twice a month. The assistant accumulates the invoices, statements, bills, and expenses in a subject file until nearing payroll day. Then, all expenses for the first half of the month are reviewed, and checks are written. The process is repeated at the end of the month.

The assistant would be wise to select a quiet time to prepare checks; interruptions may lead to errors. All statements received since the last check-writing session are taken out of the subject file. Any invoices covered by the statement are reviewed and then stapled together with the statement. If the figures are correct, the check is written for the amount of the statement; the number and date of the check are written on the part of the statement to be kept and filed. A return envelope is prepared for mailing the remittal part of the statement and check. The process is repeated until all expenses for the time period have been answered.

The collection of prepared checks are paper clipped to their envelopes and placed on the dentist's desk for signatures. If the assistant feels there may be a question regarding any of the checks, it may be wise to include the statement and invoices in the paper clip with the check for the dentist's inspection.

After the checks have been signed and returned, the assistant places each in its envelope, seals them, applies postage, and mails them. The statement stubs and invoices, which have been marked with check number and date of payment, are filed under their specific title. The checkbook is put away until the next writing session.

Just as the dental office may have a one write system for incoming funds, there is a one write system for outgoing monies (Figure 11–18). A sheet of checks is placed on a master card and the dates, payees, and amounts are filled in. The checks are sent, and the master sheet is retained as a record, similar to a stub or a check register in a private account. Checks from this system fit into a window envelope, save time, and permit fewer transposing errors.

For offices using a checkbook stub method, the first step in writing a check is to fill in the stub. The assistant uses a pen to write in the date, the name of the person receiving the check, the reason, and the amount of the check in the stub area. The balance brought forward from the last check is added together with any deposits made since the last check was written and then totaled for a new balance. The amount of the check being written is subtracted from the new balance, which in turn gives another new balance brought forward. All math may be completed in pencil until the checking account has been reconciled. In this way, any corrections may be made and then marked over with pen for permanent keeping (Figure 11–19).

Once the stub has been filled in, the check may be written. A check that has been completed on a typewriter is more professional than a handwritten one. Since a business prepares more checks a month than a personal account, business checks are printed three to a page. After the assistant has filled in the stubs for the page, the check page may be ripped off, placed in the typewriter and filled in, making sure to match the check number with the stub number.

The date is filled in first. It is more professional to type out the name of the month than to use abbreviations or month numbers. The next line is the **payee** line. The payee is the person or company receiving the check payment. The name is typed in as close to the left margin as possible, to prevent any insertions or alterations. At the end of that same line is a dollar sign and a blank where the amount of the check is typed in, using figures.

The middle line of the check is the place to type out the figure in letters. The first figure is capitalized and the rest are not, except where the check is written out for an amount under a dollar. The dollars are spelled out, then the word "and" is typed before the cents amount. The cents may be written out as forty three cents, 43/100, or 43/xx.

On the bottom, there is a "for" or "memo" line on which the assistant may write in the reason for the check, such as supplies or December statement. The signature line is left blank for the dentist to sign (Figure 11–19).

Making Deposits

Money is placed in the account by using a deposit form. As mentioned earlier, this process is completed at the end of each workday when the daily receipts are totaled. All paper money collected is arranged with the faces positioned the same way in a pile with the largest bill on the top, getting smaller down through the pile. The amount is totaled and written on the currency line. Any coins are totaled and wrapped, if there are enough for a wrapper.

Before inserting the checks into the bag, the assistant reviews the back of the checks for the endorsement stamp. On receipt, the assistant should stamp "For deposit only" along with the dentist's account number on every check that comes into the office. In this manner, no one may take the check and cash it. By endorsing the check for deposit only, the bank has no choice but to place the amount into the dentist's account.

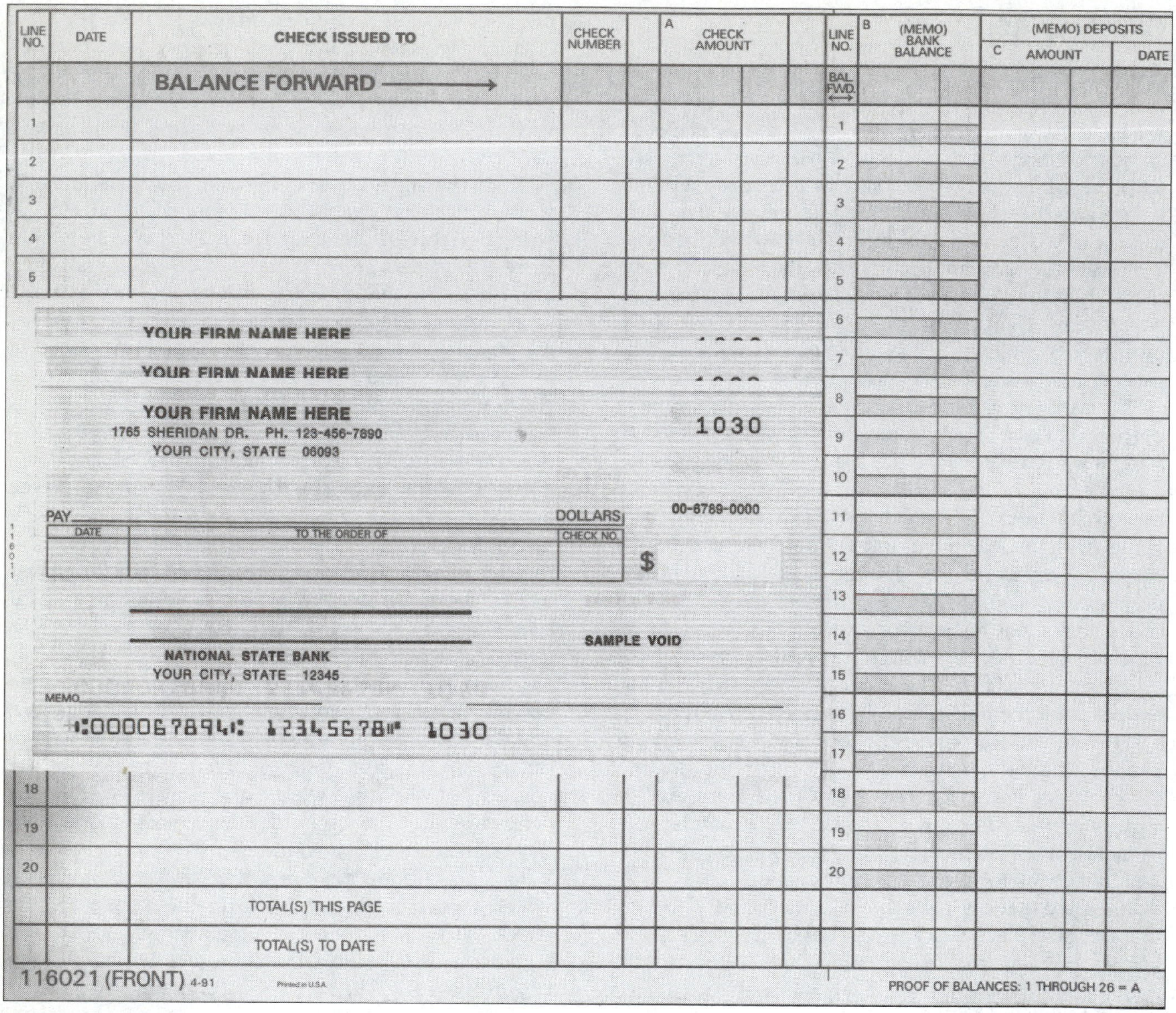

FIGURE 11-18 Some offices use a one write check system to provide fast service and few errors. (Courtesy of Colwell Systems [Deluxe Forms].)

The deposit slip and the money and checks are either placed in a deposit bag or taken directly to the bank for deposit. The teller gives the assistant a deposit receipt when receiving the money directly; if a bag is deposited, the assistant goes to the bank the next day and asks the teller for the empty deposit bag. The teller requests the assistant to sign for the bag and then presents the assistant with the bag, which is taken to the office, opened, and the deposit receipt is removed. The amount of the deposit is listed on the stub page and the receipt is placed in a file folder. It is kept there until bank statement reconciliation time.

Reconciliation

Once a month the bank returns all the checks that have been processed and a reconciliation statement. On the top of the statement, there is a review of the business that has occurred throughout the month. The beginning balance is shown. The total number and amount of deposits and the total number and amount of drafts are shown. Any charges made and the ending balance of the account are shown also.

The bottom part of the sheet shows the daily **transactions**, indicating the drafts on the left, the deposits in the middle, and the running daily total amount on the right side. The amount at the bottom of the right column is the amount the bank credits the account on the last day of the statement. This amount does not usually appear the same in the checkbook; therefore, the assistant must complete a **reconciliation** or balancing of the books.

The first process in a reconciliation is to arrange the checks in numeric order and find what checks have not cleared with the bank. These are called **outstand-**

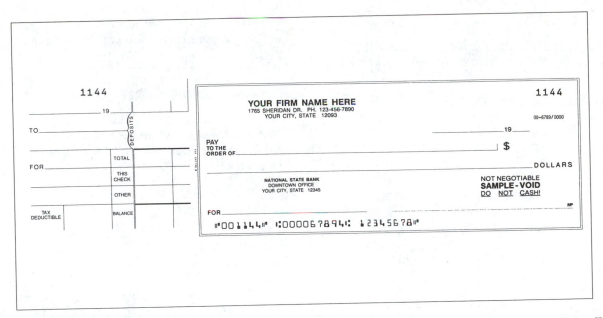

FIGURE 11-19 All information on the stub and the check must match exactly. (Courtesy of Colwell Systems [Deluxe Forms].)

ing checks. The outstanding checks are listed and totaled. The deposits are checked. Any missing deposits are listed and totaled. The assistant may turn the statement over and use the reconciliation form printed on the back or may make another form. The basic idea is to place the bank figure on one side of the page and the checkbook figure on the other. The outstanding check total is added to the checkbook account balance. Any deposits in transit total is subtracted from the checkbook account and any service charge made by the bank is subtracted from the checkbook balance. After the math has been completed, the figures should be the same and reconciliation is completed. The statement and **cancelled checks** are placed in the file. The checkbook is marked showing the outstanding checks and deposits and math to indicate where the next month's accounting will begin.

If the figures do not match, the assistant must review the checking account to find the error. Most times it is in the math. Occasionally, the assistant makes a transposition error (for example, writing the check for $14.23 and entering the amount in the stub as $14.32). The assistant may check this possibility out when reviewing for outstanding checks. The assistant may check the amount of the check with the stub amount at the beginning of the process.

The only money to go out of the office is through the checking account. Occasionally, there is need of a small amount for postage or a newspaper or whatever. A petty cash fund can be maintained to cover these small, quick expenses. The assistant makes out a check for $25 or whatever small amount the dentist prefers. This check is cashed and placed in an envelope. Whenever an amount is used for an expense, the figure is subtracted from the $25 and the voucher for the use is placed inside. This continues until the envelope needs replenishing. At that time, the assistant writes out another check, placing that amount plus any change left over into a new envelope. The original petty cash envelope is filed with the vouchers in the file cabinet. The new envelope is used for funding. In this way all expenses are accounted for.▲

THEORY RECALL

Checking Accounts

1. What is a check?

2. Whose responsibility is it to sign the checks for the dental office?

3. What is written on the statement to be filed, after the check has been written to cover the expense?

4. If the assistant feels the dentist may have a question regarding a statement, what is attached to the check to be signed?

5. What is the first step when writing a check?

6. Who is the payee in a check writing experience?

_____

7. What does the assistant do when receiving a check?

_____

8. What is checking account reconciliation?

_____

9. What kind of error is it when the figures on the check and the stub are not the same?

_____

10. Where does the assistant keep the vouchers or receipts for the petty cash money spent?

_____

For additional activities related to this lesson, turn to assignment Sheet 11.4, Checking Accounts, located in Appendix B of this text.

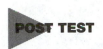

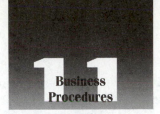

Total possible points = 100 points
80% needed for passing = 80 points

Total points this test _____ pass _____ fail _____

MULTIPLE CHOICE: Circle the correct answer. Each question is worth 4 points for a total of 100 points.

1. When calling a patient to inquire about the condition following surgery, the assistant is making which type of phone call?
   a. followup   b. inquiry   c. confirmation   d. emergency

2. What should be done with mail that is marked "personal"?
   a. Open it and place it on top of the mail pile.   c. Leave it unopened and place it on the dentist's desk.
   b. Open it and answer it as best you can.   d. Wait until the dentist asks for the personal mail.

3. When dividing a title into little sections for filing purposes, what are the sections called?
   a. sections   b. word divisions   c. index units   d. file areas

4. Which of the following information is *not* usually placed on the appointment card?
   a. the doctor's name and address   c. the time and day of the appointment
   b. the patient's name   d. the procedure planned for the appointment

5. What is meant by the term "maintaining records confidentiality"?
   a. Keep all records and information gathered private.
   b. Keep all records and information in good working order.
   c. Keep all records and information up to date.
   d. Type or print in bold type to show confidence.

6. When paying a statement by check, which line on the check is used to show who is receiving the payment?
   a. the payee line   b. the signature line   c. the amount line   d. the "for" line

7. What is an appointment call list?
   a. a confirmation call list
   b. a list of patients to call when an appointment time becomes available
   c. a list of items to order
   d. a person who called in for an appointment time

8. Who signs the assignment of benefits line on an insurance claim form?
   a. DDS   b. patient   c. subscriber   d. insurance agent

9. How many copies of the superbill are given to the patient?
   a. 1   b. 2   c. 3   d. 4

10. What is *not* usually printed in the insurance benefit booklet?
    a. the patient's name and address   c. the limit of permitted expenses
    b. the type of coverage for patient   d. the effective dates of the insurance

11. In a recall appointment the patient
    a. calls for the first visit.   c. makes a future appointment.
    b. completes current treatment.   d. makes up an appointment for one the patient didn't recall or remember.

12. How soon should a phone be answered?
    a. on the first ring   c. on the fifth ring
    b. after a while so the patient knows the dentist is busy   d. it does not matter when the phone is answered

13. Which type of call is the most frequently placed call by an assistant?
    a. an emergency call   b. an inquiry call   c. a confirmation call   d. a call to order supplies

14. What does the assistant do when receiving a check for payment on account?
    a. places it in the drawer
    b. places it in the deposit bag
    c. shows the dentist
    d. endorses the back of the check

15. In coordination of benefits, which company pays first for the services given the worker member?
    a. the spouse's insurance
    b. the dependent's insurance
    c. the subscriber's insurance
    d. none of the above

16. Who is responsible for signing the checks used to pay the office invoices and bills?
    a. the dentist   b the dental hygienist   c. the dental assistant   d. the office manager

17. Insurance coverage for a husband and wife is considered which type of insurance?
    a. independent   b. family   c. dependent   d. company

18. Which of the daily totals must match the figure on the deposit slip?
    a. charge business
    b. amount received business
    c. mail business
    d. the total of all business transactions

19. Where does the dental assistant find the current balance of a patient's account?
    a. on the ledger card
    b. on the patient's statement
    c. on the charge list
    d. in the file case

20. Which is *not* considered an accepted manner for filing records?
    a. numeric   b. chronologic   c. alphabetic   d. selective

21. After answering the phone, what is the first thing an assistant must do?
    a. tell the caller about the good work the dentist does
    b. ask if the caller has insurance
    c. identify the reason for the call
    d. determine the caller's mood

22. What are ADA insurance procedure codes?
    a. code letters among professionals
    b. numbers for the patients
    c. insurance code for treatment procedure
    d. code letters used to find the proper insurance company to pay account

23. What form is used to place money into the office's checking account?
    a. deposit   b. check   c. savings   d. withdrawal

24. Before placing a caller on hold, what should the assistant do?
    a. Ask what type of music the patient likes.
    b. Tell the patient to "wait a second."
    c. Ask if the patient minds being placed on hold.
    d. Don't ask, just push the button.

25. What item should be placed near the phone to help the assistant talk correctly and nicely?
    a. gum   b. a pencil for chewing   c. candy to sweeten the voice   d. a mirror

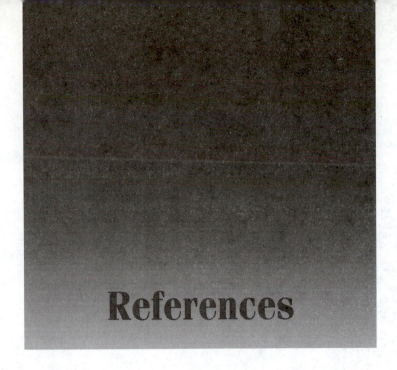

References

Anderson, P. C., & Burkard, M. R. (1994). *The dental assistant* (6th ed.). Albany: Delmar Publishers.

Anderson, P. C., & Clifford, S. B. (1981). *Dental radiography*. Albany: Delmar Publishers.

Bloodborne infections: A practical guide to OSHA compliance. (1992). Arlington, TX: Johnson and Johnson.

Castano, F. A. & Allen B. (1973). *Handbook of expanded dental auxiliary practice*. Philadelphia: J. B. Lippincott.

Chasteen, J. E. (1989). *Essentials of clinical dental assisting* (6th ed.). St Louis: C. V. Mosby Company.

Chernega, J. B. (1994). *Emergency guide for dental auxiliaries* (2nd ed.). Albany: Delmar Publishers.

Community CPR. (1993). American Red Cross. St. Louis: Mosby Lifeline.

Controlling occupation exposure to bloodborne pathogens in dentistry. (1992). U.S. Department of Labor. OSHA.

deLyre, W. & Johnson, A. N. (1990). *Essentials of dental radiography for dental assistants and hygienists* (4th ed.). Englewood Cliffs: Prentice-Hall, Inc.

Dental dam procedures (9th ed.). (1992). Akron, OH: Hygienic Corporation.

Ehlrich, A. & Torres, H. (1990). *Essentials of dental assisting* (4th ed.). Philadelphia: W. B. Saunders Company.

Emergency response workbook. (1993). American Red Cross. St. Louis: Mosby Lifeline.

Flight, M. (1988). *Law, liability, and ethics for medical office personnel*. Albany: Delmar Publishers.

Intraoral radiography with Rinn XCP/BAI instruments. (1989). Elgin, IL: Rinn Corporation.

Kelly, M. C. (January/February 1994). Infection control: Handpiece sterilization. *The Journal of Practical Hygiene*, 3(1), 8–9.

Keir, L., Wise, B. A., & Krebs-Shannon, C. (1993). *Medical assisting: Clinical and administrative competencies* (2nd ed.). Albany: Delmar Publishers.

Littrell, J. J. (1984). *From school to work*. South Holland, IL: Goodheart-Willcox Company, Inc.

National Institute of Health. (January 1993). Clinical evaluation and public health aspects of high blood pressure. *Dental Hygienist News*, 6(4), 3–5.

Paarmann, C. (January/February 1993). Finishing, recontouring, and polishing amalgam restorations. *The Journal of Practical Hygiene*, 2(1) 9–15.

Schwarzrock, S. & Jensen, J. (1982). *Effective dental assisting* (6th ed.). Dubuque, IA: Wm. C. Brown Company.

Simmers, L. (1993). *Diversified health occupations* (3rd ed.). Albany: Delmar Publishers.

Sterilization in the medical and dental office. (1988). Erie, PA: AMSCO.

Torres, H. O. & Ehrich, A. (1990). *Modern dental assisting*. Philadelphia: W. B. Saunders.

Wasserman, D. (July/August 1993). The hygiene olympiad: A step by step checklist. *Practical Hygiene*. 2(4), 31–33.

X-rays in dentistry. (1985). Rochester, NY: Eastman Kodak Company.

Young, J. (March/April 1994). Dental handpieces and the clinician. *Dental Teamwork*. 7(2), 33–36.

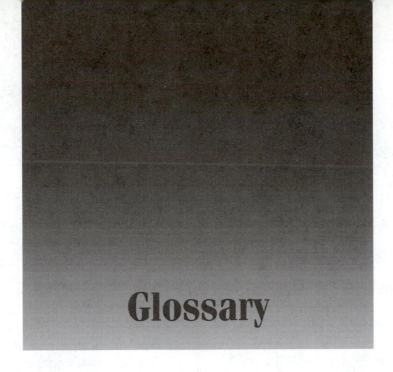

Glossary

abrasive—condition of being rough; grinding or wearing away
Abrasive wheels are used to smooth and polish dental appliances.

abutment—prepared tooth that is part of a fixed bridge
The **abutment** may hold a crown, inlay, or onlay and be part of a fixed bridge.

accelerate—chemical or material speeding up or hastening a reaction
Some chemicals or products need another chemical to **accelerate** setting up.

acclimate—to become accustomed to; to get used to
The patient's mouth must **acclimate** to the new appliance.

accommodate—to fit in or make room for
There must be enough room in the preparation to **accommodate** the fixed bridge.

acrylic—plastic type of material frequently used in dental appliances
Care must be taken when cleaning the **acrylic** denture.

activator—appliance or chemical that speeds up or helps a reaction occur
Some cements need an **activator** to get hard.

adjacent—nearby; next to; touching
The central incisors are **adjacent** to each other.

aggravate—to irritate; to annoy
Eating or drinking hot or cold foods could **aggravate** a sensitive tooth.

ALARA (As Low As Reasonably Achievable)—lowest possible amount of x-ray exposure
ALARA practices or techniques should be used by all in the dental office.

alginate—an elastic type of impression material used mostly for study models
An **alginate** impression is usually taken when teeth are present in the arch.

alignment—row or line; arrangement
The orthodontist tries to move the teeth into **alignment**.

alphabetic—filing or lining up arrangement determined by alphabetic letters
Most records are filed in an **alphabetic** arrangement in the file drawer.

alveolar—pertaining to the bony crest on top of the jawbones
When a tooth is extracted, the **alveolar** plate wears down from trauma and use.

alveolitis—dry socket; loss of or condition of not having a blood clot form
The treatment for **alveolitis** is to stimulate bleeding for a new clot.

alveoplasty—surgery of the alveolar bony plate
When a group of teeth are removed, the surgeon may do an **alveoplasty**.

amalgam—restoration material; mixture of metals, mainly mercury and silver
Amalgam restorations are commonly called "silver fillings."

amalgamator—mechanical device used to unite mercury and metals for amalgam

The assistant used an **amalgamator** to prepare the restorative material.

ambidextrous—for use of both hands with ease and comfort

Many examination gloves are **ambidextrous** and do not need matching.

ambu bag—an air-forcing balloon device found on emergency trays

The **ambu bag** is used to force air into the patient's lungs when needed.

anaphylactic—type of shock reaction, resulting from allergic reactions

Anaphylactic reactions are somewhat common in the dental office.

anatomic—shape of body parts, resembling a natural form

Many dental charts show **anatomic** representations of the teeth.

anesthesia—state of being without feeling

Many people request **anesthesia** for dental treatments.

antimicrobial—against microbes or germs; an agent or chemical to kill microbes

The assistant should use an **antimicrobial** soap to wash hands.

apical—pertaining to the tip or end of a tooth's root

An abscess may form near the **apical** foramen of the tooth.

appliance—a device used to replace, restore, or aid body functions

A dental bridge is considered an **appliance** that restores chewing functions.

applicant—a person applying for a job

The **applicant** fills in an application blank and goes to job interviews.

arch—upper or lower half of a dentition; horseshoe arrangement of teeth

An individual has a maxillary and mandibular **arch**.

articulator—device to simulate jaw movements, used in appliance construction

The technician prepares the teeth arrangement using an **articulator**.

asepsis—condition of being without pathogenic microbes or germs

The assistant should practice techniques to maintain **asepsis** in the office.

aspirate—to suction; to remove by vacuum

The assistant will **aspirate** the mouth many times during a dental procedure.

associate degree—two-year degree usually granted in community colleges

Some assistants earn an **associate degree** when studying dental assisting.

attributes—qualities or characteristics possessed by an individual

The resume should stress the positive **attributes** of an applicant.

automatic—performed without thinking, from habit or mechanical setting

An **automatic** film processor can save processing time for an assistant.

avulsed—ripped, knocked, or torn off or out of the human body

Sometimes the **avulsed** tooth can be replaced.

axillary—pertaining to the underarm area of the body, armpit

Axillary temperature may be taken by placing the thermometer in the armpit.

barrier—agent or device used to block, keep out, or protect from

The PPE worn by an assistant is one method of **barrier** protection.

base form—lower part or support part of study models

The **base form** of the study models is added to make the models look natural.

beaker—glass container used as auxiliary cleaning unit in ultrasonic cleaner

The scratched, etched **beaker** is not used because waves cannot travel through.

bicuspid—premolar fourth and fifth permanent tooth back from the midline of the face

The two **bicuspid** teeth are situated between the cuspids and molars.

biodegradable—capable of dissolving or breaking down by biologic means

Some products are **biodegradable**, given the proper time and conditions.

biohazard—any material, item, or agent harmful to humans or the environment

The assistant will place a **biohazard** label on caustic or poisonous materials.

biomechanical—combined use of body and mechanical forces

The endodontist uses **biomechanical** techniques to clean the root canal.

biopsy—small sample of tissue removed for microscopic study

The oral surgeon may send a **biopsy** from a questionable area to the lab.

bisecting angle technique—radiographic technique using imaginary angles and teeth axis lines

The **bisecting angle technique** requires more precision than the paralleling technique.

bite registration—replica of the patient's bite while in occlusion
The **bite registration** is used to align the poured impressions for trimming.

bloodborne—method of transmission or carriage of pathogens through blood products
The assistant must be careful of **bloodborne** infections.

brachial—pertaining to the brachial artery situated in the elbow area
The assistant listens to the **brachial** artery with a stethoscope.

brackets—orthodontic hooks or devices used for attaching the arch wires
Brackets may be cemented directly on the tooth or on a band around the tooth.

buccal—toward the cheek
The posterior teeth have a **buccal** surface that touches the cheek.

buccal tubes—devices placed on the buccal surface to hold arch wires
The **buccal tubes** hold the ends of the arch wire in place.

buffer—device used to polish or smooth a surface
A **buffer** wheel is one item used when polishing.

calcification—quality of becoming hard or calcified
Newly erupted teeth take a while to undergo final **calcification.**

calculus—hard excrustations of plaque and material that adhere to tooth surfaces
The hygienist removes **calculus** during prophylaxis.

cancelled checks—checks that have been processed by the bank
Cancelled checks are returned to the office and kept for records.

canine (also cuspid)—third tooth back from the midline of the face
A **canine** tooth also may be called a dog, fang, or vampire tooth.

cardiogenic—one type of shock arising from heart problems
Cardiogenic shock is very serious and needs immediate attention.

cardiopulmonary—combination of heart and lungs
The assistant should be aware of the **cardiopulmonary** process while doing CPR.

cariogenic—start or beginning of caries or decay
Some foods, such as caramels, are considered more **cariogenic** than others.

carotid—pertaining to the artery in the neck
The **carotid** artery may be used to take a patient's pulse.

carpule—a glass container of anesthetic solution
The **carpule** tip should be wiped off with an alcohol swipe before use.

cartridge—device to carry, measure, or dispense a material or solution
Some impression materials come in a self-mixing **cartridge**.

cassette—device to hold objects (film for x-ray, instruments for cleaning)
The **cassette**, holding instruments, can be lowered into the ultrasonic cleaner.

catalyst—agent that hastens or causes action
Some materials need a **catalyst** to work.

caustic—acid in nature; burning or corrosive
Care must be taken when working with **caustic** materials.

cavitate—to cause bubbles or a bubbling effect
The ultrasonic unit makes the solution **cavitate**.

cementum—tissue covering of the root section of the tooth
The **cementum** surface is rough so that fibers may attach and hold the tooth.

central—midline tooth; front tooth; largest incisor
The **central** incisor is the tooth that gives the face the most character.

cephalometric—pertaining to the head or skull; radiograph or head measure
The orthodontist uses the **cephalometric** radiograph to measure growth.

cervix—neck of the tooth; area where enamel and cementum tissues meet
Some people have sensitivity at the **cervix** area.

chronologic—filing arrangement according to time or sequence
Job experiences are listed in **chronologic** order, with most recent as first.

classified ad—a business or commercial ad placed in a newspaper
The job applicant seeks work opportunities in the **classified ads**.

clinical attire—dress or uniform worn in dental setting
The **clinical attire** is supplied by the dentist and not worn home.

competent—to have the ability, talent, and knowledge to complete a task
The assistant must be trained to be **competent** to complete procedures.

compliance—acceptance and following of rules and regulations
OSHA officials may visit a dental facility to determine rules **compliance**.

composite—resin or plastic type of material
Light-colored restorations are composed of a **composite** material.

compress—press to make smaller; make condensed; dressing for wound
One method of controlling bleeding is to **compress** the wound.

condense—pack or shove in; stow
The amalgam plugger is used to **condense** the material in the preparation.

confidential—private; personal and business matters
Confidentiality is the act of keeping all records and business **confidential**.

confirmation calls—phone calls made to remind patients of upcoming appointments
Confirmation calls lessen the amount of "no show" appointments.

consent—written, oral, or understood agreement or permission for treatment
A written **consent** is required before some surgery and treatment for children.

consistency—condition of thickness or smoothness of material
Cement must be mixed to a smooth, creamy **consistency**.

consultant—authority of a subject of interest or need
The dentist may hire a **consultant** to review the practice and make suggestions.

contaminated—condition of being exposed and possible condition of sepsis
If there is any doubt an item has been **contaminated**, sterilize it.

contour—shape or form of an object; to make something into a certain shape
The dental technician will **contour** the denture base for an exacting fit.

coordination of benefits—insurance payment with two or more company coverage
The patient will receive more benefits with a **coordination of benefits**.

correspondence—written communication
The assistant makes sure the **correspondence** is clean, correct, and neat.

counteract—to work against or balance; to nullify an action
Some drugs **counteract** other drugs and cause reactions or problems.

courtesy—polite action; consideration of others' feelings
All dental patients should be treated with **courtesy**.

cover letter—letter sent with the resume
A **cover letter** explains to the employer why the resume is being sent.

crosscut—two-way cutting
Some dental burs have a **crosscut** action.

cross-reference—method to keep track of numeric filing material
The assistant keeps a **cross-reference** book with the numbers and matching names.

crown—part of tooth covered by enamel; the upper or top part of the tooth
The **crown** is covered by enamel tissue.

culture—a medium used to grow microbes for microscopic study
A **culture** of the pulp chamber may be taken to determine if there is infection.

cumulative effect—condition of receiving too much radiation or too often
The assistant should question the patient to avoid a radiation **cumulative effect**.

curettage—scraping or removal of necrotic tissue and deposits from tooth
The hygienist will perform a **curettage** on deep-seated periodontal pockets.

cuspid (also canine)—third tooth back from midline, strongest anterior tooth
The **cuspid** is a tearing tooth, used to grasp and tear food.

custom tray—special impression tray made from a patient's study models
A **custom tray** gives more detail and form than a commercial tray.

DDS or **DMD**—Doctor of Dental Surgery or Doctor of Medical Dentistry
The **DDS** or **DMD** must complete many years of study and training.

debride—remove foreign, necrotic matter from a wound
The dentist must **debride** the wound before treatment can begin.

deciduous—falling out or primary; first teeth
The **deciduous** teeth are replaced by permanent teeth.

deductible—amount subscriber must pay before insurance company pays
The benefit booklet states if a **deductible** is required.

degenerative—breaking down; destructive; tissue decay
Decay is a **degenerative** process affecting tooth tissue.

dental assistant—person who aides, helps, and assists the dentist
The **dental assistant** is a very valuable member of the dental team.

dental crown—artificial cover for natural tooth crown surface

A **dental crown** may be constructed from different materials.

dental equipment serviceperson—individual trained to service dental machines
The **dental equipment serviceperson** is called to repair or install equipment.

dental hygienist—person who performs prophylaxis and teaches prevention
The **dental hygienist** monitors the patient's home care progress.

dentin—inner tissue that gives bulk and shape to tooth
Dentin is present both in the crown and root sections.

denture—artificial tooth replacement of an entire arch
The **denture** replaces the patient's natural dentition.

deodorize—to eliminate or diminish presence of odors and smells
The suction lines are flushed after use to **deodorize** the tubes.

dependents—those who rely on others for support and care
The family insurance policy provides for coverage for **dependents**.

deposit—to put in; add to
The assistant will make a bank **deposit** each workday.

detail or salesperson—one employed by commercial business to sell and promote a product
The **detail or salesperson** keeps the office informed of new products.

deteriorate—break down or lose effectiveness
Gypsum products will **deteriorate** if too much moisture is absorbed.

developer—chemical solution used in processing radiographs
The radiographs are placed in the **developer** before the fixer solution.

diaphragm—flat, hollow circle in stethoscope used to accent sound
The **diaphragm** of the stethoscope is used to hear the blood pressure sounds.

diastolic—flow of blood in artery while the heartbeat or pulse is at rest
The **diastolic** reading is the lower reading in a blood pressure quote.

dilated—enlarged or opened up; the opening is made larger
The pupils of the eyes will **dilate** if oxygen to the brain becomes scarce.

disinfection—action taken to lessen pathogenic microbes from an object
There is a difference between **disinfection** and sterilization.

disparaging—unkind, untruthful, mean, or poor taste remark
The assistant does not make **disparaging** remarks about the employer or staff.

distal—toward the back; far off
The molar teeth are **distal** to the bicuspids.

dosimeter—device used to monitor the amount of radiation received
The assistant must wear a **dosimeter** when exposing or coming near film exposure.

dry socket—condition arising from loss of clot or from clot not forming
A **dry socket** can be very painful.

edentulous—without teeth, loss or lack of natural teeth
An arch that wears a denture is considered **edentulous** or without teeth.

effervescent—a bubbling action of a solution caused by chemical reactions
When some chemicals combine they produce an **effervescent** action.

embrasure—V-shaped area formed by the neck (cervix) indents
The gingiva in the **embrasure** area resorbs as the person ages.

enamel—hardest tissue in body; covers crown of tooth
Fluoride products help strengthen the tooth **enamel**.

endodontist—dentist specialist concerned with pulp tissue
The **endodontist** performs root canals and tooth bleachings.

esthetic—beauty; good looks
The denture must have **esthetic** quality as well as proper function.

ethics—moral code placed on members of a profession by the members of the profession
Ethics is the code of behavior that a professional person practices.

eugenol—oil of cloves; material used in dental cements and restorations
Eugenol is the liquid used to make a ZOE preparation.

evacuation—removal; aspiration or suction of a substance
One of the assistant's duties during procedures is moisture **evacuation**.

exfoliate—to become loose or fade away
The deciduous teeth will **exfoliate** and be replaced by secondary teeth.

expiration—time used up; over; finished; elimination of air from lungs
The **expiration** date of a product must be checked before use.

exposure—amount of time for radiation ioning an object

The assistant follows safety rules when performing an x-ray **exposure**.

extirpation—removal of tissue or organ, such as dental pulp

In root canal therapy, the dentist will perform an **extirpation** of the pulp.

extraoral—exposure of radiographic film situated outside the mouth

The panoramic film is an example of an **extraoral** exposure.

exudate—necrotic; infectious material; pus from wound

The **exudate** is removed by inserting a suction tip into the incision.

fabrication—construction; making or building of

The **fabrication** of a denture may be performed by a commercial lab.

festoon—smooth, shape, round out

The technician will **festoon** the wax rims after attachment to the base plate.

fixer—chemical solution used to process radiographic films

The **fixer** solution can easily stain clothes if splashing occurs.

fluoride—chemical compound helpful for strong enamel

The dentist may prescribe **fluoride** vitamins for children living in rural areas.

foramen—hole or opening in a bone

The mandibular nerve branch runs through the mental **foramen**.

frenum—muscle or tissue lip or cheek attachment to mouth areas

The lingual **frenum** is located under the tongue in the floor of the mouth.

functional—useful; productive or practical

The dental appliance must be **functional**, comfortable, and pleasant to look at.

gauge—degree of thickness around a round object

The needle's **gauge** is indicated by the color on the sheath.

gingiva—gum tissue; membrane covering the root and surrounding the teeth

The unhealthy **gingiva** looks red and swollen and may bleed when touched.

gypsum—rock quarry product used in dental study models and lab work

Gypsum products are supplied in various colors, types, and classes.

hazardous—condition of being in peril; danger; unhealthy

OSHA is concerned with **hazardous** conditions facing workers.

hemorrhage of **hemorrhagic**—excessive bleeding; loss of blood

Some chemicals can be used to treat pulp **hemorrhage**.

Hg—symbol for mercury

The assistant lets the mercury column drop at a rate of 2 mm **Hg** per second.

holistic—entire body involvement; health including all systems

Many dentists use a **holistic** approach to dental care.

homogeneous—mixture of two products into one evenly mixed preparation

Impression materials must be mixed to a **homogeneous** state before use.

HVE—high vacuum evacuation

The assistant uses **HVE** to remove fluids from the mouth.

hyperactive—overactive; sensitive; excited

A **hyperactive** pulp may cause a severe toothache.

I & D—Incision and drainage process of incising and letting a wound drain

The dentist may place a dental dam drain in the incision during an **I & D** procedure.

immunization—acquired immunity either by natural or given toxins

Each dental worker must receive a hepatitis **immunization** before employment.

impregnated—filled up with; absorbed into

Some dental flosses are **impregnated** with fluoride or baking soda.

incisor—cutting type of tooth; anterior tooth with sharp edge

The **incisor** teeth have sharp, cutting edges to bite into food.

increment—bit by bit; small amount

The amalgam material is placed in the preparation one **increment** at a time.

incubation—period of growing time

The culture tube is placed in **incubation** to determine if infection is present.

indentation—marks or dents left from biting edges of teeth

The **indentation** areas of an impression are filled first.

indexing—process of dividing name or title into divisions for filing

A person's name must be **indexed** before placing the record in a file.

infectious—condition of being able to infect or give disease or malady
Each patient must be treated as a possible **infectious** source.

infiltration—type of local anesthesia, usually given in maxillary arch
The patient received **infiltration** anesthesia before the restoration procedure.

inflate—to enlarge, blow up, or make full
The assistant will **inflate** the blood pressure cuff to get a reading.

ingested—taken into the body, as food or drink
Fluoride, which is placed in the city water supply, is **ingested** by patients.

inject/injection—to stick in; to insert under
The dentist will **inject** the anesthetic solution before beginning the procedure.

inquiry—questioning; asking
An assistant may receive an **inquiry** phone call about a patient's bill.

inspiration—inhaling air during the breathing process
The assistant counts one **inspiration** and expiration of air as a respiration count.

intensifying—increasing the potential or making something larger or stronger
An **intensifying** screen in a radiographic cassette increases the ray exposure to film.

intensity—deepness; strength; great amount
The **intensity** of the operatory light may be changed for different procedures.

interproximal—area between two sides; area between nearby teeth
Dental floss is used in the **interproximal** areas to remove debris and plaque.

interview—questioning talk between two or more people
An **interview** helps the employer and applicant discuss the job opening.

intraoral—radiographic exposure of film placed inside the mouth
The periapical x-ray is considered an **intraoral** exposure type of film.

inverted—turning inward, tucking edges under
The dental dam edges must be **inverted** to keep mouth moisture out.

ionize—effect of radiation upon tissue contents
Radiographic rays have the ability to **ionize** human cells.

irreversible—cannot be changed back; remains in set condition
Some alginate impression materials have an **irreversible** set.

irrigation—washing out; flushing with water
The root canal debris is removed by **irrigation** and drying of the canal.

isolation—placing apart from; setting aside
Dental dam places the affected tooth in **isolation**.

job application form—document requesting information regarding the applicant
A **job application form** is filled out in a neat and correct manner.

jurisprudence—science of laws and regulations affecting professional acts
State dental practice laws are a concern in dental **jurisprudence**.

kilovoltage (kVp)—controls the speed of the electrons of a radiographic beam
Contrast of a radiograph is affected by the **kilovoltage** control.

laboratory technician—person who is employed to do dental lab work
The **laboratory technician** may work in an office or commercial lab.

lateral—side; next to; nearby; also, second tooth from the midline
The **lateral** incisor is distal to the central incisor.

ledger card—business chart where patient and financial matters are recorded
The **ledger cards** should be placed in a safe area overnight.

liability—legal responsibility
An accident in the office may cause a **liability** claim to be filed.

license—legal permission to perform designated professional duties
The dentist must have a **license** to work in the state where the practice occurs.

lingual—relating to the tongue; tooth surface that touches the tongue
The back surface of the teeth that touches the tongue is called **lingual**.

lute/luting—cementing together of two different substances
Some parts of a dental appliance are constructed by **luting** the pieces.

mallet—surgical or operative hammer
To remove bone around an impaction, the dentist taps the chisel with a **mallet**.

malocclusion—state of having poor or improper occlusion
The orthodontist treats various types and degrees of **malocclusion**.

malpractice—improper professional performance; negligence

A **malpractice** suit can be placed on a dentist for improper professional service.

mandibular—pertaining to the lower jaw or mandible
All teeth present in the lower jaw are termed **mandibular** teeth.

mandrel—device used to hold the wheels, disk, and stones used in polishing
A **mandrel** with an attached wheel or disk may be placed in a slow handpiece.

manual—completed by hand, without machines; forethought and effort are required
Processing radiographs with a **manual** technique involves a lot of time.

matrix—artificial stainless steel or mylar wall; substitute for missing side
A stainless steel **matrix** is placed around a preparation before amalgam insertion.

maxillary—pertaining to upper jaw or maxillae bone areas
The teeth situated in the upper jaw are called **maxillary** teeth.

maximum—most; upward limit
Most insurance policies have a yearly **maximum** for patient coverage.

medicament—solution, preparation, or material used for treatment
Some offices color code bottles to help identify the enclosed **medicament**.

mesial—toward the center or midline
The surface of the tooth closest to the midline or center is called **mesial**.

metabolic—living process reaction; taking and giving energy
Some individual's **metabolic** rate may be faster than other individuals.

milliamperage (mA)—measurement of amount of electrons in electric current; affects the intensity of radiation beam
Adjusting the **milliamperage** control affects the density of the radiograph.

misalignment—improper arrangement; out of place
The **misalignment** of teeth can cause decay and poor oral hygiene.

mobility—condition of being mobile; moving or loose
Two instrument handles are used to test tooth **mobility**.

modification—change or alteration of item; procedure or action
Some instruments or techniques must undergo **modification** to perform properly.

molar—multicusped tooth; grinding tooth; most posterior tooth

Maxillary **molars** have three roots while mandibular ones have two.

monitor—to watch over or observe; supervise
The assistant should **monitor** a patient who has just received anesthesia.

monomer—one of the two materials needed to produce an acrylic product
The **monomer** is added to the polymer to make an acrylic tray.

multitufted—having many tufts or many bristles
Many dentists prefer a patient to use a **multitufted** toothbrush.

necrotic—state of being infected; dying or dead tissue; pus affected
The **necrotic** tissue is removed before treatment.

negligence—lack of attention or proper treatment through concern or care
A dentist who does not follow up a surgical procedure may be guilty of **negligence**.

networking—procedure in which applicant tells everyone about seeking a job
Many jobs can be found for a person who attempts **networking** the situation.

neurogenic—condition caused by nervous reaction or stressful state.
Fainting can be a symptom of **neurogenic** shock.

numeric—arrangement by use of sequential numbers
Radiographs may be filed and stored using **numeric** filing systems.

obligation—due; debt; responsibility
The assistant has an **obligation** to properly sterilize all instruments.

occlusal—chewing surface of posterior teeth
Sealants are placed on the **occlusal** surface to protect the teeth.

occlusion—state of grinding; teeth meeting for chewing or biting
The new restoration is checked for high spots by checking the **occlusion**.

on-the-job training (OJT)—situation in which employee learns duties after employment
Some dental assistants must learn the profession through **on-the-job training (OJT)**.

ora-evac (oral evacuation)—a machine or device used to remove mouth fluid
The **ora-evac** machine is cleaned after each use.

oral and maxillofacial surgeon—specialist for surgical repair extraction, and fractures
An **oral and maxillofacial surgeon** is a member of a cleft palate reconstruction team.

oral pathologist—specialist dealing with diseases of the mouth

Many **oral pathologists** are employed by local, state, and federal governments.

orthodontist—specialist concerned with the alignment of teeth and jaws
The **orthodontist** places brackets, tubes, and wires to rearrange the teeth.

outstanding—deposits or checks written on an account that bank is not aware of; special or excellent
The **outstanding** checks are totaled before reconciliation of the checkbook.

palpate/palpation—feel by touch, tapping, or light pressure by finger or hand
The dentist will **palpate** the neck looking for lymph nodes.

panoramic—wide view, radiographic exposure of entire lower area of skull
Panoramic radiographs expose impactions, missing teeth, cysts, and fractures.

papilla/papillae—gingival tissue mounds present in the embrasure areas
Red, irritated **papillae** indicate possible gingivitis.

para-dental professionals—those whose training is related to or aids dentistry
Many **para-dental professionals** are called on in various situations.

parallel—technique for exposing x-rays with the film and tooth axis parallel
A different type of PID is used for the **parallel** exposure technique.

pathogens—disease- or sickness-causing microbe or germ
Sterilization and disinfection are completed to destroy all **pathogens**.

payee—person designated on a check to receive funds
The "pay to the order of" line is filled with the name of the **payee**.

pediatric dentistry—specialty concerned with dental care for children
The **pediatric dentist** is concerned with the child's teeth.

penetrate—enter into; go through; affect deeply
Radiography rays can **penetrate** tissues and bones.

percussion—tapping or beating on an object with an instrument or finger
The **percussion** test can help determine if an abscess is present.

periapical—around the apex of the tooth
A group of **periapical** films makes up a full-mouth study of the dentition.

periodontist—specialist concerned with the gingival tissues

The **periodontist** tries to eliminate gingival problems and restore dental health.

periodontium—gingival tissues made up of alveolar plate; periodontial fibers; gingiva
The dental hygienist is concerned with the **periodontium**.

peripheral—area around; nearby section; encircling space
Radiographs can expose the tooth and **peripheral** areas.

permanent—secure, final, secondary, meant to stay, adult teeth
The adult patient should develop 32 **permanent** teeth.

placement—locality; position; set area
The applicant is looking for a job **placement**.

placing—act of arrangement into sequence; put in order; set into
Business files undergo the **placing** procedure when filed in the cabinet.

plastic filling instrument (**PFI**)—flat-bladed instrument
The **PFI** is useful to carry cement and other materials.

pliable—movable; flexible; soft and easy to situate
Wax can be warmed until it is **pliable** and in condition to use.

polymer—one of the two materials needed to make acrylic material
In most acrylic combination situations, the **polymer** is supplied in powder form.

polymerization—action of the union of monomer and polymer to make product
The two materials are united and undergo **polymerization** to form an acrylic pad.

pontic—artificial tooth in fixed bridge that replaces a missing tooth
The **pontic** is united with the bridge through soldering or welding.

position indicating device (**PID**)—used to align or focus radiographic rays
The assistant should know how to change the **PID** on the radiographic machine.

posting—listing; arranging; bringing forth to receive attention
At least once a month the assistant will perform **posting** duties.

postsecondary—after high school; formal education after high school
Many dental assisting programs are completed in **postsecondary** schools.

pre-authorized—approved for procedure prior to service
Many insurance companies insist on **pre-authorized** permission for treatment.

preliminary—first; beginning; start of; first appointment of a series
The first appointment is considered the **preliminary** visit.

pressurized—item or article that has been subjected to outside or external forces
The steam in an autoclave has been **pressurized** in the machine's chamber.

preventive—action used to prevent or deter disease
Education in home care of the teeth is considered **preventive** dentistry.

primary—first; early; before secondary; deciduous teeth
The deciduous teeth are called **primary** teeth.

prophylaxis—removal of calculus and deposits with cleaning and polishing
The dental hygienist performs the **prophylaxis** in many offices.

prosthodontist—specialist in artificial teeth and replacement appliances
The **prosthodontist** is a specialist who prepares and delivers dentures.

protrude—sticking out; forward thrust of jaw; mandible anterior to maxilla
Protrusion of the lower jaw is a symptom of one type of malocclusion.

proximal—nearby; at the side; adjacent to
When two teeth touch, they are **proximal** to each other.

psychogenic—caused by thought; arising from thinking; fear or internal ego
One type of shock caused from nervousness is called **psychogenic** shock.

public health dentist—specialist in community and public dentistry
Most **public health dentists** work for government agencies.

pulp—living section of tooth; inner tooth tissue
The **pulp** gives vitality and life to the tooth.

pulverized—smashed into powder; very finely ground
Gypsum rock is **pulverized** and then treated to remove moisture.

quadrant—one fourth section of mouth dentition; half of one arch
Each permanent **quadrant** should contain eight teeth.

radial—pertaining to the radial artery found in the wrist
The pulse is taken at the **radial** artery site.

radiograph—x-ray; film exposed and processed to show internal body conditions
The operator must be trained to expose a **radiograph**.

reconciliation—a balancing of figures; getting together
Checkbook **reconciliation** must be performed once a month.

reconstruction—repair; rebuilding; restoring to original condition
Some patients need extensive **reconstruction** of the mouth for good health.

reference—someone who will attest to good character of another person
The applicant should ask permission to list a person as a **reference**.

regulates—controls by rules or laws; gauges; measures to a certain amount
The professional acts performed are **regulated** by the State Dental Practice Act.

relativity—related to a subject; akin to
Some records are filed according to their **relativity** to a subject.

remittal—money turned in for payment of a bill; received on account (ROA)
A **remittal** may be requested when the patient is finishing the appointment.

replenishing—act of restoring or freshening by additional solution
X-ray developer requires **replenishing** each work day.

replica—a duplicate; a look alike; similar in shape and form
The study model is a **replica** of the patient's dentition.

reproduction—a similarity; a duplicate; construction of a new object to substitute or replace
A denture is a **reproduction** of the patient's dentition.

restoration—make like new; replace; restore to its original condition
A dental **restoration** can save a patient from further decay and tooth problems.

resume—collection of data regarding job applicant; vita; personal information
A **resume** will tell the employer about the applicant's qualifications.

resuscitation—process of breathing or filling lungs of an unconscious victim
The rescuer will try to restore oxygen to the victim by **resuscitation**.

retractor—device or instrument used to retract or pull away
The evacuation tip may be used as a **retractor**.

retruded—pulled back; underdeveloped jaw; mandible posterior to maxilla
A **retruded** jaw is a symptom of one type of malocclusion.

revitalization—reconstruction or growth of tissue; redevelopment

Some tooth tissues may repair themselves through **revitalization**.

rhythm—beat; regularity; same sequence; pattern
The **rhythm** of the pulse is noted when taking vital signs.

roots—bottom section of tooth; submerged part of tooth; anchor area
The **root** section of the tooth is covered with cementum.

rotary—rotating motion; moving around; circular; type of instrument
The handpiece is a **rotary** instrument used to affect tooth tissue.

safelight—filtered or colored light used in darkroom procedures
The **safelight** is used when the films are placed on the developing rack.

saliva ejector—machine or device used to evacuate mouth fluids
The **saliva ejector** tip is used to remove small amounts of fluids.

sanitation—act of cleaning instrument item or area
Each office should have a **sanitation** procedure sheet and schedule.

scaling—removal of hard deposits from surfaces of tooth in prophylaxis
Calculus above and below the gum line is removed in the **scaling** procedure.

schedule of benefits—printed notification of what is covered by insurance
The **schedule of benefits** is listed in the policy handbook.

sealant—hard, acrylic protective cover painted on newly erupted teeth
Sealant material can be supplied in clear or tinted colors.

secondary—to come behind; to follow; to be second; of lesser value
The permanent teeth are said to be **secondary** teeth.

sensitivity—reaction to stimulus; activated feeling
Sensitivity to temperature or sweetness may indicate possible decay.

septic—pertain to presence of sepsis or microbes
Treatment is postponed when a **septic** condition is present.

sequence—series of events or happenings; order of occurrences
Some treatment plans are arranged in a **sequence** of appointments.

shank—body of bur; part that inserts into handpiece; shaft part of an instrument
The **shank** of the bur determines the type of handpiece placement.

sorting—arranging by number, alphabet, or time; putting into place
When preparing to file, the assistant performs a **sorting** of the indexes.

spatula—flat-bladed instrument mainly used for mixing materials
There are different types of **spatulas** used in the dental office.

specialist—someone trained in a specialty; expert in a field or profession
There are several different types of dental **specialists**.

sphygmomanometer—mercury or air pressure device used to measure blood pressure
The **sphygmomanometer** cuff is placed around the patient's arm.

spicule—sharp, hard, needlelike splinter, usually of bone tissue
Bone **spicules** may work through the gingiva after alveolar surgery.

State Dental Practice Act—legal regulation regarding the practice of dentistry
The dentist must abide by the **State Dental Practice Act**.

statistical—according to records; related or involved numbers
Public health dentists deal with **statistical** information.

statutes—government laws or regulations
The State Dental Practice Act determines the dental **statutes** of the state.

sterilization—removal of all forms of life
All living matter is destroyed in the **sterilization** process.

sternum—chest bone; bone between the ribs
The rescuer compresses the **sternum** in CPR.

stethoscope—device for listening to heart and pulse noises
The **stethoscope** is used to hear the blood pressure readings.

study models—gypsum replicas of the teeth and mouth conditions
The **study models** are used to determine treatment and prepare appliances.

subscriber—person to whom insurance coverage is granted
The employee is usually the **subscriber** on the insurance policy.

sulcus—gingiva-free marginal area around the neck of the tooth
The toothbrush is inserted into the **sulcus** to clean the area.

supernumerary—over the amount of; extra; more than the normal amount of teeth
Some patients have **supernumerary** teeth that may be removed.

supervision—watching over; direction of; taking responsibility for

Supervision of dental personnel can be direct or indirect.

supine—position in which the patient is resting on the back with the face up

The patient is placed in a **supine** position during dental treatment.

supragingival—area above the gingival margin or crest

Calculus that is easily seen is said to be **supragingival** calculus.

symmetry—balance; alike on one side and the other

During the exam, the dentist will check the patient's face for **symmetry**.

syncope—fainting, loss of consciousness due to lack of brain oxygen

Syncope is the most common dental emergency.

systemic—throughout the system; in the network

Fluoride ingested through city water is said to be a **systemic** application.

systolic—force of blood in artery during beat wave or pulse

The upper number of the blood pressure reading is the **systolic** reading.

techniques—procedures or methods to perform a task or job

Each dentist will have a personal **technique** for a procedure.

(TMJ)— pertaining to union of temporal and mandibular bones

Clicking of the jaws is an indication of trouble in the **TMJ.**

topical—on top of; surface part; situated on upper part

Before injecting the anesthesia, a **topical** anesthetic is used to lessen the pain.

transaction—a business deal; a business event or occurrence

The receptionist or business manager performs many office **transactions**.

transillumination—act of shining light through a tooth to look at the inner side

Transillumination of a tooth may sometimes show an inflamed pulp or cracked tooth.

transposition—to move to another area; to replace to a new section

In orthodontics, a tooth may undergo **transposition** to improve occlusion.

traumatic—hurtful; severe or excessive damage or injury

A blow to a tooth may cause **traumatic** pulpal damage.

tuberosity—natural growth or rounded area at the end of the maxillary arch

The denture must fit over the maxillary **tuberosity** for a proper fit.

tympanic—pertaining to the tympanic or inner membrane in the ear

The ear thermometer registers the heat of the **tympanic** membrane.

UCR (usual, customary, and reasonable)—type of insurance coverage

Some insurance companies pay claims under **UCR** coverage.

ultrasonic—a device used to bubble or cavitate debris from submerged articles

Ultrasonic action breaks up and helps remove debris from objects.

ultrasonic cleaner—method of cleaning using high-pitched sound waves

The **ultrasonic cleaner** removes microscopic dirt from instruments.

ultrasonic handpiece—a prophylactic device used to cavitate or remove calculus and stains from tooth surfaces

The **ultrasonic handpiece** eliminates much of the traumatic force and pressure of hand prophylactic instruments.

universal precautions—theory assuming that every patient is infectious

Assistants use **universal precautions** when dealing with patients.

vasoconstrictor—chemical used to constrict blood vessels

Anesthesia that contains a **vasoconstrictor** decreases bleeding.

verification—to test the accuracy of; to prove to be true

Radiographs are one form of diagnosis **verification**.

vibrator—instrument used to vibrate or shake air bubbles from gypsum mixes

The gypsum mixture is placed on the **vibrator** before being put in the mold.

vitality—life; functional ability of a tooth

A root canal treatment may be performed on a tooth with no **vitality**.

void—nothing; opening or hole in material or object

Large bubbles in the gypsum mix can cause **voids** in the model.

xiphoid—cartilage extension at the bottom of the sternum

The rescuer is careful not to compress the **xiphoid** process during CPR.

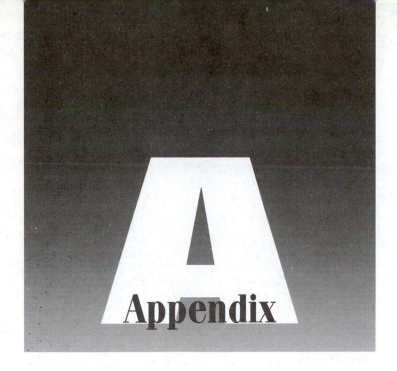

Appendix A

ANSWERS TO THEORY RECALLS, POST TESTS, AND ASSIGNMENT SHEETS

UNIT 1 THE DENTAL PROFESSION

Theory Recall:
The Professional Dental Team

1. The dentist is ultimately responsible for the actions of the personnel in the office.
2. Before beginning practice in a particular state, the dentist must fulfill the requirements and successfully pass the written and clinical state boards of the state where the practice will reside.
3. There are eight recognized dental specialties.
4. The primary duty of the dental hygienist is in prevention of dental disease.
5. Before working in a practice in a particular state, the hygienist must successfully pass the dental tests of the state dental board which mandates the duties and responsibilities of that profession.
6. The dental assistant may receive on-the-job training or go to a vocational school or community college.
7. The assistant may assist at chairside, laboratory, reception, support, or in expanded-duties assistance.
8. The American Dental Assistants Association is the name of the national professional organization for dental assistants.
9. The dental laboratory technician assists the dentist by performing the laboratory tasks.
10. The dentist may call upon a pharmacist, nutritionist, medical laboratory assistant, or dental office consultant.

Assignment Sheet 1.1
The Professional Dental Team

A. 1. prosthodontics, periodontics, oral pathology, oral and maxillofacial surgery, orthodontics, endodontics, pedodontics, public health dentistry
   2. a. dentist—provides treatment and dental care for patients
      b. dental hygienist—concerned with the prevention of dental disease
      c. dental assistant—assists dental personnel with delivery of dental care
      d. dental lab technician—completes dental laboratory services
   3. Dental detail or salespersons may acquaint the dental personnel of new products and equipment and changes in supplies and provide the office with sales products.
   4. Dental equipment servicepersons may repair office equipment, install new treatment equipment, calibrate radiation machines, or assist with relocation of dental units.
   5. Related professionals who may be called on to assist the dentist in providing care and treatment are physicians, pharmacists, laboratory technicians, dietitians, and other health care providers.
B. Bulletin boards may offer an individual's personal impression of dental care personnel. Boards may be judged on accuracy, originality, color, neatness, and interpretation.

Theory Recall:
The Role of the Dental Assistant

1. The initials OJT mean on-the-job training.
2. A person may be educated to be a dental assistant by OJT, vocational school, or junior or community colleges.
3. A dental assistant may find employment in a dental office, private and commercial medical and or dental clinics, hospitals, mobile dental units, nursing homes, research, and specialist's offices.
4. The clinical support dental assistant may sterilize and disinfect, seat patients, and perform duties that keep the flow of patients moving.
5. The dental laboratory assistant may pour, trim and articulate impressions, prepare laboratory materials and appliances, and perform general lab work.
6. The American Dental Assistants Association is the national organization that represents dental assistants.
7. The three levels of membership are local, state, and national.
8. The Dental Assisting National Board (DANB) certifies dental assistants.
9. Infection control (ICE), radiation health and safety (RHS), oral and maxillofacial surgery assisting (COMSA), dental practice management assisting (CDPMA), and orthodontic assisting (COA).
10. State certification is valid in the state where it is issued.

Assignment Sheet 1.2
The Role of the Dental Assistant

A. 1. Answers may include on-the-job training, vocational schools, community college programs, proprietary schools, correspondence classes
2. Answers may include the following (placement order is personal choice): dental offices, clinics, hospitals, schools, military bases, specialty offices, research facilities, mobile dental units
3. a. Expanded duty assistants may perform coronal polishing, exposure of radiographs, finishing and polishing of restorations, placement of dental dams and restorative materials, impressions, and other duties as permitted by the State Dental Practice Act.
   b. Chairside assistants perform all types of assisting procedures as permitted by the State Dental Practice Act and the assistant's ability.
   c. Clinic support assistants may seat and prepare patients, remove used equipment and materials, sterilize, and prepare operatories for the next procedures. They may also maintain inventory and order supplies.

d. Receptionist or manager assistants maintain the business office matters for the dental practice, including duties such as bookkeeping, telephone and appointment control, insurance filing, record control, banking procedures, recalls, and other office procedures.
   e. Dental laboratory assistants provide laboratory services including fabrication of study models, prosthodontic appliance and materials, crowns, prostheses, bite planes, and other lab articles.
4. The dental assistant may become involved in the local, state, and national levels of ADAA membership.
5. a. CDA (certified dental assistant) —involves all areas of dental assisting
   b. CDPMA (certified dental practice management)—office business matters
   c. (COMSA (certified oral and maxillofacial surgical assistant)—oral surgery
   d. COA (certified orthodontic assistant)—orthodontics
   e. ICE (infection control exam)—sterilization and asepsis
   f. RHS (radiation health and safety)—dental radiation
B. The posterboard showing variety in the dental assistant profession will be a reflection of the student's concept of the dental career. The board should be judged on originality, message, variety, neatness, and color.

Theory Recall:
Qualities of the Dental Assistant

1. Patient records consist of information and data collected as well as business and financial recordings and transactions.
2. The dental assistant may demonstrate an interest by recognizing the needs, emotions, and feelings of others.
3. Patient records should be maintained accurately and neatly.
4. To be considered reliable, the dental assistant should have consistent attendance and perform work correctly.
5. The dental assistant may appear professional by wearing clean, professional clothes and shoes, wearing hair back and well groomed, keeping nails short and snag free, and using good posture.
6. The dental assistant can improve communication skills by speaking clearly, avoiding slang, and using a calm voice.
7. The dental assistant can exhibit good job qualities by being willing to learn, accept criticism, and adapt to situations.

8. The dental assistant protects self and patient.
9. The dental assistant can observe safety by avoiding shortcuts, following safety rules, looking up hazard controls, and being careful.
10. The dental assistant can become a team member by being a willing worker, concerned with the welfare of the practice, dentist, and patient.

Assignment Sheet 1.3
Qualities of the Dental Assistant

A. 1. Answers may include the following reasons:
   a. Information must be kept confidential for legal and personal reasons, liability, and violation of patient's rights can occur.
   b. Showing an interest in the patient's welfare will establish a bonding and confidence with the patient as well as provide information.
   c. Following instructions carefully prevents mistakes and errors.
   d. Recognizing the needs of others provides for more personal care and develops a respect between patient and staff.
   e. Practicing the Golden Rule develops mutual consideration between the assistant and others.
   f. Performing only delegated duties ensures that the care given a patient is legal and within the practice ability of the operator.
   2. Answers may include the following reasons:
   a. Dependability and honesty make an assistant reliable and someone who can be counted on.
   b. Being well groomed and having good hygiene indicate the assistant's personal reflection on cleanliness and self-respect.
   c. Showing a healthy appearance indicates a good outlook on life and a zest or interest in living.
   d. Using good posture indicates a person who is self-assured and confident.
   e. Projecting a confident self-image indicates an accomplished person who people will find reliable and able.
   f. Having good communication skills helps to establish relations with staff and others.
   3. Answers may include the following reasons:
   a. A willingness to learn indicates a team person with an open mind who will be a cooperative worker and aide.
   b. Persons who can adapt to situations help to lessen conflicts, make the office more pleasant, and encourage others with their example.
   c. An assistant who can accept criticism is an intelligent person who will learn from mis-

takes and become more knowledgeable in the practice.
   d. Following safety rules will help protect the well-being of not only the assistant but the patients, staff, and others.
B. A one-page paper on the dental assisting qualities can be a personal expression of the student.

Theory Recall:
Ethics for the Dental Assistant

1. Ethics is a code of discipline, a statement of moral obligations.
2. Professional organizations develop their own standards of conduct.
3. Each person practicing the art of a profession should follow that profession's code of ethics.
4. The "Code of Ethics of the American Dental Assistants Association" is a formal statement of conduct.
5. The Golden Rule demands the action of treating others as you wish to be treated.
6. All details of the professional dental services should be held in confidence.
7. The assistant should avoid disparaging remarks about the dentist or profession.
8. The assistant can increase skills and efficiency through education.
9. The assistant should take part in and support the profession of dental assisting.

Assignment Sheet 1.4
Ethics for the Dental Assistant

A. 1. Answers may include the following reasons:
   a. Ethics expresses a code of discipline by obligating the person to act and perform in a manner that is accepted in the dental profession.
   b. Ethics is a statement of moral obligations by setting forth examples of responsibilities for conduct and performance for the assistant to follow.
   c. Ethics is a professional and self-imposed code determined by the profession it serves and the persons who embrace the art of dental healing. The code is an expression of the ideals of these people.
   d. Ethics is required to help maintain high standards and confidences in the profession and the persons who maintain the ethical obligations.
   2. Answers may include the following reasons:
   a. By performing the Golden Rule, the assistant gives the highest and most appersonal service that is expected. Treating others as you wish

to be treated provides superior limits of service.

b. An assistant who is honest, loyal, and willing to serve is a team or cooperative worker that people wish to be around and work with.

c. By holding professional matters confidential, the assistant proves loyalty and intelligence. Lack of concern for privacy can cause lawsuits and perhaps a serious harmful conclusion.

d. Refraining from performing illegal or incompetent services not only protects the assistant from legal involvement, but it safeguards the quality of service given to the patient.

e. An assistant who avoids disparaging remarks avoids issuing statements that can hurt and destroy. When the assistant finds a situation uncomfortable, some attempt to quietly discuss the matter with the person should be attempted instead of grumbling and complaining.

f. When the assistant increases skills and efficiency the worker becomes more talented and valuable to self and the dental practice.

g. By joining professional organizations, the assistant will learn of new developments, share experiences, and acquire a deeper interest in the dental profession.

B. Designs relating aspects of the Code of Ethics will reflect the student's interests.

Theory Recall: Dental Jurisprudence— Legal Considerations

1. Dental jurisprudence is the application of legal statutes and regulations covering the practice of dentistry.
2. The dentist must obtain a federal narcotics stamp yearly.
3. The State Dental Board regulates and monitors the dental practice of the state.
4. A person illegally practicing dental acts may be fined and imprisoned.
5. Malpractice may occur from performing an act or failure to correctly perform a service that results in an injury to the patient.
6. Reasons for a malpractice suit may be: did not perform "standard of treatment," improperly performed a service, did not fully instruct patient, did not seek competent care, lack of treatment, did not diagnose properly, violated the patient's privacy, did not give attention to symptoms or complaints, did not fulfill contract with patient.
7. The assistant may do assigned duties thoroughly and correctly and perform only trained and legal services.

8. The assistant must maintain correct, neat, and clear records. Mark off mistakes and get written permission for sending records out.
9. The assistant gives clear instructions to the patient or the patient's guardian or companion. Give out printed instructions for take home use.
10. The assistant should keep emergency skills fresh; avoid comments about an emergency, the dentist, or dental professionals.

Assignment Sheet 1.5 Dental Jurisprudence—Legal Considerations

A. 1. Federal narcotics stamp
   2. Answers may include the following reasons:
      a. The State Dental Practice Act (SDPA) has the duty to govern and supervise the amount, type, and effectiveness of the art of dentistry within the state boundaries.
      b. To maintain control of the quality of the dental treatment within the state, the SDPA regulates the competence of the dental professionals through the licensing and certification processes.
      c. By requiring the practitioner to display the license and renewal stamp, the SDPA informs the patients of the operator's certification.
      d. The SDPA monitors developments in the dental profession and makes recommendations to the state legislature for passage of legal statutes.
      e. By maintaining a board of dental examiners and state office, the SDPA provides a watchful concern for dental care and professional treatment.
      f. When infractions of the law occur, the SDPA may suspend or revoke a dental professional license. The courts may impose fines or prison sentences.
   3. a. duties—perform only duties legally able or permitted; complete assigned tasks properly and competently (such as sterilizing and maintaining asepsis)
      b. record keeping—maintain confidentiality of patient's records; when making corrections, mark through original, inscribe new material, and initial
      c. instructions—gives full and complete instructions to patient; give written instructions to sedated patient; make sure patient understands instructions before dismissal
      d. actions—be alert and look for possible hazards; maintain ethical standards and avoid slander and libel
B. Students should provide a presentation indicating their legal interests.

Theory Recall:
Job Sources

1. The Sunday edition of the newspapers usually contains the most want ads.
2. The job-seeking assistant should read all ads in the classified section to avoid missing one placed in an unusual statement or division.
3. A school placement office seeks jobs in local businesses and receives inquiries about placement for students in local facilities.
4. A former instructor may be a good source for employment because the instructor has relationships with local dentists and facilities and may place a reference.
5. Networking is telling everyone that a job is desired and needed.
6. Attending local professional meetings may help continue education and also establish contacts in the dental world.
7. The state government offers free employment services for its residents.
8. When dealing with a commercial placement agency, the assistant should be sure the agency is licensed and keeps records confidential. Fee payment requirements and schedules should be in the contract, and all contracts should be carefully read and understood before signing.
9. Employment in a temporary placement service keeps the assistant's knowledge and skills current and also establishes contacts for employment.
10. After leaving a resume in an office, the assistant should wait a week before calling back to inquire into the status of the resume.

Assignment Sheet 1.6
Job Sources

Answers for these questions depend on the student's choices, location, and instructional facility. Student's answers are personal and related to individual situations.

Theory Recall:
Composing a Resume and Cover Letter

1. A resume is a fact sheet describing the experiences and education of an applicant applying for a job.
2. The correctness and appearance of the resume are important because it is the first impression made upon the employer.
3. A resume should be short and brief, usually one page long.
4. The employer becomes aware of the applicant's goals and objectives, which are stated on the resume.
5. The functional resume stresses skills and educational experiences.

6. All work and educational experiences are listed from the most recent to the least recent in the chronological resume.
7. References need not be placed on the resume; but if the applicant feels that the references are particularly strong, they may be included.
8. A cover letter explains the reason for the resume.
9. Paragraph one of the cover letter should explain why the letter and resume were sent. Paragraph two describes the strengths of the applicant, and paragraph three states the desire and availability of the applicant for an interview.
10. Photographs are not included in the letter, but copies of certificates and related awards may be enclosed.

Assignment Sheet 1.7
Composing a Resume and Cover Letter

The assignment sheet indicates a point system to evaluate the student's resume and cover letter.

Theory Recall:
Completing a Job Application Form

1. A job application form is given to a potential employee when the applicant arrives for an interview, or it may be requested at the place of employment.
2. Job application forms differ from form to form. Some are simple; others are quite complicated.
3. The applicant can be prepared for the questions by taking along a written card with the information usually requested on an application.
4. Being prepared with the information may prevent erasures or blanks.
5. Before filling out the form, the applicant should read it over and follow directions.
6. If the question does not apply to the applicant, "NA" (not applicable) should be written in the blank.
7. All answers should be truthful because employers check references and former places of employment.
8. If there is a question the applicant does not understand, the applicant should ask for an explanation.
9. The appearance of the application form indicates the type of work the potential employee can contribute.

Assignment Sheet 1.8
Completing a Job Application Form

The assignment sheet suggests a point system to evaluate the student's ability to complete a job application form.

Theory Recall:
Demonstrating Job Interview Skills

1. During this early arrival time, the assistant may appraise the office, looking at the staff-patient relationships and the atmosphere.
2. If the assistant is not sure of the office location, he or she should go there the night before.
3. The assistant should come to the interview alone to avoid giving the impression of dependence and fear.
4. The assistant should be neat and clean and dressed in a business style of clothing.
5. The assistant should wear pleasant, light perfume or cologne and daytime makeup.
6. When seated, the assistant should avoid any irritating mannerisms.
7. The grammar of the office staff projects the office image to the patients.
8. The assistant can show a positive attitude by saying only good things and avoiding negative items.
9. If the assistant is not aware of a certain procedure, a quick "I am willing to learn" will help.
10. The thank-you letter should thank the person for the interview, restate the interest in the job, and indicate availability for another interview.

Assignment Sheet 1.9
Demonstrating Job Interview Skills

The assignment sheet suggests a point system for evaluation of the student's job interview skills.

Post Test

MATCHING: 1.c 2.j 3.i 4.a 5.b 6.g 7.h 8.d 9.e 10.f
TRUE OR FALSE: 1. false 2. false 3. true 4. false 5. true
MULTIPLE CHOICE: 1.a 2.d 3.d 4.c 5.a 6.a 7.b 8.a 9.c
10.a 11.b 12.c 13.d 14.b 15.d 16.c 17.c 18.c 19.d 20.c

UNIT 2 EMERGENCY CARE AND FIRST AID

Theory Recall:
Emergency Care Preparation

1. The most effective and efficient way of dealing with an emergency is to be prepared.
2. Practicing emergencies helps each member of the dental team become familiar with his or her duties.
3. The dental assistant may be the first to notice distress because the assistant monitors and remains with the patient after injections and surgery and stressful situations.

4. The first rule an assistant must follow in an emergency is to remain calm.
5. The patient may become more stressful when witnessing panic.
6. One way to summon aid without unnecessary excitement is to develop a special code word to signify an emergency.
7. While the assistant is waiting for aid, a quick look for medical identification tags or a check of the medical history may be made.
8. Numbers for emergency assistance should be placed near each phone in the dental office.
9. The assistant should check the timeliness of all materials on the emergency tray, especially the expiration date of the drugs.
10. The assistant may aid in administering oxygen by obtaining the tank and mask and regulating the flow of the oxygen.
11. An ambu bag is a pressurized, forced-air mask and bag used to push air into the patient's lungs.
12. When an emergency has passed, the assistant records the date, time, symptoms, treatment, medications used, and any other data the dentist requests.

Assignment Sheet 2.1
Emergency Care Rules

A. Answers may include some of the following reasons:
1. By monitoring the patient's health history, we can be alerted to possible health hazards and cautions and help prevent emergencies from occurring.
2. By watching the patient and being alert for emergency signals, we can give emergency treatment at the onset and prevent further or progressive damage.
3. By remaining calm in an emergency, we can avoid distressing the patient, avoid intensifying the problem, and work more smoothly.
4. By seeking assistance, we can give undivided attention to the patient and start treatment while help is arriving.
5. When we review the patient's records, we may discover silent or unnoticed health hazards or conditions that may be involved in the emergency.
6. If emergency room or care phone numbers are readily available for use, time may be saved and assistance can be obtained more quickly.
7. By being familiar with the emergency tray, the assistant may more quickly and efficiently serve the dentist during an emergency.
8. Knowing how to administer oxygen may be a necessity during an emergency because so

many conditions are eased or treated with the administration of oxygen.

9. Being able to assist the dentist with emergency care will be an asset as it will permit faster and better care to the victim.

10. Recording important data after an emergency can be useful for future treatment and also may be used in any legal case following an episode.

B. Students may enact an emergency of choice and simulate proper use of emergency care rules.

Theory Recall:
Measuring and Recording Vital Signs

1. Pulse, respirations, blood pressure, and body temperature compose the vital signs.
2. Pulse is an indication of blood flow within an artery.
3. The pulse is felt by placing gentle pressure against the artery to feel the "beat."
4. The quality and rhythm of the pulse also is recorded with the count.
5. The index and third fingers are used to feel the radial pulse.
6. The normal pulse range for an adult is 60 to 80 beats per minute; a child's range is 80 to 110 beats per minute.
7. The assistant must count one full inhale and exhale to make up one respiration.
8. The assistant does not caution the patient when taking respiration readings so that the patient does not alter the count.
9. The normal range of respirations per minute for an adult is 14 to 18; for a child the normal range is 18 to 24 per minute.
10. Diastolic pressure is the force of the blood flow when the vessel is at rest.
11. The assistant places the sphygmomanometer cuff around the brachial artery when taking a blood pressure reading in the dental office.
12. The diaphragm of the stethoscope is placed over the brachial artery when taking a blood pressure reading.
13. The systolic pressure reading is taken when the first heartbeat sound is heard.
14. A high systolic reading is anything over 140 mm Hg and a high diastolic reading is over 90 mm Hg.
15. The oral cavity and the ear canal may be used to take a body temperature in the dental office.
16. The glass oral thermometer is kept in the oral cavity for three minutes.
17. A sterile, plastic probe cover is placed over the probe of the electric thermometer when taking a temperature.
18. The infrared scanner senses the body heat of the tympanic membrane in the ear.
19. A clear barrier shield is placed over the probe end of the infrared scanner to keep the optic scanner clean and sanitary.
20. The infrared scanner takes about five seconds to record the heat of the tympanic membrane.

Theory Recall:
Assisting the Choking Victim

1. Some symptoms of choking are inability to speak or make a noise, patient grasps neck, terror-filled eyes, panic.
2. The assistant should say to the patient "Are you choking?"
3. The first thing an assistant must do with a choking victim is to stay calm and seek assistance.
4. If an assistant must contact the emergency squad operator, the assistant should identify the caller, the emergency, and the place, and remain on the line until the operator has enough information.
5. The patient is positioned in front of the rescuer in the standing Heimlich maneuver.
6. The fist is placed above the belt line and below the rib cage in the standing Heimlich maneuver.
7. The assistant straddles the victim who is on the floor.
8. The pregnant woman needs modification in the placement of the fist in the Heimlich maneuver. The fist is placed in the midsection of the sternum instead of above the belt line and below the rib cage.
9. Enough thrusts are given to the victim to remove the object. Many times one or two are enough. Sometimes it may take ten or more.
10. Any sweep of the oral cavity should be from side to side and not straight into the cavity.
11. If the victim begins to cough, the assistant should cease the thrusts until the victim coughs up the object.
12. After the item is dislodged, the assistant should remain with the patient and perhaps offer oxygen and reassurance until the stress has passed.
13. When the patient leaves, the emergency, the treatment and any other data the dentist wishes to note are written on the patient's chart.

Theory Recall:
Cardiopulmonary Resuscitation

1. CPR designates cardiopulmonary resuscitation, which is restoring the functions of the heart and lungs.
2. The air inflation of the lungs and the beat of the heart are functions that CPR imitates.
3. When finding an unconscious victim, the assistant shakes and tries to arouse the patient.

4. The assistant checks for breathing by listening for air, feeling for exhalations, and watching the rise and fall of the chest.
5. The assistant determines if the heart is beating by feeling the carotid artery.
6. If the attempt to inflate the lungs is unsuccessful, the assistant attempts the Heimlich maneuver to expel any object.
7. If the airway is open, the assistant must check the carotid artery to determine if the heart is beating. If present, no CPR compression is given.
8. The heel of the palms is placed on the victim's sternum, two fingers above the sternum tip (xiphoid process).
9. The assistant compresses the chest 1½ to 2 inches deep.
10. In one-person CPR, the rate of breaths and compressions is 2 breaths per 15 compressions.
11. The assistant checks the carotid artery after every four cycles of breath and compression exchanges.
12. When two persons are available for CPR, the rate of breaths and compressions is one breath for five compressions.
13. Rescuer two, the person doing the chest compressions, gives the order to exchange positions in CPR.
14. CPR is continued until aid arrives or a doctor pronounces death.
15. When the emergency is over, the assistant records the date, day, and time of the emergency, the symptoms, the treatment, and any timing notes. The summary is reviewed with the dentist.

Theory Recall:
Assisting with a Shock Emergency

1. Shock is a sign of the body functions undergoing undue stress and damage.
2. The most common type of shock found in the dental office is fainting or syncope.
3. Anaphylactic shock is shock caused from an allergic reaction.
4. A patient who chokes on an object may go into respiratory shock.
5. Patients who are taking insulin may go into metabolic shock.
6. Visible signs of shock are pale or bluish skin, cool and clammy skin, excessive perspirations, anxiety, nervousness, rapid and weak pulse, and rapid respirations.
7. To treat shock, remain calm, seek assistance, remove the cause of shock, restore the body functions, keep the patient warm, and remain with the patient demonstrating a reassuring attitude.
8. Syncope is fainting.

9. Spirits of ammonia is administered to a syncope or fainting victim.
10. An anaphylactic shock victim may wheeze, show a rash, or complain of a thick tongue.
11. An antihistamine or epinephrine is given to the anaphylactic shock victim.
12. The heart attack or cardiogenic shock victim is the most dangerous type.
13. If a heart patient becomes unconscious, the assistant should check the breathing and the carotid artery. If no breathing and pulse is found, CPR is started.
14. The dentist may give the heart patient a nitroglycerine pill to place under the tongue to ease the pain.
15. If the patient has suffered an anaphylactic shock due to a medication in the dental office, the medication is noted on the patient's chart in big red letters so it will not be given in the future.

Post Test

FILL IN: 1. ventilator 2. carotid 3. vital signs 4. tympanic
MATCHING: 1.e 2.g 3.b 4.h 5.c 6.f 7.d 8.a
MULTIPLE CHOICE: 1.b 2.d 3.a 4.d 5.c 6.c 7.d 8.a 9.b 10.b 11.d 12.a 13.a 14.d 15.a 16.a 17.b 18.c 19.b 20.a

UNIT 3 INFECTION CONTROL AND HAZARD MANAGEMENT

Theory Recall:
Hand-washing Technique

1. Hand washing begins the chain of asepsis series.
2. Antimicrobial soap removes dirt and germs and retards the growth of pathogens.
3. Hands should be washed at the beginning and end of workday and between each procedure.
4. The blunt end of a cuticle or orange stick may be used to remove matter.
5. A paper towel placed between the hand and faucet is used to work the faucets.
6. Antimicrobial soap, disposable towels, cuticle or orange stick, nail brush, and a sink are needed for a hand-wash procedure.
7. Rings can hide microbes and tear rubber gloves.
8. The nail brush is used in a circular motion on knuckles and nails.
9. The hands are held downward during the rinsing cycle.
10. The assistant does not touch the container.

Theory Recall:
Barrier Attire

1. The dental office or facility is responsible for office laundry.
2. Clothing used in office wear should be moisture resistant.
3. Eyeglasses are for protection from pathogens and flying debris and objects.
4. The face shield should be cleaned after each use.
5. The face mask should be changed when it is wet and for each patient.
6. The four types of gloves used in the dental facility are rubber surgical, latex examination, vinyl overglove, and rubber or nitryl utility.
7. After use gloves are placed in disposal bags marked biohazard and contaminated material.
8. Gloves used in cleaning should be heavy rubber or nitryl utility.
9. Dirty attire is placed in a properly marked laundry bag.
10. The laundry bag is held by the outside and folded over on top.

Theory Recall:
Ultrasonic Cleaning

1. The ultrasonic cleaner is one of the most effective cleaners.
2. The ultrasonic cleaner uses cavitation (bubbling action).
3. Chemical action may be added in the type of solution.
4. The manufacturer has printed charts to aid with determining solutions and time.
5. The band regulates the seating depth of the beaker into the main tank.
6. The burs are placed in the bur basket for cleaning.
7. Instruments are placed in sequential order.
8. The condition of the solution and the cleaning schedule for the unit determines how often the solution is changed.
9. Etched beakers are discarded because scratches interfere with sonic wave transmission.
10. Placing lids during use prevents scattering of solution and pathogens. Placing lids during storage helps keep the solution clean and avoids evaporation.

Theory Recall:
Sterilization by the Autoclave Method

1. To be sterilized, all forms of life, pathogenic or not, must be destroyed.
2. The most effective method of sterilization is autoclaving.
3. To perform correct sterilization through autoclaving, the assistant must avoid overcrowding, tilt jars, open hinges, and remove lids.
4. Distilled water is used in the autoclave to produce steam.
5. The thermostat activates the heat and is used until the amber light is off.
6. The desired conditions are 15 pounds of pressure, 250°F, and 20 minutes.
7. When the timer bell goes off, the assistant turns the dial to the vent position.
8. The pressure and temperature dials must indicate zero before opening the door of the warm autoclave.
9. The assistant waits a few minutes before emptying the autoclave to allow for final evaporation and moisture to escape.
10. With higher pressure and heat, the time is lessened.

Theory Recall:
Dry Heat Sterilization

1. There is no rusting with dry heat. Rusting is possible with an autoclave.
2. One disadvantage is the dry heat sterilizer takes longer than the autoclave.
3. The amount of temperature determines the time requirement for dry heat sterilization.
4. Time requirements are one hour for 340°F and two hours for 320°F.
5. Aluminum foil can be used as a wrap for dry heat sterilization.
6. Avoid overcrowding. Permit the heat to circulate.
7. The temperature will drop when cool instruments are placed in the chamber. Allow the temperature to rise to the proper temperature again.
8. Inserting new objects into a dry oven sterilizer during a sterilizing process ruins the present cycle.
9. Instruments are put away in their proper places after sterilization.
10. New loads may be started immediately.

Theory Recall:
Chemicals as Disinfectants and Sterilizers

1. Spores are pathogens that can build protective coatings around them.
2. Chemicals used in the office should have seals from the EPA and ADA.
3. Distilled water is used to dilute chemicals.
4. Sterilization takes hours of immersion; disinfection takes minutes.
5. Shelf or active life is the amount of time a chemical product is effective.
6. Sodium hypochlorite must be prepared daily.

7. Indicators reflect when effectiveness is weakening or gone.
8. Ratio determines if solution is to be used as sterilizer or disinfectant.
9. When working with chemicals avoid spills and splashes on the body or clothing. Flush affected areas with water. Read the manufacturer's precautions. Use transfer forceps, and avoid inserting fingers into solutions. Do not rush or move in a hurried manner.
10. The assistant has the responsibility to read the manufacturer's directions, use chemicals in the proper manner, test effectiveness, and record test results.

Theory Recall:
Cleanup of Operatory and Equipment Techniques

1. Handpieces are operated to move the water through the hoses.
2. The assistant uses suction to aspirate a disinfecting and deodorizing solution through the hoses.
3. Handpieces that cannot be sterilized should be disinfected or discarded.
4. Solutions should remain on the surfaces as long as recommended by the manufacturer.
5. Sharp objects are given attention first on an instrument tray.
6. They must be cleaned, checked for function, wrapped, and prepared.
7. They are placed in a marked disposal bag.
8. The floor is checked and any spills or splashes are wiped up.
9. The gloves are washed, rinsed, disinfected, and placed on a rack to dry.
10. Sterile transfer forceps are used to transport unwrapped instruments.

Theory Recall:
Hazard and Fire Control

1. The assistant must label the small bottle to indicate the contents.
2. The manufacturer supplies a manufacturer's safety data sheet (MSDS).
3. Chemical hazards can come in any size bottle.
4. When working around chemicals, the assistant should identify the materials, wear PPE, keep MSDS references, investigate new products, keep bottles and jar lids on and tight, know first aid for materials, have good ventilation, keep chemicals away from flame, store products according to the manufacturer's plan, and clean up messes.
5. Gloves, eyeglasses, and, in some cases, masks should be worn when working with chemicals.

6. The assistant must wear eye protection when working on a trimmer.
7. The assistant should start work on a dental lathe on slow speed.
8. The electrical cord should be placed behind the appliance.
9. Some heat hazard sources are: sterilizers, Bunsen burners, and alcohol torches.
10. The best preparation for a fire emergency is to stay calm, know emergency numbers, and know the location, type, and use of the fire extinguisher.

Assignment Sheet 3.1
Hazard and Fire Control

A. Answers may include the following reasons or definitions:
1. Ten rules to use when working with chemicals are:
   know the identity of the chemical in use
   wear protective garments
   keep MSDSs on file for reference
   investigate contents of new products
   keep bottles and jars capped when not in use
   know first-aid for contact with hazardous materials
   have good ventilation when working with chemicals
   keep flames and heat sources away from chemicals
   store products according to the manufacturers' directions
   clean up messes immediately, dispose of residue properly
2. Some rules to follow when working with the power trimmer are:
   wear safety glasses when in use
   pull and tie back hair
   roll up sleeves, remove bracelets
   keep electrical cord behind and out of the way of the machine
   plug in the cord just before use
   remain with machine after turn off until fully stopped
   keep sufficient water supply on trimmer abrasive wheel
   trim only gypsum products on trimmer wheel
   use moderately firm pressure when in use
   keep models on tray for stability during trimming
   concentrate on the job at hand
   always leave the wheel clean
   brush or clean wheel only when fully stopped and unplugged
3. Some rules to follow when working with power equipment in general are:

wear glasses, tie hair back, remove jewelry

check the electrical cord, place it behind the machine

check the sturdiness of the machine

start action in slow speed, increase later if necessary

remain with machine until fully stopped

clean machine only when stopped and unplugged

concentrate on the job at hand

4. General rules to be followed when working with hazards are:

avoid clutter, pick up and put things away after use

close all drawers and file cabinet shelves when not in use

keep electrical cords behind machines

read directions before using machines and equipment

maintain a watchful eye for possible hazards

B. Student may simulate an emergency fire situation of choice and dramatize what actions to take.

Post Test

MATCHING: 1.f 2.h 3.i 4.j 5.a 6.c 7.g 8.e 9.b 10.d
MULTIPLE CHOICE: 1.d 2.d 3.d 4.c 5.a 6.d 7.b 8.b 9.a
10.b 11.b 12.d 13.a 14.a 15.d 16.a 17.a 18.a 19.b 20.a

UNIT 4 BASIC DENTAL FUNDAMENTALS

Theory Recall:
Tooth Anatomy

1. Teeth are for chewing (mastication), speaking (articulation), and looks (esthetics).
2. Four types of teeth are:
   incisors—used to cut food
   canines/cuspids—used to tear food
   bicuspids/premolars—used to break up and crush food
   molars—used to grind and pulverize food
3. Mandibular signifies lower jaw; maxillary signifies upper jaw.
4. Adults develop permanent or secondary teeth; children develop primary or deciduous teeth.
5. Adults develop bicuspids or premolars and third molars, which children do not.
6. The half section of an arch is a quadrant.
7. Anatomic landmarks of a tooth are:
   cusp—round or hilly growth or projection
   ridges—elevations in a tooth
   pits—small depressions in tooth surface

fissures—developmental grooves between lobes

grooves—linear depressions running between cusps

cingulum—lobe on lingual side of maxillary incisors

lobes—bumps or lumps arising from surface

8. The three major tissues of the periodontium are the alveolar plate, periodontal ligaments, and gingiva.
9. The area between the attached and loose gingiva is called the sulcus.
10. The interdental papilla is gingival tissue that mounds up between the interproximals of the teeth.

Assignment Sheet 4.1
Tooth Anatomy

A. 1. The permanent teeth in a quadrant are the central incisor, lateral incisor, canine or cuspid, first premolar or first bicuspid, second premolar or second bicuspid, first molar, second molar, and the third molar. The primary teeth in a quadrant are the central incisor, lateral incisor, canine or cuspid, first molar, second molar, and the third molar.

2. The anterior teeth are the central and lateral incisors and cuspids or canines. The posterior teeth are the first and second premolars or bicuspids and the first, second, and third molars.

3. The four tissues and their functions are:
   a. enamel—provides cover and protection for tooth
   b. dentin—gives bulk and shape to tooth
   c. pulp—provides nourishment and sensation for tooth
   d. cementum—provides cover for root and anchorage for periodontal tissues.

B. 1.d, 2.e, 3.a, 4.b, 5.c, 6.f, 7.i, 8.j, 9.g, 10.h

Theory Recall:
Tooth Surfaces

1. Knowledge of tooth surfaces is necessary for charting teeth, posting treatment and charges, writing insurance claims, and other dental work.
2. The cutting edge of the anterior teeth is called incisal.
3. The grinding surface of the posterior teeth is called occlusal.
4. The surfaces of the teeth that touch the tongue are called lingual.
5. The surfaces of the teeth touching the cheek are called facial or buccal surfaces.

354

6. The teeth touch together at the proximal area.
7. The side of the tooth closer to the midline is the mesial.
8. The side of the tooth farther from the midline is the distal.
9. Occlusal is O or Occ; Buccal is B or Buc; Distal is D.
10. MODL or MODLi is the abbreviation, and it would be written mesio-occluso-disto-lingual.

Assignment Sheet 4.2
Tooth Surfaces

A. 1. Six surfaces of the tooth and its location are:
  a. mesial—closest side surface to midline of face
  b. distal—side of tooth away from midline of face
  c. buccal or facial—side of posterior tooth touching cheek tissue
  labial or facial—side of anterior tooth touching lip tissue
  d. lingual—surface of tooth touching tongue
  e. incisal—cutting surface of anterior tooth
  occlusal—chewing surface of posterior tooth
  f. apical—root tip surface
2. Abbreviations are: labial—Lab, facial—F, occlusal—O or Occ, incisal—I, mesial—M, distal—D, lingual—L or Li, buccal—B
3. Terms for the following abbreviations are: a. MOD—mesio-occlusodistal, b. MO—mesio-occlusal, c. MOL—mesio-occlusolingual, d. MI—mesioincisal, e. MID—mesioincisodistal, f. DOB—disto-occlusobuccal
B. Students may use clinic chart to color designated tooth surfaces.

Theory Recall:
Tooth Numbering Systems

1. The Universal numbering system starts numbering in the maxillary right quadrant.
2. Deciduous teeth are identified by the letters A–T.
3. They are numbered 1 because they are closest to the midline.
4. Brackets are used to designate quadrants.
5. Prefixes are added to the Palmer tooth number.
6. In the Palmer method, the deciduous teeth have letters, while in the Federation Dentaire Internationale system, they have numbers.

Assignment Sheet 4.3
Tooth Numbering Systems

	Universal Number	Palmer Number	Federation Number
A. Permanent teeth			
Max. rt. third molar	1	8|	18
Max. rt. second molar	2	7|	17
Max. rt. first molar	3	6|	16
Max. rt. second bicuspid or premolar	4	5|	15
Max. rt. first bicuspid or premolar	5	4|	14
Max. rt. canine or cuspid	6	3|	13
Max. rt. lateral	7	2|	12
Max. rt. central	8	1|	11
Max. lt. central	9	|1	21
Max. lt. lateral	10	|2	22
Max. lt. canine or cuspid	11	|3	23
Max. lt. first bicuspid or premolar	12	|4	24
Max. lt. second bicuspid or premolar	13	|5	25
Max. lt. first molar	14	|6	26
Max. lt. second molar	15	|7	28
Max. lt. third molar	16	|8	28
Man. lt. third molar	17	|8	38
Man. lt. second molar	18	|7	37
Man. lt. first molar	19	|6	36
Man. lt. second bicuspid or premolar	20	|5	35
Man. lt. first bicuspid or premolar	21	|4	34
Man. lt. canine or cuspid	22	|3	33
Man. lt. lateral	23	|2	32
Man. lt. central	24	|1	31
Man. rt. central	25	1|	41
Man. rt. lateral	26	2|	42
Man. rt. canine or cuspid	27	3|	43
Man. rt. first bicuspid or premolar	28	4|	44
Man. rt. second bicuspid or premolar	29	5|	45
Man. rt. first molar	30	6|	46
Man. rt. second molar	31	7|	47
Man. rt. third molar	32	8|	48
Deciduous teeth			
Max. rt. second molar	A	E|	55
Max. rt. first molar	B	D|	54
Max. rt. canine or cuspid	C	C|	53
Max. rt. lateral	D	B|	52
Max. rt. central	E	A|	51
Max. lt. central	F	|A	61
Max. lt. lateral	G	|B	62
Max. lt. canine or cuspid	H	|C	63

Max. lt. first molar	I	D	64
Max. lt. second molar	J	E	65
Man. lt. second molar	K	E	75
Man. lt. first molar	L	D	74
Man. lt. canine or cuspid	M	C	73
Man. lt. lateral	N	B	72
Man. lt. central	O	A	71
Man. rt. central	P	A	81
Man. rt. lateral	Q	B	82
Man. rt. canine or cuspid	R	C	83
Man. rt. first molar	S	D	84
Man. rt. second molar	T	E	85

B. Give numbering system letter for each tooth listed below:

	Universal Number	Palmer Number	Federation Number
Permanent max. rt. first molar	3	6	16
Permanent man. lt. central	24	1	31
Deciduous max. rt. central	E	A	51
Permanent max. lt. second premolar	13	5	25
Deciduous man. lt. first molar	L	E	75
Permanent man. rt. canine or cuspid	27	3	43
Permanent man. lt. second premolar	20	5	35
Deciduous max. rt. canine	C	C	53
Permanent man. lt. lateral	23	2	32
Deciduous max. rt. lateral	D	B	52

Theory Recall: Charting Teeth

1. The mandibular left first molar, #19, is missing and not replaced.
2. The fixed bridge is located in the maxillary left quadrant.
3. The mandibular right first molar needs to be extracted.
4. RCT means root canal treatment.
5. The restoration of tooth #27 is Class V.
6. The restoration on the maxillary right first molar is on the buccal or facial surface.
7. Tooth #18 is drifting mesially.
8. A striped crown indicates gold material is used.
9. Zigzag lines indicate fractured roots or tooth.
10. The mouth used in this exercise is an adult dentition.

Assignment Sheet 4.4 Charting Teeth

Patient A

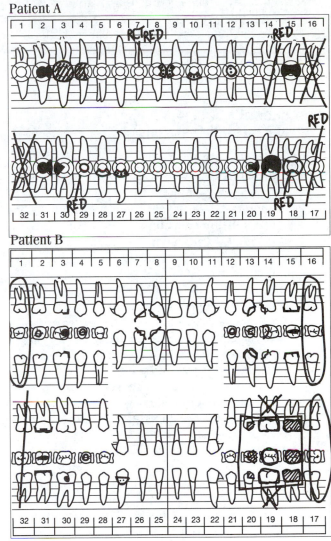

Patient B

(Courtesy of Medical Arts Press, 1-800-328-2179.)

Theory Recall: Operative Hand Instruments

1. Instruments are divided according to their work task.
2. The assistant may read the manufacturer's name, composition material of the instrument, code number of the instrument, and name of instrument.
3. Three parts are shaft or handle, shank or neck, and blade or nib.
4. The shaft or handle may be round or eight- or six-sided; smooth, rough, or scored; or oversized.
5. Some groups of instruments are basic, cutting, condensing, burnishing, plastic filling, carving, and miscellaneous.
6. The cotton plier tips may be plain or serrated.

7. Instruments are arranged in their order of use on a dental tray.
8. Plastic means the material is movable, soft, and pliable.
9. A burnisher may be purchased in a ball, oval, football, beaver-tail, or round shape.
10. The cleoid end of the discoid/cleoid instrument is pointed.

Assignment Sheet 4.5
Operative Hand Instruments

A. The function of the following instruments is:
   1. amalgam carrier—to transport amalgam while in plastic shape to tooth prep
   2. explorer—to locate and define carious lesions and tooth imperfections; may also be used to spoon out decay during restoration preparation
   3. discoid/cleoid—to carve tooth restorative material while in plastic stage
   4. mirror—to view mouth interior, reflect light, and retract tongue or tissue
   5. burnisher—to smooth and adapt restoration margins of newly placed material
   6. condenser—to condense or compact plastic restorative material into prep
   7. PFI (plastic filling instrument)—to carry materials to site, smooth edges
   8. pick up or college pliers—to carry, transport, or pick up materials or objects
   9. scaler—to scale or remove deposits from surface of tooth
   10. hatchet—to remove carious tooth tissues during tooth restoration prep
   11. curette—to remove or scale deep-seated deposits from teeth
   12. carver—to prepare restorative surface, carve form into restoration
   13. excavator—to remove carious tooth tissue during restoration prep

B. Instruments listed in appropriate family:
   1. amalgam carrier—plastic filling
   2. explorer—basic
   3. discoid/cleoid—cutting
   4. mirror—basic
   5. burnisher—plastic filling
   6. condenser—plastic filling
   7. PFI—plastic filling
   8. pick up or college pliers—basic
   9. scaler—prophylaxis
   10. hatchet—cutting
   11. curette—prophylaxis
   12. carver—plastic filling
   13. excavator—cutting

Theory Recall:
Transfer of Instruments

1. The assistant must have a working knowledge of the instruments.
2. Two basic groups of instruments are the pen grasp (mouth mirror, explorer, scaler, curette, excavator, hatchet, burnisher, condensor), and the palm grasp (anesthetic syringe, dental dam clamp holder, punch, elevator, pliers, forceps, scissors).
3. Don't transfer over the patient's face.
   Await signal for transfer.
   Keep passing zone close to face.
   Arrange instruments in sequential order and working position.
   Pass instrument with working part faced toward work site.
   Use left hand for passing and receiving.
   Place double-ended instruments with the working area away from the assistant.
   Be prepared to move double-ended instruments as needed.
   Be alert and prepared.
4. The assistant picks up an instrument with the thumb and forefinger of the left hand.
5. The little finger is used to retrieve used instruments.
6. The used instrument is placed back on the tray in proper order.
7. The palm-thumb grasp reception is in the fingers of the palm. The palm grasp is in the full palm.
8. Forceps, dental dam clamp holders, and hinged instruments may be used.
9. The working end of the instrument is placed toward the operator.
10. The operator uses a palm grasp finger type of instrument in a wedge or pushing motion.

Theory Recall:
Dental Rotary Instruments

1. The four functions of a bur are cut, reduce, finish, and polish teeth, restorations and appliances.
2. The three parts of the dental bur are head, neck, and shank.
3. The size and shape of the head determine the bur's number.
4. Crosscut burs have extra cuts on the blade edge, are faster cutting, and are more abrasive.
5. HP denotes handpiece; LT denotes latch type; FG denotes friction grip.
6. Diamond heads do not have cutting or blade edges.
7. Water keeps the tip cool and prevents clogging the surface.
8. Stones are used for finishing and polishing.

9. Surgical burs are used in larger areas, such as alveolar plates, impacted molars, and maxillary and mandibular bones.
10. Disks, cups, and wheels are attached to provide for finishing and polishing.

Post Test

MATCHING: 1.i 2.g 3.h 4.b 5.c 6.d 7.a 8.j 9.f 10.e
TRUE OR FALSE: 1. false 2. false 3. false 4. true 5. false
MULTIPLE CHOICE: 1.a 2.b 3.b 4.c 5.d 6.b 7.d 8.c 9.b 10.b 11.d 12.d 13.c 14.b 15.a

UNIT 5 CHAIRSIDE FUNDAMENTALS

Theory Recall:
Preparing and Dismissing the Patient

1. The preparation begins the day before by pulling charts and preparing.
2. The receptionist normally pulls the charts for the coming day.
3. The chairside assistant makes sure all needed materials are present, sets up the tray, and covers the tray for the coming appointment.
4. The chairside assistant escorts the patient to the operatory.
5. When working on the upper arch, the chair is placed in a supine position. For the lower arch, the chair back is at a 30 to 40 degree angle with the floor.
6. The assistant must always caution the patient when making chair movement.
7. Particular attention is given to any medication changes.
8. The operatory light is about 36 inches from the work site.
9. The assistant reviews postoperative instructions before dismissing the patient.
10. After the exam gloves are removed and the hands are washed, the assistant records the procedure on the patient's chart.

Theory Recall:
Evacuate and Rinse

1. Evacuation of fluids makes for better observation, more comfort for the patient, and less gagging.
2. A saliva ejector is smaller than an HVE tip, rounded on tip, gentle and disposable. An HVE tip is larger and has more force than a saliva ejector, and may be disposable or reused after proper sterilization.
3. Lines must be flushed, cleaned, and sanitized.

4. Ora-evac solutions dissolve gross debris and are biodegradable, pleasantly scented, and nonfoaming.
5. The Environmental Protection Agency (EPA) approves ora-evac system solutions.
6. Saliva ejector tips "hang" on the lower jaw, out of the work area site.
7. HVE tips should be kept distal to the work site. HVE tips should be held ¼ inch above or below the occlusal plane. HVE tip openings should be pointed to the source of fluids.
8. A triple syringe is used to rinse, spray and air dry the mouth.
9. The three functions of the triple syringe are air, water, and spray flow.
10. The assistant may gently pull out or extend the cheeks or lip into a cup shape.

Theory Recall:
Administration of Local Anesthesia

1. The area is dried and receives topical anesthesia before injection.
2. The anesthetic needles are 1 inch and $1\frac{5}{8}$ inches, the 1-inch needle is used for maxillary infiltration and the $1\frac{5}{8}$ for mandibular block.
3. The rubber plunger colors denote the presence and concentration of a vasoconstrictor.
4. The assistant should examine the cartridge for cracks, the condition of the plunger, the size of the air bubbles, and the clearness of the solution.
5. After the injection, the assistant monitors the patient's respirations and general health and behavior.
6. The assistant grasps the anesthetic syringe on the barrel after the injection.
7. The assistant replaces the sheath with one hand. The needle is placed in the sheath on the table, tilted upright, and snapped closed.
8. The assistant cautions the patient not to bite on the numbed lip.
9. The needle and sheath are placed in the sharps disposal after use.
10. The local anesthetic procedure is recorded on the patient's chart after the latex exam gloves are removed and the hands are washed.

Theory Recall:
Preparing Dental Liners and Cements

1. Some dental cements may be used as cements, bases, or temporary or permanent restorations.
2. The type of procedure, the depth of preparation, the pulpal involvement, and the choice of restorative material dictate the choice of material.

3. Capsule form helps cut down on cross contamination, and keeps dosage and preparation regulated.
4. Among the answers are: follow directions, don't mix manufacturer's materials with others, keep containers clean, recap immediately, check expiration dates, level scoops and measurements, fluff and shake before use, and clean up as soon as possible.
5. Zinc phosphate cement may be used as cement, base, or temporary restoration.
6. Zinc phosphate is mixed on a glass slab to absorb some heat from the mix.
7. Calcium hydroxide may be used under all restorations.
8. Type I glass ionomer materials are used for luting purposes.
9. Type II glass ionomer materials may be used in Class V erosion, small Class III restorations, and in pediatric restorations.
10. Materials that release fluoride help promote secondary dentin growth.

Theory Recall:
Placement and Removal of the
Tofflemire Retainer

1. The matrix band gives support and provides resistance while the amalgam is being placed.
2. A matrix band retainer keeps the matrix band in place.
3. The matrix band retainer is prepared by turning the outer knob to retract the spindle pin head to provide room for band insertion.
4. The assistant will assess the tooth involved and the tooth preparation.
5. The wing tips of the matrix band are situated toward the gingiva.
6. The head slot is directed toward the gingiva in a proper placement.
7. The spindle head pin presses against the band ends to hold the band in the retainer.
8. On a maxillary right quadrant tooth, the loop is placed through the gate side where there is no attachment.
9. The wedge holder with a wedge is passed to the dentist after the matrix is in place.
10. The wedge helps the matrix band adapt to the tooth, forms the contour of the tooth restoration, and helps avoid overhanging restorations.

Post Test

MULTIPLE CHOICE: 1.b 2.b 3.d 4.d 5.b 6.a 7.d 8.a 9.a 10.b 11.d 12.a 13.c 14.c 15.c
MATCHING: 1.g 2.a 3.c 4.f 5.b 6.h 7.e 8.d 9.j 10.i

UNIT 6 CHAIRSIDE ASSISTING

Theory Recall:
The Preliminary Examination

1. The first dental examination of a new patient establishes the professional relationship and determines the patient's general health and future treatment.
2. Setup includes: basic setup, periodontal probe, dental floss, forms, charts, pens, alginate impression setup, radiograph setup, vital signs setup, and miscellaneous setup as needed.
3. The assistant may take the new patient on a quick walking tour of the facility to acquaint the patient.
4. The dental exam begins with a thorough health history.
5. The patient's blood pressure is taken to discover hidden health problems.
6. The assistant records the findings accurately, neatly, and legibly during the physical exam.
7. An offensive mouth odor may represent poor dental health or diabetes.
8. The dentist checks the condition of the glands and nodes under the neck and chin.
9. The dentist may request the mirror, explorer, or periodontal probe during an exam.
10. The assistant dries a tooth area to prevent moisture reflection from distorting the view of the tooth surface.

Theory Recall:
Alginate Impressions

1. Alginate that turns from gel to solid and cannot be changed back to a gel is called irreversible.
2. Bumps or growths become dents or depressions (the opposite).
3. The assistant dons overgloves to gather or assemble any extra items.
4. The patient removes appliances and rinses mouth, and the upcoming procedure is explained.
5. Disposable trays receive a coat of adhesive to help hold the alginate.
6. The alginate is placed on the tray in more than one increment to avoid air bubbles.
7. If the patient has difficulty breathing during an impression taking, the patient is advised to bend over and take shallow breaths.
8. The impression is wrapped in a disinfectant moistened towel after it is removed from the mouth.
9. The bite should include the occlusal surfaces of the premolars and the first molar.
10. The impressions should be rinsed under tap water and sprayed with disinfectant before placing in a plastic bag.

Theory Recall:
Dental Prophylaxis

1. The tooth surfaces are scaled.
2. Teamwork and observation will help with the anticipation and familiarization of routines.
3. The assistant passes and receives instruments when called for or signaled.
4. The gauze may be held near the work site so the operator may wipe off the prophy instrument during the procedure.
5. The ultrasonic handpiece works on the same principle as the ultrasonic cleaner—cavitation.
6. Water is used to cool the ultrasonic tip.
7. Hard materials, tartar, calculus, and stain have been scraped off the crowns of the teeth.
8. Polishing of the crowns of the teeth follows the scaling procedure.
9. Prophylaxis pastes differ in grit, flavor, size, color, and container.
10. After polishing, the teeth are dental flossed.

Theory Recall:
Topical Fluoride Protection

1. Fluoride strengthens the enamel to make it more resistant to decay.
2. Topical fluoride is applied to the teeth. Systemic fluoride is acquired from ingesting fluoride in the water system.
3. Fluoride is applied after the teeth have been cleaned and the plaque is removed.
4. Topical fluoride comes in pastes, foams, gels, and liquid solutions.
5. The manufacturer's directions are included with the product.
6. Saliva and moisture may interfere with medicine touching the surfaces or dilute the medication.
7. The assistant discusses the treatment to allay the anxiety of the patient.
8. Overgloves prevent contamination to the mixing or supply bottles.
9. The mouth is packed with cotton rolls, and the saliva ejector removes moisture.
10. The patient is advised not to eat or drink for 30 minutes.

Theory Recall:
Application of Sealants

1. A sealant is a special epoxy resin material painted onto a tooth surface for protection of the occlusal surface.
2. As an advantage, sealants protect new teeth. As a disadvantage, sealants may provide a false security and they may become cracked or chipped.
3. Nonfluoridated prophylaxis paste is used.
4. The tooth to be treated is isolated by dental dam or cotton rolls.
5. The acid remains on the tooth the length of time directed by the manufacturer, which is usually one minute.
6. The enamel surface is a dull white.
7. The two types of sealants are self-curing and light-curing
8. The dentist probes the new surface with an explorer.
9. After the sealant proves to be successful, isolation is removed.
10. A round bur in a handpiece and articulating paper are used to finish the sealant.

Theory Recall:
Brushing and Flossing Techniques Instruction

1. Plaque is an invisible film that collects on the teeth and contains bacteria, which feed on the sugars in the mouth.
2. The teeth surfaces have been cleaned and do not contain any plaque for discoloring.
3. Encourage the patient to establish a routine in which all surfaces are cleaned.
4. The patient must get all tooth surfaces clean.
5. Flossing removes the interproximal matter.
6. A dentist may prefer waxed floss to get between hard or overlapping areas. Unwaxed floss does not leave any residue behind.
7. The patient wiggles and works the floss in between the teeth.
8. Interdental stimulators are inserted interproximally and rotated around to stimulate the tissues.
9. A bridge cleaner or loop could be used to clean a fixed appliance.
10. Each person must be treated as an individual and work with the patient to discover that person's best technique to clean the teeth.

Theory Recall:
Diet and Nutrition Counseling

1. A good diet and nutrition provide good health and control decay.
2. The counselor and patient need to establish feelings of teamwork and mutual understanding.
3. The lesson begins with an explanation of the decay process.
4. The counselor may draw three interlapping circles, which represent teeth, bacteria, and sugar (food).
5. There are many printed lists available to help show hidden sugars.

6. The patient can lift a spoonful of sugar from a bowl to represent each hidden spoonful or sugar in a favorite food or drink.
7. A cariogenic food is food that may encourage the growth of decay.
8. The patient should make out a diet diary to determine what types of foods are being consumed.
9. The assistant may circle cariogenic foods with red and substitute foods with blue.
10. The patient should become happier and healthier with less dental decay.

Theory Recall: Dental Dam Application

1. A dental dam isolates for sanitation, decreases moisture in work site, controls mouth tissue and tongue movement, and increases access and visibility.
2. Dental dam frames may be supplied in stainless steel, nylon, or plastic.
3. A dental dam stamp or template may be used to locate the hole's position.
4. The assistant must take into account missing teeth and malpositioned teeth.
5. Ragged holes tend to tear and pull apart.
6. A dental dam clamp holds the material on the anchor tooth.
7. The operator looks for any missing spots or pieces of material.
8. Tucking in dental dam material is called inversion. It is done to prevent moisture from seeping into the area.
9. A saliva ejector is used to empty the patient's mouth.
10. The assistant removes the napkin, rinses and evacuates the mouth, and massages the gingival area.

Theory Recall: Anterior Restorations

1. Anterior restorations can be present in any cavity classification except Class II (marginal or proximal walls of posterior tooth).
2. The choice of anterior restorative material may be based on such factors as the patient's age or habits, and the size, shape, and location of the preparation.
3. The choice of bases and liners depends on the restorative material used.
4. The assistant reviews the patient's health history after seating, draping, and positioning the patient.
5. The assistant helps to maintain visibility by clearing the mirror with air and holding the HVE tip at the work site to capture spray.
6. The assistant holds the prepared liner and base

mixes near the operative site for the dentist's use.
7. After the prep is overfilled, the assistant passes the anterior matrix and wedges.
8. The assistant holds the visible light tip next to the material, which needs the rays for setting.
9. The dentist uses abrasive stones, disks, and finishing burs to finish anterior restorations.
10. Treatment items such as type and quantity of anesthetic, type of base, and liners, type and class of restorative material are noted.

Theory Recall: Amalgam Posterior Restoration

1. Amalgam is the most common material used for posterior restorations.
2. Composite restorations may be finished and polished at the original appointment; amalgam restorations must have 24 to 48 hours to harden before finishing and polishing.
3. The dental dam, if used, is placed after the anesthetic has been administered.
4. The assistant aids in a light-curing process by holding the light tip near the work site and holding the safety shield.
5. After the matrix has been placed, the assistant passes a wedge holder or hemostat with wedge.
6. If there is no dental dam, cotton rolls are used to isolate a prep.
7. While the dentist carves the restoration, the assistant aspirates the shavings with the HVE.
8. The assistant passes college pliers to the dentist to gently remove the matrix band.
9. The assistant gives postoperative instructions to the patient before dismissal from the operatory.
10. Before lowering the chair, the assistant cautions the patient regarding the movement.

Theory Recall: Composite Posterior Restoration

1. The composite and amalgam restorations are similar in the following aspects: anesthesia, dental dam, and cavity preparation.
2. Calcium hydroxide, glass ionomer, and polycarboxylates may be placed under a composite restoration.
3. A clear mylar strip and a clear wedge are used in a light-cured composite.
4. A composite may be finished and polished at the original appointment.
5. To avoid discoloring, the dentist uses plastic or composite instruments when working with composite.
6. The assistant either passes or uses the air syringe to spray and dry the etching solution.

7. When mixing and preparing a composite material, the assistant follows the manufacturer's directions.

8. The assistant holds the curing light whenever an increment is placed or the material is soft.

9. When the dentist wishes to check the occlusion height of a new restoration, the assistant holds the articulating paper holder with paper over the occlusal biting surface.

10. The dentist may use composite points, stones, finishing bur, sandpaper strips, and dental floss to finish and polish a restoration.

Theory Recall:
Finishing and Polishing of Amalgam Restorations

1. Final finishing and polishing is done at least 24 to 48 hours after placement.

2. Finishing and polishing of a restoration is done to permit a more thorough contouring and polishing of the restoration.

3. An explorer is passed to the dentist to check the integrity of the restoration.

4. The most abrasive disk or point is used first.

5. The blue trace from the articulating paper indicates a high spot.

6. Dental floss or tape is passed through the interproximal space to check contact points.

7. The assistant passes a mirror and slow handpiece with rubber cup and pumice.

8. The brown, then green, then green with yellow band are used, in that order.

9. The abrasive strip is used to refine the interproximal spaces.

10. The assistant may place a slurry of pumice on the dental floss to aid in smoothing the interproximal spaces.

Theory Recall:
Tooth Bleaching Appointments

1. The two methods of bleaching are office and home bleaching.

2. Teeth stained from food or tobacco are the easiest to bleach.

3. Patients with periodontal problems must seek treatment for this problem before the bleaching process.

4. Large resin or porcelain restorations may not bleach and may need to be replaced because they do not match the new tooth shade.

5. The impression is poured into study models upon which a tray is built.

6. The acrylic tray is trimmed closely so that gingiva is not exposed to the bleach gel.

7. The teeth must be cleaned and isolated before gel placement.

8. The gel may be applied from a syringe or placed in a tray.

9. The shade guide indicates the change in color that is taking place.

10. The lips are elevated from the bleach site to avoid tissue irritation.

Post Test

MULTIPLE CHOICE: 1.a 2.d 3.c 4.d 5.a 6.d 7.b 8.b 9.b 10.a 11.d 12.c 13.a 14.d 15.b 16.a 17.b 18.c 19.a 20.a 21.c 22.b 23.a 24.a 25.a 26.b 27.c 28.c 29.d 30.d 31.b 32.b 33.a 34.a 35.b 36.b 37.d 38.a 39.a 40.c 41.d 42.d 43.c 44.a 45.a 46.c 47.b 48.b 49.d 50.a

UNIT 7 CHAIRSIDE SPECIALTIES

Theory Recall:
Pediatric Dentistry

1. Pediatric dentistry is the branch of dentistry that deals with children.

2. A mouth with primary and secondary teeth present is said to be a mixed dentition.

3. An assistant must be prepared and rehearsed but not abrupt or fast moving to worry the patient.

4. Three reasons that dental care is a necessity for the child patient may be: to maintain function of teeth for chewing, speaking, and looks; to maintain normal jaw growth and integrity of teeth movement; and to avoid pain and discomfort for the child patient.

5. Fluoride is applied to teeth to assist with decay prevention.

6. The methods of fluoride application in the dental office are rinse, gel, or foam application and liquid solution application.

7. The root is not fully formed on a newly erupted tooth and the calcification of the tissues is not complete.

8. The assistant can make the child more comfortable by explaining the operatory, equipment, and procedures.

9. The surfaces of properly etched teeth have a white, milky, or chalky appearance.

10. The teeth to receive sealant material may be isolated by dental dam or cotton rolls.

Theory Recall:
Pulp Therapy and Protective Crowns

1. The three treatments are pulp capping, pulpotomy, and pulpectomy.

2. Calcium hydroxide is placed over the pulpal exposure in a pulp capping. This medicine soothes the pulp and promotes secondary dentin formation.

3. The aseptic technique is needed because the bloodstream is entered.

4. The dentist may call for calcium hydroxide or ZOE.

5. A protective crown may be used: when a tooth is too broken down, when a tooth crown has been fractured, as part of an appliance, over pulpal therapy, in hypoplasia, or as a temporary restoration.

6. Crowns may be made of chrome, stainless steel, aluminum, or resin.

7. The assistant passes a boley gauge or a millimeter rule to measure the protective crown.

8. Zinc phosphate is mixed for cementation under the protective crown.

9. The assistant holds articulating paper on the occlusal surface to test the occlusal height of the new crown.

10. The assistant reviews the postoperative instructions with the parents.

Theory Recall: Space Maintainers

1. Two types of space maintainers are removable and fixed.

2. The space maintainer keeps the area open for the unerupted tooth that is to enter into the area.

3. The space maintainer is kept in place until the permanent tooth erupts.

4. The three types of space maintainers are band and loop or band-bar, distal shoe bar, and spring-activated appliances.

5. The band and loop type of appliance is most commonly used.

6. A distal shoe bar appliance is used in a one-sided area of the mouth.

7. A band or protective crown may serve as coverage on the anchor tooth.

8. The larger of the two teeth involved in the missing site is chosen.

9. Space maintainers will save costly orthodontic care caused by malocclusion from drifting teeth.

10. All three people—a dentist, a pediatric dentist, and an orthodontist—may apply space maintainers.

Theory Recall: Endodontics

1. The series of tests can indicate the degree of pulpal degeneration and the future treatment to the dentist.

2. The medication and antibiotic reaction part of the health questionnaire is most important in endodontics.

3. The dentist palpates the neck and gland areas looking for infection.

4. Using the mirror and explorer, the dentist can perform the clinical exam, the percussion test, and the mobility test.

5. The assistant dons overgloves while processing the radiographs.

6. Ice and hot gutta percha points may be used in thermal testing.

7. The nonfluoridated paste serves as a conductor in the vitality test.

8. The assistant checks that the gauge is set on zero when starting the vitality testing.

9. The patient is taken to the consultation room after testing.

10. The assistant takes the records, findings, and radiographs to the consultation room with the patient.

Theory Recall: Endodontic Root Canal Treatment

1. The patient is requested to wear protective eyeglasses for protection from caustic chemicals.

2. The tooth is isolated during treatment for better vision, as a safety precaution against swallowing objects and chemicals, and to maintain a sterile field.

3. The sizes of the reamers and files are either color coded or marked on the base.

4. A glass bead sterilizer may be used to chairside sterilize instruments during root canal therapy.

5. Small cotton pellets are used to carry and hold medicine in the root canal.

6. Gutta percha points or silver points or a combination of the two are used.

7. A temporary stopping material, such as cavit, is used between visits.

8. Stoppers are used in root canal therapy to show how deep the instrument should be inserted into the canal.

9. The permanent restoration used after root canal therapy is determined by the dentist and patient, and may be a composite resin or permanent crown.

10. X-rays taken during root canal therapy are kept in the patient's record file.

Theory Recall: Removable Prosthodontics (Visit 2)

1. Removable appliances may be any artificial tooth, group of teeth, or an entire dentition that may be placed and removed by the patient.

2. The impression taking of a partial and complete denture may differ in the choice of impression materials and certain techniques.

3. A custom tray is constructed on the study cast from the first visit.
4. The dentist may require radiographs, photographs, and any mouth preparations that may be done.
5. A person receiving a partial appliance may need restorative work, abutment work, or root canal therapy.
6. The assistant prepares the lighter viscous elastic impression material first and then the heavier.
7. A dentist may prefer a zinc oxide paste impression material for a denture impression.
8. When the tray is taken from the mouth the assistant rinses the impression, disinfects it, and places it in a plastic bag.
9. The shade guide is dipped into water and the light is moved so that the shade guide reflects like the original tooth and the light is as natural as living conditions.
10. The dentist may request the patient to bring old photos to show the original shape and size of the patient's teeth, especially if no original teeth are present.

Theory Recall: Try in and Delivery Appointments

1. The third appointment is for a try in of the temporary appliance.
2. The actual teeth of the new denture are placed in the wax try in denture.
3. The try in appliance or dentures are returned to the dental lab for construction of the final appliance or denture.
4. The patient's old dentures or appliance are placed in a denture cup filled with cool water.
5. The dentist may request a boley gauge or millimeter rule to measure alteration depth.
6. Whenever the appliance is taken out of the mouth for adjustment, it is moistened before reinsertion.
7. Before the try in appliance or denture is returned to the dental lab, it is disinfected.
8. Before the delivery appointment, the assistant must be sure the appliance or denture has been delivered by the lab. It is disinfected and rinsed before the try in.
9. The assistant passes or holds articulating paper to test the new bite.
10. The patient is instructed to wash the new appliance or denture in cool water over a sink full of water.

Theory Recall: Fixed Prosthodontics

1. Fixed prosthodontia involves the placement of artificial teeth or an appliance that the patient cannot remove.

2. The four procedures that may be performed at the first visit are impression for temporary crown, tooth preparation, final impression, and construction and cementation of a temporary crown cover.
3. A soft piece of wax is placed in the blank space in a bridge impression.
4. During the tooth preparation, the assistant sprays water on the work site and maintains visibility.
5. The gingiva is retracted before the final impression.
6. Acrylic cover material is mixed for a temporary crown.
7. The cover is washed and dried before cementation.
8. Cotton rolls are passed for isolation in cementation.
9. Dental floss is used to remove cement from the interproximal spaces.
10. Dental floss in a threader is used to remove dry cement from under a temporary bridge.

Theory Recall: Fixed Crowns (Final Visit)

1. On the final visit, the completed crown is fitted and cemented to the prepared tooth.
2. The adjustments are completed before the patient is dismissed.
3. A crown remover is passed to the dentist to remove the temporary crown.
4. The patient bites on a wooden bite stick to seat the crown.
5. The dentist may call for a mallet to seat the crown.
6. The crown is checked for dents and rough edges after removal.
7. Hydrogen peroxide is used to clean and disinfect the crown before applying cement.
8. Permanent cement, zinc phosphate, is used to cement the permanent crown.
9. While the cement is setting, the assistant places a saliva ejector in the patient's mouth for moisture control.
10. When the cement has set, the assistant hands a mirror and explorer for examination.

Post Test

MULTIPLE CHOICE: 1.b 2.a 3.d 4.a 5.a 6.a 7.c 8.c 9.d 10.d 11.a 12.b 13.b 14.d 15.a 16.b 17.a 18.b 19.a 20.a
MATCHING: 1.d 2.e 3.b 4.h 5.i 6.j 7.g 8.f 9.a 10.c

Unit 8 Dental Specialties

Theory Recall:
Orthodontics

1. Orthodontics is the branch of dentistry concerned with tooth alignment and jaw structure.
2. A variety of diagnostic procedures are needed to determine the treatment plan for a patient.
3. The preliminary examination is a preparatory examination.
4. The State Dental Practice Act determines the amount and type of assistance that an assistant may give.
5. A consultation appointment is given after the preliminary one.
6. Future orthodontic appointments are centered around the information gathered in the preliminary exam.
7. The preliminary exam begins with an interview in the consultation room.
8. The patient holds clear cheek retractors during the photo session.
9. The assistant tries to establish a casual but businesslike atmosphere.
10. The orthodontist requires intraoral, occlusal, panoramic, and cephalometric radiographs.

Theory Recall:
Placement of Orthodontic Bands

1. Orthodontic treatment and facial recontouring is completed by the use of push and pull forces.
2. Pressure applied to the tooth eventually compresses and resorbs the periodontal bone.
3. Appliances may be attached by banding or bonding the teeth.
4. Tubes are usually placed on molar bands.
5. Brackets and tubes are placed on the facial side of the band.
6. Lugs and buttons used for seating the band are placed on the lingual side.
7. Separators may be purchased in rubber, plastic, or metal.
8. The patient is advised not to eat, chew candy or gum, and not to worry if separators fall out prematurely.
9. The assistant helps with the fitting of the bands, the preparation of the bands, the cementation of the bands, cleaning up the patient, and giving instructions to the patient.
10. The assistant gives instructions in care of appliances, oral hygiene, and nutrition.

Theory Recall:
Bonding Brackets

1. Direct bonding is preferred for better hygiene, appearance, faster application, and less fitting trauma.
2. DB brackets are supplied in metal, plastic, and porcelain.

3. Plastic brackets must be preconditioned before bonding.
4. Before the etching process, the orthodontist polishes the tooth surfaces.
5. The etching gel is placed on the facial surface of the tooth to be bonded.
6. The activator material is placed on the etched surface and the back of the bracket.
7. The assistant dons overgloves to prevent or lessen contamination of the material syringes.
8. The approximate time for the bonding material to set is 35 to 45 seconds.
9. The assistant hands a scaler to the orthodontist for removal of excess bonding material.
10. Arch wires may be placed after the final set of the bonding material (approximately four minutes).

Theory Recall:
Arch Wire and Ligature Placement

1. Before the arch wire and ligatures are placed, the bands and tubes must be securely in place.
2. The study cast from the initial appointment is used to preform the arch wire.
3. Ligature tying pliers are passed for tying of ligatures.
4. The ligature wire cutting instrument is passed for cutting the ligatures.
5. The orthodontist cuts the ligatures approximately 3 to 4 millimeters close.
6. The assistant passes the ligature direction instrument to push the ligatures aside.
7. The orthodontist uses the ligature tucking or Schure instrument to tuck under the cut edges.
8. The patient is requested to run a tongue around the mouth to find raw or sharp edges.
9. The patient is rescheduled for an appointment for approximately three to four weeks later.
10. The assistant copies the notes to avoid placing contaminated records in the patient's file.

Theory Recall:
Arch Wire, Band, and Bracket Removal

1. When alignment is reached, a band removal appointment is scheduled.
2. All intraoral appliances are removed, cement is cleaned off, and the teeth are polished. An impression is taken for study casts.
3. A patient may wear a retainer for one or two years.
4. The study casts are used for comparison with the initial bite and also for fabrication of a retainer.
5. The patient is requested to wear safety glasses at the band removal appointment.

6. The scaler or Schure instrument is passed to expose ends.
7. A needleholder and ligature cutters are passed for removal of ligatures.
8. The cement is removed after the bands and brackets are taken off.
9. A scaler, hand or ultrasonic, is used to remove cement.
10. The teeth are polished after the cement is removed.

Theory Recall: Oral Surgery Procedures

1. The oral surgeon removes teeth, repairs fractures, and completes bone reduction and reconstruction, implantation, and other procedures.
2. Patients with compromising health problems may be referred to the oral surgeon.
3. The referring dentist sends recent x-rays, dental records, and a prescription or recommendation for surgery.
4. During the exam, the oral surgeon and patient discuss the treatment plan, financial cost, and the recuperative stage.
5. The oral surgery assistant must prepare by making sure all x-rays, records, and the treatment plan are present. Pre-set trays are prepared. Equipment is checked, and emergency trays are placed nearby.
6. The patient may be premedicated and draped, and the face may be scrubbed prior to surgery.
7. Alveoplasty is the term used for smoothing and contouring bony ridges.
8. The assistant dabs the wound site to avoid aspirating the clot.
9. The assistant gives postoperative instructions to the patient and the patient's companion.
10. The patient returns for suture removal four to seven days after surgery.

Theory Recall: Minor Tissue Surgery

1. Severe and lasting pain a few days after surgery are symptoms of a dry socket.
2. A dry socket occurs when the clot is removed or washes away.
3. The surgeon uses a curette to debride the wound and stimulate new blood flow for a new clot.
4. The assistant must be sure not to aspirate the wound site to avoid disturbing the clot.
5. Accumulation of pus, lymph, dead cells, and matter causes the pain, heat, and swelling in an infection.
6. The surgeon may use nitrous oxide analgesia or premedication with local anesthesia for pain control.
7. Local anesthesia is difficult in infection because of the presence of exudate.

8. The dental dam material is permitted to remain to provide drainage opening.
9. A biopsy is a surgical removal of tissue for microscopic examination.
10. After surgery, the assistant checks the laboratory orders, notes the name and date, prepares the bottle for shipment, and records the treatment on the patient's chart.

Theory Recall: Periodontics

1. Periodontics is the branch of dentistry that deals with the treatment of diseased tissues around the tooth.
2. One of the most important procedures for the periodontist is the exam.
3. The assistant's main duty in the interview is to take accurate notes.
4. The diet and nutrition level may affect treatment and regeneration of tissue.
5. Habits could affect the tissue and teeth position of the mouth.
6. Notes recorded in the patient's words may indicate the patient's intensity or desire for treatment.
7. Radiographs show individual areas as well as the alveolar crest.
8. The periodontist makes six readings per tooth or three facial and three lingual.
9. Class III is the class for moderate periodontitis.
10. During the scaling, curettage, and root planing, the assistant may aid the operator by rinsing and evacuating; spraying air to dry pockets; and disinfecting, passing, and exchanging instruments.

Theory Recall: Gingivectomy and Removal of Periodontal Packing

1. The need for a gingivectomy is indicated when there is necrotic tissue that does not respond to treatment.
2. The procedure is to remove the unattached, inflamed necrotic tissue, remove irritating deposits, and pack the area with a soothing material.
3. The periodontal pocket markers are placed into the diseased pocket.
4. The scalers and curettes are passed to the periodontist to remove exposed deposits.
5. The assistant dons overgloves before mixing periodontal packing.
6. The consistency of the periodontal packing material should be like stiff dough.
7. The facial sides of the teeth are packed with gingival packing first.
8. The periodontist may place foil or clear plastic wrap over the packing until it is dry.
9. The patient may be cautioned to drink cool drinks, avoid smoking, avoid hot and spicy and rough foods, brush other teeth regularly but rinse

the operative site, and expect some bleeding and pieces of packing to break away.

10. A large scaler or excavator is used to loosen and remove the packing.

Post Test

MATCHING: 1.g 2.j 3.i 4.h 5.e 6.c 7.b 8.d 9.f 10.a
MULTIPLE CHOICE: 1.a 2.d 3.c 4.d 5.d 6.b 7.b 8.a 9.d 10.b 11.d 12.d 13.d 14.a 15.d 16.a 17.d 18.b 19.b 20.b

UNIT 9 DENTAL LABORATORY PROCEDURES

Theory Recall:
Fabrication of Study Models

1. The two types of gypsum products found in the dental office are laboratory plaster and dental stone.
2. The formula for preparation of plaster of Paris (laboratory plaster) is 60 ml of water to 100 grams of plaster.
3. The formula for preparation of dental stone is 30 ml of water to 100 grams of dental stone.
4. Gypsum is stored in a tight container, in a dry place.
5. Gypsum materials can set up under water and clog pipes.
6. Room-temperature water permits correct mixing and setting time.
7. Disinfection must be performed before starting to work on a lab case.
8. Voids or holes may be present where drops were.
9. Start pouring the gypsum in the extreme rear of the impression, retromolar area or maxillary tuberosity.
10. The dentist may request study models to plan or measure services.

Theory Recall:
Separation of Models and Impression

1. The models and impression must be separated.
2. Urgency is determined by the work planned and the patient's next scheduled appointment.
3. The assistant wears safety glasses to avoid flying chips from entering the eyes.
4. Excess and overhanging impression material is removed from the tray.
5. The tip is inserted to permit air to get between the two items.
6. The model is removed in a straight up and off motion.
7. The models teeth can break off during an improper removal.
8. Lower anterior incisors are prone to snap off in rough separation.
9. Models are marked with the patient's name and date after separation.

10. The models will be trimmed after separation from the impression.

Theory Recall:
Trimming Gypsum Models

1. Gypsum models are trimmed to make them more functional and esthetic.
2. The electric model trimmer is used to trim models.
3. Overgloves are worn to protect against cross contamination.
4. A constant water flow over the trimmer wheel is necessary to prevent clogging of the abrasive wheel.
5. Safety glasses prevent damage from flying debris.
6. The anterior maxillary cut is trimmed to a point.
7. The anterior mandibular cut is trimmed to be rounded.
8. Rough scratch marks may be removed by using sandpaper or a rasp to finish up a model.
9. Soap solutions serve two purposes, which are easy separation and a shiny appearance.
10. Models can be identified by patient's name, date, and sometimes the case number.

Theory Recall:
Articulating Gypsum Models

1. Study models are mounted on laboratory articulators.
2. Study models are mounted to imitate the jaw functions and show the teeth in occlusion.
3. The bite registration form indicates the proper position for model placement during the mounting process.
4. Laboratory plaster is used to attach the study models to the articulators.
5. A soap solution painted on the top and bottom surfaces of the models permit easy removal of the models when needed.
6. A large elastic band or sticky wax can be used to hold the models in union when mounting.
7. Petroleum jelly can be rubbed on the articulator surfaces between uses.

Theory Recall:
Construction of Base Plates and Occlusal Rims

1. Base plates and occlusal rims are used for the construction of dentures.
2. The base plate represents the base of the denture.
3. The occlusal rims is the wax block used to hold the denture teeth.
4. The two materials used for plates are base plate wax and gutta percha material.
5. Talc or baby powder may be used to prepare the stone model.
6. The base plate wax is prepared by heating over a Bunsen burner flame or in hot water.

7. The excess wax is trimmed approximately $1/8$ to $1/4$ inch from the edge.

8. The occlusal rim is placed on the plate just over the occlusal ridge.

9. Melted excess base plate wax is used to unite and fill in the two pieces.

10. The heel cuts are made to permit up-and-down articulation movement.

Theory Recall:
Construction of Custom Trays

1. Two reasons for construction of the custom tray are the patient has an abnormal mouth and the dentist requires a final impression.

2. Custom trays are constructed in a dental laboratory or the lab room of the office.

3. Two materials used for custom tray construction are acrylic resin mixture and pelletized resin dough.

4. Acrylic resin is a mixture of a liquid and powder and is combined in a paper cup.

5. A spacer is used to leave area for final impression material.

6. Petroleum jelly may be put on fingers or gloves to prevent sticking.

7. The custom tray mixture should be about $1/16$ to $1/8$ inch thick.

8. Cutoff excess material is used to make a small handle for the tray.

9. Laboratory sandpaper or emery disks, and dental lathe trimmer wheels can be used to smooth custom trays.

10. Care in construction of trays, avoiding rough tears and cuts, will make final smoothing and polishing easier.

Theory Recall:
Fabrication of Temporary Crowns

1. The purpose of a temporary crown cover is to provide protection from sensitivity and decay.

2. No, it is not wise. Not all manufacturers process materials in the same manner.

3. The first procedure is to take an alginate impression of the quadrant.

4. The materials are united in the indentation of the preparation in the alginate impression.

5. The chemical union of monomer and polymer is called polymerization.

6. Flashing is a thin layer of mixture extending out beyond the gingival margin line.

7. Instruments used for smoothing and trimming are crown and bridge scissors (curved), sandpaper disks, round burs in a slow handpiece, and crimping pliers.

8. The impression must be treated as a separate case and disinfected.

9. A preformed resin crown cover or metal shell may be used.

10. A preformed crown is prepared basically in the same manner as the resin mixed cover.

Theory Recall:
Preparing Laboratory Cases for Shipping

1. The amount of work sent to a commercial lab depends on the dentist's available time and expertise.

2. Commercial labs are located in all areas.

3. A dentist's work order or prescription is required for work to be done in a dental laboratory.

4. The assistant may fill in the patient's name, address, sex, age, and time of next appointment.

5. The office can keep track of lab cases by keeping a lab work schedule log and recording transactions on the patient's chart.

6. The dental laboratory usually supplies the lab cartons used for shipping.

7. Five tasks the assistant must be sure to complete when preparing cases for the commercial lab are:
   ▸ All orders and information needed must be on the prescription form, complete and legible.
   ▸ All case materials relative to the procedure must be present and packed in a safe manner.
   ▸ All disinfection procedures must be indicated and noted with the case.
   ▸ The patient's records must be updated and the transaction recorded.
   ▸ The shipment must be made correctly and immediately.

Post Test

MATCHING: 1.c 2.i 3.d 4.h 5.a 6.f 7.e 8.g 9.b 10.j
MULTIPLE CHOICE: 1.b 2.a 3.d 4.c 5.c 6.a 7.b 8.d 9.b 10.a 11.d 12.c 13.c 14.c 15.b 16.b 17.a 18.a 19.b 20.d

UNIT 10 DENTAL RADIATION

Theory Recall:
Radiation Safety Knowledge

1. Dental x-rays may expose hidden decay, root tips, cysts, infection, growth irregularities, and foreign bodies.

2. Dental x-rays possess the ability to ionize or alter and harm tissues.

3. Growing or immature tissues are the most sensitive to radiation.

4. Cumulative effect occurs when radiation is not sloughed off or builds up in the tissues.

5. This law requires the states to monitor and govern the ability of the person exposing the radiation.

6. The assistant has the responsibility to look into the legality of taking x-rays in a resident state.

7. The assistant may be required to schedule safety checking of the machine or expose films for safety testing.
8. The assistant must know how to operate the on/off control, the mA, the kVp, and the timer control of a radiation machine.
9. All controls on the radiation machine may need to be adjusted in a PID change.
10. ALARA means *as low as reasonably achievable* in radiation.

Assignment Sheet 10.1 Radiation Safety Knowledge

A. Puzzle solution:

B. Student sentences containing key words will vary but should stress dental radiation safety principles.

Theory Recall: Radiation Film Knowledge

1. Dental radiographs used in the mouth are called intraoral films. Dental radiographs used outside the mouth are called extraoral films.
2. The most common intraoral film is the periapical film, size 2.
3. For an anterior shot, the film is placed in a vertical position.
4. The patient bites edge to edge in an anterior bitewing exposure.
5. The child-sized periapical film is called size 0.

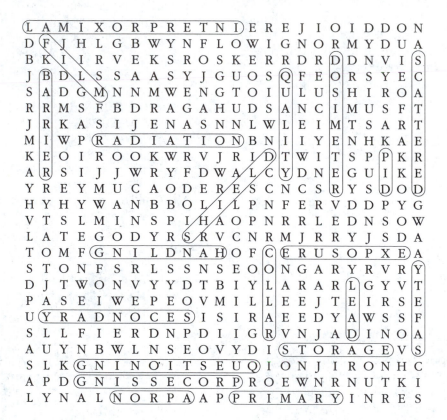

6. The occlusal film may be used intra- or extraorally.
7. A periapical film may be modified by placing the film in a film loop with the front of the packet toward the tab or by placing a tab on the front.
8. Two views per side are necessary for the modified bitewing films.
9. The occlusal film may be used extraorally for TMJ problems, bone cysts, and large trouble areas.
10. The panoramic view shows the entire mouth area.

Assignment Sheet 10.2 Radiation Film Knowledge

A. periapical film—View may show individual area with appropriate landmarks. Student should identify exposure area.
B. interproximal film—View should show wing area with crowns of both arches and appropriate landmarks. Student will identify exposure.

C. child-sized periapical film—View should show individual area with appropriate landmarks, possible mixed dentition. Student should identify exposure.
D. occlusal film—View should show larger area of mouth, perhaps entire arch, with appropriate landmarks. Student will identify exposure.

Theory Recall:
Exposure of Dental Radiographs

1. The individual states set the licensing requirements for exposing x-rays.
2. The two common methods of exposing dental x-rays are the bisecting angle technique and paralleling technique.
3. Positioning the patient's face with an imaginary line perpendicular to the floor ensures the patient's face to be centered and evenly positioned.
4. All biting edges are placed about 1/8 inch from the film edge.
5. The plain side of the film faces the tubehead.
6. The films are placed in a horizontal position for a posterior exposure.
7. Exposed and unexposed films are placed in a lead-lined box or out of exposure range.
8. The timer is preset to save time while the film is in the mouth.
9. The PID is placed next to the aiming ring.
10. The assistant stands behind the shield or six feet away from the tubehead when activating the timer button.

Theory Recall:
Processing Dental Radiographs

1. Radiographs may be processed manually or in an automatic processor.
2. Splashing or spilling may neutralize chemical solutions or predevelop radiographs.
3. Lids should be left on manual developing tanks to avoid oxidation.
4. Barrier shields may be placed on films before exposure, or the film coverings can be removed before the processing begins to reduce contamination in the darkroom.
5. The contaminated waterproof coverings are placed in the contaminated trash container.
6. The waterproof coverings are removed in a safelight situation only.
7. Separate stir rods are used to avoid mixing chemical solutions together.
8. The assistant alternates the placement of the films on the developing rack in preparation for processing.
9. The films and rack are placed under running water stream to remove any chemicals.

10. The films are placed in a dustless, air-circulating area for drying.

Theory Recall:
Mounting Dental Radiographs

1. A series of small dental x-rays is systematically placed in order to offer a total view of the mouth.
2. X-ray mounts are cardboard, plastic, or vinyl sheeting with windows that permit the placing of films.
3. Mounts come in dark black, clear, or light shades.
4. Anterior dental x-ray films are placed in a vertical position.
5. Fourteen films are needed for a full-mouth series without bitewings.
6. Commercial bitewing film is size 3.
7. The assistant will wear gloves to avoid smearing or leaving fingerprints.
8. If the dentist wishes to view the series of films from the outside of the mouth, they are mounted with the pimple facing the operator.
9. If the assistant does not wear gloves, the films are touched and handled by the edges of the film.
10. The patient's name and date are written on the mount before placing the films. If a numbering system is used, the patient's number is also written.

Theory Recall:
Analyzing Dental Radiographs

1. Three ways a film may be spoiled in handling, purchasing, or storing are out of date, exposed to heat or chemicals, scratched, or bent from handling.
2. Films may be too light and lack contrast or have too much exposure and be too dark if the machine controls are not set properly.
3. When movement occurs during exposure, a blurring effect will happen.
4. If the vertical angle of the central ray is incorrect, elongation or foreshortening may occur.
5. If the horizontal angle of the central ray is incorrect, overlapping will occur.
6. If the central ray misses the edge of the film, conecutting occurs.
7. If developer drips onto a film before processing, a dark spot will occur.
8. A partial radiographic image may indicate that the film was not covered with developing solution during the processing procedure.
9. If a film is opened to a white light and then processed, it will be black.
10. Films that have or develop a yellowish-brown stain indicate they were not properly washed during the processing procedure.

Assignment Sheet 10.3
Exposure of Dental Radiographs

Students should supply and analyze radiographs displaying five different technical errors and state the method to correct the mistake. Some errors could be foreshortening, movement, conecutting, over or under exposure, improper film placement, overlapping, processing mistakes, or storage problems.

Post Test

MATCHING: 1.f 2.d 3.g 4.a 5.b 6.c 7.h 8.i 9.j 10.e

MULTIPLE CHOICE: 1.d 2.d 3.a 4.d 5.c 6.b 7.a 8.b 9.d 10.b 11.d 12.d 13.b 14.a 15.b 16.b 17.b 18.c 19.a 20.d

UNIT 11 BUSINESS PROCEDURES

Theory Recall:
Opening and Closing the Dental Office

1. Good opening and closing procedures in the dental office provide for office efficiency.
2. The first duties the receptionist performs in the morning are opening the office, turning on the lights, adjusting the air conditioner or heater, and checking the answering machine or service and fax machines.
3. Four types of incoming mail and where they may be placed follow:
   personal—on the doctor's desk
   lab cases—to the lab area
   bills—to reception area
   payments—reception area
   journals—to doctor's desk
   magazine—reception room
   junk—where needed
4. The receptionist makes confirmation calls of the next day's schedule before leaving for the day.
5. Outgoing mail may consist of laboratory cases, statements, payments, correspondence, referrals, or records.
6. A hardcopy of the day's business must be made before the computer is turned off at night.
7. The duties of the chairside assistant are centered around the operatory, laboratory, and darkroom areas.
8. Before preparing for the day, the chairside assistant checks the daily appointment schedule.
9. When closing for the day, the assistant dons utility gloves and PPE before disinfecting all areas and surfaces; removing barrier shields; flushing lines; disinfecting, changing, or cleaning the filter traps to hoses; and removing trash.
10. The contaminated trash bundles are placed at a designated place for pick up service. The contaminated laundry is placed in a marked bag and taken to a designated spot for pick up or to the office laundry area away from the operatory area.

Theory Recall:
Telephone Techniques

1. The assistant must always remain calm in an emergency call.
2. It is important to get the name, address, and phone number of a new patient so the office may contact that person in the event of a change.
3. After making an appointment and before hanging up, the assistant restates the date, day, and time of the appointment.
4. Before placing a caller on "hold," the assistant asks for permission to do so.
5. If a professional is calling the dentist about a patient, the assistant gathers the patient's records and gives them to the dentist.
6. An on-call list is a list of people who prefer to be called for an appointment on short notice.
7. Before placing an order, the assistant gathers all needed information.
8. Before placing a collection call, the assistant reviews the case with the dentist.
9. The results of the collection call are noted on the patient's chart.
10. A followup call is a call placed to the patient the day after the visit to inquire about the patient's condition.

Theory Recall:
Appointment Scheduling

1. Bad scheduling can cause idle, unproductive days or days in which patients are overcrowded.
2. The time sections are called units.
3. The first thing the dental assistant does with a new appointment book is block or mark off times when the dentist will not be in the office.
4. When making an appointment, the patient's name, phone number, and work procedure planned are marked down.
5. The phone number of a new patient is important to have handy if any changes in the appointment occur.
6. The amount of time reserved is indicated by the name line and the arrow descending from the name line.
7. The new assistant may use an office manual to determine how much time to reserve for a specific procedure.
8. Young children are scheduled for work in the mornings before nap time.
9. Buffer time is a unit or two set aside toward mid-morning or lunch. It may be used for emergencies or to catch up or prepare.
10. The appointment card contains the patient's name, date and day of appointment, and time scheduled. The doctor's name, address, and phone number are also on the card, if needed.

Assignment Sheet 11.1
Appointment Scheduling

A and B.

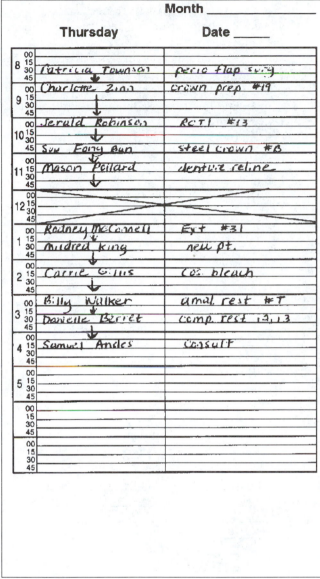

Month _____	
Thursday	**Date** ____

8 00 15 30 45 — Patricia Townson / perio flap surg
9 00 15 30 45 — Charlotte Zinn / crown prep #19
10 00 15 30 45 — Jerald Robinson / RCT1 #13
11 00 15 30 45 — Sue Fong Ann / steel crown #B
Mason Pollard / denture reline
12 00 15 30 45 — (X)
1 00 15 30 45 — Rodney McConnell / Ext #31
Mildred King / new pt.
2 00 15 30 45 — Carrie Gillis / cos. bleach
3 00 15 30 45 — Billy Walker / amal. rest #T
Danielle Berret / comp. rest 12,13
4 00 15 30 45 — Samuel Andes / consult
5 00 15 30 45 —

C. Students have choice of patients to make out appointment cards.

Theory Recall:
Patient Dental Records

1. The name of a new patient is starred or circled in the appointment book.
2. The new patient is requested to arrive early for the first appointment so that registration papers and health history forms may be completed.
3. The dentist determines what information is needed for the dental records.
4. The two methods used to collect information are to give the papers to the patient to fill out and

transfer the data, or directly question the patient and use the data to complete the forms.
5. The dental assistant should never show shock or lose patience when questioning a patient.
6. When the data has been collected, the assistant may offer a tour of the office and make the patient feel welcomed.
7. The dentist's clinical exam, charting, and x-ray findings as well as study models, photographs, and slides may be part of the file.
8. Any information collected regarding the patient is placed in the patient's file.
9. The patient's records are the property of the dentist.
10. To the dental assistant, "maintaining confidentiality of the patient's records" means not to discuss or relate any information regarding the patient.

Assignment Sheet 11.2
Patient Dental Records

WELCOME TO OUR OFFICE

CATHERINE C. COLE, D.D.S.
100 West Mifflin St.
Best Town, US 12345
(123) 456-7890

DATE July 5, 19XX

To help us serve you better, please print the needed information below: All replies are treated as confidential information.

Patient's Name: Mary Ellen Young | Birthdate: 5-11-XX | Marital Status: Married
Address: 3 Pellican Way | City: Coastown | State: MD | ZIP: 12345 | Phone: (302)555-8272
Social Security Number: 123-45-5678 | Physician's Name and Address/Phone Number: Thomas Payne, Towers Bldg. Suite 2000 5th and 7th Ave, Largetown, MD 12344 (302)555-3630
Spouse's Name: Harold Allen Young | Birthdate: 2-16-XX | Social Security Number: 234-56-7890
Name of Patient's Employer: Belcar Communications | Address: 199387 Power Ave, Largetown, MD 12344 | Phone: (302)555-3783 ext. 205
Dental Insurance Plan: Dentcare, Inc. | Group: Belmed | Number: 445566 | Effective Date: 9-10-90
Name of Spouse's Employer: Self-employed | Address: Home address | Phone: Home Phone
Dental Insurance Plan: None | Group: — | Number: — | Effective Date:
Children's First Name: Tim | Last Name: Young | Birthdate: 10-12-XX

Name of person who referred you to our office: Susan Livingstone

RELEASE OF INFORMATION:
I authorize the release of any dental information necessary to process this claim.
Mary Ellen Young / 7-5-XX
(Patient's Name) / (Date)

ASSIGNMENT OF BENEFITS:
I authorize payment of dental benefits directly to the named provider for professional services rendered.
Mary Ellen Young / 7-5-XX
(Subscriber's Name) / (Date)

B. Students' answers will vary.

Theory Recall:
Records Management-Filing

1. The four methods of filing materials are alphabetic, numeric, chronologic, and subject matter.
2. Dental x-rays, study models, or photos may be filed numerically in the dental office.
3. When filing material numerically, it is important to maintain a cross-reference.
4. Recall patients and patients on a payment plan may have names in a chronologic file.
5. The assistant may maintain a subject file for invoices, supply orders, correspondence to be completed, and insurance inquiries.
6. When an item falls into more than one category, an assistant makes a cross-reference card.
7. Color coding helps to locate files that have been placed incorrectly.
8. The three procedures for filing preparation are indexing, sorting, and placing.
9. Hyphenated names are treated as one name.
10 The most important rule in filing is *nothing* is filed before *something*.

Assignment Sheet 11.3 Records Management

A. Names to be filed

Indexing Order

	Unit 1	Unit 2	Unit 3	Unit 4
1. National Caregivers Assoc.	National	Caregivers	Assoc.	
2. Miss Barbara Lou Black	Black	Barbara	Lou	Miss
3. Jeffrey Jones, Sr.	Jones	Jeffrey		Sr.
4. Mr. Woody Hollows	Hollows	Woody		Mr.
5. Hewitt-Merill Computer Co.	Hewitt-Merill	Computer	Co.	
6. Martha Ann Miller	Miller	Martha	Ann	
7. St. Louis Dental Society	St. Louis	Dental	Society	
8. Mrs. Michele Zinn (Tim)	Zinn	Michele		(Mrs. Tim)
9. Mr. James Da Mocco	Da Mocco	James		Mr.
10. 5th Avenue Supply Co.	5th	Avenue	Supply	Co.
11. Mrs. Paul Pleasant (Kerri)	Pleasant	Kerri		(Mrs. Paul)
12. ABC Cleaners	ABC	Cleaners		
13. Michael Louis Le Paul	Le Paul	Michael	Louis	
14. Carol's Gift Shop	Carol's	Gift	Shop	
15. Jeffrey Jones, Jr.	Jones	Jeffrey		Jr.
16. Kristin Gill, DDS	Gill	Kristin		DDS
17. Mrs. Sam Pleasant (Kathleen)	Pleasant	Kathleen		Mrs. Sam
18. Miss Ivy Lans-Worthy	Lans-Worthy	Ivy		Miss
19. W. W. Hollows	Hollows	W.	W.	
20. Ms. Laura Jones-Martin	Jones-Martin	Laura		Ms.
21. John Collen Gilbert	Gilbert	John	Collen	
22. Kristin Gill	Gill	Kristin		
23. John William Gilbert	Gilbert	John	William	
24. Southeast Airline	Southeast	Airline		
25. John Gilbert	Gilbert	John		

B. The alphabetic order of the titles and names:

1. 12	6. 22	11. 5	16. 20	21. 17
2. 2	7. 16	12. 19	17. 18	22. 11
3. 14	8. 25	13. 4	18. 13	23. 7
4. 9	9. 21	14. 15	19. 6	24. 24
5. 10	10. 23	15. 3	20. 1	25. 8

Theory Recall: Bookkeeping Procedures

1. The bookkeeping procedures may be completed using a programmed computer or manually using a pegboard system.
2. The pegboard system offers one entry, saving time and lessening transposition errors.
3. The first shingle of the receipt or charge slip is placed on the first working line.
4. The number of the first shingle should follow the number of yesterday's last shingle.
5. The patient's balance due is taken from the ledger card.
6. When the charge slip has been filled out, it is placed on the patient's file, which goes to the operatory.
7. The ledger card is inserted under the receipt card on the master sheet.
8. If the patient requests a superbill, it is placed on the next working line after the shingle sheet is removed.
9. The total of the deposit slip column matches the amount received for the day.
10. The master sheet for the day is removed from the pegboard and placed in a loose-leaf index over yesterday's master sheet.

Theory Recall: Dental Insurance

1. A new patient who has dental insurance is requested to bring his or her identification card and benefit booklet.
2. A pre-authorization form is a request to do the services; a claim form is a statement of services rendered.
3. Family coverage covers the subscriber and dependents; individual coverage includes the subscriber only.
4. The two payment methods used by dental insurance companies are a schedule of allowances and UCR.
5. In a coordination of benefits, the primary (subscriber's) company pays first.
6. The first section of the claim requests information regarding the patient.
7. Procedure codes are ADA numbers to indicate specific treatment.
8. The patient, or guardian, signs the release of information line.
9. The subscriber signs the assignment of benefits line.
10. The assistant may keep track of insurance claims by placing the name and claim on an insurance log and marking the progress until completed.

Assignment Sheet 11.4 Checking Accounts

A.

(Courtesy of Colwell Systems [Deluxe Forms].)

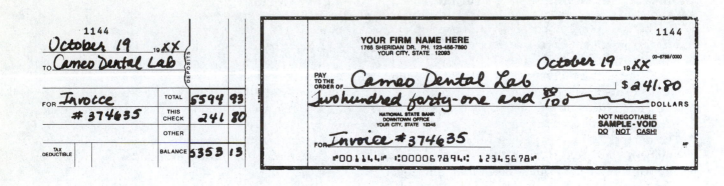

B.

Bank Balance		Account Balance
9,934.90		9,651.25

Outstanding Checks	
#	Amount
309	304.11
311	77.19
313	122.35
Total	503.65

9,934.90
503.65 —Oustanding Checks Total

9,431.25 Bank Balance

9,651.25

—Less Bank Charges	20.00 safe box
New Account Balance	9,631.25
—Outstanding Deposit	200.00
Account Balance	9,431.25

Theory Recall: Checking Accounts

1. A check is a written order to the bank to pay a certain amount to a specific person or company.
2. It is the dentist's responsibility to sign the checks in the dental office.
3. When the check has been written for the statement, the check number and date are written on the statement part, which is kept in the office.
4. If the assistant feels the dentist may have a question regarding a check, the assistant paper clips the statement and invoice to the check for the dentist to review.
5. The first step in writing a check is to fill in the stub.
6. The payee is the person to whom the check is being written.
7. When the assistant receives a check, it is immediately stamped for deposit only with the dentist's account number.
8. Checkbook reconciliation is the balancing of the checkbook account with the bank statement.
9. When the figure on a check and the figure in the stub are not the same, a transposition error is said to have occurred.
10. The receipts or vouchers for petty cash spending are kept inside the petty cash envelope.

Post Test

MULTIPLE CHOICE: 1.a 2.c 3.c 4.d 5.a 6.a 7.b 8.c 9.b 10.a 11.c 12.a 13.c 14.d 15.c 16.a 17.b 18.b 19.a 20.d 21.c 22.c 23.a 24.c 25.d

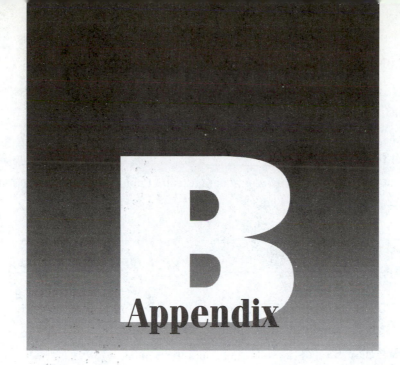

B Appendix

Assignment Sheet 1.1 The Professional Dental Team

Name _____ Date _____ Grade _____

OBJECTIVE: To demonstrate knowledge of the necessary education, training, and responsibilities of the various members of the dental team.

INSTRUCTIONS: Review the material on the professional dental team. Completely answer the following questions.

A. 1. List the eight recognized dental specialties:

a. _____   e. _____

b. _____   f. _____

c. _____   g. _____

d. _____   h. _____

2. State the primary goal of each of the following dental personnel:

a. dentist—_____

b. dental hygienist—_____

c. dental assistant—_____

d. dental lab technician—_____

3. Give an example of how a dental detail or salesperson may be of assistance in a dental facility.

_____

4. What type of dental equipment found in a dental practice may require the services of a dental equipment serviceperson?

_____

5. List two related professional individuals who may be called on to assist the dentist in providing good health care to a patient.

a. _____   b. _____

B. Many dental facilities exhibit a bulletin board in the reception area. It is used to inform and educate the patients and visitors. The themes are changed from time to time and stress important health issues and information.

Prepare a bulletin board introducing the public to the various members of the dental team. Indicate the specific members, their training, responsibilities, and primary contributions to the patient's dental health. Prepare the display and deliver the message using accuracy, neatness, color, and attraction.

Assignment Sheet 1.2 The Role of the Dental Assistant

Name _____ Date _____ Grade _____

OBJECTIVE: To demonstrate knowledge of the education, employment positions, duties and responsibilities, opportunities, and professional organizations of the dental assistant.

INSTRUCTIONS: Review material regarding the role of the dental assistant. Completely answer the following questions.

A. 1. List three educational opportunities for studying the dental assisting profession.

a. _____   b. _____   c. _____

2. Describe four employment opportunities for the trained dental assistant. List them in order of personal preference.

a. _____   c. _____

b. _____   d. _____

3. Give an example of a duty required of a/an:

a. expanded duty assistant—_____

b. chairside assistant—_____

c. clinic support assistant—_____

d. receptionist or manager—_____

e. dental laboratory assistant—_____

4. Name the three basic levels of ADAA involvement for a dental assistant.

a. _____   b. _____   c. _____

5. State the areas of concern involving the following DANB certifications.

a. CDA—_____

b. CDPMA—_____

c. COMSA—_____

d. COA—_____

e. ICE—_____

f. RHS—_____

B. Many assistants are called on to present a display or discussion about the dental assisting profession. Prepare a posterboard presentation, which may be shown at a junior or senior career day exhibit, showing the role of the dental assistant. Make the display neat, colorful, and attractive. Provide the students with a knowledge of the dental assisting career.

Assignment Sheet 1.3 Qualities of the Dental Assistant

Name _____ Date _____ Grade _____

OBJECTIVE: To demonstrate knowledge of the necessary attributes for professional and job qualities of the dental assistant.

INSTRUCTIONS: Review material about the professional and job qualities that are needed by a competent dental assistant. Completely answer the following questions.

A. 1. Give a reason for the importance of performing the following:

   a. keeping information confidential
   _____

   b. showing an interest in the patient's welfare
   _____

   c. following instructions carefully
   _____

   d. recognizing the needs of others
   _____

   e. practicing the Golden Rule
   _____

   f. performing only delegated knowledgeable skills
   _____

   2. State how the following personal qualities help a dental assistant:

   a. dependability and honesty
   _____

   b. being well-groomed, having good hygiene
   _____

   c. showing a healthy appearance
   _____

   d. using good posture
   _____

   e. projecting a confident self-image
   _____

   f. having good communication skills
   _____

   3. Give an example how the dental assistant can display good job qualities in the following situations:

   a. willing to learn
   _____

   b. adapting to situations
   _____

   c. accepting criticism
   _____

   d. following safety rules
   _____

B. Compose a one-page report indicating the importance of possessing and using good dental assisting personal, professional, and job qualities. Explain how you, as a student, could develop and practice these attributes.

Assignment Sheet 1.4 Ethics for the Dental Assistant

Name _____ Date _____ Grade _____

OBJECTIVE: To demonstrate knowledge of the meaning of ethics and the ethical standards expected of the dental assistant.

INSTRUCTIONS: Review material. Completely answer the following questions.

A. 1. Explain how the term "ethics'" expresses:

       a. code of discipline

       _____

       b. statement of moral obligations

       _____

       c. professional and self-imposed code

       _____

       d. need for maintaining code

       _____

   2. State the need for the dental assistant to uphold the following terms of the Dental Assistant's Code of Ethics:

       a. to perform the Golden Rule

       _____

       b. to be honest, loyal, and willing to serve

       _____

       c. to hold all professional matters in confidence

       _____

       d. to refrain from performing illegal or incompetent services

       _____

       e. to avoid disparaging remarks

       _____

       f. to increase skills and efficiency

       _____

       g. to join professional organizations

       _____

B. Many assistants display their diploma, certification (with current active registration card), and other significant awards on an office wall to inform the patient of their ability and competence.

    Complete a suitable printing or wall design showing the dental assistant's principles of the Code of Ethics. Place this design in a frame to be hung with pride near the other awards of distinction.

Assignment Sheet 1.5 Dental Jurisprudence—Legal Considerations

Name _____ Date _____ Grade _____

OBJECTIVE: To demonstrate the knowledge of various types of legal restrictions and statutes regarding the practice of dentistry and how a dental assistant may conform to these standards.

INSTRUCTIONS: Review material. Completely answer the following questions.

A. 1. To legally prescribe medicines, the dentist must first obtain and yearly renew what federal control?
    _____

    2. Discuss the importance of the State Dental Practice Act enactment of the following regulations:

        a. govern practice of dentistry within the state
        _____

        b. right to license and certify dental personnel
        _____

        c. require display of current license and renewal
        _____

        d. suggesting statutes to state legislature
        _____

        e. monitoring the practice of dentistry in the state
        _____

        f. imposing fines or prison on illegal practitioners
        _____

    3. State two methods the dental assistant may use to avoid legal claims for malpractice or personal injury in the following modes:

        a. duties
        _____

        b. record keeping
        _____

        c. instructions
        _____

        d. actions
        _____

B. Select a partner or construct a small team of fellow students to prepare and present a role-playing situation offering a scenario depicting a potential occurrence that may result in either a malpractice or personal injury claim. After presentation of this action, present a corrected version of the previous scene.

Assignment Sheet 1.6 Job Sources

Name _____ Date _____ Grade _____

OBJECTIVE: To demonstrate the ability to determine various methods and avenues of obtaining information for job placement as a dental assistant.

INSTRUCTIONS: Review material. Complete the following job source worksheet.

1. Compose or locate specific advertisements of job openings for each of the following types of ads. Print the information or cut out the advertisement and paste it in the space provided.

    fully stated ad   blind ad   commercial agency ad

2. Name a person who serves as a placement officer for this institution/school.

    _____

3. Name an instructor who may assist in a job placement.

    _____

4. List three friends or relatives who may serve as good networking agents.

    _____

    _____

    _____

5. Name the local professional organizations where you may attend meetings and state a desire for employment.

    _____

    _____

6. Write the address of the local state employment office.

    _____

7. Write the names and addresses of two local commercial employment services.

    _____

    _____

8. Name a local agency that places personnel for temporary employment.

    _____

9. Name two local facilities that you may telephone to inquire of possible dental assistant employment.

_____

_____

10. Name two local facilities or offices where you may enter and place a resume for dental assistant employment.

_____

_____

Assignment Sheet 1.7 Composing a Resume and Cover Letter

Name _____ Date _____ Grade _____

OBJECTIVE: To demonstrate the ability to compose an effective resume and cover letter requesting employment as a dental assistant.

INSTRUCTIONS: Review material. Using the check-list that follows, compose and prepare (A) a personal resume and (B) a cover letter seeking employment as a dental assistant. When completed, evaluate both items.

A.   Resume construction (appearance evaluation):
_____ bonded, white or neutral shaded paper
_____ contents typed in dark ink, professional script
_____ brief, one-page report
_____ correct spelling and punctuation
_____ no use of abbreviations
_____ correct margins, letter well-balanced on page
_____ overall neatness

Resume construction (contents evaluation):
_____ relative personal data included
_____ goals or objective stated
_____ positive attributes and skills listed
_____ chronologic facts in proper order
_____ functional facts stress employment and experience
_____ information complete and correct
_____ references furnished on request listed

B.   Cover letter construction (appearance evaluation):
_____ bonded, white or neutral shaded paper
_____ typed contents in dark ink, professional script
_____ short, brief contents, one page
_____ correct margins, letter centered
_____ spelling and punctuation correct
_____ letter style consistent
_____ no abbreviations

Cover letter construction (contents evaluation):
_____ correct addresses and titles
_____ paragraph one relates reason for letter
_____ paragraph two relates applicant's strengt desires, and abilities
_____ paragraph three indicates how to reach a icant for an interview
_____ closing and signature are neat and correctly spaced

Assignment Sheet 1.8 Completing a Job Application Form

Name _____ Date _____ Grade _____

OBJECTIVE: To demonstrate the ability to correctly complete a job application form for employment as a dental assistant.

INSTRUCTIONS: Review material. Using a sample job application form supplied by the instructor, properly fill out the form. When finished, use the following checklist for evaluation.

A.   Job application form appearance:

_____ instructions followed

_____ neat writing or printing

_____ no abbreviations used

_____ correct spelling and punctuation

_____ neat, wrinkle- and smudge-free paper

_____ no scratched out areas

B.   Job application form contents:

_____ all lines and questions answered completely

_____ work experience in proper chronologic order

_____ education experiences in proper chronologic order

_____ complete information on references

_____ information correct and truthful

Assignment Sheet 1.9 Demonstrating Job Interview Skills

Name _____ Date _____ Grade _____

OBJECTIVE: To demonstrate proper job interviewing skills for a position as a dental assistant.

INSTRUCTIONS: Review material. With a partner, practice role-playing a job interview for a dental assisting position. Practice as both applicant and interviewer. When prepared, role-play a job interview using the evaluation provided (Part A). Complete a thank-you letter for the interviewer. Evaluate using list provided (Part B).

A.   Role-playing job interview situation evaluation:

_____ arrival on time, alone

_____ neat, clean, appropriate dress and appearance

_____ good physical movements: smiles on entrance, shakes hands, uses names, stands and sits erect, does not fidget

_____ uses good grammar: no slang, uses clear voice, no mumbling, uses full sentences, voice is level and pleasant

_____ good attitude: positive, enthusiastic approach, willing to work, cooperative

_____ knowledge of work area: prepared, has researched work site, knowledgeable about work duties required for the job

_____ good questioning skills: lets interviewer take the lead, answers questions, asks questions

_____ good closing: recognizes the end of the interview, expresses thanks, does not linger

B.   Followup letter

_____ good physical form of letter: use of good paper, dark ink, professional script, correct margins, smudge and error free

_____ paragraph one expresses thanks for the interview

_____ paragraph two restates interest and ability to do the job

_____ paragraph three states availability for another interview

_____ pleasant closing

Assignment Sheet 2.1 Emergency Care Preparation

Name _____ Date _____ Grade _____

OBJECTIVE: To demonstrate the ability to use basic emergency care rules for assistance during emergency procedures.

INSTRUCTIONS: Review material. Discuss the importance of each emergency care rule for office emergency procedure (Part A). With partner, prepare a role-playing episode of an emergency procedure. During care and treatment plan, follow basic steps for emergency care (Part B).

A.   Discuss the importance of using each of the following basic emergency care steps:

1.   Monitor the patient's health history

    _____

2.   Be alert for emergency signals

    _____

3.   Remain calm during an emergency

    _____

4.   Seek assistance

    _____

5.   Review health and medical records

    _____

6.   Know emergency phone numbers

    _____

7.   Be familiar with the emergency tray

    _____

8.   Know how to administer oxygen

    _____

9.   Assist with care giving

    _____

10.   Record data

    _____

B.   In a role-playing situation with a partner, simulate a typical emergency that may occur during dental treatment. Offer assistance and care following the emergency care rules. When comfortable with the care-giving procedure, request evaluation from a peer or an instructor.

Assignment Sheet 3.1 Hazard and Fire Control

Name _____ Date _____ Grade _____

OBJECTIVE: Demonstrate knowledge of precautions to use when dealing with chemical, mechanical and fire hazards in the professional office.

INSTRUCTIONS: Review the material on hazard control and fire safety.

A. Completely answer the following questions.

1. List ten general rules to follow when working with chemicals.

_____   _____

_____   _____

_____   _____

_____   _____

_____   _____

2. List ten rules to follow when working with a model trimmer.

_____   _____

_____   _____

_____   _____

_____   _____

_____   _____

3. List seven rules for dealing with power equipment.

_____   _____

_____   _____

_____   _____

_____

4. List five general rules for dealing with hazards.

_____   _____

_____   _____

_____

B. In a role-playing situation, simulate a fire emergency. Demonstrate what action should be taken to obtain assistance. In a simulated activity, role-play obtaining a fire extinguisher and indicate what cautions should be observed. When prepared, ask the instructor for an evaluation of your fire control procedure.

Assignment Sheet 4.1 Tooth Anatomy

Name _____ Date _____ Grade _____

OBJECTIVE: To demonstrate knowledge of different types and names of teeth along with general tooth anatomy
and morphology.

INSTRUCTIONS: Review material. Fill in answers to questions in section A. Match letter of tooth with best descriptions
listed in list B.

A. 1. List the permanent and primary teeth in a quadrant.

Permanent   Primary

_____   _____

_____   _____

_____   _____

_____   _____

_____   _____

_____

_____

2. Name the anterior and posterior teeth.

Anterior   Posterior

_____   _____

_____   _____

_____

3. Name and state the function of the four tissues of a tooth.

a. _____

b. _____

c. _____

d. _____

B. Match the letter of the tooth in column B with the best description in column A.

Column A

_____ 1. three-rooted tooth
_____ 2. fourth tooth posterior from midline
_____ 3. another name for premolar tooth
_____ 4. baby or child's tooth
_____ 5. two-rooted molar tooth
_____ 6. tooth touching midline
_____ 7. tooth in upper jaw
_____ 8. smallest tooth in mouth
_____ 9. tooth in lower jaw
_____ 10. third anterior tooth in upper jaw

Column B

a. bicuspid tooth
b. deciduous tooth
c. mandibular second molar
d. maxillary molar tooth
e. first bicuspid or premolar tooth
f. central incisor
g. mandibular tooth
h. maxillary canine or cuspid
i. maxillary tooth
j. mandibular central incisor

Assignment Sheet 4.2 Tooth Surfaces

Name _____ Date _____ Grade _____

OBJECTIVE: To demonstrate knowledge of the surfaces of a tooth and the abbreviations used to designate single and multiple surfaces.

INSTRUCTIONS: Review material. Completely answer the questions in Part A. Complete the project indicated in Part B.

A.   1.   List the six surfaces of the tooth and state where they are positioned in the mouth.

   a. _____

   b. _____

   c. _____

   d. _____

   e. _____

   f. _____

   2.   Give the abbreviations for the following surfaces.

   labial _____   facial _____   occlusal _____   incisal _____

   mesial _____   distal _____   lingual _____   buccal _____

   3.   Write in the term for the following abbreviated surface combinations:

   MOD _____   MI _____

   MO _____   MID _____

   MOL _____   DOB _____

B.   Using a dental chart supplied by the instructor, color all surfaces on the chart using the following pattern:
   mesial surfaces—blue
   distal surfaces—yellow
   occlusal surfaces—red
   buccal surfaces—green
   incisal surfaces—black
   lingual surfaces—orange
   labial surfaces remain white

Assignment Sheet 4.3 Tooth Numbering Systems

Name _____ Date _____ Grade _____

OBJECTIVE: Demonstrate knowledge of the Universal, Palmer, and Federation Dentaire Internationale tooth numbering systems.

INSTRUCTIONS: Review material. Fill in designated numbering systems for teeth listed in each section of Part A. Give all three numbering systems for the teeth listed in Part B.

	Universal Number	Palmer Number	Federation Number
A. Permanent teeth			
Max. rt. third molar	_____	_____	_____
Max. rt. second molar	_____	_____	_____
Max. rt. first molar	_____	_____	_____
Max. rt. second bicuspid or premolar	_____	_____	_____
Max. rt. first bicuspid or premolar	_____	_____	_____
Max. rt. canine or cuspid	_____	_____	_____
Max. rt. lateral	_____	_____	_____
Max. rt. central	_____	_____	_____
Max. lt. central	_____	_____	_____
Max. lt. lateral	_____	_____	_____
Max. lt. canine or cuspid	_____	_____	_____
Max. lt. first bicuspid or premolar	_____	_____	_____
Max. lt. second bicuspid or premolar	_____	_____	_____
Max. lt. first molar	_____	_____	_____
Max. lt. second molar	_____	_____	_____
Max. lt. third molar	_____	_____	_____

Man. lt. third molar   _____   _____   _____

Man. lt. second molar   _____   _____   _____

Man. lt. first molar   _____   _____   _____

Man. lt. second bicuspid or premolar   _____   _____   _____

Man. lt. first bicuspid or premolar   _____   _____   _____

Man. lt. canine or cuspid   _____   _____   _____

Man. lt. lateral   _____   _____   _____

Man. lt. central   _____   _____   _____

Man. rt. central   _____   _____   _____

Man. rt. lateral   _____   _____   _____

Man. rt. canine or cuspid   _____   _____   _____

Man. rt. first bicuspid or premolar   _____   _____   _____

Man. rt. second bicuspid or premolar   _____   _____   _____

Man. rt. first molar   _____   _____   _____

Man. rt. second molar   _____   _____   _____

Man. rt. third molar   _____   _____   _____

Deciduous teeth

Max. rt. second molar   _____   _____   _____

Max. rt. first molar   _____   _____   _____

Max. rt. canine or cuspid   _____   _____   _____

Max. rt. lateral   _____   _____   _____

Max. rt. central   _____   _____   _____

Max. lt. central   _____   _____   _____

Max. lt. lateral   _____   _____   _____

Max. lt. canine or cuspid   _____   _____   _____

Max. lt. first molar   _____   _____   _____

Max. lt. second molar   _____   _____   _____

Man. lt. second molar   _____   _____   _____

Man. lt. first molar   _____   _____   _____

Man. lt. canine or cuspid   _____   _____   _____

Man. lt. lateral   _____   _____   _____

Man. lt. central   _____   _____   _____

Man. rt. central   _____   _____   _____

Man. rt. lateral   _____   _____   _____

Man. rt. canine or cuspid   _____   _____   _____

Man. rt. first molar   _____   _____   _____

Man. rt. second molar   _____   _____   _____

B.   Give the numbering system letter for each tooth listed below:

	Universal Number	Palmer Number	Federation Number
Permanent max. rt. first molar	_____	_____	_____

Permanent man. lt. central   _____   _____   _____

Deciduous max. rt. central   _____   _____   _____

Permanent max. lt. second premolar   _____   _____   _____

Deciduous man. lt. first molar   _____   _____   _____

Permanent man. rt. canine or cuspid   _____   _____   _____

Permanent man. lt. second premolar   _____   _____   _____

Deciduous max. rt. canine   _____   _____   _____

Permanent man. lt. lateral   _____   _____   _____

Deciduous max. rt. lateral   _____   _____   _____

Assignment Sheet 4.4 Charting Teeth

Name _____ Date _____ Grade _____

Objective: To demonstrate the method for charting mouth conditions, using symbols and dental markings.

Instructions: Review material. Using the dental charts supplied by the instructor, chart and record the following conditions.

Patient A (Universal numbering system): 1. OK, 2. MO amalgam restoration, 3. full gold crown, 4. $^3/_4$ gold crown, 5. OK, 6. OK, 7. RCT needed, 8. M composite restoration, 9. mesial composite restoration, 10. lingual composite restoration, 11. OK, 12. O composite restoration, 13. OK, 14. to be extracted, 15. MOD amalgam restoration, 16. missing, 17. to be extracted, 18. MOD caries, 19. MODL amalgam restoration, 20. DO amalgam restoration, 21. OK, 22 to 26. OK, 27, Class V composite restoration on facial surface, 28. OK, 29. O caries, 30. OD amalgam restoration, 31. MO amalgam restoration, 32. missing

Patient B: 1. fully impacted, 2. O caries, 3. MO amalgam, 4. O composite restoration, 5. OK, 6. OK, 7. fractured MI corner, 8. fractured DI corner, 9. OK, 10. OK, 11. OK, 12. O caries, 13. DO caries, 14. MO caries, 15. MOD amalgam restoration, 16. fully impacted, 17. partially impacted on distal third, 18. full gold crown that is part of a fixed three-unit bridge, 19. missing and replaced with pontic from three-unit bridge, 20. DO gold inlay that is part of a three-unit bridge, 21 to 26. OK, 27, facial composite restoration on gingival third, 28. OK, 29. O caries, 30. buccal amalgam restoration, 31. MOD amalgam restoration, 32. needs extracting

Assignment Sheet 4.5 Operative Hand Instruments

Name _____ Date _____ Grade _____

Objective: To demonstrate knowledge of operative hand instruments used in dental procedures.

Instructions: Review material. State the function of the instruments listed in Part A. Determine which grouping or family the instruments listed in Part B belong.

A.   State the function of the following instruments:

1.   amalgam carrier—_____

2.   explorer—_____

3.   discoid/cleoid—_____

4.   mirror—_____

5.   burnisher—_____

6.   condenser—_____

7.   PFI—_____

8.   pick up or college pliers—_____

9.   scaler—_____

10.   hatchet—_____

11.   curette—_____

12.   carver—_____

13.   excavator—_____

B.   Place the instruments listed in Part A into one of these families or groups: basic, prophylaxis, cutting, or plastic filling:

1. _____   8. _____

2. _____   9. _____

3. _____   10. _____

4. _____   11. _____

5. _____   12. _____

6. _____   13. _____

7. _____

Assignment Sheet 10.1 Radiation Safety Knowledge

Name _____ Date _____ Grade _____

OBJECTIVE: To demonstrate knowledge of the various types of radiation and the methods to provide safety for the patient and operator.

INSTRUCTIONS: Review material about radiation safety. Complete the word search problem below which contains key words for safety and radiation terms (Part A). Using the words given in the puzzle, write a sentence about radiation safety containing one word per sentence (Part B).

A. Words contained in puzzle are: apron, barrier, collar, dosimeter, exposure, film, handling, interproximal, lead, PID, primary, processing, quality, questioning, radiation, safety, scattered, secondary, shield, storage.

```
L A M I X O R P R E T N I E R E J I O I D D O N
D F J H L G B W Y N F L O W I G N O R M Y D U A
B K I I R V E K S R O S K E R R D R D D N V I S
J B D L S S A A S Y J G U O S Q F E O R S Y E C
S A D G M N N M W E N G T O I U L U S H I R O A
R R M S F B D R A G A H U D S A N C I M U S F T
J R K A S I J E N A S N N L W L E I M T S A R T
M I W P R A D I A T I O N B N I I Y E N H K A E
K E O I R O O K W R V J R I D T W I T S P P K R
A R S I J J W R Y F D W A L C Y D N E G U I K E
Y R E Y M U C A O D E R E S C N C S R Y S D O D
H Y H Y W A N B B O L I L P N F E R V D D P Y G
V T S L M I N S P I H A O P N R R L E D N S O W
L A T E G O D Y R S R V C N R M J R R Y J S D A
T O M F G N I L D N A H O F C E R U S O P X E A
S T O N F S R L S S N S E O O N G A R Y R V R Y
D J T W O N V Y Y D T B I Y L A R A R L G Y V T
P A S E I W E P E O V M I L L E E J T E I R S E
U Y R A D N O C E S I S I R A E E D Y A W S S F
S L L F I E R D N P D I I G R V N J A D I N O A
A U Y N B W L N S E O V Y D I S T O R A G E V S
S L K G N I N O I T S E U Q I O N J I R O N H C
A P D G N I S S E C O R P R O E W N R N U T K I
L Y N A L N O R P A A P P R I M A R Y I N R E S
```

B. Write a radiation safety sentence using each word from the puzzle in Part A.

Assignment Sheet 10.2 Radiation Film Knowledge

Name _____ Date _____ Grade _____

OBJECTIVE: Demonstrate knowledge of dental radiation film use and purpose.

INSTRUCTIONS: Review the material on dental radiation films. Identify film shapes. State the kind of film and its purpose on the line preceding the drawing. Select one exposure for each film shape and either draw or write in the teeth and landmarks that would be found in that exposure. On the line following the space, identify that exposure.

A. _____

B. _____

Exposure _____

Exposure _____

C. _____

D. _____

Exposure _____

Exposure _____

Assignment Sheet 10.3 Analyzing Dental Radiographs

Name _____ Date _____ Grade _____

OBJECTIVE: To demonstrate the ability to discover errors on dental radiographs and to state the methods to eliminate such errors.

INSTRUCTIONS: Review material on radiograph errors. Select radiographs that display five different technique errors (may be care and handling, exposure or processing errors). Paste the radiograph to this paper. In the space preceding the radiograph, state what error is present in the film. In the line under the film, state the method to correct this error. ℘ If films are not available for use, draw view of proper exposure in area provided.

1. Diagnosis of error _____.

  Correction procedure _____.

2. Diagnosis of error _____.

  Correction procedure _____.

3. Diagnosis of error _____.

  Correction procedure _____.

4. Diagnosis of error _____.

   Correction procedure _____.

5. Diagnosis of error _____.

   Correction procedure _____.

Assignment Sheet 11.1 Appointment Scheduling

Name _____ Date _____ Grade _____

OBJECTIVE: To demonstrate the ability to prepare an appointment sheet and schedule a variety of patients for a typical day in a dental facility.

INSTRUCTIONS: Complete the three work projects that follow. Use the blank appointment sheet provided (page 401).

A. Prepare an appointment sheet for this typical day: Office hours are from 8:30 AM to 5 PM. Lunch is from 12:00 to 1:00 PM and a buffer period of one unit is maintained at 11:45 AM. The facility operates on a 4U per hour system. There are no special events happening today so nothing else needs to be marked off.

B. Schedule the following patients for the appointment page just prepared: The time needed for each procedure (units) is given with the needed work.

Patient	Age	Phone Number	Work Description	Best Time
Samuel Andes	36	101-343-7463	consultation 3U	afternoon
Carrie Gillis	33	101-344-2649	cosmetic bleach (max) 3U	afternoon
Jerald Robinson	41	101-343-6563	root canal visit 1 #13 3U	AM
Danielle Berret	45	233-927-7652	composite #12DO, #13MO, 3U	PM
Suu Fong Bun	5	101-344-1246	steel crown #B 2U	open
Mildred King	38	233-927-2467	new patient 3U 403 Main St.	afternoon
Rodney McConnell	29	233-433-8765	extraction #31 2U	open
Mason Pollard	73	233-433-1246	denture reline 2U	AM
Patricia Townson	18	233-927-4836	perio-flap surgery 2U	AM
Billy Walker	7	101-343-4726	O amal rest #T 2U	open
Charlotte Zinn	51	233-433-0987	crown prep #19 4U	AM

C. Select two patients scheduled on the appointment page and make out an appointment card for each.

Your dental appointment is scheduled for: _____ at_____ AM _____ PM **CATHERINE C. COLE, D.D.S.** 100 West Mifflin St. Best Town, US 12345 (123) 456-7890	**Your dental appointment is scheduled for:** _____ at_____ AM _____ PM **CATHERINE C. COLE, D.D.S.** 100 West Mifflin St. Best Town, US 12345 (123) 456-7890

Month _____

Thursday

Date _____

8	00		
	15		
	30		
	45		
9	00		
	15		
	30		
	45		
10	00		
	15		
	30		
	45		
11	00		
	15		
	30		
	45		
12	00		
	15		
	30		
	45		
1	00		
	15		
	30		
	45		
2	00		
	15		
	30		
	45		
3	00		
	15		
	30		
	45		
4	00		
	15		
	30		
	45		
5	00		
	15		
	30		
	45		
	00		
	15		
	30		
	45		
	00		
	15		
	30		
	45		

Assignment Sheet 11.2 Patient Dental Records

Name _____ Date _____ Grade _____

OBJECTIVE: To demonstrate the ability to transpose patient information to a registration form and to interview a person for health history data.

INSTRUCTIONS: Using the following information, complete the blank registration form provided.

A. Mrs. Mary Ellen Young was referred to our office by one of our patients, Mrs. Susan Livingstone. Mary Ellen is married to Harold Allen Young. They have recently moved here from 119 Bright Way in Hopewell, NJ 01032. They and their 14-year-old son, Tim, whose birthday is October 12, live at 3 Pellican Way, Coastown, MD 12345. Their home phone number is 302-555-8272.

Mary Ellen works for Belcar Communications located at 199387 Power Avenue in Largetown, MD 12344. Her work phone number is 302-555-3783, extension 205. Mary Ellen was 38 years old last May 11th. Her social security number is 123-45-5678. Her husband, whose social security number is 234-56-7890, was born 40 years ago on February 16th. He is self-employed as a wireless consultant and works out of the home. He does not carry family medical or dental insurance, but Mary Ellen has dental insurance through her company with an organization called Dentcare Inc., located at 300 Howell Building in Largetown, MD 12344. She is in the Belmed group and her policy number is 445566, effective 9-10-90. She wishes to be responsible for her own account and prefers late afternoon appointments.

Mary Ellen's physician's name is Thomas Payne and his office is located in the Towers Building Suite 2000 at 5th and 17th Avenue in Largetown, MD 12344. His phone number is 302-555-3630.

B. Use the health history form shown in Figure 11.6 to interview another person and record the given data on the health history form.

WELCOME TO OUR OFFICE

CATHERINE C. COLE, D.D.S.
100 West Mifflin St.
Best Town, US 12345
(123) 456-7890

DATE _____

To help us serve you better, please print the needed information below:
All replies are treated as confidential information.

Patient's Name	Birthdate	Marital Status

Address	City	State	ZIP	Phone

Social Security Number	Physician's Name and Address/Phone Number

Spouse's Name	Birthdate	Social Security Number

Name of Patient's Employer	Address	Phone

Dental Insurance Plan	Group	Number	Effective Date

Name of Spouse's Employer	Address	Phone

Dental Insurance Plan	Group	Number	Effective Date

Children's First Name	Last Name	Birthdate

Name of person who referred you to our office _____

RELEASE OF INFORMATION:

I authorize the release of any dental information necessary to process this claim.

_____   _____
(Patient's Name)   (Date)

ASSIGNMENT OF BENEFITS:

I authorize payment of dental benefits directly to the named provider for professional services rendered.

_____   _____
(Subscriber's Name)   (Date)

Assignment Sheet 11.3 Records Management

Name _____ Date _____ Grade _____

OBJECTIVE: To demonstrate method for indexing of names and titles and arrange a list of given names and titles in alphabetic order.

INSTRUCTIONS: Use the following list of names and titles. Index each name or title (Part A). Arrange each title or name into alphabetic order and place the number of the title or name number in order (Part B).

A. Names to be filed

	Indexing Order			
	Unit 1	Unit 2	Unit 3	Unit 4
1. National Caregivers Assoc.				
2. Miss Barbara Lou Black				
3. Jeffrey Jones, Sr.				
4. Mr. Woody Hollows				
5. Hewitt-Merill Computer Co.				
6. Martha Ann Miller				
7. St. Louis Dental Society				
8. Mrs. Michele Zinn (Tim)				
9. Mr. James Da Mocco				
10. 5th Avenue Supply Co.				
11. Mrs. Paul Pleasant (Kerri)				
12. ABC Cleaners				
13. Michael Louis Le Paul				
14. Carol's Gift Shop				
15. Jeffrey Jones, Jr.				
16. Kristin Gill, DDS				
17. Mrs. Sam Pleasant (Kathleen)				
18. Miss Ivy Lans-Worthy				
19. W. W. Hollows				
20. Ms. Laura Jones-Martin				
21. John Collen Gilbert				
22. Kristin Gill				
23. John William Gilbert				
24. Southeast Airline				
25. John Gilbert				

B. The alphabetic order of the titles and names:

1. _____	6. _____	11. _____	16. _____	21. _____
2. _____	7. _____	12. _____	17. _____	22. _____
3. _____	8. _____	13. _____	18. _____	23. _____
4. _____	9. _____	14. _____	19. _____	24. _____
5. _____	10. _____	15. _____	20. _____	25. _____

Assignment Sheet 11.4 Checking Accounts

Name _____ Date _____ Grade _____

OBJECTIVE: To demonstrate the ability to complete a check writing exercise and perform a checking account reconciliation using a set of given figures.

INSTRUCTIONS: Complete Part A by writing three checks for the given payees. In Part B reconcile the checking account.

A.   Using today's date, the forms provided, a bank balance brought forward of $5,744.26, and a deposit of $386.00 to be made this afternoon, write out three checks and the stubs for the following:

Downtown Dental Supply for last month's statement	$457.33
Mr. George Yannick for a patient refund	78.00
Cameo Dental Laboratory for invoice #374635	241.80

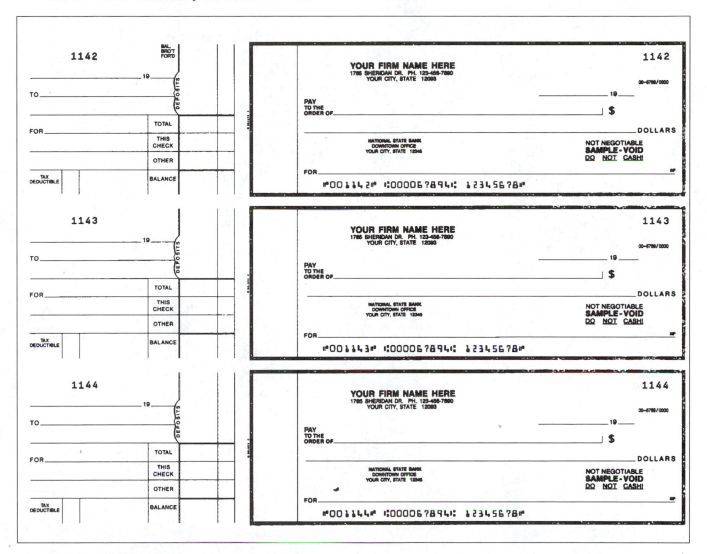

Courtesy of Colwell Systems [Deluxe Forms].)

B. Using the provided form and given figures, complete a checking account reconciliation. The account balance is $9,651.25 with outstanding checks #309 for $304.11, check #311 for $77.19, and check #313 for $122.35. The bank balance is $9,934.90, and there was a $20 charge for a safe deposit box. There is one outstanding deposit for $200.

Bank Balance   Account Balance

_____

                                       Outstanding Checks
                                  #   Amount

                                  _____

                                  _____

                             Total _____

_____ –Outstanding Checks Total

                                                                         _____

                                        –Less Bank Charges _____
                                        New Account Balance _____
                                        –Outstanding Deposit _____
_____ Bank Balance   Account Balance _____

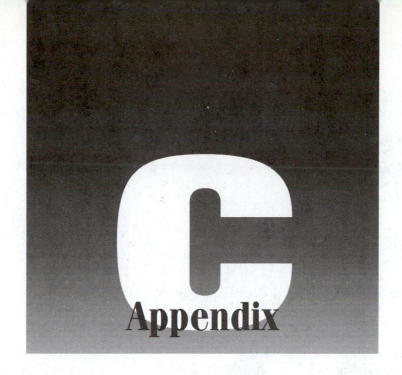

Appendix

COMPETENCY EVALUATION SHEETS FOR PROCEDURES 1–65

COMPETENCY EVALUATION SHEET

PROCEDURE 1

Measuring and Recording Vital Signs

Student Name _____ Date _____

GRADING PROTOCOL: Student is awarded the number of points indicated on the evaluation sheet for completing steps successfully.

Total possible points = 100 points
80% needed for passing = 80 points

Total points this test _____   pass _____   fail _____

	PEER REVIEW	TEACHER REVIEW

POINTS

1 Complete Preparations (2 points)

(2) _____ gather necessary items   _____   _____

2 Measure and Record Pulse (15 points)

(2) _____ explain procedure
(2) _____ identify site
(2) _____ place fingers on radial pulse
(2) _____ apply gentle pressure to feel pulse
(2) _____ establish timing

(2) _____ count beat and note rhythm
(3) _____ record pulse count and condition or rhythm _____ _____

3 Measure and Record Respirations (15 points)

(2) _____ identify inspiration (chest rise)
(2) _____ identify exhalation (chest fall)
(2) _____ establish timing
(2) _____ avoid detection of procedure
(2) _____ count respirations
(2) _____ determine respiration quality
(3) _____ record findings _____ _____

4 Measure and Record Blood Pressure (30 points)

(2) _____ explain procedure
(2) _____ prepare arm for sphygmomanometer attachment
(2) _____ wrap deflated cuff over brachial artery
(2) _____ check tubing position
(2) _____ locate radial pulse
(2) _____ inflate cuff until no radial pulse, note reading
(2) _____ deflate cuff
(2) _____ locate brachial pulse site
(2) _____ position diaphragm over pulse site
(2) _____ inflate cuff slightly over noted systolic area
(2) _____ open valve, release pressure (2 mm Hg per second)
(2) _____ note mercury or dial level at 1st sound (systolic)
(2) _____ note mercury or dial reading at last sound (diastolic)
(2) _____ deflate cuff, remove, record findings (even numbers)
(2) _____ restore arm clothing, replace equipment _____ _____

5 Measure and Record Temperature (30 points)

Oral temperature (10 points)
(1) _____ explain procedure for oral thermometer
(1) _____ ask if ate, drank, or smoked in last 15 minutes
(1) _____ check that mercury shook down to bulb tip
(1) _____ caution patient not to bite hard on thermometer
(1) _____ place sterilized thermometer into patient's mouth, under tongue
(1) _____ maintain thermometer under tongue for three minutes, remove
(1) _____ wipe thermometer with cotton roll, read temperature
(2) _____ record temperature on chart
(1) _____ wash, sterilize, and replace thermometer _____ _____

Electric thermometer (10 points)
(1) _____ explain procedure for electric thermometer
(1) _____ question patient regarding eating, drinking, or smoking
(1) _____ insert probe into sterile probe cover
(1) _____ caution patient not to bite hard on probe
(1) _____ place probe cover under tongue, hold in place
(1) _____ at buzzing sound, remove probe, note LED temperature printout
(1) _____ release used probe cover into a contaminated trash container
(1) _____ replace probe rod into carrier
(2) _____ record temperature _____ _____

Ear thermometer or Ototemp (10 points)
(1) _____ explain procedure (tympanic infrared scanner thermometer)
(1) _____ demonstrate process, activate thermometer

(1) _____ show patient reading of table top
(1) _____ apply clean barrier cover over probe tip
(1) _____ insert tip and cover into ear canal, rotate
(1) _____ find deepest section, activate thermometer
(1) _____ hold tip in ear canal until removal signal
(1) _____ remove, read, and record temperature
(1) _____ remove barrier shield, place in trash container
(1) _____ replace equipment   _____   _____

6 Replace the Equipment (8 points)

(2) _____ sterilize oral thermometer
(2) _____ deflate blood pressure cuff
(2) _____ wipe earpieces with disinfectant swab
(2) _____ replace equipment   _____   _____

(100)   Total points   _____   _____

COMPETENCY EVALUATION SHEET

Assisting the Choking Victim

Student Name _____ Date _____

GRADING PROTOCOL: Student is awarded the number of points indicated on the evaluation sheet for completing steps successfully.

Total possible points = 100 points
80% needed for passing = 80 points

Total points this test _____ pass _____ fail _____

	PEER REVIEW	TEACHER REVIEW

POINTS

1 Be Alert (9 points)

(3) _____ look for signals
(2) _____ observe patient
(2) _____ ask "Are you choking?"
(2) _____ watch for cough or speaking   _____ _____

2 Seek Assistance (6 points)

(2) _____ summon help
(2) _____ call emergency assistance
(2) _____ give complete data to emergency operator   _____ _____

3 Prepare for the Heimlich Maneuver (4 points)

(2) _____ assist patient to stand
(2) _____ position patient for assistance   _____ _____

4 Administer the Heimlich Maneuver (Standing Victim) (20 points)

(2) _____ support patient
(2) _____ move to patient's rear
(2) _____ explain procedure to patient
(2) _____ place arms around patient
(3) _____ close hands into fist with thumb against patient's front
(3) _____ position fist above beltline, under ribcage
(2) _____ lean patient slightly over fists
(2) _____ administer quick thrust with fist inward and upward
(2) _____ continue until object loose and expelled or until patient is coughing   _____ _____

5 Administer the Heimlich Maneuver (Patient on the Floor) (14 points)

(2) _____ supine position body
(2) _____ straddle patient
(3) _____ place heel of hand against abdomen, between the ribcage and belt
(3) _____ place second hand over palm's heel
(2) _____ give quick thrust, inward and upward
(2) _____ continue until object loose and expelled or patient is coughing   _____ _____

6 Administer the Heimlich Maneuver (Seated Patient) (8 points)

(2) _____ complete questioning
(2) _____ position patient and rescuer as if standing
(2) _____ apply pressure in same method as standing technique
(2) _____ continue until object dislodged or patient coughing   _____   _____

7 Administer the Heimlich Maneuver (Pregnant or Obese Person) (15 points)

(2) _____ question victim
(2) _____ position victim and rescuer in normal stance
(3) _____ place fist on sternum midsection
(3) _____ support fist with other hand
(3) _____ perform quick thrust backward and inward
(2) _____ continue thrust until object dislodges or patient is coughing   _____   _____

8 Search the Oral Cavity (8 points)

(2) _____ grasp tongue and lower jaw, lift jaw
(2) _____ slide finger down inside cheek
(2) _____ curve finger into C and do finger sweep
(2) _____ do finger sweep only on child if object visible   _____   _____

9 Monitor the Recovered Patient (9 points)

(3) _____ reassure patient
(3) _____ administer oxygen to relieve stress
(3) _____ remain with patient until recovered   _____   _____

10 Record Emergency Treatment on the Patient's Chart (7 points)

(2) _____ note date and time
(2) _____ note treatment, outcome
(3) _____ review summary with dentist   _____   _____

(100)   Total points   _____   _____

COMPETENCY EVALUATION SHEET

P R O C E D U R E   3

Cardiopulmonary Resuscitation

Student Name _____ Date _____

GRADING PROTOCOL: Student is awarded the number of points indicated on the evaluation sheet for completing steps successfully.

Total possible points = 100 points
80% needed for passing = 80 points

Total points this test _____ pass _____ fail _____

	PEER REVIEW	TEACHER REVIEW

POINTS

1 Examine the Patient (12 points)

(2) _____ shake or try to rouse patient
(2) _____ summon assistance
(2) _____ tilt head to open airway
(2) _____ search for breathing
(2) _____ attempt inflation of lungs
(2) _____ check carotid pulse   _____   _____

2 Position the Patient (10 points)

(3) _____ place patient in supine position on hard surface
(3) _____ retilt head to open airway
(2) _____ attempt to breathe into lungs, two breaths
(2) _____ look for chest rising   _____   _____

3 Attempt to Relieve Blockage (12 points)

(2) _____ examine oral cavity
(2) _____ do finger sweep for unconscious adult, child with visible blockage
(2) _____ retilt head to open airway
(2) _____ attempt breaths
(2) _____ perform Heimlich maneuver
(2) _____ retest airway, repeat until clear   _____   _____

4 Perform CPR (One Person) (20 points)

(2) _____ check carotid artery
(2) _____ give two slow, full breaths
(2) _____ if no pulse, locate sternum and xiphoid process
(2) _____ position heel of hands on lower $2/3$ of sternum
(2) _____ compress chest $1\frac{1}{2}$ to 2 inches for 15 times
(2) _____ maintain rhythm of compressions
(2) _____ return to give two breaths
(2) _____ return to give chest compression 15 times
(2) _____ repeat process for four rotations
(2) _____ check carotid artery   _____   _____

5 Continue CPR (6 points)

(2) _____ continue cycles of 2 breaths to 15 compressions
(2) _____ test carotid artery every four cycles
(2) _____ continue process until help arrives, scene unsafe, or doctor
             pronounces death   _____   _____

6 Perform CPR (Two Persons) (16 points)

(2) _____ rescuer two seeks assistance, if needed
(2) _____ rescuer two positions self at victim's side
(2) _____ rescuer one completes compresses and gives two breaths
(2) _____ rescuer two locates sternum and xiphoid process
(2) _____ places hand heel and gives five compressions
(2) _____ rescuer one checks pulse while compressions are occurring
(2) _____ rescuer one gives one breath for every five compressions
(2) _____ both rescuers continue cycles until help appears   _____   _____

7 Exchange Rescuers (14 points)

(2) _____ rescuer two (compressor) orders change during count
(2) _____ rescuer two (compressor) compresses and counts to five
(2) _____ rescuer two (compressor) moves to head
(2) _____ rescuer one (ventilator) gives breath after count five, moves
(2) _____ rescuer two (new ventilator) checks pulse, reopens airway, and inflates lungs
(2) _____ rescuer one (new compressor) gives compressions
(2) _____ both rescuers continue rhythm until help arrives   _____   _____

8 Record the Emergency on the Patient's Chart (10 points)

(2) _____ record date, day, and time
(2) _____ record emergency symptoms
(2) _____ record CPR treatment
(2) _____ estimate and record time of unconsciousness and CPR
(2) _____ review summary notes with dentist   _____   _____

(100)   Total points   _____   _____

COMPETENCY EVALUATION SHEET

PROCEDURE 4

Assisting with a Shock Emergency

Student Name _____   Date _____

GRADING PROTOCOL: Student is awarded the number of points indicated on the evaluation sheet for completing steps successfully.

Total possible points = 100 points
80% needed for passing = 80 points

Total points this test _____   pass _____   fail _____

	PEER REVIEW	TEACHER REVIEW

POINTS

1 Discuss Various Types of Shock and Causes (10 points)

(5) _____ name types of dental office shock emergencies
(5) _____ name types of general shock emergencies   _____   _____

2 State General Symptoms of Shock (15 points)

(5) _____ list skin and surface symptoms
(5) _____ list behavior symptoms
(5) _____ list vital sign symptoms   _____   _____

3 Give General Rules for Care of a Shock Patient (6 points)

(2) _____ eliminate reason for shock
(2) _____ restore body functions
(2) _____ maintain vital signs   _____   _____

4 Demonstrate Care of a Fainting Victim (Syncope) (22 points)

(2) _____ state reason for reaction
(4) _____ position body
(4) _____ administer spirits of ammonia
(4) _____ restore oxygen intake
(4) _____ take and record vital signs
(4) _____ reassure and remain with patient   _____   _____

5 Demonstrate Care of an Anaphylactic Shock Victim (18 points)

(2) _____ state reason for shock
(2) _____ list anaphylactic shock symptoms
(2) _____ summon assistance
(2) _____ position patient
(2) _____ administer antihistamine (epinephrine) preparation
(2) _____ administer oxygen preparation
(2) _____ take and record vital signs
(2) _____ maintain body functions
(2) _____ reassure and remain with patient   _____   _____

6 Demonstrate Care of a Heart Attack Shock Victim (12 points)

(2) _____ state cardiogenic shock symptoms
(2) _____ summon assistance
(2) _____ administer oxygen preparation
(2) _____ be prepared for CPR
(2) _____ keep victim warm
(2) _____ reassure and remain with patient   _____   _____

7 Record the Emergency on the Patient's Chart (17 points)

(5) _____ record date, day, and time of emergency
(5) _____ record symptoms
(4) _____ record treatment and outcome
(3) _____ review data with dentist for completeness and accuracy   _____   _____

(100)   Total points   _____   _____

COMPETENCY EVALUATION SHEET

PROCEDURE 5

Hand-washing Technique

Student Name _____ Date _____

GRADING PROTOCOL: Student is awarded the number of points indicated on the evaluation sheet for completing steps successfully.

Total possible points = 100 points
80% needed for passing = 80 points

Total points this test _____ pass _____ fail _____

	PEER REVIEW	TEACHER REVIEW

POINTS

1 Assemble Equipment and Materials (5 points)

(5) _____ all materials and equipment present   _____   _____

2 Remove Jewelry and Watch (5 points)

(5) _____ jewelry and watch removed, put away   _____   _____

3 Hold Paper Towel to Turn On Faucet (15 points)

(5) _____ wet hands and wrists
(5) _____ adjust flow and temperature of water
(5) _____ use paper toweling on faucet, if not automatic   _____   _____

4 Apply Antimicrobial Soap Solution (10 points)

(5) _____ work up lather on hands
(5) _____ work lather onto wrist   _____   _____

5 Work Up a Lather (15 points)

(4) _____ palms of one hand lather back of other
(4) _____ extend palm-rubbing action to include wrists
(4) _____ rub fingertips into palm of other hand
(3) _____ reverse order   _____   _____

6 Work Lather Around Hands (5 points)

(5) _____ interlace fingers for scrub   _____   _____

7 Use Cuticle Stick and Brush (10 points)

(4) _____ use cuticle stick under fingernails (blunt end)
(4) _____ use brush on nail tips and knuckles (circular motion)
(2) _____ perform at start and end of day and whenever needed   _____   _____

8 Rinse Hands (10 points)

(5) _____ hold hands downward while rinsing
(5) _____ rinse brush and cuticle stick, set aside   _____   _____

9 Dry Hands with a Paper Towel (10 points)

(5) _____ dispose of towel properly
(5) _____ do not touch sides of container   _____   _____

10 Turn Off the Faucet with a Paper Towel (15 points)

(5) _____ use fresh towel to clean sink area
(5) _____ dispose of towel in proper container
(5) _____ do not touch sides of sink or container   _____   _____

(100)   Total points   _____   _____

COMPETENCY EVALUATION SHEET

PROCEDURE 6

Donning and Disposing Clinical Attire

Student Name _____ Date _____

GRADING PROTOCOL: Student is awarded the number of points indicated on the evaluation sheet for completing steps successfully.

Total possible points = 100 points
80% needed for passing = 80 points

Total points this test _____   pass _____   fail _____

	PEER REVIEW	TEACHER REVIEW

POINTS

Donning

1 Gather Personal Protection Equipment (PPE) (5 points)

(5) _____ assemble all necessary items   _____   _____

2 Remove Jewelry and Wash Hands (5 points)

(3) _____ place removed jewelry in secure area
(2) _____ use correct hand-washing method   _____   _____

3 Don Clinical Attire (10 points)

(2) _____ check for cleanliness, stains, tears
(2) _____ have proper size and fit
(2) _____ remove or cover personal clothing
(2) _____ don personal protection attire
(2) _____ button, tie, or velcro closures   _____   _____

4 Don Clinical Footwear (5 points)

(1) _____ don clean hosiery
(2) _____ observe cleanliness, condition of shoes
(2) _____ have proper fit and support   _____   _____

5 Prepare for Procedure (10 points)

(2) _____ ready operatory
(2) _____ greet patient
(2) _____ seat and position patient
(4) _____ review health history   _____   _____

6 Apply Mask (5 points)

(1) _____ fresh, dry, and new each time
(2) _____ cover nose and mouth
(1) _____ tie or slip elastic over head/ears (loops)
(1) _____ adjust for comfort   _____   _____

7 Don Eyeglass Protection (5 points)

(2) _____ check cleanliness
(2) _____ have proper fit
(1) _____ side shields in place   _____   _____

8 Don Face Shield, if Desired (5 points)

(1) _____ place visor edges over temples
(2) _____ check for extension below chin
(1) _____ check for cleanliness
(1) _____ have wraparound face protection   _____   _____

9 Don Gloves (5 points)

(2) _____ new pair each time
(1) _____ proper type for procedure
(1) _____ proper fit, no tears or holes
(1) _____ prepare overgloves   _____   _____

Disposing

10 Remove Instruments to Sterilizing Room (5 points)

(2) _____ take all removable equipment and items
(2) _____ discard faceshield for disinfection
(1) _____ flush lines   _____   _____

11 Remove Gloves (5 points)

(1) _____ place gloved fingers under outside cuff of other glove
(1) _____ lift and pull down on glove keeping glove in fingers of pulling hand
(1) _____ insert freed hand inside gloved hand and pull down and out on second glove
(1) _____ second glove is removed inside out over glove from first hand
(1) _____ both gloves dropped into marked disposal bag   _____   _____

12 Remove Face Coverings (5 points)

(2) _____ remove eyeglasses for disinfection
(2) _____ remove mask, touch on ties or elastic on back of head or ears and
lift up and over
(1) _____ dispose of mask in disposal bag   _____   _____

13 Remove Clinical Attire (15 points)

(1) _____ unbutton, untie, or open velcro closures
(1) _____ remove first arm
(3) _____ unwrap gown, dress, or coat around body with contaminated side folded inside
(2) _____ slip out other arm and fold inside
(2) _____ fold article in half having inside exposed and contaminated surfaces tucked in
(2) _____ drop into marked laundry bag or, if paper, into marked disposal bag
(2) _____ pull pants and tops off inside out, fold in half and drop into disposal bag
(1) _____ removal done slowly to avoid spreading germs
(1) _____ redon personal clothing   _____   _____

14 Remove Clinical Footwear (10 points)

(1) _____ step out of shoes
(2) _____ remove stockings inside out and place into marked laundry bag
(2) _____ wipe off shoes with disposable, wet, disinfected towelette while not touching with hands
(2) _____ dispose of towel into marked disposal bag
(1) _____ check condition of shoes and laces, polish
(1) _____ wash or dispose of laces if necessary
(1) _____ redon personal footwear   _____   _____

15 Wash Hands and Remove Laundry Bag (5 points)

(1) _____ close and tie laundry bag
(2) _____ perform thorough hand wash
(1) _____ redon jewelry
(1) _____ remove laundry bag to proper area   _____   _____

(100)   Total points   _____   _____

COMPETENCY EVALUATION SHEET

PROCEDURE 7

Ultrasonic Cleaning

Student Name _____ Date _____

GRADING PROTOCOL: Student is awarded the number of points indicated on the evaluation sheet for completing steps successfully.

Total possible points = 100 points
80% needed for passing = 80 points

Total points this test _____ pass _____ fail _____

	PEER REVIEW	TEACHER REVIEW

POINTS

1 Prepare for the Procedure (5 points)

(2) _____ wash and dry hands, don PPE
(3) _____ assemble materials and equipment   _____   _____

2 Preclean the Items (If Not Cassette) (12 points)

(2) _____ soak, rinse, scrub instruments, burs, and all washable items
(2) _____ use brush to remove debris
(2) _____ brush hinges, serrations, edges
(2) _____ brush burs and small objects
(2) _____ rinse, drain on towel, pat dry with towels
(2) _____ dispose of towel in proper container   _____   _____

3 Prepare the Ultrasonic Machine (10 points)

(3) _____ check solution in ultrasonic tank
(2) _____ check condition of solution
(2) _____ check level of solution, add or change solution, if needed
(3) _____ engage electrical plug into outlet   _____   _____

4 Immerse the Instruments into the Solution (15 points)

(2) _____ read manufacturer's directions for solution and time
(2) _____ place instruments for general cleaning in wire basket
(3) _____ totally submerge instruments or articles
(2) _____ place burs in bur basket in solution
(3) _____ avoid overloading, allow for circulation of bubbles
(2) _____ place lid on tank, avoid spreading pathogens
(1) _____ set timer for proper cycle   _____   _____

5 Immerse Small or Special Items into the Beakers (10 points)

(2) _____ read manufacturer's directions for correct solution and time
(1) _____ select proper beaker and solution
(2) _____ submerge beaker correctly into solution, adjust beaker band if needed, avoid beaker touching sides or bottom
(1) _____ submerge articles in beakers of correct solution

(2) _____ avoid overcrowding
(1) _____ place lid on beaker to avoid spreading pathogens
(1) _____ set timer for proper cycle _____ _____

6 Drain the Articles (10 points)

(1) _____ drip excess from articles in wire or bur basket into tank
(1) _____ carry baskets to sink
(1) _____ rinse and drain articles in baskets
(2) _____ remove/toss from basket and pat dry
(2) _____ remove from beakers using transfer forceps, rinse, pat dry
(2) _____ check for cleanliness and function
(1) _____ dispose of towels in proper container _____ _____

7 Use the Ultrasonic Cassette (15 points)

(1) _____ return exposed instruments, items to cassette
(1) _____ place small items in boxes or blocks in cassette
(2) _____ place in sequential order
(2) _____ take to sterilizing area, immerse in tank
(2) _____ make sure cassette tray is totally covered with solution
(1) _____ activate timer
(2) _____ remove from unit, rinse cassette and all
(1) _____ permit cassette to drip dry
(1) _____ replace disposables, check condition of items, lubricate
(2) _____ insert sterilizing indicator strip _____ _____

8 Prepare Articles for Sterilization (8 points)

(2) _____ wrap instruments, cassette in paper, wrap sleeves
(2) _____ foil wrap or leave bare for dry heat
(2) _____ arrange burs in bur tray
(2) _____ mark all wraps with date and contents _____ _____

9 Clean Up the Area and Equipment (10 points)

(1) _____ drain main tank if need be
(1) _____ scrub and wipe dry
(1) _____ refill with fresh general-purpose solution
(1) _____ check beakers for cracks or excessive scratches
(1) _____ polish exterior
(1) _____ change solutions, if needed
(2) _____ replace equipment, lids
(2) _____ unplug machine _____ _____

10 Remove PPE (5 points)

(2) _____ wash, dry, and disinfect gloves
(1) _____ remove gloves
(2) _____ wash hands _____ _____

(100) Total points _____ _____

COMPETENCY EVALUATION SHEET

P R O C E D U R E   8

Operation of an Autoclave

Student Name _____ Date _____

GRADING PROTOCOL: Student is awarded the number of points indicated on the evaluation sheet for completing steps successfully.

Total possible points = 100 points
80% needed for passing = 80 points

Total points this test _____ pass _____ fail _____

	PEER REVIEW	TEACHER REVIEW

POINTS

1 Prepare for the Procedure (10 points)

(2) _____ wash hands
(2) _____ don utility gloves
(3) _____ assemble cleaned instruments and materials
(3) _____ wrap and mark if desired   _____   _____

2 Prepare the Autoclave (10 points)

(2) _____ check reservoir water level and condition
(2) _____ fill with distilled water, if needed
(2) _____ engage electrical plug into socket
(2) _____ turn on power, check gauges
(2) _____ open door   _____   _____

3 Load the Autoclave Chamber (10 points)

(3) _____ open hinged instruments
(3) _____ do not overcrowd or overfill
(2) _____ pack loosely to allow for flow of steam in chamber
(2) _____ remove lids and tilt jars   _____   _____

4 Fill the Chamber with Water (10 points)

(3) _____ turn control dial counterclockwise to "fill"
(3) _____ allow water to cover water plate in chamber
(2) _____ turn control dial to "sterilize" to stop flow
(2) _____ check gasket, close door securely   _____   _____

5 Adjust the Thermostat (10 points)

(5) _____ raise or lower temperature as needed, amber light is off when
           gauge indicates 250°F
(5) _____ monitor that temperature is regular   _____   _____

6   Set the Timer (If Not Automatic) (10 points)

(10) _____ set timer for 20 minutes after proper conditions have been obtained (15 lbs. at 250°F)

_____   _____

7   Vent the Autoclave (10 points)

(4) _____ after timer goes off, turn control dial to "vent"
(4) _____ allow temperature and pressure to drop to zero
(2) _____ turn control dial to "off"

_____   _____

8   Open the Autoclave Door (10 points)

(4) _____ don safety glasses to release and open door
(4) _____ stand at side and "crack open" door
(2) _____ allow final evaporation for 4 to 5 minutes

_____   _____

9   Remove the Contents (10 points)

(2) _____ remove pack from chamber
(2) _____ use sterile forceps to transfer bare items
(2) _____ store contents, rotate packs in storage
(2) _____ cover sterile items in proper area
(2) _____ remove plug from outlet

_____   _____

10   Clean Up the Area (10 points)

(2) _____ wipe chamber and exterior (after machine cools)
(2) _____ close door on autoclave
(2) _____ wipe up area
(2) _____ wash, dry, disinfect utility gloves
(2) _____ wash and thoroughly dry hands

_____   _____

(100)   Total points

_____   _____

COMPETENCY EVALUATION SHEET

P R O C E D U R E   9

Operating a Dry Heat Sterilizer

Student Name _____ Date _____

GRADING PROTOCOL: Student is awarded the number of points indicated on the evaluation sheet for completing steps successfully.

Total possible points = 100 points
80% needed for passing = 80 points

Total points this test _____ pass _____ fail _____

	PEER REVIEW	TEACHER REVIEW

POINTS

1 Prepare for the Procedure (10 points)

(5) _____ wash and dry hands
(5) _____ don utility gloves   _____   _____

2 Assemble the Equipment and Materials (10 points)

(3) _____ gather contaminated material and items
(4) _____ preclean items
(3) _____ wrap items for sterilization, if desired   _____   _____

3 Prepare the Dry Heat Sterilizer (10 points)

(3) _____ engage electrical plug into socket
(3) _____ check gauges for temperature
(4) _____ read manufacturer's directions   _____   _____

4 Heat the Sterilizer (10 points)

(5) _____ turn power on to heat sterilizer
(5) _____ monitor thermometer for proper heat   _____   _____

5 Load the Dry Heat Sterilizer (10 points)

(2) _____ use handle to open door carefully
(2) _____ adjust handle to tray, remove tray
(1) _____ place instruments on tray
(2) _____ check for circulation, avoid overcrowding
(1) _____ insert loaded tray into sterilizer
(2) _____ use handle to carefully close door   _____   _____

6 Complete the Sterilization Cycle (10 points)

(2) _____ monitor temperature for desired cycle time
(3) _____ adjust thermostat, if needed
(3) _____ set timer according to temperature
(2) _____ avoid adding any new items   _____   _____

7 Remove the Articles (10 points)

(4) _____ at timer signal, use handle to open door
(4) _____ remove loaded tray, place on top of sterilizer
(2) _____ permit items to cool   _____   _____

8 Store the Sterilized Items (10 points)

(2) _____ place wrapped packages in place
(3) _____ use sterile transfer forceps to move bare items
(2) _____ place all articles in proper storage area
(3) _____ rotate items, newer to front   _____   _____

9 Clean Up the Area (10 points)

(3) _____ use handle to carefully open door
(3) _____ replace tray in oven
(2) _____ when machine is cool, wipe out interior
(2) _____ polish outside, remove plug from wall   _____   _____

10 Remove the PPE (10 points)

(5) _____ wash, dry, disinfect, and remove gloves
(2) _____ wash and dry hands thoroughly
(3) _____ make sure area is clean and neat   _____   _____

(100)   Total points   _____   _____

COMPETENCY EVALUATION SHEET

P R O C E D U R E   1 0

Using Chemicals as Disinfectants and Sterilizers

Student Name _____ Date _____

GRADING PROTOCOL: Student is awarded the number of points indicated on the evaluation sheet for completing steps
successfully.

Total possible points = 100 points
80% needed for passing = 80 points

Total points this test _____   pass _____   fail _____

	PEER REVIEW	TEACHER REVIEW

POINTS

1 Assemble the Necessary Items (10 points)

(5) _____ assemble chemical and containers
(5) _____ gather equipment   _____   _____

2 Don PPE (10 points)

(3) _____ don utility gloves
(4) _____ don eyeglasses or safety goggles
(3) _____ don mask if working with caustic or vaporous chemicals   _____   _____

3 Prepare Disinfectant Spray (10 points)

(3) _____ read manufacturer's directions
(7) _____ dilute to proper ratio, or activate chemicals, or mix solutions as
             per directions   _____   _____

4 Record Active Life (10 points)

(3) _____ mark expiration date on bottle
(3) _____ mark down procedure and chemical
(4) _____ record procedure in log book   _____   _____

5 Fill the Spray Bottle (10 points)

(2) _____ check for cleanliness and condition of spray bottle
(3) _____ fill spray bottle, test working condition
(3) _____ tighten top and lock spray
(2) _____ place prepared spray bottles in storage   _____   _____

6 Prepare Chemical Solutions for Sterilization (10 points)

(2) _____ read manufacturer's directions
(2) _____ prepare as indicated
(1) _____ obtain clean, proper style sterilizer with close-fitting lid
(2) _____ fill to marked fill line
(2) _____ wipe sterilizer, close lid and mark expiration date or active life
(1) _____ place sterilizer in proper working area   _____   _____

7 Use the Disinfecting Spray (10 points)

(2) _____ spray counter or working area
(2) _____ wipe area of debris and matter with disposable towel
(2) _____ dispose towel in proper container
(2) _____ spray area again, wait recommended time for disinfection
(2) _____ blot up any excess after disinfection   _____   _____

8 Use the Chemical Sterilizer (15 points)

(1) _____ check sterilizer for effectiveness and proper solution
(1) _____ clean instruments or articles, pat dry
(2) _____ submerge totally with all working areas exposed
(2) _____ avoid overcrowding
(1) _____ mark time of immersion into solution
(1) _____ raise, drain articles in tray, after time cycle is completed
(2) _____ take tray with articles to sink, rinse and drain on sterile towel or
           rinse with sterile water
(1) _____ pat dry articles with sterile towel
(2) _____ transfer sterile articles with sterile transfer forceps to storage area
(2) _____ clean up area with towels, dispose of towels   _____   _____

9 Storage and Disposal of Chemicals (10 points)

(3) _____ read manufacturer's recommendations
(2) _____ store in cool, dark area, unless otherwise noted
(2) _____ rotate stock, use older, ineffective solutions first
(3) _____ dispose of solutions in manner recommended by manufacturer
           and local regulations   _____   _____

10 Clean Up the Area (5 points)

(1) _____ replace equipment
(1) _____ wipe up spill on counters, floors
(1) _____ dispose towel into container
(1) _____ wash, disinfect, remove gloves
(1) _____ wash and thoroughly dry hands   _____   _____

(100)   Total points   _____   _____

COMPETENCY EVALUATION SHEET

P R O C E D U R E   1 1

Cleanup of Operatory and Equipment Techniques

Student Name _____ Date _____

GRADING PROTOCOL: Student is awarded the number of points indicated on the evaluation sheet for completing steps successfully.

Total possible points = 100 points
80% needed for passing = 80 points

Total points this test _____ pass _____ fail _____

	PEER REVIEW	TEACHER REVIEW

POINTS

1 Clean up the Operatory (12 points)

(3) _____ flush lines, run handpieces for 30 seconds to flush water, remove to tray
(3) _____ run syringes to drain line, remove to tray
(2) _____ run ultrasonic handpieces, remove to tray
(2) _____ suction deodorizing or disinfecting solution into suction line
(2) _____ remove suction tip and handle, place on tray   _____   _____

2 Gather Items for Sterilization (8 points)

(2) _____ gather instruments, place on tray
(2) _____ gather disposables, place on tray
(2) _____ remove all records, x-rays, and charts
(2) _____ remove all materials and assemble in sterilizing room   _____   _____

3 Don PPE (5 points)

(1) _____ remove examination gloves
(1) _____ wash hands
(2) _____ check gloves for holes, cracks, or openings
(1) _____ don utility gloves   _____   _____

4 Disinfect the Operatory (10 points)

(3) _____ spray-wipe-spray all surfaces, counters, chairs, units, x-ray
(2) _____ disinfect all handles, switches, and tubing
(2) _____ disinfect any other objects used in operatory
(3) _____ replace barrier protectors   _____   _____

5 Remove the Sharps (10 points)

(2) _____ return to sterilizing area
(2) _____ pick up sharp instruments with utility gloves
(2) _____ place needle and sheath as one unit into sharps container
(2) _____ remove sharps with device, outward motion from body
(2) _____ place sharps into proper container   _____   _____

6 Remove the Disposables (10 points)

(5) _____ pick up disposables, deposit into disposal containers
(5) _____ use steady motion to avoid spreading pathogens   _____   _____

7 Prepare the Handpieces (10 points)

(2) _____ follow manufacturer's directions for care
(3) _____ wash with detergent, pat dry, dispose towel properly
(2) _____ lubricate, if designated by manufacturer
(3) _____ wrap or sleeve for sterilization   _____   _____

8 Prepare the Instruments (15 points)

(2) _____ place instruments into holding or disinfection solution
(2) _____ brush instruments to remove debris and pathogens
(2) _____ rinse instruments, dump spill onto toweling
(2) _____ pat instruments dry on paper towel
(2) _____ place instruments into ultrasonic cleaner, check manufacturer's directions for time and solution, set timer
(2) _____ rinse instruments, dump or spill, pat dry on paper towel
(1) _____ dispose of towel in contaminated container
(2) _____ prepare instruments for sterilization   _____   _____

9 Sterilize the Instruments (10 points)

(4) _____ load and set autoclave, if desired
(3) _____ load and set dry heat sterilizer, if desired
(3) _____ load and set chemical vapor sterilizer, if desired   _____   _____

10 Clean Up the Area (10 points)

(2) _____ dispose of any towels and debris into containers
(2) _____ clean and disinfect counter tops
(2) _____ clean up and disinfect floor, if necessary
(2) _____ wash, clean, disinfect, and remove utility gloves
(2) _____ place gloves on rack to dry, wash hands   _____   _____

(100)   Total points   _____   _____

COMPETENCY EVALUATION SHEET

PROCEDURE 12

Transfer of Instruments

Student Name _____ Date _____

GRADING PROTOCOL: Student is awarded the number of points indicated on the evaluation sheet for completing steps successfully.

Total possible points = 100 points
80% needed for passing = 80 points

Total points this test _____ pass _____ fail _____

	PEER REVIEW	TEACHER REVIEW

POINTS

1 Prepare for the Procedure (10 points)

(2) _____ gather pen grasp instruments
(2) _____ gather palm grasp instruments
(2) _____ gather palm-thumb grasp instruments
(1) _____ don personal protective equipment
(1) _____ arrange in proper sequential order
(1) _____ arrange in proper position for transfer
(1) _____ summon operator partner   _____   _____

2 Perform the Pen Grasp Transfer (20 points)

(3) _____ place instrument on tray properly
(2) _____ await signal for transfer
(2) _____ use correct passing zone
(3) _____ release instrument in working position
(3) _____ restore instrument to tray in proper position
(3) _____ perform transfer with no exchange
(4) _____ perform transfer with exchange of instruments   _____   _____

3 Perform the Palm Grasp Transfer (20 points)

(3) _____ place instrument on tray properly
(3) _____ await signal for transfer
(3) _____ use correct passing zone
(3) _____ release instrument in working position
(3) _____ restore instrument to tray in proper position
(2) _____ perform palm grasp with no exchange
(3) _____ perform palm grasp with exchange of instruments   _____   _____

4 Perform the Palm-thumb Grasp Transfer (20 points)

(3) _____ place instrument on tray properly
(3) _____ await signal for transfer
(3) _____ use correct passing zone
(3) _____ release instrument in working position
(3) _____ restore instrument to tray in proper position

(2) _____ perform palm-thumb grasp with no exchange
(3) _____ perform palm-thumb grasp with exchange of instruments   _____   _____

5 Perform Alternating Transfers (20 points)

(2) _____ place instruments on tray properly
(2) _____ await signal for transfer
(2) _____ use correct passing zone
(2) _____ release instrument in working position
(3) _____ restore instrument to tray in proper position
(3) _____ perform palm-thumb transfer with pen grasp exchange
(3) _____ perform pen grasp transfer with palm grasp exchange
(3) _____ perform palm grasp transfer with pen grasp exchange   _____   _____

6 Cleanup Procedures (10 points)

(1) _____ remove instruments to sterilizing room
(1) _____ remove exam gloves, wash hands
(1) _____ don utility gloves
(2) _____ clean instruments, ultrasonic also
(1) _____ prepare instruments for sterilization
(2) _____ sterilize instruments
(1) _____ wash and disinfect gloves
(1) _____ remove gloves and wash hands   _____   _____

(100)   Total points   _____   _____

COMPETENCY EVALUATION SHEET

PROCEDURE 13

Dental Rotary Instruments

Student Name _____ Date _____

GRADING PROTOCOL: Student is awarded the number of points indicated on the evaluation sheet for completing steps successfully.

Total possible points = 100 points
80% needed for passing = 80 points

Total points this test _____ pass _____ fail _____

	PEER REVIEW	TEACHER REVIEW

POINTS

1 Assemble Equipment and Materials (5 points)

(2) _____ wash hands
(1) _____ prepare equipment
(2) _____ don PPE   _____   _____

2 Demonstrate Background Knowledge of Dental Burs (10 points)

(3) _____ identify parts of dental bur
(2) _____ give significance of shank ends
(2) _____ give significance of carbide markings
(3) _____ explain numbering system   _____   _____

3 Demonstrate Ability to Place Burs in Handpieces (15 points)

(5) _____ place HP bur in proper handpiece
(5) _____ place LT bur in proper handpiece
(5) _____ place FG bur in proper handpiece   _____   _____

4 Explain Operative Procedure Function of Burs (10 points)

(2) _____ round bur function
(2) _____ inverted cone bur function
(2) _____ straight fissure plain and crosscut bur function
(2) _____ tapered fissure plain and crosscut bur function
(2) _____ end cutting bur function   _____   _____

5 Explain Sterilizing and Care Instructions for Burs (5 points)

(2) _____ steel bur care
(3) _____ carbide bur care   _____   _____

6 Demonstrate Knowledge of Diamond Instruments (10 points)

(4) _____ types of diamond instruments
(3) _____ function of diamond instruments
(3) _____ care and sterilization of diamond instruments _____   _____

7 **Demonstrate Knowledge of Dental Rotary Stones (10 points)**

(3) _____ identify dental stones
(2) _____ explain function of dental stones
(5) _____ place rotary stone in proper handpiece   _____   _____

8 **Demonstrate Knowledge of Surgical Burs (10 points)**

(3) _____ explain larger operative head of surgical bur
(2) _____ explain sterilization of surgical bur
(5) _____ place surgical bur in proper handpiece   _____   _____

9 **Demonstrate Knowledge of Mandrels (10 points)**

(2) _____ explain function of mandrels
(3) _____ identify head attachments and function of each
(3) _____ identify and mount mandrel with disk, wheel
(2) _____ place mandrel with attachment into handpiece   _____   _____

10 **Demonstrate Knowledge of Handpiece Sterilization (10 points)**

(1) _____ identify slow- and high-speed handpieces
(3) _____ demonstrate sterilization method of slow handpiece
(3) _____ demonstrate sterilization method of high-speed handpiece
(3) _____ demonstrate sterilization method for contra or right angle   _____   _____

11 **Clean Up the Area (5 points)**

(3) _____ clean instruments, sterilize
(2) _____ replace equipment   _____   _____

(100)   Total points   _____   _____

COMPETENCY EVALUATION SHEET

PROCEDURE 14

Preparing and Dismissing the Patient

Student Name _____ Date _____

GRADING PROTOCOL: Student is awarded the number of points indicated on the evaluation sheet for completing steps successfully.

Total possible points = 100 points
80% needed for passing = 80 points

Total points this test _____ pass _____ fail _____

	PEER REVIEW	TEACHER REVIEW

POINTS

1 Prepare for the Appointment (6 points)

(2) _____ review charts
(2) _____ disinfect operatory
(2) _____ assemble necessary equipment and materials   _____   _____

2 Prepare the Patient (22 points)

(2) _____ greet patient
(2) _____ assist patient into chair
(3) _____ lower armrest
(3) _____ position headrest
(3) _____ position patient
(3) _____ drape and bib patient
(3) _____ offer patient tissue and eyeglasses for safety
(3) _____ open sterile packs, place cup and tips   _____   _____

3 Take the Health History (6 points)

(3) _____ update old histories
(3) _____ review new histories   _____   _____

4 Prepare for the Procedure (18 points)

(3) _____ arrange stools
(3) _____ arrange work tray or table
(3) _____ don mask
(3) _____ wash hands
(3) _____ don exam gloves
(3) _____ don eyeglasses or shield   _____   _____

5 Adjust the Operatory Light (8 points)

(2) _____ have proper beam intensity
(2) _____ turn on light in low position
(2) _____ adjust to patient's mouth area
(2) _____ place 36 inches from face or work area   _____   _____

▆6 Clean Up and Dismiss the Patient (20 points)

(2) _____ move work tray and tables out
(2) _____ clean patient's face
(2) _____ remove bib and drape
(2) _____ review postoperative instructions
(2) _____ lower chair
(2) _____ raise arm of chair
(2) _____ assist patient from chair
(2) _____ return packages and purse
(2) _____ give patient charge slip
(2) _____ escort patient from operatory   _____   _____

▆7 Cleanup Procedures (20 points)

(2) _____ collect contaminated equipment and materials
(2) _____ remove to sterilizing room
(2) _____ remove exam gloves, wash hands
(2) _____ record procedures on patient's chart
(2) _____ take chart to front desk or place in appropriate area
(2) _____ don sterilizing apparel
(2) _____ disinfect operatory, flush lines
(2) _____ sterilize instruments and equipment
(2) _____ wash and disinfect utility gloves
(2) _____ wash hands   _____   _____

(100)   Total points   _____   _____

COMPETENCY EVALUATION SHEET

P R O C E D U R E   1 5

Evacuate and Rinse

Student Name _____ Date _____

GRADING PROTOCOL: Student is awarded the number of points indicated on the evaluation sheet for completing steps successfully.

Total possible points = 100 points
80% needed for passing = 80 points

Total points this test _____   pass _____   fail _____

	PEER REVIEW	TEACHER REVIEW

POINTS

1 Prepare for the Procedure (8 points)

(2) _____ gather saliva ejector tip and HVE tip
(2) _____ gather triple syringe tip
(2) _____ place all tips into position in presence of patient
(2) _____ bend saliva ejector tip   _____   _____

2 Demonstrate Use of Saliva Ejector (12 points)

(2) _____ insert tip into hose
(2) _____ check working condition
(2) _____ hang on mandibular jaw on correct side
(2) _____ monitor fluid retention in entire mouth
(2) _____ move to troublesome area
(2) _____ replace to original site   _____   _____

3 Prepare HVE Tip (6 points)

(3) _____ set up HVE tip in handpiece
(3) _____ test regulator dial and force of HVE   _____   _____

4 Assist with HVE in Maxillary Quadrants (14 points)

(2) _____ place tip in mouth, gently retracting cheek
(2) _____ hold tip distal to work site
(2) _____ hold opening to source of fluids
(2) _____ hold tip parallel to floor for maxillary left side
(2) _____ hold tip at 45-degree angle to floor for right side
(2) _____ hold tip ¼ inch below occlusal plane
(2) _____ regulate evacuation force with dial or button   _____   _____

5 Assist with HVE in Mandibular Quadrants (15 points)

(2) _____ insert tip, gently retract cheek
(2) _____ hold tip parallel to floor
(3) _____ hold tip opening to source of flow
(3) _____ hold tip distal to work site

440

(3) _____ hold tip ¼ inch above occlusal plane
(2) _____ regulate evacuation force with dial or button _____ _____

6 Assist with HVE in Anterior Region (16 points)

(4) _____ hold tip opening ¼ inch from incisal plane
(4) _____ hold tip distal to work site
(4) _____ hold opening toward force of flow
(4) _____ regulate evacuation force with dial or button _____ _____

7 Monitor Mouth Area (4 points)

(2) _____ observe for fluid pockets
(2) _____ aspirate fluid accumulations _____ _____

8 Demonstrate Use of Triple Syringe (15 points)

(5) _____ spray four quadrants with air
(5) _____ spray four quadrants with water
(5) _____ spray four quadrants with water spray _____ _____

9 Cleanup Procedure (10 points)

(1) _____ remove contaminated materials and gloves
(1) _____ wash hands, record treatment
(1) _____ don utility gloves, return to operatory
(1) _____ flush HVE tip and lines with water
(1) _____ flush lines with ora-evac or disinfecting solutions
(1) _____ take tips to sterilizing room for disposal or sterilization
(1) _____ spray-wipe-spray lines, replace barriers
(1) _____ clean trap on cleaning schedule
(1) _____ clean up area and replace equipment
(1) _____ wash, dry, disinfect, remove utility gloves, wash hands _____ _____

(100) Total points _____ _____

COMPETENCY EVALUATION SHEET

P R O C E D U R E   1 6

Assisting with Local Anesthesia Administration

Student Name _____ Date _____

GRADING PROTOCOL: Student is awarded the number of points indicated on the evaluation sheet for completing steps successfully.

Total possible points = 100 points
80% needed for passing = 80 points

Total points this test _____ pass _____   fail _____

	PEER REVIEW	TEACHER REVIEW

POINTS

1 Complete the Preparations (7 points)

(3) _____ obtain orders for desired cartridge and syringe
(2) _____ wash hands
(2) _____ assemble needed materials and equipment   _____   _____

2 Load the Syringe (16 points)

(2) _____ wipe cartridge with alcohol
(2) _____ unwrap syringe
(3) _____ drop cartridge into barrel
(2) _____ engage harpoon (if aspirating syringe)
(2) _____ remove protective cap
(3) _____ insert needle into diaphragm center
(2) _____ cover syringe on tray   _____   _____

3 Assist with Topical Anesthesia (24 points)

(4) _____ greet, seat, and drape patient
(4) _____ review health history
(4) _____ wash hands, don PPE
(4) _____ rinse and evacuate mouth
(4) _____ dry injection area with gauze
(4) _____ place topical anesthesia applicator on site   _____   _____

4 Assist with Local Anesthesia Injection (23 points)

(2) _____ summon dentist
(3) _____ receive applicator, pass syringe to dentist, retain sheath
(4) _____ guard patient's arms for defense
(4) _____ receive syringe
(4) _____ recap syringe using one-handed technique or recap device
(4) _____ observe patient respiration and general health
(2) _____ assist with operative procedure   _____   _____

5 Dismiss the Patient (10 points)

(2) _____ clean up patient
(2) _____ remove bib and drape
(2) _____ caution against numbed lip
(2) _____ give patient charge slip
(2) _____ assist from chair and operatory   _____   _____

6 Cleanup Procedure (20 points)

(2) _____ gather all contaminated equipment, remove to sterilizing room
(2) _____ remove latex exam gloves, wash hands
(2) _____ record on patient's chart
(2) _____ place chart on front desk or designated area
(2) _____ don utility gloves
(2) _____ place needle and sheath into sharps container
(2) _____ dispose of sundry and disposables in proper container
(2) _____ clean and sterilize instruments
(2) _____ disinfect operatory and equipment
(2) _____ wash and disinfect gloves, wash hands   _____   _____

(100)   Total points   _____   _____

COMPETENCY EVALUATION SHEET

P R O C E D U R E   1 7

Preparing Dental Liners and Cements

Student Name _____ Date _____

GRADING PROTOCOL: Student is awarded the number of points indicated on the evaluation sheet for completing steps
successfully.

Total possible points = 100 points
80% needed for passing = 80 points

Total points this test _____ pass _____ fail _____

	PEER REVIEW	TEACHER REVIEW

POINTS

1 Assemble Equipment and Materials (10 points)

(4) _____ gather necessary items
(3) _____ group items for particular task
(3) _____ don exam gloves (for practice)   _____   _____

2 Prepare Cavity Varnish (10 points)

(2) _____ state use of cavity varnish
(2) _____ uncap and recap bottle immediately
(2) _____ demonstrate saturation of pellet with varnish
(2) _____ demonstrate expressing excess varnish
(1) _____ demonstrate method to thin varnish
(1) _____ demonstrate cleanup method   _____   _____

3 Prepare Zinc Phosphate Material (15 points)

(2) _____ state uses for ZnP as cement and base
(5) _____ prepare ZnP for use as cement
　　　　　_____ fluff powder and measure powder
　　　　　_____ dispense liquid
　　　　　_____ mix materials using smallest powder pile
　　　　　_____ mix to creamy mixture over large area
(5) _____ prepare ZnP for use as base
　　　　　_____ mix in same manner with larger amount of powder
　　　　　_____ mix to stiff consistency
(3) _____ demonstrate cleanup method   _____   _____

4 Prepare Zinc Oxide Eugenol Material (15 points)

(2) _____ state uses for ZOE
(4) _____ prepare ZOE as cement
　　　　　_____ measure powder and liquid
　　　　　_____ mix to creamy consistency using larger powder pile
　　　　　_____ mix on paper pad
(4) _____ prepare ZOE as base
　　　　　_____ place powder and liquid on pad
　　　　　_____ draw large amount of powder into liquid
　　　　　_____ mix to heavy dough consistency

444

(4) _____ prepare ZOE as temporary restoration
_____ place powder and liquid on paper pad
_____ draw large amount of powder into liquid
_____ incorporate powder into mixture as much as possible
_____ mix to stiff consistency
(1) _____ demonstrate clean up method   _____   _____

5 Prepare Calcium Hydroxide Material (10 points)

(2) _____ state use for calcium hydroxide paste
(4) _____ demonstrate preparation of calcium hydroxide
(4) _____ demonstrate cleanup method for calcium hydroxide   _____   _____

6 Prepare Glass Ionomer Material (10 points)

(2) _____ state use for glass ionomers
(1) _____ fluff powder, uncap, scoop or spatulate
(1) _____ disperse powder on paper pad
(1) _____ dispense liquid in upright position
(1) _____ place drops near powder, recap immediately
(1) _____ incorporate powder into liquid in small area
(2) _____ complete mix in approximately one minute
(1) _____ demonstrate cleanup method   _____   _____

7 Prepare Polycarboxylate Cement Material (10 points)

(2) _____ state uses for polycarboxylate cement
(1) _____ fluff powder, uncap, scoop measured amount
(1) _____ divide powder in halves
(1) _____ shake bottle, dispense required drops or proper dosage from calibrated syringe
(1) _____ quickly mix powder into liquid
(2) _____ mix to desired consistency
(2) _____ demonstrate cleanup method   _____   _____

8 Prepare Resin Cement (10 points)

(2) _____ state use for resin cement
(2) _____ pass acid etch brush to operator
(2) _____ receive brush or pass syringe for tooth dry
(2) _____ mix resin materials to homogeneous mixture
(1) _____ use light source, if needed
(1) _____ demonstrate cleanup method   _____   _____

9 Cleanup Procedure (10 points)

(3) _____ clean all equipment
(2) _____ remove disposables
(3) _____ replace materials
(2) _____ remove gloves, wash hands   _____   _____

(100)   Total points   _____   _____

COMPETENCY EVALUATION SHEET

P R O C E D U R E   1 8

Placement and Removal of the Tofflemire Retainer

Student Name _____ Date _____

GRADING PROTOCOL: Student is awarded the number of points indicated on the evaluation sheet for completing steps
successfully.

Total possible points = 100 points
80% needed for passing = 80 points

Total points this test _____   pass _____   fail _____

	PEER REVIEW	TEACHER REVIEW

POINTS

1 Complete Preparations (10 points)

(10) _____ assemble equipment: supply of assorted bands, selected
Tofflemire matrix retainer, typodont with tooth preparation   _____   _____

2 Prepare Matrix Retainer (10 points)

(5) _____ rotate outer knob to retract spindle pin
(5) _____ head clear of head slot   _____   _____

3 Position Band in Retainer (10 points)

(2) _____ observe preparation and tooth size
(4) _____ select proper size and type of band
(4) _____ place band with wing tips facing gingiva   _____   _____

4 Insert Band into Retainer (10 points)

(3) _____ hold matrix with head slot facing gingiva
(2) _____ fold tips together
(3) _____ place band through proper gate for restoration
(2) _____ place ends through head slot, approximately $1/16$ inch   _____   _____

5 Stabilize Band in Retainer (10 points)

(5) _____ rotate outer knob clockwise to close
(5) _____ spindle pin tip onto wing tips for anchorage   _____   _____

6 Adapt Band Size (5 points)

(5) _____ rotate inner knob to form loop, press loop open   _____   _____

7 Adapt Loop Shape (5 points)

(5) _____ insert mirror handle into loop to adapt shape   _____   _____

■8 Pass Matrix Retainer and Band to Dentist (10 points)

(5) _____ pass retainer and band
(5) _____ pass burnisher, if requested   _____   _____

■9 Pass Wedge Holder and Wedge to Dentist (15 points)

(5) _____ select proper size wedge
(5) _____ insert wedge into holder, pass to dentist
(5) _____ be prepared to pass second wedge for stability   _____   _____

■10 Removal of Tofflemire Retainer and Matrix Band (15 points)

(4) _____ pass wedge holder, hemostat, or cotton pliers to dentist
(4) _____ accept wedges, retainer, and band; return items to tray
(4) _____ receive holder, hemostat, or cotton pliers; pass instrument of choice
(3) _____ complete restoration   _____   _____

(100)   Total points   _____   _____

COMPETENCY EVALUATION SHEET

P R O C E D U R E   1 9

Assisting with the Preliminary Examination

Student Name _____ Date _____

GRADING PROTOCOL: Student is awarded the number of points indicated on the evaluation sheet for completing steps successfully.

Total possible points = 100 points
80% needed for passing = 80 points

Total points this test _____ pass _____ fail _____

	PEER REVIEW	TEACHER REVIEW

POINTS

1 Complete the Preparations (10 points)

(2) _____ assemble equipment and necessary materials
(2) _____ greet patient
(2) _____ introduce patient to office areas
(4) _____ seat patient in dental chair   _____   _____

2 Complete the Health History (10 points)

(2) _____ take health history
(2) _____ assist patient with health questionnaire
(2) _____ review answers
(2) _____ stress answers to allergies, medications, and present treatment
(2) _____ indicate interest in patient's welfare   _____   _____

3 Complete Vital Signs (15 points)

(5) _____ take and record blood pressure
(5) _____ take and record temperature, if requested
(5) _____ take and record pulse and respiration   _____   _____

4 Don PPE (5 points)

(1) _____ summon dentist
(2) _____ don equipment
(2) _____ assume position on assistant's stool   _____   _____

5 Record Physical Exam Findings (10 points)

(5) _____ write neatly and legibly
(5) _____ write complete descriptions   _____   _____

6 Assist with Oral Tissue Examination (10 points)

(3) _____ pass and receive instruments as needed
(3) _____ pass and receive gauze as needed
(4) _____ record findings   _____   _____

7 Record Findings of Neck and TMJ Examination (5 points)

(3) _____ write neatly and legibly
(2) _____ pass and receive stethoscope, if needed

8 Assist with Oral Exam and Charting of Teeth (15 points)

(3) _____ pass and receive mirror and explorer when indicated
(2) _____ pass periodontal probe when requested
(3) _____ record findings correctly and neatly
(2) _____ use office coding and colors for charting
(3) _____ pass or use triple syringe as requested
(2) _____ pass dental floss as requested

9 Complete Exam as Requested by Dentist (10 points)

Be prepared to assist with:
(3) _____ taking alginate impressions
(3) _____ radiographs
(3) _____ photographs
(1) _____ miscellaneous testing

10 Cleanup Procedures (10 points)

(2) _____ remove contaminated equipment and materials
(1) _____ remove exam gloves, wash hands
(2) _____ record procedures on patient's chart
(1) _____ take chart to desk
(1) _____ don utility gloves
(2) _____ clean operatory, equipment, area
(1) _____ wash, dry, disinfect, and remove gloves, wash hands

(100)   Total points

COMPETENCY EVALUATION SHEET

PROCEDURE 20

Assisting with Alginate Impressions

Student Name _____ Date _____

GRADING PROTOCOL: Student is awarded the number of points indicated on the evaluation sheet for completing steps successfully.

Total possible points = 100 points
80% needed for passing = 80 points

Total points this test _____ pass _____ fail _____

	PEER REVIEW	TEACHER REVIEW

POINTS

1 Complete Preparations (5 points)

(1) _____ assemble equipment and materials
(1) _____ cover patient with plastic drape or bib, offer tissues
(1) _____ don PPE
(1) _____ prepare patient, explain procedure
(1) _____ remove appliances, rinse mouth   _____   _____

2 Prepare the Trays (5 points)

(2) _____ select and test tray size
(1) _____ wax bead edges of tray
(2) _____ spray or paint disposable tray with adhesive   _____   _____

3 Mix the Alginate (10 points)

(2) _____ select proper alginate, shake to fluff
(2) _____ measure according to manufacturer's advice and measuring scoops
(2) _____ fill water vial with cool water to measuring mark
(4) _____ blend water and alginate, stir with pressing motion and
circulation of bowl until creamy and smooth   _____   _____

4 Load the Mandibular Tray (10 points)

(4) _____ load from posterior edges of tray
(3) _____ use more than one spatula
(3) _____ smooth top of alginate with wet finger   _____   _____

5 Assist with the Insertion and Removal of the Impression Tray (10 points)

(1) _____ insert tray with rotation movement
(1) _____ center tray over and under teeth edges
(1) _____ seat tray from posterior to anterior
(1) _____ release impinged tissue or lips
(1) _____ request patient to raise tongue (mandibular)
(1) _____ hold tray stationary in mouth
(1) _____ monitor patient gagging reflex

(1) _____ smooth and contour tray edges, test for firmness
(1) _____ release tray suction, remove with rotation movement
(1) _____ rinse impression, disinfect, wrap in moist disinfectant towel _____ _____

6 Freshen the Patient's Mouth (5 points)

(2) _____ rinse patient's mouth with spray or mouthwash
(1) _____ praise patient's effort
(2) _____ explain next tray procedure _____ _____

7 Mix the Second Alginate Impression Material (5 points)

(1) _____ use clean bowl and spatula
(1) _____ follow manufacturer's recommendation and measuring scoop
(1) _____ measure cool water in manufacturer's vial
(2) _____ rapidly mix materials with pressure and rotation of bowl until mixture
is creamy and smooth _____ _____

8 Load the Maxillary Tray (10 points)

(4) _____ fill from posterior of tray
(3) _____ use more than one spatula load of alginate
(3) _____ smooth top of impression with wet finger _____ _____

9 Assist with the Insertion and Removal of the Impression Tray (10 points)

(1) _____ insert tray with rotation movement
(1) _____ center tray under teeth edges
(1) _____ seat from posterior to anterior
(1) _____ release impinged tissue or lips
(1) _____ monitor patient gagging reflex
(1) _____ smooth and contour tray edges, test for firmness
(1) _____ release suction hold of tray
(1) _____ remove tray in rotation movement
(1) _____ rinse impression, disinfect
(1) _____ wrap tray with moist disinfectant towel _____ _____

10 Freshen the Patient's Mouth (5 points)

(2) _____ rinse mouth with spray or mouthwash
(1) _____ praise patient effort
(2) _____ explain bite registration procedure _____ _____

11 Assist with Bite Registration (10 points)

(1) _____ heat wax bite in warm water
(1) _____ insert wax into mouth
(2) _____ center wax over posterior occlusal edges
(1) _____ instruct patient to bite on back teeth
(1) _____ contour wax
(1) _____ request patient to release pressure
(1) _____ remove wax in rotation movement
(1) _____ rinse, disinfect
(1) _____ insert wax in bowl of very cool water _____ _____

12 Dismiss the Patient (5 points)

(2) _____ wipe face, remove all impression material
(1) _____ rinse and freshen mouth
(1) _____ remove drape
(1) _____ dismiss patient if procedures are completed   _____   _____

13 Prepare the Impressions (5 points)

(1) _____ spray impression with disinfectant
(1) _____ open plastic bag by inserting fingers and lifting
(1) _____ place impressions into plastic bag
(1) _____ place bite registration in bag
(1) _____ do not close bag   _____   _____

14 Cleanup Procedures (5 points)

(1) _____ take disposables and contaminated materials to sterilizing room,
           remove latex gloves, wash hands
(1) _____ record procedure on patient's chart, take chart to desk or appropriate place
(1) _____ seal plastic impression bag and take to lab
(1) _____ don utility gloves and equipment, spray-wipe-spray operatory,
           flush lines clean, prepare and sterilize instruments
(1) _____ disinfect, clean gloves, remove, wash hands   _____   _____

(100)   Total points   _____   _____

COMPETENCY EVALUATION SHEET

P R O C E D U R E   2 1

Assisting with Dental Prophylaxis

Student Name _____ Date _____

GRADING PROTOCOL: Student is awarded the number of points indicated on the evaluation sheet for completing steps
successfully.

Total possible points = 100 points
80% needed for passing = 80 points

Total points this test _____ pass _____ fail _____

	PEER REVIEW	TEACHER REVIEW

POINTS

1 Complete the Preparations (10 points)

(2) _____ assemble equipment
(2) _____ prepare operatory
(1) _____ greet and seat patient
(1) _____ set out disposable items
(2) _____ review health history
(2) _____ don PPE, summon operator   _____   _____

2 Assist with Mouth Rinse and Evacuation (5 points)

(3) _____ operate evacuator
(2) _____ operate triple syringe   _____   _____

3 Assist with Scaling of Teeth (20 points)

(4) _____ pass or receive mirror and scaling instruments
(4) _____ hold gauze near work site
(4) _____ pass and receive instruments as needed or signaled
(4) _____ pass ultrasonic handpiece
(4) _____ evacuate and rinse mouth as needed   _____   _____

4 Assist with Polishing of Teeth (15 points)

(5) _____ pass and receive polishing instruments
(5) _____ pass handpiece with prophylaxis angle or sand polishing tip
(3) _____ hold prophylaxis paste near work site
(2) _____ evacuate and rinse mouth as needed   _____   _____

5 Assist with Flossing of Teeth (15 points)

(4) _____ cut floss to prescribed lengths
(3) _____ hold near work site
(4) _____ exchange as necessary or signaled
(4) _____ pass and receive flossing aids   _____   _____

6 Assist with Charting, Notations, and Instructions (15 points)

(5) _____ assist with any charting
(5) _____ make notations as needed
(5) _____ give instructions, if directed   _____   _____

7 Dismiss the Patient (10 points)

(2) _____ clean patient's face
(2) _____ remove bib and drape
(2) _____ loosen lock and turn chair, if needed
(2) _____ return packages or purse to patient
(2) _____ dismiss patient   _____   _____

8 Cleanup Procedures (10 points)

(1) _____ remove contaminated materials to sterilizing room
(1) _____ remove exam gloves, wash hands
(2) _____ record patient visit and treatment
(1) _____ don utility gloves, PPE
(2) _____ clean operatory, flush lines
(1) _____ clean equipment, instruments
(1) _____ disinfect, sterilize, clean area
(1) _____ wash, dry, disinfect, remove gloves, wash hands   _____   _____

(100)   Total points   _____   _____

COMPETENCY EVALUATION SHEET

P R O C E D U R E   2 2

Assisting with Topical Fluoride Application

Student Name _____ Date _____

GRADING PROTOCOL: Student is awarded the number of points indicated on the evaluation sheet for completing steps successfully.

Total possible points = 100 points
80% needed for passing = 80 points

Total points this test _____ pass _____ fail _____

	PEER REVIEW	TEACHER REVIEW

POINTS

1 Complete the Preparations (15 points)

(3) _____ assemble equipment and materials
(2) _____ prepare operatory
(2) _____ greet, seat, and position patient
(3) _____ review health history
(3) _____ explain procedure
(2) _____ don PPE, summon dentist   _____ _____

2 Assist with the Prophylaxis and Coronal Polish (10 points)

(5) _____ pass handpiece with prophylaxis cup and paste
(5) _____ rinse and evacuate mouth   _____ _____

3 Assist with the Isolation of the Mouth (20 points)

(5) _____ pass or place cotton rolls
(5) _____ air dry crowns of teeth
(5) _____ pass or use triple syringe to move flow of air on teeth
(5) _____ apply saliva ejector   _____ _____

4 Assist with the Topical Fluoride Application (25 points)

(6) _____ pass or apply saturated swab to area teeth or pass filled tray, seat tray on tooth surfaces
(3) _____ await prescribed time
(3) _____ amuse patient with books or stories
(3) _____ evacuate as needed
(4) _____ monitor patient
(3) _____ remove topical fluoride applicators
(3) _____ repeat process for other arch, if needed   _____ _____

5 Dismiss the Patient (15 points)

(4) _____ advise not to eat or drink for 30 minutes
(4) _____ clean patient's face

(4) _____ remove bib, lower chair
(3) _____ dismiss patient   _____   _____

6 Cleanup Procedures (15 points)

(2) _____ remove contaminated items to sterilizing room
(2) _____ remove exam gloves, wash hands
(3) _____ record treatment on chart, return chart to desk
(2) _____ don utility gloves and PPE
(2) _____ clean operatory, flush lines
(2) _____ clean, disinfect, and sterilize equipment, materials, and area
(2) _____ wash, dry, disinfect, remove gloves, wash hands   _____   _____

(100)   Total points   _____   _____

COMPETENCY EVALUATION SHEET

P R O C E D U R E   2 3

Assisting with Sealant Application

Student Name _____ Date _____

GRADING PROTOCOL: Student is awarded the number of points indicated on the evaluation sheet for completing steps successfully.

Total possible points = 100 points
80% needed for passing = 80 points

Total points this test _____ pass _____ fail _____

	PEER REVIEW	TEACHER REVIEW

POINTS

1 Complete the Preparations (10 points)

(2) _____ assemble equipment and material
(2) _____ prepare operatory
(1) _____ greet and seat patient (if not prophylaxis patient)
(2) _____ review health history
(1) _____ explain procedure
(1) _____ don personal protective equipment
(1) _____ summon dentist   _____   _____

2 Assist with Coronal Polish (10 points)

(5) _____ pass handpiece with prophylaxis cup and paste
(5) _____ rinse, evaluate as needed   _____   _____

3 Assist with Isolation of the Teeth (10 points)

(4) _____ assist with dental dam, or pass cotton rolls
(2) _____ pass air syringe
(2) _____ dry tooth or teeth to receive etching
(2) _____ place saliva ejector   _____   _____

4 Assist with Acid-Etching of the Teeth (10 points)

(3) _____ pass etching materials
(3) _____ time process
(4) _____ monitor for evacuation of moisture   _____   _____

5 Assist with Rinsing and Repacking (10 points)

(3) _____ pass syringe
(2) _____ evacuate mouth
(2) _____ pass fresh cotton rolls
(3) _____ remove cotton rolls from beneath   _____   _____

6 Assist with Sealant Placement (10 points)

(2) _____ mix self-curing pastes
(1) _____ pass applicator with paste
(1) _____ hold mixture close to work site
(3) _____ time setting process, or pass sealant applicator with material
(1) _____ hold material near work site
(1) _____ hold curing lamp near application site
(1) _____ monitor time   _____   _____

7 Assist with Examination of Sealant (10 points)

(3) _____ pass explorer
(2) _____ repeat process if not successful
(5) _____ receive cotton rolls, or remove dental dam   _____   _____

8 Assist with Finishing of Sealant (10 points)

(4) _____ pass articulating paper
(4) _____ pass round bur and handpiece
(2) _____ alternate as needed   _____   _____

9 Dismiss the Patient (10 points)

(3) _____ clean up patient
(4) _____ lower chair, as cautioning
(3) _____ dismiss patient   _____   _____

10 Cleanup Procedures (10 points)

(1) _____ remove contaminated materials to sterilizing room
(1) _____ remove exam gloves, wash hands
(2) _____ record treatment on chart
(1) _____ don utility gloves
(2) _____ clean operatory, flush lines
(2) _____ clean, disinfect, and sterilize equipment and instruments
(1) _____ wash, dry, disinfect, remove gloves, wash hands   _____   _____

(100)   Total points   _____   _____

COMPETENCY EVALUATION SHEET

PROCEDURE 24

Brushing and Flossing Techniques Instruction

Student Name _____ Date _____

GRADING PROTOCOL: Student is awarded the number of points indicated on the evaluation sheet for completing steps successfully.

Total possible points = 100 points
80% needed for passing = 80 points

Total points this test _____ pass _____ fail _____

	PEER REVIEW	TEACHER REVIEW

POINTS

1 Complete the Preparations (10 points)

(2) _____ assemble equipment and materials
(2) _____ prepare operatory
(2) _____ greet and seat patient
(2) _____ explain reason for instruction
(2) _____ assure patient comfort and cooperation   _____   _____

2 Explain Plaque Buildup (10 points)

(4) _____ describe plaque
(3) _____ explain consequences of plaque
(3) _____ explain reason for brushing and flossing   _____   _____

3 Demonstrate the Patient's Plaque (10 points)

(5) _____ administer disclosing solution
(5) _____ show patient mouth plaque   _____   _____

4 Demonstrate Brushing Technique (20 points)

(3) _____ demonstrate holding of toothbrush
(3) _____ demonstrate angle placement of bristles
(3) _____ demonstrate wiggle and brush away from sulcus
(3) _____ establish routine pattern
(2) _____ demonstrate tongue brush
(3) _____ observe patient performance of brushing
(3) _____ evaluate and reinforce patient's technique   _____   _____

5 Demonstrate Flossing Technique (15 points)

(2) _____ explain principle of flossing
(1) _____ demonstrate selection of floss
(2) _____ demonstrate finger wrap and holding of floss
(2) _____ demonstrate insertion of floss
(2) _____ demonstrate wrap of floss around tooth surfaces
(2) _____ demonstrate scrape of tooth surfaces

(1) _____ establish routine pattern of flossing
(1) _____ observe patient's performance of flossing
(2) _____ evaluate and reinforce flossing technique   _____   _____

6 Demonstrate Use of Interproximal Stimulator and Aids (15 points)

(2) _____ explain principle of stimulators
(2) _____ demonstrate placement of tip
(2) _____ demonstrate movement of tip
(1) _____ establish routine pattern necessary for stimulation
(2) _____ explain principle of aids
(2) _____ demonstrate aids use
(1) _____ establish routine necessary for aids use
(1) _____ observe patient's performance with stimulator and aids
(2) _____ evaluate and reinforce use of stimulator and aids   _____   _____

7 Review All Techniques (10 points)

(4) _____ review entire procedure
(3) _____ answer any questions
(3) _____ reassure patient   _____   _____

8 Dismiss the Patient (5 points)

(2) _____ give patient supply of home aids
(2) _____ schedule for reevaluation appointment
(1) _____ dismiss patient   _____   _____

9 Cleanup Procedures (5 points)

(2) _____ clean up area and replace equipment
(1) _____ dispose of exam gloves
(2) _____ wash hands   _____   _____

(100)   Total points   _____   _____

COMPETENCY EVALUATION SHEET

PROCEDURE 25

Diet and Nutrition Counseling

Student Name _____ Date _____

GRADING PROTOCOL: Student is awarded the number of points indicated on the evaluation sheet for completing steps successfully.

Total possible points = 100 points
80% needed for passing = 80 points

Total points this test _____   pass _____   fail _____

	PEER REVIEW	TEACHER REVIEW

POINTS

1 Complete the Preparations (5 points)

Note to instructor: This procedure will require a sample diet diary sheet. Make out a typical sheet before counseling testing.

(3) _____ assemble equipment
(1) _____ prepare area
(1) _____ make patient comfortable   _____   _____

2 Explain the Decay Process (20 points)

(8) _____ display triple circle decay process
(8) _____ show controls over each element
(4) _____ turn in demonstration paper after procedure   _____   _____

3 Review Brushing and Flossing Techniques (20 points)

(5) _____ show effect of brush and floss on germs
(5) _____ review techniques for brushing
(5) _____ review techniques for flossing
(5) _____ review techniques for interproximal aids use   _____   _____

4 Demonstrate and Display Cariogenic Foods (20 points)

(7) _____ display sugar content
(7) _____ give list of sugar content in foods
(6) _____ have patient display sugar amounts of foods   _____   _____

5 Demonstrate Diet Modification (25 points)

(5) _____ circle cariogenic foods in red
(5) _____ suggest diet change
(5) _____ suggest substitute foods
(5) _____ have patient make diet substitute choice
(5) _____ turn paper in at completion of procedure   _____   _____

6 Dismiss the Patient (5 points)

(2) _____ review appointment with patient
(1) _____ answer questions
(1) _____ assure concern for well-being
(1) _____ make return visit appointment   _____   _____

7 Cleanup Procedures (5 points)

(1) _____ clean up area
(2) _____ return equipment and material to proper places
(2) _____ wash hands   _____   _____

(100)   Total points   _____   _____

COMPETENCY EVALUATION SHEET

PROCEDURE 26

Assisting with Dental Dam Application

Student Name _____   Date _____

GRADING PROTOCOL: Student is awarded the number of points indicated on the evaluation sheet for completing steps
successfully.

Total possible points = 100 points
80% needed for passing = 80 points

Total points this test _____   pass _____   fail _____

	PEER REVIEW	TEACHER REVIEW

POINTS

1 Complete the Preparations (10 points)

(2) _____ assemble equipment and materials
(1) _____ disinfect operatory
(1) _____ examine chart for dental dam orders
(2) _____ punch prescribed holes in dental dam material
(1) _____ greet and seat patient
(1) _____ review health history
(1) _____ explain procedure to patient
(1) _____ don PPE   _____   _____

2 Assist with Dental Dam Application Preparation (10 points)

(3) _____ rinse and evacuate mouth
(2) _____ pass and receive mirror and explorer for exam
(3) _____ pass and receive dental floss
(2) _____ be prepared to clear interproximal space   _____   _____

3 Assist with Clamp Selection (10 points)

(4) _____ tie safety ligature to clamp
(2) _____ load dental dam clamp forceps
(2) _____ pass and receive dental dam clamp forceps
(2) _____ repeat as needed until fit found   _____   _____

4 Pass Dental Dam Materials (20 points)

(1) _____ place lubricant on material prepunched holes
(2) _____ put material over clamp
(2) _____ pass dental dam forceps with clamp and material to dentist
(2) _____ assist with placement of clamp and material
(1) _____ receive dental dam clamp forceps
(2) _____ pass dental dam napkin, slide over dam, spread onto face
(1) _____ arrange dental dam material over napkin
(2) _____ pass dental dam frame, hold frame under material
(2) _____ pick up material and secure to frame pins

(1) _____ rearrange material as needed for smooth fit
(1) _____ make sure safety ligature from clamp is exposed
(3) _____ pass ligatures, as needed, assist with tie off, or pass stabilizing cord pieces _____ _____

5 Assist with Dental Dam Inversion (10 points)

(2) _____ pass blunt instrument to dentist
(2) _____ air spray dam material area
(2) _____ assist with inversion
(2) _____ place saliva ejector
(2) _____ situate saliva ejector on opposite side from work site, assist with procedure _____ _____

6 Assist with Removal of Dental Dam (20 points)

(3) _____ spray and evacuate all areas of dental dam
(2) _____ pass and receive scissors
(2) _____ assist with ligature cut and removal
(3) _____ assist with holding material for interproximal cuts
(3) _____ remove saliva ejector
(3) _____ pass and receive dental dam clamp forceps
(2) _____ receive dental dam material and frame
(2) _____ examine material for missing pieces _____ _____

7 Clean Up Patient (15 points)

(3) _____ remove napkin
(3) _____ spray and evacuate mouth
(4) _____ massage gingival region
(2) _____ dismiss patient
(1) _____ remove latex gloves, wash hands
(2) _____ record procedure on patient's chart _____ _____

8 Cleanup Procedures (5 points)

(1) _____ remove contaminated materials to sterilizing room, remove
          exam gloves, wash hands
(1) _____ record procedure on patient's chart
(1) _____ don utility gloves and PPE, sterilize and disinfect equipment and materials
(1) _____ disinfect operatory, clean up area
(1) _____ wash, disinfect, and remove gloves; wash hands _____ _____

(100)   Total points _____ _____

COMPETENCY EVALUATION SHEET

P R O C E D U R E   2 7

Assisting with Anterior Restoration

Student Name _____ Date _____

GRADING PROTOCOL: Student is awarded the number of points indicated on the evaluation sheet for completing steps successfully.

Total possible points = 100 points
80% needed for passing = 80 points

Total points this test _____ pass _____ fail _____

	PEER REVIEW	TEACHER REVIEW

POINTS

1 Complete the Preparations (10 points)

(2) _____ assemble equipment and materials
(2) _____ prepare operatory and equipment
(1) _____ gather chart and records
(1) _____ greet, seat, and position patient
(2) _____ review health history
(1) _____ drape and bib patient
(1) _____ don PPE   _____   _____

2 Assist with Local Anesthesia (10 points)

(2) _____ prep patient with topical anesthesia
(3) _____ pass and receive anesthesia syringe
(3) _____ recap syringe with one-hand technique
(2) _____ monitor patient reaction to anesthesia   _____   _____

3 Assist with Dental Dam Application (If Used) (10 points)

(2) _____ floss interproximals and lubricate dam
(2) _____ pass prepared dental dam, clamp, and frame
(2) _____ pass and adjust dental dam napkin
(2) _____ assist with ligatures
(2) _____ assist with saliva ejector placement   _____   _____

4 Assist with Cavity Preparation (10 points)

(3) _____ pass and receive instruments, rotors, and triple syringe
(3) _____ rinse and evacuate as needed
(4) _____ maintain visibility by air stream on mirror and HVE tip at work site   _____   _____

5 Assist with Cavity Base and Liners or Etch (10 points)

(1) _____ obtain selection from dentist
(2) _____ mix material according to manufacturer's directions
(2) _____ pass instrument with material to dentist

(2) _____ hold material and refuse gauze close to area for dentist use
(2) _____ air dry with syringe as directed by dentist
(1) _____ pass acid etch material, if needed   _____   _____

6 Assist with Preparation of Restorative Materials (10 points)

(3) _____ assist with shade selection, if necessary
(2) _____ obtain selection from dentist
(5) _____ mix material according to manufacturer's recommendation   _____   _____

7 Assist with Placement of Restorative Materials (10 points)

(2) _____ pass lubricated matrix strip
(2) _____ pass instrument with mixture to dentist
(2) _____ hold additional material and refuse gauze near site
(2) _____ pass wedge when signaled
(1) _____ hold curing light and shield, if necessary
(1) _____ be prepared for rinsing and evacuation   _____   _____

8 Assist with Finishing of Restoration (10 points)

(3) _____ pass finishing stones and articulating paper as needed
(2) _____ remove dental dam (if applicable)
(3) _____ pass and receive finishing stones, disks, and cups on demand
(2) _____ be prepared for rinse and evacuation   _____   _____

9 Dismiss the Patient (5 points)

(2) _____ clean up patient
(2) _____ give postoperative instructions to patient
(1) _____ escort patient from operatory to front desk   _____   _____

10 Cleanup Procedures (15 points)

(1) _____ gather disposables and contaminated materials and equipment, remove
           contaminated materials from operatory to sterilizing area
(1) _____ remove exam gloves, wash hands
(2) _____ record treatment and anesthesia on patient's chart
(1) _____ place chart at front desk or appropriate place
(2) _____ don utility gloves, spray-wipe-spray items in operatory area, flush and
           disinfect all lines in operatory area
(2) _____ dispose of sharps and disposable items in proper containers
(2) _____ rinse, ultrasonically, clean, dry instruments
(1) _____ disinfect shield and glasses and other large items
(2) _____ prepare items for sterilization
(1) _____ clean up area and replace equipment, wash and disinfect utility gloves,
           remove and wash hands   _____   _____

(100)   Total points   _____   _____

COMPETENCY EVALUATION SHEET

PROCEDURE 28

Assisting with Amalgam Posterior Restoration

Student Name _____ Date _____

GRADING PROTOCOL: Student is awarded the number of points indicated on the evaluation sheet for completing steps successfully.

Total possible points = 100 points
80% needed for passing = 80 points

Total points this test _____ pass _____ fail _____

	PEER REVIEW	TEACHER REVIEW

POINTS

1 Complete the Preparations (10 points)

(2) _____ assemble materials and equipment
(2) _____ prepare operatory
(1) _____ greet, seat, and position patient
(2) _____ review health history
(1) _____ explain procedure
(2) _____ don PPE, summon dentist

2 Assist with Local Anesthesia (5 points)

(1) _____ check proposed treatment plan
(1) _____ rinse mouth and dry injection site
(1) _____ place topical anesthetic
(1) _____ pass and receive anesthetic syringe, recap anesthetic needle with one-handed technique or device
(1) _____ monitor patient reaction to anesthesia

3 Assist with Dental Dam Placement (10 points)

(4) _____ pass prepared dam, clamp, frame
(2) _____ assist with napkin placement
(2) _____ assist with ligature placement and tie offs
(2) _____ arrange saliva ejector tip

4 Assist with Cavity Preparation (10 points)

(5) _____ pass instruments and rotors as requested
(5) _____ maintain visibility with syringe and evacuation

5 Assist with Cavity Preparation Dressings (10 points)

(2) _____ pass cleansing and drying pellet
(2) _____ mix and pass varnish
(4) _____ mix and pass liner and base as requested
(2) _____ hold materials near work site

6 Assist with Matrix Placement (If Needed—Class II) (10 points)

(3) _____ pass matrix retainer with matrix band
(2) _____ pass and receive burnisher

(3) _____ pass wedge holder or hemostat with wedge

(2) _____ apply syringe air as requested _____ _____

7 Assist with Amalgam Placement (10 points)

(2) _____ prepare and set amalgamator

(2) _____ pass cotton rolls to isolate, if no dental dam

(2) _____ place plastic amalgam in well or dappen dish

(2) _____ load amalgam carrier and pass

(2) _____ alternate with carrier and condenser _____ _____

8 Assist with Carving Restoration and Matrix Removal (10 points)

(1) _____ pass and receive carving instruments

(2) _____ aspirate shavings with HVE tip

(1) _____ pass wet pellet to wipe off amalgam

(2) _____ pass and receive wedge holder or hemostat to retrieve wedge

(1) _____ pass explorer, pass college pliers to retrieve matrix band

(2) _____ receive matrix band, explorer, and retainer

(1) _____ pass carver, if requested _____ _____

9 Assist with Dental Dam Removal (5 points)

(1) _____ assist with ligature removal

(1) _____ pass and receive scissors for dam release

(1) _____ pass and receive dental dam clamp holder and clamp

(1) _____ receive frame, dental dam material, napkin

(1) _____ check dental dam for missing material _____ _____

10 Assist with Final Carving (10 points)

(2) _____ pass or receive carver or discloid/cleoid instrument

(3) _____ place articulating paper in holder on occlusal plane

(3) _____ pass college pliers with wet pellet

(2) _____ alternate as needed _____ _____

11 Dismiss the Patient (5 points)

(1) _____ wipe restoration off with wet cotton roll or pellet

(1) _____ rinse patient's mouth

(1) _____ give postoperative instructions

(1) _____ caution patient about chair movement

(1) _____ clean up and dismiss patient _____ _____

12 Cleanup Procedures (5 points)

(1) _____ gather contaminated materials and equipment, remove to sterilizing area

(1) _____ remove latex gloves, wash hands, record treatment on patient's chart and take to front desk

(1) _____ don utility gloves and PPE, spray-wipe-spray disinfect operatory, flush lines

(1) _____ dispose of sharps and wastes in proper containers, clean and prepare instruments for sterilizing, disinfect larger items, clean up area

(1) _____ wash, disinfect gloves, and remove; wash hands _____ _____

(100)   Total points _____ _____

COMPETENCY EVALUATION SHEET

PROCEDURE 29

Assisting with Composite Posterior Restoration

Student Name _____ Date _____

GRADING PROTOCOL: Student is awarded the number of points indicated on the evaluation sheet for completing steps successfully.

Total possible points = 100 points
80% needed for passing = 80 points

Total points this test _____   pass _____   fail _____

	PEER REVIEW	TEACHER REVIEW

POINTS

1 Complete the Preparations (10 points)

(2) _____ assemble materials and equipment
(2) _____ prepare operatory
(1) _____ greet and seat patient
(2) _____ review health history
(1) _____ explain procedure
(2) _____ don PPE, summon dentist   _____   _____

2 Assist with Local Anesthesia (10 points)

(1) _____ check proposed treatment plan
(1) _____ rinse mouth, dry injection site
(2) _____ apply topical application of anesthesia
(2) _____ pass and receive anesthetic syringe
(1) _____ recap needle with one-handed technique or device
(1) _____ guard against sudden movement
(2) _____ monitor patient reaction to anesthesia   _____   _____

3 Assist with Dental Dam Placement (If Requested) (10 points)

(4) _____ pass clamp holder with clamp and dam, frame
(2) _____ assist with napkin placement
(2) _____ assist with ligature placement and tie off
(2) _____ arrange saliva ejector   _____   _____

4 Assist with Cavity Preparation (10 points)

(5) _____ pass and receive rotor, cutting instruments as needed
(5) _____ maintain visibility using syringe and evacuation tip   _____   _____

5 Assist with Cavity Protective Dressings (10 points)

(3) _____ mix and pass instruments with dressings
(2) _____ hold material near work site for refill

(3) _____ hold gauze near work site for wipe of instrument
(2) _____ maintain visibility   _____   _____

6 Assist with Etching of Cavity Preparation (10 points)

(2) _____ pass prepared brush or instrument
(2) _____ pass or air spray preparation
(2) _____ receive instrument
(2) _____ repeat process, if needed
(2) _____ hold curing light, if needed   _____   _____

7 Assist with Placement of Restorative Material (10 points)

(1) _____ pass cotton rolls for isolation, if dental dam not used
(2) _____ mix composite or prepare according to manufacturer's directions
(1) _____ pass matrix strip or form, if needed
(1) _____ pass composite filling instrument with material
(1) _____ hold excess mix and gauze near site for refill and wipe
(1) _____ pass or receive composite carver
(2) _____ hold curing light and shield, if needed
(1) _____ maintain dry field and visibility   _____   _____

8 Assist with Dental Dam Removal (If Used) (5 points)

(1) _____ pass clamp holder
(2) _____ receive clamp, dam, frame, napkin
(1) _____ check dental dam material for holes and missing pieces
(1) _____ rinse patient's mouth, lightly massage area   _____   _____

9 Assist with Finishing and Polishing of Restoration (10 points)

(2) _____ pass mirror and slow-speed handpiece with finishing bur
(2) _____ maintain water spray and evacuation
(2) _____ hold articulating holder with paper for testing
(2) _____ clean area
(2) _____ pass or receive finishing and polishing items, as needed   _____   _____

10 Dismiss the Patient (5 points)

(1) _____ rinse patient mouth
(1) _____ clean patient face
(1) _____ caution lowering of chair
(1) _____ give postoperative instructions
(1) _____ dismiss patient   _____   _____

11 Cleanup Procedures (10 points)

(2) _____ gather and remove contaminated materials, take to sterilizing area
(2) _____ remove gloves, wash hands, record treatment and take chart to desk
(2) _____ don utility gloves and PPE, disinfect operatory, flush lines
(2) _____ clean and prepare instruments for sterilization, disinfect large
         articles, clean up area
(2) _____ wash, disinfect gloves, remove, wash hands   _____   _____

(100)   Total points   _____   _____

COMPETENCY EVALUATION SHEET

PROCEDURE 30

Assisting with Finishing and Polishing of Amalgam Restorations

Student Name _____ Date _____

GRADING PROTOCOL: Student is awarded the number of points indicated on the evaluation sheet for completing steps successfully.

Total possible points = 100 points
80% needed for passing = 80 points

Total points this test _____ pass _____ fail _____

	PEER REVIEW	TEACHER REVIEW

POINTS

1 Complete the Preparations (10 points)

(2) _____ assemble equipment
(2) _____ prepare operatory
(1) _____ greet and seat patient
(2) _____ review health history
(1) _____ offer safety eyeglasses to patient
(1) _____ explain procedure
(1) _____ don PPE   _____   _____

2 Assist with Evaluation of Restoration (10 points)

(4) _____ pass triple syringe for spray rinse of mouth
(4) _____ evacuate mouth with HVE
(2) _____ pass explorer and mirror to dentist   _____   _____

3 Assist with Occlusal Adjustment (15 points)

(1) _____ receive explorer
(5) _____ pass slow handpiece with small round bur
(4) _____ pass or hold articulating paper in holder
(2) _____ pass or use wet pellet on markings
(1) _____ repeat as needed
(2) _____ receive mirror and slow handpiece and bur _____   _____

4 Assist with Isolation (If Requested) (5 points)

(5) _____ pass cotton rolls, or assist with dental dam placement   _____   _____

5 Assist with Contouring of Restoration Surfaces (15 points)

(3) _____ receive mirror
(3) _____ pass slow handpiece with large round finishing bur or points
(3) _____ pass amalgam knife or file and slow handpiece with disks
(3) _____ rinse and evacuate as needed
(3) _____ aspirate with HVE tip as needed   _____   _____

6 Assist with Smoothing and Polishing of Restoration (15 points)

(3) _____ exchange handpiece with rubber cup filled with pumice
(3) _____ rinse and evacuate as needed
(3) _____ receive handpiece and exchange to stones
(3) _____ alternate impregnated stones in order of abrasiveness
(3) _____ rinse and evacuate as needed   _____   _____

7 Assist with Interproximal Surfaces (10 points)

(2) _____ receive handpiece
(3) _____ pass dental floss or tape or abrasive strip
(2) _____ place slurry of pumice on work site
(3) _____ rinse and evacuate as needed   _____   _____

8 Assist with Final Evaluation (10 points)

(1) _____ receive dental floss, pass explorer
(1) _____ remove dental dam
(2) _____ pass or hold articulating paper in holder on occlusal surface
(2) _____ receive explorer and pass what requested
(2) _____ rinse and evacuate as needed
(1) _____ clean up patient, pass mirror for viewing
(1) _____ dismiss patient   _____   _____

9 Cleanup Procedures (10 points)

(1) _____ remove contaminated materials
(1) _____ remove latex gloves, wash hands
(2) _____ record treatment on patient's chart
(1) _____ don utility gloves, PPE
(2) _____ disinfect operatory and equipment
(1) _____ clean instruments, prepare for sterilizing
(1) _____ clean up area
(1) _____ wash, disinfect gloves, remove, wash hands   _____   _____

(100)   Total points   _____   _____

COMPETENCY EVALUATION SHEET

PROCEDURE 31

Assisting with Tooth Bleaching Appointments

Student Name _____ Date _____

GRADING PROTOCOL: Student is awarded the number of points indicated on the evaluation sheet for completing steps successfully.

Total possible points = 100 points
80% needed for passing = 80 points

Total points this test _____ pass _____ fail _____

	PEER REVIEW	TEACHER REVIEW

POINTS

Visit 1

1 Complete the Preparations (5 points)

(1) _____ assemble equipment and materials
(1) _____ prepare operatory or consultation room and operatory
(1) _____ greet and seat patient, drape and bib patient
(1) _____ explain procedure
(1) _____ don PPE   _____   _____

2 Assist with Examination and Consultation (10 points)

(1) _____ pass or receive mirror and explorer
(2) _____ record findings
(2) _____ pass moistened shade guide
(1) _____ deflect operatory light
(2) _____ record shade number
(2) _____ record findings and notations of exam or consultation   _____   _____

3 Take Photographs (5 points)

(1) _____ adjust lighting to standard
(1) _____ place ID card on patient
(1) _____ insert mouth props
(1) _____ take full-face photograph
(1) _____ take side photos, if requested   _____   _____

4 Assist with Impressions (10 points)

(1) _____ pass or receive syringe for mouth rinse, evacuate
(2) _____ pass or receive tray for test fit; adapt tray, if needed
(2) _____ mix alginate material, fill tray, pass to dentist
(2) _____ receive tray, rinse, disinfect, place in plastic bag
(1) _____ rinse mouth, evacuate, repeat process for other arch
(1) _____ warm wax, pass for bite registration
(1) _____ receive registration, rinse, disinfect, place in bag   _____   _____

5 Cleanup Procedures (5 points)

(1) _____ clean patient's face, remove drape and bib, dismiss patient
(1) _____ gather equipment and material, take to sterilizing room
(1) _____ remove gloves, wash hands, record treatment on chart
(1) _____ don utility gloves, disinfect, sterilize and clean up
(1) _____ wash, disinfect, remove gloves, wash hands _____ _____

Visit 2

6 Complete the Preparations (5 points)

(1) _____ assemble equipment and materials
(2) _____ have patient's bite tray and carrying case
(1) _____ greet patient, escort to patient control room
(1) _____ explain and review procedure _____ _____

7 Assist with Coronal Polish of Teeth (5 points)

(1) _____ pass or use prophy angle with cup or brush
(2) _____ polish crowns of teeth
(2) _____ rinse and evacuate mouth _____ _____

8 Assist with Gel Placement (20 points)

(2) _____ pass cotton rolls for isolation
(2) _____ pass or insert cheek retractor for lips
(2) _____ pass dam gel material for gingiva
(2) _____ pass or use syringe for air dry of tooth surfaces
(4) _____ fill patient's tray with bleach gel, pass to dentist or pass syringe to dentist
(2) _____ place saliva ejector tip, use HVE
(2) _____ time bleaching process
(2) _____ remove trays and isolation, rinse mouth
(2) _____ remove gel dam, freshen mouth _____ _____

9 Review Instructions for Home Care (5 points)

(1) _____ check dentist's prescription for wear
(2) _____ instruct patient in precautions, wear, and care
(2) _____ demonstrate tray use and procedure _____ _____

10 Dismiss the Patient and Clean Up (5 points)

(1) _____ instruct patient in rinsing and appliance care, review instructions
(1) _____ reschedule for recall appointment, dismiss patient
(1) _____ clean up area, wash hands, don PPE, disinfect large items and surfaces
(1) _____ sterilize instruments, dispose of gauze and tissues
(1) _____ wash, dry, disinfect, remove gloves, wash hands _____ _____

Visit 3

11 Complete the Preparations (5 points)

(3) _____ assemble materials and equipment
(2) _____ greet and escort patient _____ _____

12 Assist with Assessment (10 points)

(2) _____ pass and receive mirror for exam
(2) _____ pass and receive wet shade guide indicator
(3) _____ provide natural lighting
(3) _____ record shade on patient's chart   _____   _____

13 Take Photographs (5 points)

(1) _____ adjust lighting to standard
(1) _____ place ID card on patient
(1) _____ insert cheek retractors
(1) _____ take full-face view photograph
(1) _____ take side views, if requested   _____   _____

14 Dismiss the Patient and Clean Up (5 points)

(1) _____ review home care instructions, make recall appointment for patient, dismiss patient
(1) _____ remove contaminated materials to sterilizing room, remove exam gloves, wash hands
(1) _____ record procedure on patient's chart
(1) _____ don PPE, clean up, disinfect, sterilize in the usual manner
(1) _____ wash, dry, disinfect, remove gloves, wash hands   _____   _____

(100)   Total points   _____   _____

COMPETENCY EVALUATION SHEET

```
P R O C E D U R E  3 2
```

Assisting with the Initial Exam and Preventive Techniques in Pediatric Dentistry

Student Name _____ Date _____

GRADING PROTOCOL: Student is awarded the number of points indicated on the evaluation sheet for completing steps successfully.

Total possible points = 100 points
80% needed for passing = 80 points

Total points this test _____ pass _____ fail _____

	PEER REVIEW	TEACHER REVIEW

POINTS

1 Assemble Materials and Equipment (4 points)

(2) _____ prepare operatory
(2) _____ assemble equipment and materials, needed items

2 Prepare the Patient (3 points)

(1) _____ seat and position patient
(1) _____ review health history with parent or guardian
(1) _____ explain procedure

3 Don PPE (3 points)

(1) _____ don lab coat or outerwear
(1) _____ don mask or face shield, eyeglasses
(1) _____ don exam gloves

4 Assist with Examination (10 points)

(2) _____ rinse mouth
(2) _____ pass gauze for tongue exam
(2) _____ record findings on chart
(2) _____ pass mirror and explorer for mouth exam
(2) _____ retract, evacuate, and record as needed

5 Assist with Coronal Polish (10 points)

(2) _____ pass mirror and handpiece with prophy cup and pumice
(2) _____ hold dappen dish with paste near work site
(2) _____ pass syringe or spray mouth
(2) _____ evacuate and maintain visibility
(2) _____ pass floss when requested

6 Assist with Supplemental Diagnostic Procedures (Radiological Exam) (20 points)

(2) _____ don overgloves
(2) _____ prepare patient with safety wear

(2) _____ explain procedure

(2) _____ set machine controls and timer

(2) _____ pass or insert periapical film

(2) _____ expose radiograph

(2) _____ prepare machine for panoramic exposure

(2) _____ position patient for panoramic exposure

(2) _____ expose radiograph

(2) _____ remove radiographs for processing _____ _____

7 Assist with Fluoride Treatment Supplemental Preventive Procedures (15 points)

(1) _____ don overgloves

(2) _____ pass fluoride trays to secure fit, or obtain topical applicators

(2) _____ mix fluoride materials and prepare tray

(2) _____ dry or isolate area, aid in dental dam if needed

(2) _____ pass loaded fluoride tray or topical applicators, assist with placement

(2) _____ time exposure

(2) _____ evacuate and maintain visibility and dry field

(2) _____ repeat procedure for other arch or side if single tray used _____ _____

or

Sealant Placement (20 points)

(1) _____ don overgloves

(2) _____ isolate teeth

(2) _____ pass or use syringe for air dry of teeth

(2) _____ pass acid-etch sponge for tooth etching

(2) _____ time etching period

(2) _____ pass or use syringe for rinse of teeth

(2) _____ re-isolate and remove old cotton rolls

(2) _____ pass or use syringe for air dry of surfaces

(2) _____ pass sealant material on brush

(2) _____ time sealing process

(1) _____ pass explorer for test of sealant _____ _____

8 Clean Up Patient (5 points)

(1) _____ remove isolation and dental dam, if used; lightly rinse mouth; wipe patient's face

(1) _____ give patient postoperative instructions

(1) _____ lower chair and remove drape and bib

(1) _____ review instructions with parent

(1) _____ dismiss patient _____ _____

9 Clean Up Operatory (5 points)

(1) _____ gather contaminated materials

(1) _____ remove items to sterilizing room

(1) _____ remove latex gloves, wash hands

(1) _____ record treatment on patient's chart

(1) _____ take chart to front desk or the appropriate place _____ _____

10 Clean Up Materials and Equipment (5 points)

(1) _____ don utility gloves and PPE

(1) _____ disinfect large items in operatory

(1) _____ place disposables in proper container

(1) _____ clean and prepare instruments for sterilization

(1) _____ wash and disinfect gloves, remove; wash hands _____ _____

(100) Total points _____ _____

COMPETENCY EVALUATION SHEET

PROCEDURE. 33

Assisting with Pulp Treatment and Protective Covers

Student Name _____ Date _____

GRADING PROTOCOL: Student is awarded the number of points indicated on the evaluation sheet for completing steps successfully.

Total possible points = 100 points
80% needed for passing = 80 points

Total points this test _____ pass _____ fail _____

	PEER REVIEW	TEACHER REVIEW

POINTS

1 Assemble Equipment and Prepare the Patient (5 points)

(1) _____ assemble equipment
(1) _____ prepare operatory
(1) _____ greet and seat patient
(1) _____ review history with parents
(1) _____ don PPE   _____   _____

2 Assist with Topical and Local Anesthesia (5 points)

(2) _____ rinse and dry mouth, place topical applicator
(2) _____ receive applicator, pass syringe, monitor for movement
(1) _____ receive syringe, monitor for reaction   _____   _____

3 Assist with Dental Dam (5 points)

(1) _____ pass clamp holder, clamp, material, frame
(1) _____ receive holder, pass napkin
(1) _____ pass ligatures, assist with tie in
(1) _____ pass inversion instrument
(1) _____ place saliva ejector   _____   _____

4 Assist with Tooth Preparation (10 points)

(2) _____ disinfect tooth area
(3) _____ pass handpiece with sterile round bur
(3) _____ pass hand instruments and burs as needed
(2) _____ maintain visibility and evacuation   _____   _____

5 Assist with Pulp Sterilization and Bleeding Control (10 points)

(3) _____ pass formocresol pellet
(2) _____ receive pellet
(2) _____ pass syringe
(3) _____ evacuate as needed with HVE   _____   _____

6 Assist with Protective Cover Selection (10 points)

(2) _____ pass boley gauge or millimeter rule
(3) _____ pass crown for try in

(2) _____ repeat as needed until fit

(3) _____ pass explorer for testing and marking

7 Assist with Reduction of Crown Form (10 points)

(2) _____ pass curved crown and collar scissors

(3) _____ pass slow handpiece and finishing bur

(3) _____ pass crimping pliers

(2) _____ pass explorer for testing fit and contour

8 Assist with Medication of Prepared Tooth (10 points)

(2) _____ pass syringe for air dry, repeat process

(2) _____ prepare medication for pulp, if requested

(2) _____ pass medication, hold excess near

(2) _____ pass explorer to check medication

(2) _____ perform varnish step to cover medication

9 Assist with Dental Dam Removal (5 points)

(1) _____ remove saliva ejector, pass cotton pliers, receive ligatures

(1) _____ pass dental dam clamp holder, receive holder and clamp

(1) _____ pass scissors, receive scissors and dam material

(1) _____ receive frame and napkin

(1) _____ pass and receive syringe, evacuate mouth

10 Assist with Cementation of the Crown (10 points)

(2) _____ pass cotton rolls for isolation

(2) _____ mix cement according to manufacturer's directions

(2) _____ fill crown, pass to dentist

(2) _____ pass bite stick for patient to bite

(2) _____ maintain dry field with HVE tip

11 Assist with Cleanup of Tooth (5 points)

(1) _____ pass scaler for removal of excess dry cement

(1) _____ pass explorer to test fit and cement

(1) _____ receive cotton rolls

(1) _____ hold articulating paper for occlusal test

(1) _____ pass handpiece with finishing bur

12 Assist with Polish of Crown (10 points)

(2) _____ receive handpiece, exchange to prophy cup and pumice

(2) _____ pass handpiece for polishing

(2) _____ pass or use syringe to rinse area

(2) _____ evacuate area, wipe patient's face

(2) _____ review postoperative instructions with parents, dismiss patient

13 Cleanup Procedures (5 points)

(1) _____ remove contaminated items to sterilizing room

(1) _____ remove gloves, wash hands, record patient treatment on chart, take chart to front desk

(1) _____ disinfect operatory, dispose of sharps and disposables in proper container

(1) _____ disinfect large items, clean and sterilize instruments

(1) _____ clean up area; wash; disinfect gloves, remove; wash hands

(100) Total points

COMPETENCY EVALUATION SHEET

Assisting with Space Maintainers

Student Name _____ Date _____

GRADING PROTOCOL: Student is awarded the number of points indicated on the evaluation sheet for completing steps
successfully.

Total possible points = 100 points
80% needed for passing = 80 points

Total points this test _____   pass _____   fail _____

	PEER REVIEW	TEACHER REVIEW

POINTS

Visit 1

1 Assemble Equipment and Prepare the Patient (10 points)

(1) _____ gather needed equipment and materials
(1) _____ obtain materials for impression and fitting
(1) _____ prepare operatory
(2) _____ review health history with parent or guardian
(2) _____ greet, seat, and position patient
(2) _____ explain procedure
(1) _____ don PPE, summon dentist   _____   _____

2 Assist with Band Placement (10 points)

(1) _____ pass and receive triple syringe for mouth rinse
(1) _____ evacuate mouth
(2) _____ pass and receive mirror and explorer for examination
(2) _____ pass estimated sized band for fit
(2) _____ pass band driver, continue until proper fit
(2) _____ pass explorer for etch mark of location   _____   _____

3 Assist with Alginate Impression (10 points)

(1) _____ pass and receive tray for proper fit
(1) _____ place wax on tray edges if needed
(2) _____ mix alginate material to smooth, creamy consistency
(2) _____ pass triple syringe for air dry
(2) _____ receive syringe, pass loaded tray to dentist
(2) _____ receive tray, rinse, disinfect, bag   _____   _____

4 Assist with Band and Crown Removal (10 points)

(2) _____ pass syringe for rinse
(2) _____ evacuate mouth
(2) _____ pass band remover
(2) _____ receive band remover and band
(2) _____ rinse, disinfect band, bag impression   _____   _____

5 Dismiss Patient and Clean Up (10 points)

(1) _____ clean patient's face
(1) _____ lower chair, remove bib and coverings, dismiss

(1) _____ remove gloves, wash hands
(1) _____ write procedure on patient's chart
(1) _____ take chart to front desk, make another appointment
(1) _____ seal plastic impression bag
(1) _____ gather and remove contaminated materials
(1) _____ don utility gloves, disinfect operatory
(1) _____ clean, disinfect, and sterilize equipment and materials
(1) _____ wash, dry, disinfect gloves, remove; wash hands   _____ _____

Visit 2

6 Gather Materials and Prepare the Patient (10 points)

(3) _____ assemble equipment, materials, and appliances
(2) _____ greet, seat, and position patient
(3) _____ explain procedure
(2) _____ don PPE, summon dentist   _____ _____

7 Assist with Try In of Appliance (10 points)

(2) _____ pass, receive triple syringe for mouth rinse, evacuate
(1) _____ pass and receive mouth mirror and explorer for exam
(2) _____ pass prepared appliance
(1) _____ pass and receive band driver
(2) _____ pass and receive articulating paper for testing
(2) _____ pass syringe for rinse, evacuate   _____ _____

8 Assist with Cementation (10 points)

(1) _____ pass band remover
(1) _____ receive remover and appliance
(1) _____ check appliance for roughness, distortion, smooth if needed
(1) _____ pass or use slow handpiece, prophy cup and pumice to polish
(1) _____ don overgloves or use gauze barriers to prepare cement materials
(2) _____ mix cement to creamy consistency
(1) _____ load band from gingival side, pass
(1) _____ pass explorer
(1) _____ hold wet gauze near site   _____ _____

9 Assist with Cleanup of the Appliance and the Patient (10 points)

(1) _____ pass scaler
(1) _____ evacuate debris
(2) _____ pass triple syringe for mouth rinse, evacuate
(2) _____ pass and receive explorer for testing
(2) _____ clean up patient, lower chair, summon parent
(2) _____ give postoperative instructions, dismiss   _____ _____

10 Clean Up Operatory, Disinfect, and Sterilize (10 points)

(1) _____ remove exam gloves, wash hands
(2) _____ write procedure on patient's chart, take to front desk
(1) _____ don utility gloves
(2) _____ clean up operatory area
(2) _____ disinfect and sterilize equipment and materials
(2) _____ wash, dry, disinfect gloves, remove; wash hands   _____ _____

(100)   Total points   _____ _____

COMPETENCY EVALUATION SHEET

▶ P R O C E D U R E   3 5

Assisting with the Endodontic Examination

Student Name _____ Date _____

GRADING PROTOCOL: Student is awarded the number of points indicated on the evaluation sheet for completing steps successfully.

Total possible points = 100 points
80% needed for passing = 80 points

Total points this test _____ pass _____ fail _____

	PEER REVIEW	TEACHER REVIEW

POINTS

1 Assemble Equipment (10 points)

(4) _____ gather needed equipment and material
(3) _____ prepare operatory
(3) _____ prepare radiographic equipment   _____   _____

2 Prepare the Patient and Don PPE (10 points)

(3) _____ greet and seat patient
(3) _____ take health and medical history
(2) _____ explain procedure
(2) _____ don PPE, observe sterile technique   _____   _____

3 Assist with Clinical Examination (10 points)

(3) _____ record history and clinical findings
(2) _____ pass mirror and explorer
(3) _____ record percussion results
(2) _____ record palpation results   _____   _____

4 Assist with Dental Radiographs (10 points)

(2) _____ don overgloves
(2) _____ prepare patient with safety wear
(2) _____ pass or expose radiograph
(1) _____ process radiograph
(1) _____ remove overgloves
(2) _____ record radiograph findings   _____   _____

5 Assist with Thermal Testing (10 points)

(3) _____ pass ice in gauze
(2) _____ pass applicator with vaseline to coat tooth
(3) _____ pass hot gutta percha point
(2) _____ record findings   _____   _____

6 Assist with Vitality Testing (10 points)

(2) _____ pass cotton for isolation
(1) _____ use applicator stick to apply paste or moisture to tooth
(2) _____ pass vitality tip to dentist
(2) _____ check gauge at zero
(1) _____ accelerate gauge
(1) _____ stop and record at signal
(1) _____ repeat process for all affected teeth

_____ _____

7 Assist with Transillumination (10 points)

(2) _____ pass and receive syringe for rinse
(2) _____ evacuate and blow dry area
(2) _____ pass illuminator tip to dentist
(2) _____ record findings
(2) _____ receive illuminator tip

_____ _____

8 Assist with Mobility Testing (10 points)

(4) _____ pass instrument for mobility testing
(3) _____ direct operatory light for visibility
(3) _____ record findings

_____ _____

9 Clean Up the Patient (10 points)

(2) _____ wipe patient face
(2) _____ remove drape, bib, lower chair
(2) _____ remove gloves, wash hands
(2) _____ update charts and records
(2) _____ gather records, radiographs, escort patient to consultation room

_____ _____

10 Clean Up Operatory, Disinfect, and Sterilize (10 points)

(1) _____ don utility gloves and PPE
(1) _____ remove contaminated materials and equipment to sterilizing room
(1) _____ disinfect operatory area
(1) _____ place disposables in proper containers
(1) _____ clean, wrap, and autoclave vitality and illumination tips
(1) _____ disinfect large items, replace barrier wraps
(1) _____ clean and prepare instruments for sterilization
(1) _____ clean up area
(2) _____ wash, disinfect, and remove gloves; wash hands

_____ _____

(100)   Total points

_____ _____

COMPETENCY EVALUATION SHEET

PROCEDURE 36A

Assisting with Root Canal Therapy (Visits 1 and 2)

Student Name _____ Date _____

GRADING PROTOCOL: Student is awarded the number of points indicated on the evaluation sheet for completing steps
successfully.

Total possible points = 100 points
80% needed for passing = 80 points

Total points this test _____ pass _____ fail _____

	PEER REVIEW	TEACHER REVIEW

POINTS
Visit 1

1 Assemble Equipment and Prepare the Patient (5 points)

(1) _____ complete preparation
(1) _____ assemble equipment
(1) _____ prepare patient
(1) _____ offer protective eyewear to patient
(1) _____ don PPE   _____   _____

2 Assist with Local Anesthesia (10 points)

(3) _____ administer topical anesthesia
(3) _____ prepare local anesthesia
(2) _____ receive applicator, pass and receive local anesthesia syringe
(2) _____ monitor patient reaction   _____   _____

3 Assist with Isolation of Tooth (10 points)

(2) _____ pass clamp holder and test clamp
(2) _____ pass prepared clamp, dam material, frame
(2) _____ assist with napkin placement
(2) _____ assist with ligature tie in, inversion of dam
(2) _____ place saliva ejector correctly   _____   _____

4 Assist with Disinfection of Tooth and Dam (5 points)

(3) _____ pass applicator soaked with disinfectant
(2) _____ receive applicator after disinfection   _____   _____

5 Assist with Opening of Tooth (10 points)

(4) _____ pass handpiece with round bur
(3) _____ maintain visibility and dry field
(3) _____ pass excavator and instruments as signaled   _____   _____

6 Assist with Removal of Pulpal Tissue (10 points)

(5) _____ pass sterile barbed broach instrument
(3) _____ hold gauze near site
(2) _____ maintain visibility   _____   _____

486

7 Assist with Cleaning the Pulpal Canal (20 points)

(2) _____ pass file and reamer, increase in size as requested
(2) _____ hold gauze near site to clean endo instrument
(2) _____ receive used files or reamers in gloved palm
(2) _____ pass reamers, files alternately, increase size as requested
(2) _____ assist with radiograph of tooth and reamer
(2) _____ set gauge, place stops on endo instruments
(2) _____ prepare sterile, irrigation syringes; keep solutions separate
(2) _____ pass alternate syringes when requested
(2) _____ aspirate with HVE
(2) _____ pass and receive paper points to dry canal

8 Assist with Medication of the Canal (10 points)

(3) _____ moisten sterile, small, cotton pellet
(3) _____ blot pellet to moist stage
(2) _____ pass moistened pellet in sterile pliers
(2) _____ receive pliers and pass dry cotton pellet for packing

9 Assist with Temporary Filling of Canal and Tooth (10 points)

(3) _____ prepare temporary restorative material
(3) _____ pass PFI with restorative material
(2) _____ pass carver
(2) _____ maintain visibility

10 Clean Up Patient, Area, and Instruments (10 points)

(1) _____ pass dental dam clamp holder
(1) _____ receive clamp holder and clamp, frame, napkin
(1) _____ receive ligature pieces in gauze, pass and receive scissors
(1) _____ receive dental dam material, check for holes
(1) _____ rinse mouth, hold articulating paper for occlusion testing (if needed)
(1) _____ pass and receive carver or slow handpiece with bur for adjustment
(1) _____ rinse and evacuate mouth, give postoperative instructions
(1) _____ clean patient's face, dismiss
(1) _____ clean up, disinfect, sterilize in usual manner
(1) _____ record treatment and instrument sizes

(100)   Total points

Visit 2

The instruments and materials for visit 2 are the same as visit 1. The procedure is the same with the exception of the anesthesia. Since there is no pulp, anesthesia may or may not be given.

The dentist will open the tooth, remove the dressings and enlarge and smooth the root canal area. A medicated pellet and temporary restorative material will be placed and the patient will return for a third visit.

COMPETENCY EVALUATION SHEET

P R O C E D U R E   3 6 B

Assisting with Root Canal Therapy (Visit 3)

Student Name _____ Date _____

GRADING PROTOCOL: Student is awarded the number of points indicated on the evaluation sheet for completing steps successfully.

Total possible points = 100 points
80% needed for passing = 80 points

Total points this test _____ pass _____ fail _____

	PEER REVIEW	TEACHER REVIEW

POINTS

Visit 3

11 Assemble Equipment and Prepare the Patient (10 points)

(2) _____ gather needed items
(2) _____ prepare operatory
(2) _____ greet and seat patient, review health history
(2) _____ explain procedure
(2) _____ don PPE, summon dentist   _____   _____

12 Assist with Placement of Dental Dam (10 points)

(2) _____ pass clamp holder with clamp, prepared dental dam material
(2) _____ pass napkin and frame, assist with positioning
(2) _____ pass ligatures, assist with inversion of dam
(2) _____ place saliva ejector
(2) _____ pass applicator with disinfectant   _____   _____

13 Assist with Removal of Temporary Restoration (10 points)

(2) _____ pass slow handpiece with round bur
(2) _____ receive handpiece, pass explorer
(2) _____ receive explorer and pellet
(2) _____ pass barbed broach
(2) _____ receive broach and cotton pellet   _____   _____

14 Assist with Cleaning the Canal (10 points)

(2) _____ mark stoppers on reamers and files
(2) _____ pass reamers and files as needed
(2) _____ pass irrigating syringes as requested
(2) _____ pass paper point in sterile pliers to dry canal
(2) _____ evacuate as needed   _____   _____

15 Assist with Fitting of Center Core for Canal (10 points)

(3) _____ pass silver or gutta percha point for master cone
(2) _____ prepare to pass other size points

(3) _____ assist with x-ray of canal
(2) _____ pass explorer for removal of master cone   _____   _____

16 Prepare Root Canal Cement (10 points)

(3) _____ prepare glass mixing slab
(3) _____ measure cement materials
(2) _____ mix root canal cement
(2) _____ mix to creamy consistency   _____   _____

17 Assist with Cementation and Filling of Canal (15 points)

(2) _____ roll spreader through cement, pass to dentist
(1) _____ hold slab near site for refill
(1) _____ roll master cone in cement
(1) _____ receive spreader, pass cone in sterile pliers
(2) _____ dip and pass slender gutta percha points
(1) _____ dip plugger instrument into solvent, pass
(2) _____ repeat until overfilled
(1) _____ assist with final x-ray
(2) _____ pass heated spoon excavator
(1) _____ receive ends in gauze
(1) _____ pass and receive pellet with disinfectant   _____   _____

18 Assist with Final Restoration and Cover (5 points)

(2) _____ prepare restoration of choice
(2) _____ assist with placement of restoration
(1) _____ maintain visibility   _____   _____

19 Clean Up Patient and Dismiss (10 points)

(1) _____ pass dental dam clamp holder
(1) _____ receive clamp holder, clamp, frame, and napkin
(1) _____ pass scissors, receive ligatures and scissors
(1) _____ receive dam material, check holes
(2) _____ pass or hold articulating paper
(1) _____ pass handpiece with finishing bur
(1) _____ pass articulating paper and burs, as needed
(1) _____ clean up patient, give instructions
(1) _____ dismiss patient   _____   _____

20 Clean Up Operatory and Equipment (10 points)

(1) _____ gather contaminated materials and equipment
(1) _____ take all materials and equipment to sterilizing room
(1) _____ remove latex gloves, wash hands, gather records
(2) _____ update records, place x-ray films in patient file
(1) _____ take records to the front desk
(1) _____ don utility gloves
(2) _____ disinfect and sterilize all articles
(1) _____ wash, dry, sterilize, remove gloves; wash hands   _____   _____

(100)   Total points   _____   _____

COMPETENCY EVALUATION SHEET

P R O C E D U R E   3 7

Assisting with Prosthodontic Impressions (Visit 2)

Student Name _____ Date _____

GRADING PROTOCOL: Student is awarded the number of points indicated on the evaluation sheet for completing steps successfully.

Total possible points = 100 points
80% needed for passing = 80 points

Total points this test _____ pass _____ fail _____

	PEER REVIEW	TEACHER REVIEW

POINTS

Visit 2

1 Complete Preparations (20 points)

(2) _____ gather custom tray from primary impression
(2) _____ prepare operatory
(2) _____ gather necessary equipment and materials
(2) _____ arrange impression materials (dentist's choice)
(2) _____ prepare plastic lab bag
(3) _____ drape and bib patient
(2) _____ place petroleum jelly on patient's lips
(3) _____ explain procedure
(2) _____ don PPE, assist with preliminary treatment   _____   _____

2 Prepare the Impression Tray (10 points)

(3) _____ paint tray with adhesive covering
(2) _____ adapt beading or wax rope to edges of tray
(2) _____ collect patient's denture, place in denture cup (if applicable)
(3) _____ pass or use syringe to rinse mouth, evacuate   _____   _____

3 Prepare the Impression Material (10 points)

(5) _____ mix according to manufacturer's directions
(3) _____ fill, pass, and receive impression syringe (if applicable)
(2) _____ fill and pass impression tray   _____   _____

4 Assist with the Removal of the Impression Tray (10 points)

(3) _____ receive impression in tray
(2) _____ pass syringe, rinse mouth, evacuate
(5) _____ rinse impression, disinfect, place in bag   _____   _____

5 Repeat the Procedure for the Other Arch (10 points)

(2) _____ compliment patient
(2) _____ explain impression for other arch

(3) _____ prepare materials
(3) _____ pass and receive impression materials _____ _____

6 Assist with the Bite Registration (10 points)

(2) _____ warm bite wafer or base plate wax
(2) _____ pass wafer, wax, or registration syringe
(2) _____ pass triple syringe for spray, evacuate fluids
(2) _____ receive wax bite registration
(2) _____ rinse in cool water, disinfect, place in bag _____ _____

7 Assist with Tooth Selection (10 points)

(2) _____ wet tooth shade guide
(2) _____ adjust lighting
(1) _____ record shade number
(2) _____ pass mold forms
(1) _____ record mold number
(2) _____ record any other pertinent information _____ _____

8 Clean Up, Dismiss the Patient, and Sterilize (20 points)

(2) _____ wash patient's denture and appliance
(2) _____ rinse patient's mouth
(2) _____ return wet prosthesis
(2) _____ clean up and remove impression material from patient's face
(2) _____ dismiss patient
(1) _____ gather contaminated materials and equipment
(1) _____ take to sterilizing room, remove gloves, wash hands
(2) _____ record treatment and notes on patient's chart, take to desk
(1) _____ don utility gloves, disinfect operatory
(1) _____ clean, disinfect all materials including impression containers
(1) _____ sterilize, clean up area
(1) _____ wash, disinfect, and remove gloves; wash hands
(2) _____ take impression and registration to lab or prepare for shipping _____ _____

(100) Total points _____ _____

COMPETENCY EVALUATION SHEET

PROCEDURE 38

Assisting with Try In and Delivery Appointments

Student Name _____ Date _____

GRADING PROTOCOL: Student is awarded the number of points indicated on the evaluation sheet for completing steps successfully.

Total possible points = 100 points
80% needed for passing = 80 points

Total points this test _____ pass _____ fail _____

	PEER REVIEW	TEACHER REVIEW

POINTS

Try In Appointment

1 Complete the Preparations (10 points)

(2) _____ gather required items
(1) _____ gather appliance or denture from lab
(2) _____ disinfect article and rinse
(1) _____ prepare operatory
(1) _____ greet and seat patient
(1) _____ drape and bib patient
(1) _____ explain procedure
(1) _____ don PPE   _____   _____

2 Assist with Placement of the Appliance (10 points)

(4) _____ accept patient's denture or appliance, place in denture cup
(3) _____ pass or use syringe to spray rinse patient's mouth
(3) _____ pass disinfected article to dentist for insertion   _____   _____

3 Assist with Adjustment of the Appliance (10 points)

(2) _____ pass or use articulating paper in holder
(2) _____ pass warm spatula, instruments, and pliers for adjustment
(1) _____ record adjustments made
(1) _____ redampen appliance for re-insertion
(1) _____ pass hand mirror to patient for viewing
(2) _____ repeat process as needed
(1) _____ receive appliance, rinse, disinfect, and bag   _____   _____

4 Instruct and Dismiss the Patient (10 points)

(4) _____ rinse and evacuate patient's mouth
(3) _____ wash and hand wet appliance to patient for re-insertion
(3) _____ clean up patient, dismiss   _____   _____

5 Clean Up and Sterilize (10 points)

(3) _____ gather and bring materials to sterilizing room
(2) _____ remove gloves, wash hands, record treatment

(2) _____ don utility gloves, clean up, disinfect and sterilize
(3) _____ wash, disinfect, remove gloves; wash hands   _____   _____

6 Complete the Lab Work Order (10 points)

(3) _____ complete lab prescription
(3) _____ pass order and notes to dentist for prescription
(2) _____ prepare try in appliance, registration, and prescription
(2) _____ send to laboratory   _____   _____

Delivery Appointment

7 Complete the Preparations (10 points)

(2) _____ assemble materials and equipment
(2) _____ prepare operatory
(2) _____ assemble appliance from laboratory
(2) _____ seat and prepare patient
(2) _____ don PPE   _____   _____

8 Assist with Placement (10 points)

(3) _____ accept patient's old appliance, place in denture cup
(3) _____ pass or use syringe to rinse patient's mouth
(2) _____ pass dampened appliance to dentist
(2) _____ pass hand mirror to patient   _____   _____

9 Assist with Adjustment (10 points)

(2) _____ pass or hold articulating paper in holder for testing bite
(2) _____ pass slow handpiece with finishing bur or stone
(2) _____ pass and exchange burs for finishing
(2) _____ repeat process as needed
(1) _____ wash, rinse, pass completed appliance to dentist
(1) _____ pass hand mirror to patient for viewing   _____   _____

10 Dismiss Patient, Disinfect, and Sterilize (10 points)

(1) _____ clean up patient's face
(1) _____ remove drape and bib
(2) _____ give care instructions
(1) _____ return patient's old appliance in plastic bag
(1) _____ dismiss patient
(1) _____ gather materials and equipment, take to sterilizing room
(1) _____ remove gloves, wash hands, record treatment
(1) _____ don utility gloves, clean, disinfect, sterilize
(1) _____ wash, disinfect, remove gloves; wash hands   _____   _____

(100)   Total points   _____   _____

COMPETENCY EVALUATION SHEET

PROCEDURE 39

Assisting with Fixed Crowns (Visit 1)

Student Name _____ Date _____

GRADING PROTOCOL: Student is awarded the number of points indicated on the evaluation sheet for completing steps successfully.

Total possible points = 100 points
80% needed for passing = 80 points

Total points this test _____ pass _____ fail _____

	PEER REVIEW	TEACHER REVIEW

POINTS

1 Complete Preparations (5 points)

(1) _____ assemble equipment and materials
(1) _____ prepare operatory
(1) _____ greet and seat patient, drape and bib patient
(1) _____ explain procedure
(1) _____ don PPE   _____   _____

2 Assist with the Impressions (5 points)

(1) _____ pass or use syringe for spray rinse of patient's mouth
(1) _____ pass tray for test fit, prepare tray with adhesive
(1) _____ mix alginate, fill tray, pass to dentist
(1) _____ receive tray, rinse, disinfect, moist wrap
(1) _____ repeat procedure for other arch   _____   _____

3 Assist with the Anesthesia (5 points)

(1) _____ rinse mouth, dry injection area
(1) _____ apply topical anesthesia
(1) _____ pass and receive anesthetic syringe
(1) _____ recap with one-handed motion or recap device
(1) _____ monitor patient reaction   _____   _____

4 Assist with Tooth Shade Selection (5 points)

(2) _____ dampen shade guide
(1) _____ pass to dentist
(1) _____ turn off lamp or move beam
(1) _____ record shade   _____   _____

5 Assist with Crown Preparation (10 points)

(2) _____ pass high-speed handpiece with fissure bur
(5) _____ spray work area, maintain visibility, evacuate
(3) _____ exchange burs, diamonds, disks, pass instruments as requested   _____   _____

6 Assist with Final Impression Tray or Tube Fit (5 points)

(1) _____ spray rinse, evacuate mouth
(1) _____ pass tray or tube for test fit
(2) _____ pass explorer for etch of tube (if used)
(1) _____ receive tray or copper tube (if used) _____ _____

7 Assist with Gingival Retraction Cord (10 points)

(2) _____ spray rinse, evacuate mouth
(3) _____ pass college pliers with cord
(3) _____ pass cord pusher or PFI instrument
(2) _____ receive college pliers and pusher or PFI _____ _____

8 Assist with Final Impression (10 points)

(1) _____ pass college pliers
(1) _____ receive college pliers and gingival cord
(2) _____ heat compound or mix impression material, fill tube and tray
(1) _____ pass filled tray and tube with etch mark in front
(2) _____ spray rinse to cool tube
(1) _____ receive tube or impression in tray
(2) _____ rinse, disinfect, and bag _____ _____

9 Assist with Bite Registration (5 points)

(1) _____ pass impression tray for fit
(1) _____ mix impression material, fill tray
(1) _____ pass tray or wax to dentist for impression
(1) _____ evacuate mouth, provide visibility
(1) _____ receive registration, rinse, disinfect, place in bag with final impression _____ _____

10 Assist with Temporary Cover Construction (15 points)

(2) _____ retrieve impression of prep area
(1) _____ spray rinse and evacuate mouth
(2) _____ place monomer drops into impression
(2) _____ place powder into monomer drops, repeat
(2) _____ pass varnish pellet in college pliers
(2) _____ receive pellet and college pliers, pass tray
(2) _____ evacuate as needed
(1) _____ receive tray and impression
(1) _____ rinse, evacuate mouth _____ _____

11 Assist with Finishing of the Cover (5 points)

(2) _____ pass or use curved scissors to cut off flashing
(1) _____ pass or use slow handpiece and finishing bur to smooth edges
(1) _____ pass or use slow handpiece to finish cover
(1) _____ wash, dry cover _____ _____

12 Assist with Cementation of the Cover (15 points)

(1) _____ rinse, evacuate, and dry mouth; prep
(1) _____ pass cotton rolls for isolation
(2) _____ mix cement, place in cover
(1) _____ pass cover to dentist

(1) _____ pass bite stick for patient to bite on

(1) _____ pass sponge to wipe off excess, allow to dry

(2) _____ receive stick, pass scaler for cleanup of excess cement

(2) _____ pass floss and floss holder to clean interproximal spaces

(2) _____ pass or hold articulating paper for test bite

(2) _____ pass slow handpiece with bur for adjustment, if needed; rinse and evacuate mouth   _____   _____

13 Dismiss Patient, Clean Up, Disinfect, and Sterilize (5 points)

(1) _____ clean patient's face, remove drape and bib, give care and postoperative instructions, dismiss patient with appointment for second visit

(1) _____ gather equipment and materials, take to sterilizing room

(1) _____ remove gloves, wash hands, record treatment on chart

(1) _____ don utility gloves, clean, disinfect and sterilize, wash gloves, disinfect, remove and wash hands

(1) _____ gather impressions and prescription for lab work, list disinfection procedures followed, wrap materials, send to dental lab   _____   _____

(100)   Total points   _____   _____

COMPETENCY EVALUATION SHEET

PROCEDURE 40

Assisting with Fixed Crowns (Final Visit)

Student Name _____ Date _____

GRADING PROTOCOL: Student is awarded the number of points indicated on the evaluation sheet for completing steps
successfully.

Total possible points = 100 points
80% needed for passing = 80 points

Total points this test _____ pass _____ fail _____

	PEER REVIEW	TEACHER REVIEW

POINTS

1 Complete Preparations (10 points)

(3) _____ assemble materials and equipment
(3) _____ disinfect, rinse completed crown
(2) _____ prepare patient, explain procedure
(2) _____ don PPE   _____   _____

2 Assist with the Anesthesia (10 points)

(2) _____ rinse, evacuate, dry injection site
(3) _____ place topical anesthetic on injection site
(3) _____ pass and receive anesthetic syringe, recap with one hand
(2) _____ monitor patient reactions   _____   _____

3 Assist with Temporary Crown Cover Removal (12 points)

(2) _____ pass crown remover
(2) _____ receive instrument and crown
(2) _____ rinse and evacuate mouth
(2) _____ pass explorer for exam
(2) _____ pass scaler for cement removal
(1) _____ receive instruments
(1) _____ rinse and evacuate   _____   _____

4 Assist with Permanent Crown Try In (12 points)

(4) _____ pass disinfected and cleaned crown
(4) _____ pass and receive bite stick for patient to bite on
(4) _____ pass mirror and explorer for exam   _____   _____

5 Assist with the Crown Adjustment (12 points)

(3) _____ pass or use articulating paper for patient to bite on
(2) _____ pass slow handpiece with finishing bur
(2) _____ retest with articulating paper, adjust as needed
(3) _____ pass crown remover
(2) _____ receive crown remover and crown   _____   _____

6 Assist with the Crown Cementation (14 points)

(1) _____ polish and smooth crown
(2) _____ clean out crown with hydrogen peroxide soaked cotton pellet
(1) _____ pass cotton rolls for isolation
(2) _____ pass and receive varnish-moistened pellet in college pliers
(2) _____ mix zinc phosphate cement, load crown
(2) _____ pass PFI with cement to dentist, hold excess nearby
(1) _____ receive PFI, pass crown
(1) _____ pass and receive bite stick
(1) _____ pass and receive gauze to wipe off excess wet cement
(1) _____ place saliva ejector to control moisture   _____   _____

7 Assist with the Final Crown Adjustment (15 points)

(2) _____ remove cotton rolls and saliva ejector
(1) _____ pass explorer and mirror for check
(2) _____ receive explorer, pass scaler to remove excess cement
(2) _____ check occlusion with articulating paper
(2) _____ pass slow handpiece with finishing bur, if needed
(1) _____ repeat with articulating paper and finishing burs and stones
(2) _____ pass slow handpiece with prophy cup with polish
(1) _____ receive handpiece, pass syringe, evacuate
(1) _____ receive mirror, pass dental floss for interproximal spaces
(1) _____ rinse and evacuate mouth   _____   _____

8 Clean Up Patient, Disinfect, and Sterilize (15 points)

(1) _____ clean up patient's face
(1) _____ pass hand mirror to patient for viewing
(1) _____ review hygiene instructions with patient
(1) _____ remove drape and bib
(1) _____ dismiss patient
(2) _____ gather contaminated equipment and materials
(1) _____ take items to sterilizing room
(2) _____ remove gloves, wash hands
(2) _____ record treatment on patient's chart
(1) _____ don utility gloves and PPE
(1) _____ clean up, disinfect, and sterilize
(1) _____ wash, disinfect, remove gloves; wash hands   _____   _____

(100)   Total points   _____   _____

COMPETENCY EVALUATION SHEET

P R O C E D U R E   4 1

Assisting with the Orthodontic Preliminary Examination

Student Name _____ Date _____

GRADING PROTOCOL: Student is awarded the number of points indicated on the evaluation sheet for completing steps successfully.

Total possible points = 100 points
80% needed for passing = 80 points

Total points this test _____ pass _____ fail _____

	PEER REVIEW	TEACHER REVIEW

POINTS

1 Assist with Interview and Preparation (5 points)

(1) _____ prepare consultation area
(2) _____ assemble equipment and materials
(2) _____ prepare operatory

2 Assist with or Expose Photographs (15 points)

(5) _____ prepare identification plate
(5) _____ expose lateral view photographs
(5) _____ expose face view photographs

3 Prepare the Patient (15 points)

(4) _____ seat patient in operatory chair
(3) _____ drape and bib patient
(4) _____ establish rapport with patient
(4) _____ don PPE

4 Assist with Clinical Examination (15 points)

(3) _____ record health and medical history findings
(3) _____ record facial and occlusion classification
(3) _____ pass and receive mirror and explorer
(3) _____ pass and receive syringe as signaled
(3) _____ record and chart mouth and teeth findings

5 Assist with or Expose Radiographs (15 points)

(3) _____ assist with or expose intraoral radiograph
(4) _____ assist with or expose panoramic radiograph
(4) _____ assist with or expose occlusal radiograph
(4) _____ assist with or expose cephalometric radiograph

6 Assist with or Take Full-mouth Alginate Impressions (15 points)

(2) _____ assist with tray selection
(2) _____ adapt tray with wax, if needed

(2) _____ assist with impression mixture and load of tray
(3) _____ pass or take impression
(2) _____ repeat for other arch
(2) _____ assist with bite registration
(2) _____ wash, disinfect, and bag impressions   _____   _____

7 Dismiss the Patient (10 points)

(3) _____ clean up patient
(3) _____ lower chair, remove drape and bib
(2) _____ dismiss patient
(2) _____ make return appointment   _____   _____

8 Clean Up, Disinfect, and Sterilize (10 points)

(1) _____ gather contaminated materials and equipment
(1) _____ remove to sterilizing area
(1) _____ clean up operatory area
(1) _____ remove gloves, wash hands
(2) _____ record treatment, close bag, take impression to lab
(1) _____ don PPE
(1) _____ disinfect and sterilize equipment and materials
(1) _____ clean up area
(1) _____ wash, disinfect gloves, remove; wash hands   _____   _____

(100)   Total points   _____   _____

COMPETENCY EVALUATION SHEET

P R O C E D U R E 4 2

Assisting with Placement of Orthodontic Bands

Student Name _____ Date _____

GRADING PROTOCOL: Student is awarded the number of points indicated on the evaluation sheet for completing steps successfully.

Total possible points = 100 points
80% needed for passing = 80 points

Total points this test _____ pass _____ fail _____

	PEER REVIEW	TEACHER REVIEW

POINTS

1 Prepare for Banding Appointment (10 points)

(4) _____ assemble equipment and materials
(3) _____ assemble assorted orthodontic bands
(3) _____ prepare operatory area   _____   _____

2 Seat the Patient (5 points)

(1) _____ greet and seat patient
(2) _____ review health history
(1) _____ explain procedure
(1) _____ don PPE   _____   _____

3 Assist with Selection of Bands (25 points)

(1) _____ pass and receive explorer
(1) _____ pass and receive instrument to remove separators, if present
(2) _____ pass and receive air syringe for drying area
(2) _____ pass try in band, repeat until fit
(1) _____ pass and receive banding instruments as signaled
(2) _____ pass explorer for marking fitted band
(1) _____ pass and receive band remover
(2) _____ receive band, place in designated slot or pin on block
(1)_____ repeat procedure until all designated teeth are fitted
(1) _____ pass and receive air and water syringes as needed
(1) _____ maintain visibility and dry field
(2) _____ prepare patient rest period
(2) _____ check patient comfort
(2) _____ gather materials for lab
(2) _____ don overgloves
(1) _____ give reading or game material to occupy time
(1) _____ explain procedure, excuse self   _____   _____

4 Assist with Preparation of Bands (15 points)

(2) _____ prepare bands for cementation
(2) _____ smooth all band edges

(2) _____ place brackets on marked spot
(2) _____ polish bands
(2) _____ insert wax or pins in bracket openings
(2) _____ lubricate outside of bands
(3) _____ recheck band selection alignment   _____ _____

5 Assist with Crown Polish (10 points)

(2) _____ return materials and bands from lab, summon dentist
(2) _____ remove overgloves
(2) _____ pass handpiece with prophy cup and paste
(2) _____ pass or use syringe for rinse
(2) _____ pass and receive scaler, if needed   _____ _____

6 Assist with Cementation of Bands (15 points)

(2) _____ pass cotton rolls or loaded cotton roll holder
(2) _____ mix zinc phosphate cement according to manufacturer's directions
(2) _____ load band from gingival edge
(2) _____ place band on tape, pass to orthodontist
(2) _____ pass band pushing instruments, as needed
(2) _____ use wet sponge to clean instruments
(2) _____ repeat until all bands are seated
(1) _____ maintain visibility and clean field   _____ _____

7 Clean Up Patient and Dismiss (10 points)

(1) _____ monitor patient during setting time
(1) _____ remove isolation
(1) _____ check for permanent set, summon orthodontist
(1) _____ pass and receive scaler for cement removal
(1) _____ pass syringe for rinse
(1) _____ evacuate mouth with HVE
(1) _____ clean up patient's face
(1) _____ summon parent (if patient is child)
(1) _____ give hand mirror to patient for viewing bands, give postoperative and care
         instructions to patient and parent, demonstrate oral hygiene technique
(1) _____ dismiss patient   _____ _____

8 Clean Up, Disinfect, and Sterilize (10 points)

(1) _____ gather contaminated materials, take to sterilizing room
(1) _____ remove gloves, wash hands
(1) _____ record treatment, band sizes on patient's chart, take the chart to front desk
(1) _____ clean up instruments and materials
(1) _____ don utility gloves and PPE
(1) _____ disinfect large articles in operatory area
(1) _____ place disposables in proper container
(1) _____ clean and prepare instruments and bands for sterilization
(1) _____ clean up area
(1) _____ wash, disinfect gloves, remove; wash hands   _____ _____

(100)   Total points   _____ _____

COMPETENCY EVALUATION SHEET

P R O C E D U R E   4 3

Assisting with Cementation of Brackets

Student Name _____ Date _____

GRADING PROTOCOL: Student is awarded the number of points indicated on the evaluation sheet for completing steps successfully.

Total possible points = 100 points
80% needed for passing = 80 points

Total points this test _____ pass _____ fail _____

	PEER REVIEW	TEACHER REVIEW

POINTS

1 Assemble Equipment (10 points)

(4) _____ gather needed orthodontic appliances
(3) _____ assemble etching and cement materials
(3) _____ prepare operatory area

2 Prepare the Patient (10 points)

(3) _____ greet and seat patient
(3) _____ review health history
(2) _____ explain procedure
(2) _____ don PPE

3 Assist with Bonding Preparation (15 points)

(2) _____ pass and receive explorer to orthodontist for exam
(2) _____ pass handpiece with prophy angle and paste
(2) _____ pass or use syringe to spray rinse mouth
(2) _____ use HVE to evacuate mouth
(2) _____ pass syringe to air dry teeth
(3) _____ pass cotton rolls or loaded cotton roll holder for isolation
(2) _____ maintain visibility and dry field

4 Assist with Acid-Etch (20 points)

(3) _____ don overgloves for syringe use
(4) _____ prepare material, load applicator
(4) _____ pass applicator tip with gel etch
(3) _____ monitor timing
(3) _____ pass syringe for spray rinse
(3) _____ evacuate mouth, remove cotton rolls

5 Assist with Bracket and Tube Bonding (20 points)

(2) _____ pass cotton rolls for isolation
(2) _____ prepare activator material
(2) _____ pass brush with activator to orthodontist for tooth surface

(1) _____ hold syringe material to brush for refill
(2) _____ place activator material on bracket
　　　*If using plastic bracket, precondition.
(2) _____ place paste on bracket back
(2) _____ pass college pliers with bracket to orthodontist
(1) _____ receive college pliers and pass scaler to remove excess
(2) _____ repeat process for all brackets
(1) _____ remove overgloves and isolation
(1) _____ pass syringe for rinse spray
(2) _____ evacuate mouth　　　　　　　　　　　　　　　_____　_____

6 Clean Up Patient (10 points)

(2) _____ pass scaler for removal of excess bonding material
(1) _____ pass explorer for check
(2) _____ rinse and evacuate mouth
(1) _____ summon parent (if child patient)
(1) _____ give hand mirror to patient for viewing brackets
(2) _____ give instructions regarding care, hygiene, and nutrition
(1) _____ dismiss patient (if not applying arch wires)　　　_____　_____

7 Clean Up Operatory (5 points)

(1) _____ gather contaminated materials and equipment
(1) _____ remove to sterilizing area
(1) _____ remove gloves, wash hands
(1) _____ record treatment on patient's chart
(1) _____ take chart to front desk　　　　　　　　　　　_____　_____

8 Disinfect and Sterilize (10 points)

(1) _____ don utility gloves and PPE
(2) _____ disinfect operatory
(1) _____ discard disposables in proper container
(2) _____ clean and prepare instruments for sterilization
(1) _____ disinfect large articles
(2) _____ clean up area
(1) _____ wash, disinfect gloves, remove; wash hands　　_____　_____

(100)　　　Total points　　　　　　　　　　　　　　　　_____　_____

COMPETENCY EVALUATION SHEET

P R O C E D U R E   4 4

Assisting with Arch Wire and Ligature Placement

Student Name _____   Date _____

GRADING PROTOCOL: Student is awarded the number of points indicated on the evaluation sheet for completing steps successfully.

Total possible points = 100 points
80% needed for passing = 80 points

Total points this test _____   pass _____   fail _____

	PEER REVIEW	TEACHER REVIEW

POINTS

1 Assemble Equipment and Material (10 points)

(3) _____ gather necessary materials and equipment
(3) _____ prepare operatory area
(4) _____ review health history

2 Prepare the Patient (5 points)

(2) _____ greet and seat patient
(2) _____ review procedure
(1) _____ don PPE

3 Assist with Arch Wire Insertion (20 points)

(5) _____ pass and receive mirror for mouth exam
(8) _____ pass preformed arch wire in Howe pliers
(7) _____ maintain visibility and dry field

4 Assist with Ligature Placement (20 points)

(4) _____ receive Howe pliers
(4) _____ pass ligature wire
(4) _____ pass ligature tying pliers
(4) _____ receive ligature tying pliers
(4) _____ repeat process until all ligatures tied

5 Assist with Ligature Cut and Tuck (15 points)

(3) _____ pass ligature cutting pliers
(4) _____ receive ligature ends
(3) _____ pass ligature tucker or Schure tucker
(2) _____ receive ligature tucker
(1) _____ pass pliers for crimping ends
(2) _____ maintain visibility and dry field

6 Clean Up Patient (10 points)

(2) _____ rinse and evacuate mouth
(2) _____ give hygiene instructions

506

(2) _____ review nutrition and care instructions
(2) _____ reschedule for 3 to 4 weeks
(2) _____ dismiss patient   _____   _____

7 Clean Up Operatory, Disinfect, and Sterilize (20 points)

(2) _____ gather contaminated materials and equipment
(2) _____ take to sterilizing room
(2) _____ remove gloves, wash hands
(2) _____ record treatment on patient's chart
(2) _____ take chart to front desk
(2) _____ don utility gloves and PPE
(1) _____ disinfect operatory
(1) _____ dispose of contaminated disposables properly
(1) _____ disinfect large items
(2) _____ clean and prepare for sterilizing
(2) _____ clean up area
(1) _____ wash, disinfect gloves, remove; wash hands   _____   _____

(100)   Total points   _____   _____

COMPETENCY EVALUATION SHEET

PROCEDURE 45

Assisting with Arch Wire, Band, and Bracket Removal

Student Name _____ Date _____

GRADING PROTOCOL: Student is awarded the number of points indicated on the evaluation sheet for completing steps successfully.

Total possible points = 100 points
80% needed for passing = 80 points

Total points this test _____ pass _____ fail _____

	PEER REVIEW	TEACHER REVIEW

POINTS

1 Assemble Equipment and Materials, Prepare the Patient (10 points)

(2) _____ gather needed materials and equipment
(1) _____ prepare operatory
(1) _____ greet and seat patient
(2) _____ review health history
(1) _____ fit patient with protective glasses
(1) _____ explain procedure
(2) _____ don PPE, summon orthodontist   _____   _____

2 Assist with Ligature Wire Removal (15 points)

(3) _____ pass and receive mirror for mouth exam
(3) _____ pass scaler or hemostat instrument to recover ends
(2) _____ receive scaler and instrument
(2) _____ pass needleholder and wire-cutting instrument
(3) _____ hold gauze near site to accept wire pieces
(2) _____ receive needleholder and ligature wire cutters   _____   _____

3 Assist with Arch Wire Removal (10 points)

(3) _____ pass scaler or Schure instrument for arch wire release
(2) _____ receive scaler and Schure instrument
(2) _____ pass Howe pliers for arch wire removal
(3) _____ receive arch wire and Howe pliers   _____   _____

4 Assist with Band and Bracket Removal (15 points)

(5) _____ pass ligature cutter pliers for bracket removal; hold gauze near site to receive brackets
(5) _____ pass band removal pliers; hold gauze near site to receive bands
(3) _____ pass Schure instrument
(2) _____ receive bands   _____   _____

5 Assist with Cement Removal (10 points)

(1) _____ pass syringe for spray rinse
(2) _____ evacuate mouth with HVE

(2) _____ pass scaler for cement removal
(1) _____ pass tuned ultrasonic scaler, if requested
(1) _____ maintain visibility and dry field
(1) _____ pass slow handpiece with prophy cup and fluoridated paste
(2) _____ rinse and evacuate mouth   _____   _____

6 Assist with Impression (15 points)

(1) _____ pass trays for selection
(1) _____ adapt trays with wax
(2) _____ mix material as specified
(2) _____ fill tray and pass to orthodontist
(2) _____ receive tray and pass syringe for rinse
(2) _____ rinse, disinfect tray, store in plastic bag
(1) _____ repeat process for other arch
(2) _____ soften base plate wax, pass for bite registration
(1) _____ receive wax, rinse, disinfect, and store in bag
(1) _____ pass syringe for spray rinse, evacuate   _____   _____

7 Assist with Photographs (10 points)

(3) _____ place prepared ID card on patient's neck
(2) _____ insert cheek retractors
(2) _____ expose full face view
(3) _____ repeat procedure for each side view   _____   _____

8 Clean Up and Dismiss Patient (5 points)

(1) _____ clean patient's face
(1) _____ give mirror for patient to view teeth
(2) _____ review hygiene instructions
(1) _____ dismiss patient   _____   _____

9 Clean Up, Disinfect, and Sterilize (10 points)

(1) _____ gather contaminated instruments and materials, take to sterilizing room
(1) _____ remove gloves, wash hands, copy notes and treatment onto patient's
           chart, take chart to front desk
(2) _____ don utility gloves and PPE
(2) _____ disinfect operatory area
(1) _____ place disposables in proper container, disinfect large items
(2) _____ clean and prepare instruments for sterilization, clean up area
(1) _____ wash, disinfect gloves, remove; wash hands   _____   _____

(100)   Total points   _____   _____

COMPETENCY EVALUATION SHEET

PROCEDURE 46

Assisting with Multiple Extractions and Suture Removal

Student Name _____ Date _____

GRADING PROTOCOL: Student is awarded the number of points indicated on the evaluation sheet for completing steps
successfully.

Total possible points = 100 points
80% needed for passing = 80 points

Total points this test _____   pass _____   fail _____

	PEER REVIEW	TEACHER REVIEW

POINTS

Multiple Extractions

1 Assemble Equipment and Materials (10 points)

(2) _____ prepare operatory
(2) _____ use aseptic technique
(1) _____ check equipment
(1) _____ gather emergency equipment
(2) _____ place x-rays on viewer
(2) _____ review surgical plan   _____   _____

2 Prepare the Patient (10 points)

(1) _____ seat and position patient
(1) _____ review health and medical history
(1) _____ administer premedication
(1) _____ drape and bib patient
(1) _____ surgical scrub patient's face
(1) _____ explain procedure
(1) _____ don surgical coat, mask, eyewear
(2) _____ perform surgical scrub of hands
(1) _____ don sterile surgical gloves   _____   _____

3 Assist with Anesthesia (5 points)

(2) _____ administer topical anesthesia
(1) _____ summon surgeon
(1) _____ receive applicators, pass and receive anesthetic syringe
(1) _____ monitor patient reaction to injection   _____   _____

4 Assist with Extraction of Teeth (10 points)

(1) _____ pass and receive explorer to surgeon to test anesthetic stage
(1) _____ pass elevator for loosening of teeth
(1) _____ evacuate area of blood and debris
(1) _____ receive elevator

(1) _____ pass correct forceps for tooth extraction
(1) _____ receive forceps and tooth
(1) _____ aspirate socket and area
(1) _____ pass other forceps as signaled
(1) _____ repeat processes
(1) _____ maintain visibility and dry field   _____ _____

5 Assist with Alveoplasty (10 points)

(2) _____ pass scalpel to surgeon to incise gingiva
(2) _____ receive scalpel, pass periosteal elevator to retract tissues
(1) _____ aspirate area to maintain visibility and fluid control
(2) _____ receive elevator, pass rongeurs to remove bone crests, or receive elevator,
           pass handpiece with surgical bur
(1) _____ receive rongeurs or handpiece, pass bone file for smoothing
(1) _____ pass or use hemostat to retrieve bone spicules
(1) _____ aspirate or dab with sterile gauze   _____ _____

6 Assist with Artificial Clot Material (If Needed) (5 points)

(2) _____ pass cotton pliers with artificial clot material
(2) _____ hold medicine cup with excess material near site for refill
(1) _____ receive cotton pliers   _____ _____

7 Assist with Suturing (10 points)

(1) _____ dab surgical area with sterile gauze
(1) _____ aspirate throat for fluid control
(2) _____ pass tissue forceps and loaded needleholder
(2) _____ hold suture thread tails high off patient's face
(2) _____ use scissors to cut where indicated
(2) _____ repeat procedures until suturing finished   _____ _____

8 Clean Up and Dismiss Patient (5 points)

(1) _____ pass syringe for spray rinse, evacuate area
(1) _____ pass gauze pads for patient to bite on
(1) _____ wipe patient's face, remove drape and bib, summon patient's companion
(1) _____ give postoperative instructions to patient and friend
(1) _____ dismiss patient   _____ _____

9 Clean Up, Disinfect, and Sterilize (10 points)

(2) _____ gather material and equipment, remove to sterilizing room
(2) _____ remove gloves; wash hands, record treatment, medications, and sutures
           on patient's chart; take chart to front desk
(2) _____ don utility gloves and PPE
(2) _____ disinfect, sterilize, clean up
(2) _____ wash gloves, disinfect, remove; wash hands   _____ _____

Removal of Sutures

10 Assemble Materials and Equipment, Prepare the Patient (5 points)

(1) _____ prepare operatory
(1) _____ check patient's chart, prepare patient

(1) _____ review health history
(1) _____ explain procedure
(1) _____ don PPE   _____   _____

11 Remove Sutures (10 points)

(1) _____ inspect surgical area
(1) _____ rinse mouth
(1) _____ disinfect area with wet applicator
(1) _____ use pick ups to locate suture ends
(1) _____ insert suture scissors under suture near gingiva
(1) _____ incise away from knot, near gingiva
(1) _____ use pick ups to lift suture from area
(1) _____ repeat until all removed
(1) _____ inspect site, count sutures
(1) _____ rinse mouth   _____   _____

12 Clean Up the Patient, Area, Equipment, and Materials (10 points)

(2) _____ clean patient's face
(1) _____ pass mirror to surgeon for exam
(1) _____ dismiss patient
(1) _____ gather instruments, remove to sterilizing room
(1) _____ remove gloves, wash hands, record treatment on chart
(1) _____ don utility gloves and PPE
(2) _____ disinfect, sterilize, clean up
(1) _____ wash, disinfect, and remove gloves; wash hands   _____   _____

(100)   Total points   _____   _____

COMPETENCY EVALUATION SHEET

PROCEDURE 47

Assisting with Minor Tissue Surgery

Student Name _____ Date _____

GRADING PROTOCOL: Student is awarded the number of points indicated on the evaluation sheet for completing steps
successfully.

Total possible points = 100 points
80% needed for passing = 80 points

Total points this test _____ pass _____ fail _____

	PEER REVIEW	TEACHER REVIEW

POINTS

Dry Socket (Alveolitis)

1 Complete Preparations (5 points)

(2) _____ assemble equipment and materials
(1) _____ maintain sterile technique
(1) _____ prepare patient
(1) _____ don PPE   _____   _____

2 Assist with Local Anesthesia (6 points)

(1) _____ rinse mouth, gauze dry injection site
(1) _____ administer topical anesthesia
(1) _____ receive applicators
(1) _____ pass and receive anesthetic syringe
(1) _____ recap needle with one-handed motion or
              recap device
(1) _____ monitor patient reaction   _____   _____

3 Assist with Curettage (10 points)

(2) _____ pass and receive mirror for examination
(2) _____ pass syringe of saline or peroxide
(1) _____ aspirate area
(2) _____ pass curette for excavation
(1) _____ aspirate if signaled or dab area with sterile gauze
(2) _____ receive curette, pass cotton pliers with artificial clot   _____   _____

4 Assist with Suturing (6 points)

(2) _____ pass tissue forceps, needleholder with suture
(1) _____ hold suture thread off patient's chin
(1) _____ cut thread when and where indicated
(1) _____ receive tissue forceps, needleholder, and suture needle
(1) _____ blot area with sterile gauze   _____   _____

5 Clean Up the Patient, Area, and Equipment (5 points)

(1) _____ place sterile gauze pad on site
(1) _____ instruct patient to bite on pad
(1) _____ give postoperative instructions
(1) _____ clean patient's face, dismiss
(1) _____ clean up in usual manner   _____ _____

Incision and Drainage (I&D)

6 Complete Preparations (5 points)

(2) _____ assemble equipment and materials
(1) _____ maintain sterile technique
(1) _____ prepare patient
(1) _____ don PPE   _____ _____

7 Assist with Anesthesia (5 points)

(1) _____ rinse mouth, gauze dry injection area
(1) _____ swab surrounding area with topical anesthetic
(1) _____ pass and receive anesthetic syringe
(1) _____ recap needle with one-handed motion or recap device
(1) _____ monitor patient reaction   _____ _____

8 Assist with Incision and Drainage (10 points)

(1) _____ pass and receive mirror for exam
(2) _____ pass and receive scalpel for incision
(2) _____ pass and receive hemostat for opening enlargement
(2) _____ aspirate exudate and matter from wound
(2) _____ pass college pliers with drain material to surgeon
(1) _____ receive college pliers   _____ _____

9 Assist with Suturing (5 points)

(1) _____ pass tissue forceps and needleholder with suture
(2) _____ assist with suturing of drain
(1) _____ cut suture thread
(1) _____ receive tissue forceps, needleholder, and suture needle   _____ _____

10 Clean Up the Patient, Area, and Equipment (6 points)

(1) _____ aspirate and empty mouth
(1) _____ rinse mouth
(2) _____ give postoperative instructions
(1) _____ clean up patient, dismiss
(1) _____ clean up in usual manner   _____ _____

Biopsy

11 Complete Preparations (5 points)

(2) _____ assemble materials and equipment
(1) _____ maintain sterile technique
(1) _____ prepare patient
(1) _____ don PPE   _____ _____

12 Assist with Anesthesia (6 points)

(1) _____ rinse mouth, gauze dry injection area
(1) _____ administer topical anesthesia
(1) _____ pass and receive anesthetic syringe
(1) _____ recap needle with one-handed motion or recap device
(1) _____ pass indelible pencil for marking
(1) _____ monitor patient reaction   _____   _____

13 Assist with Biopsy (10 points)

(1) _____ pass and receive mirror for examination
(1) _____ rinse and evacuate mouth
(2) _____ pass tissue forceps and scalpel
(1) _____ aspirate as needed
(2) _____ collect specimen in bottle
(2) _____ receive tissue forceps and scalpel
(1) _____ assist with suturing, if needed   _____   _____

14 Clean Up Patient, Area, and Equipment (6 points)

(1) _____ swab area with sterile gauze
(1) _____ pack area with sterile gauze
(2) _____ give postoperative instructions
(1) _____ clean up patient, dismiss
(1) _____ clean up, disinfect, and sterilize as usual   _____   _____

15 Prepare Biopsy for Laboratory (10 points)

(2) _____ check labeling on bottle
(2) _____ fill out biopsy form
(1) _____ complete all information
(2) _____ wrap form with bottle, encase
(1) _____ take or send biopsy to lab
(1) _____ record treatment and shipment on patient's chart
(1) _____ place patient name and date on biopsy sheet   _____   _____

(100)   Total points   _____   _____

COMPETENCY EVALUATION SHEET

P R O C E D U R E   4 8

Assisting with Periodontal Exam and Prophylaxis

Student Name _____ Date _____

GRADING PROTOCOL: Student is awarded the number of points indicated on the evaluation sheet for completing steps successfully.

Total possible points = 100 points
80% needed for passing = 80 points

Total points this test _____ pass _____ fail _____

	PEER REVIEW	TEACHER REVIEW

POINTS

Examination

1 Complete Preparations (5 points)

(2) _____ assemble equipment and materials
(1) _____ prepare operatory
(2) _____ prepare patient   _____   _____

2 Assist with Interview (10 points)

(2) _____ record health and medical history
(2) _____ record diet and nutrition questionnaire
(2) _____ record lifestyle and habits
(2) _____ don plastic gloves
(2) _____ expose intra- and extraoral photographs   _____   _____

3 Assist with Clinical Examination (10 points)

(2) _____ don PPE
(2) _____ rinse and evacuate mouth
(2) _____ pass mirror, record oral tissue survey
(2) _____ record plaque index
(2) _____ record calculus rating   _____   _____

4 Assist with Radiographs (10 points)

(5) _____ pass or expose radiographs, as requested
(5) _____ don overgloves, process radiographs   _____   _____

5 Assist with Periodontal Probing (10 points)

(2) _____ pass periodontal probe
(2) _____ pass or use syringe for air spray, as requested
(3) _____ record findings
(3) _____ plot crest line   _____   _____

6 Assist with Mobility Testing (5 points)

(2) _____ record tooth finding
(1) _____ receive mirror and probe

(1) _____ rinse and dry with syringe, as requested
(1) _____ evacuate as needed   _____   _____

Prophylaxis

7 Assist with Anesthesia (5 points)

(1) _____ pass mouthwash solution
(4) _____ swab area with local anesthesia solution, or pass and
receive anesthetic syringe, recap   _____   _____

8 Assist with Scaling (10 points)

(2) _____ swab area with disinfectant
(1) _____ pass mirror and scaler (hand or "tuned" ultrasonic)
(2) _____ exchange disinfected instrument or tips, as requested
(2) _____ evacuate as needed
(1) _____ pass or use air syringe as requested
(2) _____ rinse and evacuate as requested   _____   _____

9 Assist with Curettage (10 points)

(2) _____ receive scaler, pass curette
(2) _____ exchange instruments as requested
(2) _____ disinfect instruments on exchange
(2) _____ pass or use syringe for air dry and rinse
(2) _____ evacuate as needed   _____   _____

10 Assist with Root Planing (10 points)

(5) _____ pass instruments as requested
(3) _____ maintain visibility and dry field with syringe
(2) _____ rinse and evacuate mouth   _____   _____

11 Assist with Polish of Teeth (5 points)

(1) _____ pass handpiece with prophy angle and paste, hold excess paste close to work site
(1) _____ pass air polisher handpiece and tip
(1) _____ rinse and evacuate as needed
(1) _____ pass and receive dental floss or tape for interproximals
(1) _____ pass or receive perio-aids as requested   _____   _____

12 Clean Up and Dismiss Patient (5 points)

(1) _____ rinse and evacuate mouth, pass mouthwash
(1) _____ give postoperative instructions
(1) _____ give home hygiene instructions
(1) _____ clean patient's face
(1) _____ dismiss patient   _____   _____

13 Clean Up Area, Disinfect, and Sterilize (5 points)

(1) _____ gather contaminated materials and equipment, take to sterilizing room, remove gloves, wash hands
(1) _____ record treatment on patient's chart
(1) _____ don utility gloves, PPE
(1) _____ clean, disinfect, sterilize
(1) _____ wash, disinfect gloves, remove; wash hands   _____   _____

(100)   Total points   _____   _____

COMPETENCY EVALUATION SHEET

PROCEDURE 49

Assisting with Gingivectomy and Removal of Periodontal Packing

Student Name _____   Date _____

GRADING PROTOCOL: Student is awarded the number of points indicated on the evaluation sheet for completing steps successfully.

Total possible points = 100 points
80% needed for passing = 80 points

Total points this test _____   pass _____   fail _____

	PEER REVIEW	TEACHER REVIEW

POINTS

Packing Placement

1 Complete Preparations (10 points)

(1) _____ prepare operatory, preset trays
(1) _____ check equipment
(1) _____ prepare patient
(1) _____ premedicate patient (if prescribed)
(1) _____ seat and position
(1) _____ scrub patient's face
(1) _____ explain procedure
(1) _____ don PPE
(1) _____ surgical scrub
(1) _____ don surgical gloves   _____   _____

2 Assist with Anesthesia (10 points)

(2) _____ rinse mouth, gauze dry injection site
(2) _____ administer topical anesthesia
(3) _____ pass and receive local anesthetic syringe
(2) _____ recap with one-handed technique or appliance
(1) _____ adjust mask for analgesia (if needed)   _____   _____

3 Assist with Gingivectomy Procedure (15 points)

(1) _____ pass mirror for exam and explorer to test anesthesia
(2) _____ receive explorer and pass indelible pencil for marking, or pass periodontal pocket marker
(1) _____ receive pencil or marker, pass gauze for packing area
(2) _____ pass gingival knife or scalpel
(1) _____ aspirate fluids, maintain visibility
(2) _____ receive knife, pass periosteal elevator
(1) _____ use hemostat to pick tissue flaps
(2) _____ pass cotton pliers, tissue scissors
(1) _____ receive tissue instruments
(2) _____ pass scaler, curette instruments as requested, blot and aspirate as needed   _____   _____

4 Prepare Periodontal Packing Material (5 points)

(1) _____ don plastic overgloves
(2) _____ mix materials, knead, roll
*Sutures may be requested, if heavy bleeding occurs.

(1) _____ pass needleholder with suture, tissue pick ups
(1) _____ use suture scissors to cut suture   _____ _____

5 Assist with Placement of Packing Material (10 points)

(1) _____ aspirate and blot dry with gauze
(1) _____ pass dressing roll
(2) _____ pass PFI instruments
(1) _____ evacuate mouth, maintain visibility
(1) _____ pass gauze for adaptation
(2) _____ pass scaler for dressing trim
(2) _____ aspirate mouth, remove excess packing   _____ _____

6 Clean Up and Instruct Patient (10 points)

(2) _____ pass foil or plastic wrap for covering
(2) _____ pass burnisher for adaptation
(1) _____ rinse mouth, evacuate
(2) _____ clean up patient
(2) _____ give postoperative instructions
(1) _____ dismiss patient   _____ _____

7 Clean Up Area, Disinfect, and Sterilize (10 points)

(3) _____ gather instruments and materials
(2) _____ remove gloves, wash hands, record treatment on chart
(3) _____ don utility gloves; clean, disinfect, and sterilize
(2) _____ wash, disinfect, remove gloves; wash hands   _____ _____

Packing Removal

8 Complete Preparations (5 points)

(2) _____ assemble equipment and materials
(2) _____ prepare patient
(1) _____ don PPE   _____ _____

9 Assist with Removal of Packing (15 points)

(2) _____ pass mirror for exam
(3) _____ pass or use syringe for rinse, evacuate
(3) _____ pass scaler for removal of packing
(3) _____ receive packing pieces
(2) _____ pass or use syringe for spray rinse and evacuate
(2) _____ remove sutures if previously placed   _____ _____

10 Clean Up Patient, Disinfect, and Sterilize (10 points)

(2) _____ wash patient face
(1) _____ dismiss patient
(2) _____ gather instruments to sterilizing room
(2) _____ remove gloves, wash hands, record treatment on chart
(2) _____ don utility gloves; disinfect, sterilize, and clean up
(1) _____ wash gloves, disinfect, remove; wash hands   _____ _____

(100)   Total points   _____ _____

COMPETENCY EVALUATION SHEET

PROCEDURE 50

Fabrication of Study Models

Student Name _____ Date _____

GRADING PROTOCOL: Student is awarded the number of points indicated on the evaluation sheet for completing steps successfully.

Total possible points = 100 points
80% needed for passing = 80 points

Total points this test _____ pass _____ fail _____

	PEER REVIEW	TEACHER REVIEW

POINTS

1 Assemble Equipment and Materials (10 points)

(3) _____ gather bagged impressions and registration
(4) _____ assemble materials and equipment
(3) _____ obtain vibrator, mixing slabs   _____ _____

2 Don PPE (5 points)

(2) _____ don gloves
(1) _____ don mask if using spray
(2) _____ wear apron or lab coat   _____ _____

3 Disinfect Impressions and Bite Registration (15 points)

(4) _____ remove items slowly from bag
(4) _____ spray surfaces or immerse in disinfectant
(4) _____ check for cleanliness; mix slurry, if needed
(3) _____ dab dry moisture   _____ _____

4 Mix Gypsum Product (15 points)

(2) _____ select proper gypsum material
(3) _____ select correct water and powder ratio
(2) _____ dampen mixing bowl, fill with measured water dose
(3) _____ measure powder and add to water, allow for absorption
(2) _____ mix materials to smooth consistency
(3) _____ vibrate material   _____ _____

5 Pour Gypsum into Impression (15 points)

(3) _____ hold impression tray at angle on vibrator or table top
(3) _____ use spatula to carry mixture to area behind last molar
(3) _____ flow mixture into teeth indentations forcing air forward
(3) _____ continue flow pattern until all teeth indentations are filled
(3) _____ fill remainder of impression   _____ _____

6   Make Art Base Form (15 points)

(3) _____ place base former on vibrator, fill; or place remaining gypsum mixture on slab in pile slightly larger than poured impression

(3) _____ invert impression tray, filled with gypsum mixture, onto pile or into center of filled base former

(3) _____ keep impression tray handle parallel to floor

(3) _____ smooth edges, unite two mixes

(3) _____ keep tray clean of excess wet gypsum mixture   _____   _____

7   Repeat Process for Other Arch (10 points)

(10) _____ smooth out tongue space or fill in space on mandibular arch   _____   _____

8   Identify Study Models (5 points)

(3) _____ mark with identification tags

(2) _____ set aside to harden   _____   _____

9   Clean Up Work Site and Equipment (10 points)

(2) _____ dispose of excess gypsum mixture in waste receptacle

(2) _____ wash and disinfect equipment, return to proper location

(1) _____ wipe up area with paper towels

(2) _____ spray area with disinfectant and wipe with towels

(1) _____ dispose of towels and litter in proper waste bag

(1) _____ wash eyeglasses with soap and water, spray disinfectant

(1) _____ remove and dispose of gloves, wash hands   _____   _____

(100)   Total points   _____   _____

COMPETENCY EVALUATION SHEET

PROCEDURE 51

Separation of Models and Impression

Student Name _____ Date _____

GRADING PROTOCOL: Student is awarded the number of points indicated on the evaluation sheet for completing steps successfully.

Total possible points = 100 points
80% needed for passing = 80 points

Total points this test _____ pass _____ fail _____

| | PEER REVIEW | TEACHER REVIEW |

POINTS

1 Assemble Materials and Equipment (10 points)

(3) _____ gather gypsum models
(3) _____ check temperature and hardness
(4) _____ assemble equipment

2 Don PPE (15 points)

(5) _____ don lab coat or apron
(5) _____ don safety glasses
(5) _____ don overgloves

3 Examine Models (15 points)

(5) _____ wait for at least one hour from pour up
(5) _____ test temperature of gypsum surface
(5) _____ attempt knife tip puncture to test firmness

4 Release Gypsum and Impression Materials (15 points)

(4) _____ clean off excess gypsum material from tray
(4) _____ insert knife tip between model and impression, twist
(4) _____ permit air pocket between materials
(3) _____ insert knife tip at various angles to loosen materials

5 Remove Impression Material (15 points)

(5) _____ raise impression material up from model
(5) _____ avoid twisting to prevent breaking off teeth
(5) _____ use knife tip to remove any impression debris from interproximal areas

6 Identify Models (15 points)

(5) _____ write patient's name on models
(5) _____ inspect for correctness and suitability
(5) _____ prepare for trimming, set aside

7 Cleanup Procedures (15 points)

(2) _____ wipe up gypsum debris, place in waste receptacle
(2) _____ clean impression tray with knife to remove impression material
(2) _____ wash impression tray and prepare for sterilization
(3) _____ wipe up table tops with disinfectant and paper towel
(2) _____ dispose of papers and litter properly
(2) _____ wash eyeglasses, gloves
(2) _____ remove gloves, wash hands   _____   _____

(100)   Total points   _____   _____

COMPETENCY EVALUATION SHEET

PROCEDURE 52

Trimming Gypsum Models

Student Name _____ Date _____

GRADING PROTOCOL: Student is awarded the number of points indicated on the evaluation sheet for completing steps successfully.

Total possible points = 100 points
80% needed for passing = 80 points

Total points this test _____ pass _____ fail _____

	PEER REVIEW	TEACHER REVIEW

POINTS

1 Assemble Materials and Equipment (5 points)

(2) _____ assemble equipment, trimmer
(3) _____ gather rough study models, bite registration   _____   _____

2 Don PPE (5 points)

(2) _____ don safety glasses
(1) _____ remove jewelry
(1) _____ tie hair back
(1) _____ don overgloves   _____   _____

3 Prepare Model Trimmer (5 points)

(1) _____ set trimming table parallel to floor
(2) _____ turn on machine
(2) _____ adjust water flow   _____   _____

4 Trim Maxillary Base Cut (5 points)

(1) _____ $1\frac{1}{2}$ times anatomic portion
(1) _____ set biting edge on table
(1) _____ mark base line edge evenly around art base
(1) _____ place on trimming table, remove excess gypsum to line
(1) _____ check for smoothness and straightness   _____   _____

5 Trim Maxillary Posterior Cut (10 points)

(1) _____ set model on table top with teeth side up
(2) _____ place plain compass point interproximal of centrals
(2) _____ extend compass to $\frac{1}{4}$ inch beyond molars, mark in tuberosity area
(1) _____ draw line out from central occlusal groove of molars to form X
(2) _____ draw straight line between two Xs
(2) _____ trim to line, should be smooth and straight   _____   _____

6 Trim Maxillary Lateral Cuts (10 points)

(2) _____ set model on trimmer tray with teeth side up
(3) _____ mark central occlusal grooves of premolars with pencil or stick
(3) _____ trim lateral gypsum parallel to mark $\frac{1}{8}$ to $\frac{1}{4}$ inch of fold
(2) _____ do both sides, should be even, smooth, and straight   _____   _____

7 Trim Maxillary Heel Cuts (5 points)

(1) _____ set model on trimmer tray with teeth up
(1) _____ place posterior corner of model next to trim wheel

(1) _____ trim to ¼ inch of molar area perpendicular to opposite canine
(1) _____ trim other corner in the same manner
(1) _____ check for smoothness and straightness

8 Trim Maxillary Anterior Cut (10 points)

(2) _____ set model on trimmer tray with teeth side up
(2) _____ mark from facial center of canines
(2) _____ mark from central interproximals of facial side
(2) _____ trim in straight line from canine to central to canine
(2) _____ form anterior arch, should be smooth and straight

9 Trim Mandibular Posterior Cut (5 points)

(1) _____ place models in occlusion, use bite registration form
(1) _____ mark mandibular model ½ inch longer than maxillary posterior
(1) _____ trim excess gypsum to first cut line
(1) _____ occlude models again, mark mandibular same as maxillary back
(1) _____ trim in occlusion, should be smooth and straight

10 Trim Mandibular Base Cut (5 points)

(1) _____ set models in occlusion with maxillary on bottom
(2) _____ compass mark line parallel to table, even distance from maxillary
(2) _____ trim to line, should be smooth and straight

11 Trim Mandibular Lateral Cuts (5 points)

(2) _____ set models in occlusion
(3) _____ trim to match, should be smooth and straight

12 Trim Mandibular Heel Cuts (5 points)

(2) _____ set models in occlusion
(3) _____ trim to match, even on both corners, smooth and straight

13 Trim Mandibular Anterior Cut (5 points)

(1) _____ set mandibular model on trimmer with teeth up
(2) _____ rotate anterior edge to form smooth arch between canines
(2) _____ trim smoothly and evenly

14 Finish Models (10 points)

(1) _____ remove overhangs and bumps with knife
(2) _____ sandpaper scratch and rough areas
(2) _____ smooth tongue area with knife, rasp, or sandpaper
(2) _____ fill in voids and holes with gypsum material
(1) _____ soak in soap solution for 30 minutes (after gypsum patch is dry)
(2) _____ rinse and buff with smooth cloth

15 Identify Models (5 points)

(2) _____ mark with patient's name
(2) _____ mark with date
(1) _____ write case number (if applicable)

16 Cleanup Procedures (5 points)

(1) _____ clean all equipment and sterilize impression trays
(2) _____ clean model trimmer
(1) _____ clean work area and return materials and equipment
(1) _____ wash hands, replace jewelry, loosen hair

(100) _____ Total points

COMPETENCY EVALUATION SHEET

PROCEDURE 53

Articulation of Study Models

Student Name _____ Date _____

GRADING PROTOCOL: Student is awarded the number of points indicated on the evaluation sheet for completing steps successfully.

Total possible points = 100 points
80% needed for passing = 80 points

Total points this test _____   pass _____   fail _____

	PEER REVIEW	TEACHER REVIEW

POINTS

1 Assemble Equipment and Materials (10 points)

(4) _____ gather models, bite registration
(3) _____ assemble clean articulator
(3) _____ gather gypsum materials and equipment

2 Soap Model Bases (10 points)

(10) _____ paint bottom of model bases for separation or soak in pan of soap solution

3 Stabilize Models (15 points)

(3) _____ place models in occlusion using bite registration
(3) _____ bond teeth in occluded pattern
(3) _____ check alignment
(6) _____ place sticky wax drops to hold teeth in occlusion, or band models
while in occlusion

4 Assemble Articulator (10 points)

(5) _____ prepare maxillary plate, check for cleanliness and function
(5) _____ prepare mandibular plate, check for same

5 Prepare Gypsum Mixture (15 points)

(8) _____ mix gypsum to heavy, creamy consistency
(7) _____ mix for smooth texture, no large air bubbles

6 Place Models on the Articulator (20 points)

(4) _____ place gypsum pile on mandibular tray, plate, or ring
(4) _____ engage mandibular model in gypsum pile, should be even and
parallel to the floor
(2) _____ measure maxillary plate to fit articulating model
(4) _____ place wet gypsum on top of maxillary model
(4) _____ engage maxillary tray, plate, or ring into gypsum mixture
(2) _____ smooth all soft gypsum, remove excess

7 Test Articulation (10 points)

(2) _____ models parallel to table top
(2) _____ models evenly set
(2) _____ elastic band cut off
(2) _____ remove bite registration
(2) _____ check articulation pattern and function   _____   _____

8 Cleanup Procedures (10 points)

(4) _____ place excess unused gypsum mix in waste, not sink
(2) _____ clean work area, replace equipment
(2) _____ set marked articulated models aside to dry
(2) _____ wash hands   _____   _____

(100)   Total points   _____   _____

COMPETENCY EVALUATION SHEET

PROCEDURE 54

Construction of Base Plates and Occlusal Rims

Student Name _____ Date _____

GRADING PROTOCOL: Student is awarded the number of points indicated on the evaluation sheet for completing steps
successfully.

Total possible points = 100 points
80% needed for passing = 80 points

Total points this test _____ pass _____ fail _____

	PEER REVIEW	TEACHER REVIEW

POINTS

1 Assemble Equipment and Material (5 points)

(3) _____ gather material and equipment
(2) _____ tie hair back   _____   _____

2 Prepare the Edentulous Models (5 points)

(2) _____ check for any specific instructions from dentist
(1) _____ check model for smoothness
(1) _____ mark indelible pencil line for denture fit
(1) _____ powder model for easy wax removal   _____   _____

3 Adapt the Base Plate to the Edentulous Model (10 points)

(4) _____ heat wax to pliable, soft state
(3) _____ drape sheet wax over edentulous model
(3) _____ finger press or pressure wax to fit form   _____   _____

4 Trim Excessive Wax (10 points)

(5) _____ cut wax ⅛ to ¼ inch from edge of model
(5) _____ bend excess flap upward   _____   _____

5 Contour Wax Sheet into Muccobuccal Fold (10 points)

(4) _____ use pencil eraser edge, push excess wax close to model in fold
(3) _____ fold remainder wax and press against base plate
(3) _____ check for inside smoothness of base plate   _____   _____

6 Place Occlusal Rim on the Plate (10 points)

(4) _____ soften commercial occlusal rim in warm water, or construct rim by
folding base plate wax to rim dimensions
(3) _____ shape occlusal rim to contour of base plate
(3) _____ center rim over bite ridge of base plate   _____   _____

530

7. Fill Space Between the Rim and Plate (10 points)

(5) _____ melt trimmed excess base plate wax to fill gaps and spaces between rim and plate

(5) _____ smooth sides of plate and rim to even surface   _____   _____

8. Cut Heel Slant (10 points)

(2) _____ warm knife for smooth cut

(3) _____ use knife to slice off back edge of rim

(5) _____ cut on diagonal   _____   _____

9. Level Occlusal Surface (5 points)

(2) _____ heat glass slab or large surface putty knife

(3) _____ set heated glass slab on occlusal surface, parallel to floor   _____   _____

10. Finish Plate and Occlusal Rims (10 points)

(4) _____ smooth all sides of rims with warm spatula

(4) _____ buff wax rims and plate to gloss finish

(2) _____ check inside of plate for any roughness   _____   _____

11. Prepare Opposite Arch in Similar Manner (10 points)

(3) _____ construct base plate for opposite arch

(3) _____ construct occlusal rims for opposite arch

(4) _____ complete set in same manner   _____   _____

12. Cleanup Procedures (5 points)

(2) _____ clean up area and replace equipment

(2) _____ leave lab area in proper condition

(1) _____ wash hands   _____   _____

(100)   Total points   _____   _____

COMPETENCY EVALUATION SHEET

P R O C E D U R E   5 5

Construction of Custom Trays

Student Name _____ Date _____

GRADING PROTOCOL: Student is awarded the number of points indicated on the evaluation sheet for completing steps successfully.

Total possible points = 100 points
80% needed for passing = 80 points

Total points this test _____ pass _____ fail _____

| | PEER REVIEW | TEACHER REVIEW |

POINTS

1 Assemble Materials and Equipment (10 points)

(4) _____ have ventilated area
(3) _____ gather equipment
(3) _____ assemble materials and models   _____   _____

2 Prepare Models (10 points)

(2) _____ note any instruction for adaptation from dentist
(4) _____ mark denture base plate line with indelible pencil
(4) _____ dust model with powder   _____   _____

3 Place Spacer on Model (10 points)

(2) _____ warm base plate wax to softened condition
(2) _____ drape wax over edentulous model and contour to form
(2) _____ trim excess wax from sides to indelible mark
(2) _____ paint spacer with foil cote or separating medium
(2) _____ place stops if desired by dentist   _____   _____

4 Prepare Tray Material (10 points)

(3) _____ warm dough in hot water, compress into shape, or measure liquid and add to measured acrylic powder
(3) _____ use stick to moisten and mix materials
(2) _____ let mixture set to doughy stage
(2) _____ use greased fingers to form wafer   _____   _____

5 Contour Acrylic Wafer (10 points)

(2) _____ drape wafer over edentulous model
(3) _____ press onto model with wax plate for tight fit
(3) _____ trim excess pressed material off edge with lab knife
(2) _____ finger smooth edges to avoid roughness   _____   _____

6 Attach Handle (10 points)

(3) _____ form trimmed excess material into small handle shape
(3) _____ bend handle to allow space for lip closure
(3) _____ attach handle onto tray material while soft and pliable
(1) _____ allow material to harden   _____   _____

7 Remove Tray from Model (10 points)

(5) _____ check dentist's order to remove or not remove spacer
(5) _____ check for roughness, overhangs, thickness, voids   _____   _____

8 Smooth Tray Edges (10 points)

(4) _____ don safety glasses
(3) _____ use bench engine, slow handpiece, or dental lathe with acrylic
             burs and wheels
(3) _____ use sandpaper, emery cloth, or disks to smooth   _____   _____

9 Identify Trays (10 points)

(5) _____ mark with patient's name and date
(5) _____ clean tray for future use   _____   _____

10 Cleanup Procedures (10 points)

(4) _____ clean up area, material, and equipment
(3) _____ restore lab to proper condition
(3) _____ wash hands   _____   _____

(100)   Total points   _____   _____

COMPETENCY EVALUATION SHEET

P R O C E D U R E   5 6

Assisting with Fabrication of Temporary Crowns

Student Name _____ Date _____

GRADING PROTOCOL: Student is awarded the number of points indicated on the evaluation sheet for completing steps
successfully.

Total possible points = 100 points
80% needed for passing = 80 points

Total points this test _____ pass _____ fail _____

	PEER REVIEW	TEACHER REVIEW

POINTS

1 Complete the Preparations (10 points)

(3) _____ assemble equipment and materials
(2) _____ prepare operatory
(2) _____ greet, seat, and position patient
(3) _____ don protective attire and equipment   _____   _____

2 Assist with Alginate Impression (10 points)

(4) _____ prepare impression mixture
(3) _____ insert mixture into tray, pass to dentist
(3) _____ receive impression, disinfect, store   _____   _____

3 Assist with Crown Preparation and Impression (10 points)

(2) _____ assist with local anesthesia
(4) _____ assist with crown preparation, gingival retraction
(2) _____ assist with impression of prepared tooth
(2) _____ receive impression, disinfect, store   _____   _____

4 Prepare Acrylic Crown (10 points)

(1) _____ retrieve alginate impression of original site
(2) _____ drop liquid into prep area indentation
(2) _____ shake small amount of powder into liquid
(1) _____ repeat until all powder particles are wet
(2) _____ fill until ¾ full
(2) _____ wait for dough texture stage of mixture   _____   _____

5 Pass Tray and Mix to Dentist (10 points)

(5) _____ assist with seating of tray
(5) _____ receive cover impression   _____   _____

6 Clean Acrylic Crown Cover Prep (10 points)

(3) _____ remove blood, debris, saliva
(2) _____ air dry
(3) _____ disinfect
(2) _____ if removing from operatory, don overgloves   _____   _____

7 Finish Acrylic Crown Cover (10 points)

(2) _____ remove flashing with curved crown and bridge scissors
(3) _____ gently crimp margins inward
(3) _____ trim and smooth edges of cover with disks, burs in slow handpiece
(2) _____ wash and clean trimmed crown cover   _____   _____

8 Return Finished Crown Cover to Dentist (10 points)

(2) _____ assist with remainder of appointment
(3) _____ fit and cementation
(3) _____ give postoperative instruction to patient
(2) _____ reschedule patient   _____   _____

9 Prepare Crown Prep Impression for Lab (10 points)

(2) _____ record procedure on patient's chart
(3) _____ place prescription for lab work with order
(2) _____ place disinfection procedures completed in order
(3) _____ prepare shipment box   _____   _____

10 Cleanup Procedures (10 points)

(5) _____ clean equipment, disinfect, sterilize
(5) _____ remove PPE, wash hands   _____   _____

(100)   Total points   _____   _____

Note: If dentist prefers to use preformed crown cover, complete trimming and finishing procedure in same manner as acrylic resin mixed covers. No construction is necessary, but patient must be measured and fitted for preformed covers.

COMPETENCY EVALUATION SHEET

PROCEDURE 57

Preparing Laboratory Cases for Shipping

Student Name _____ Date _____

GRADING PROTOCOL: Student is awarded the number of points indicated on the evaluation sheet for completing steps successfully.

Total possible points = 100 points
80% needed for passing = 80 points

Total points this test _____ pass _____ fail _____

	PEER REVIEW	TEACHER REVIEW

POINTS

1 Assemble Materials and Equipment (10 points)

(3) _____ gather work order
(2) _____ write out disinfectant procedure used
(3) _____ prepare items to be sent to lab
(2) _____ assemble box and packing material   _____   _____

2 Don Utility PPE (10 points)

(5) _____ don overgloves
(5) _____ don mask if spray disinfecting   _____   _____

3 Gather Impression or Item to be Sent to the Commercial Lab (10 points)

(3) _____ check patient's chart
(3) _____ write due dates and completion times
(4) _____ recheck that all items are present   _____   _____

4 Disinfect the Item (10 points)

(4) _____ disinfect all items
(3) _____ check for cleanliness
(3) _____ pat item dry   _____   _____

5 Bag the Item (10 points)

(4) _____ label bag with patient's name, date
(3) _____ place in plastic or supplied bag
(3) _____ seal bag   _____   _____

6 Clean PPE and Wash Hands (10 points)

(3) _____ remove overgloves, mask
(4) _____ dispose of items in proper place
(3) _____ wash hands   _____   _____

7 Fill Case Carton (15 points)

(3) _____ place wrapped bagged item in box
(3) _____ isolate and protect with bubble paper or pellets
(3) _____ insert dentist's work order and prescription
(3) _____ insert disinfection procedures taken list
(3) _____ recheck all items present   _____ _____

8 Prepare Case Carton (15 points)

(5) _____ seal carton
(5) _____ attach postage or address label
(5) _____ call for pickup or send to post office   _____ _____

9 Record Transaction on Patient's Chart (10 points)

(5) _____ record transaction on patient's chart
(5) _____ record transaction on lab work schedule paper   _____ _____

(100)   Total points   _____ _____

COMPETENCY EVALUATION SHEET

P R O C E D U R E   5 8

Exposure of Intraoral Radiographs—Bisecting and Paralleling Techniques

Student Name _____ Date _____

GRADING PROTOCOL: Student is awarded the number of points indicated on the evaluation sheet for completing steps successfully.

Total possible points = 100 points
80% needed for passing = 80 points

Total points bisecting angle technique _____ pass _____ fail _____
Total points paralleling technique _____ pass _____ fail _____

POINTS		TEACHER REVIEW BISECT	TEACHER REVIEW PARALLEL

1 Assemble Materials and Equipment (5 points)

(2) _____ assemble equipment and materials
(1) _____ prepare operatory
(2) _____ review radiograph orders   _____   _____

2 Prepare the Patient (5 points)

(1) _____ greet and seat patient
(1) _____ question patient re: latest radiograph
(1) _____ drape and collar patient
(2) _____ position patient-max=chin down, mand=chin up   _____   _____

3 Prepare for Procedure (5 points)

(1) _____ don radiographic dosimeter
(1) _____ prepare films
(1) _____ wash hands, don exam gloves
(1) _____ offer rinse or spray rinse patient's mouth
(1) _____ examine mouth   _____   _____

4 Practice Operator Safety Precautions (6 points)

(1) _____ observe safety rules throughout procedure
(1) _____ operator stay behind shield when activating machine or six feet off
(1) _____ caution patient to hold still and close eyes during exposure
(1) _____ check exposure chart for time and angles
(1) _____ place exposed film in lead-lined container or out of range
(1) _____ set exposure timer before film placement   _____   _____

5 Bitewing Exposure (24 points)

	L	R
Expose bitewing (molar)		
(2) _____ coronal view of both arches	____	____
(2) _____ centered on three-molar area	____	____
(2) _____ occlusal plane center of film	____	____

	L	R

(1) _____ distal of second premolar/bicuspid
(1) _____ pimple or raised dot toward mesial
(1) _____ plain side of film toward tooth surface
(1) _____ central ray toward center of film
(1) _____ film in horizontal position
(1) _____ proper exposure time set
Expose bitewing (premolar/bicuspid)
(2) _____ coronal view both arches
(2) _____ occlusal plane center of film
(2) _____ both bicuspids, first molar area
(1) _____ distal of canine/cuspid
(1) _____ partial view second molar
(1) _____ pimple or raised dot toward mesial
(1) _____ central ray toward center of film
(1) _____ film in horizontal position
(1) _____ proper exposure time set
Total points for bitewing (interproximal) exposures

6 Expose Maxillary Radiographs (24 points)

Expose maxillary incisors
(1) _____ two large central incisors, mesials of laterals
(1) _____ film in vertical position in holding blocks
(1) _____ crowns and roots covered
(1) _____ plain side of film toward tooth
(1) _____ PID in position to aiming ring, rod
(1) _____ proper exposure time set
Expose maxillary canine/cuspid
(1) _____ crown and root fully covered
(1) _____ distal part of lateral, full view of canine, first premolar/bicuspid
(1) _____ film in vertical position in holding block
(1) _____ plain side of film toward tooth
(1) _____ PID positioned next to aiming ring, rod
(1) _____ proper exposure time set
Expose maxillary bicuspid/premolar
(1) _____ crowns and roots of both premolars
(1) _____ film horizontal in holding block
(1) _____ distal part of canine, mesial view of first molar
(1) _____ indicator rod and aiming ring in place
(1) _____ PID is position next to aiming ring
(1) _____ proper time exposure set
Expose maxillary molar
(1) _____ crowns and roots three-molar area
(1) _____ film horizontal in holding block
(1) _____ indicator rod and aiming ring in place
(1) _____ PID in position next to aiming ring
(1) _____ second premolar and distal first premolar
(1) _____ proper time exposure set
Total points for maxillary exposures

7 Expose Mandibular Radiographs (24 points)

Expose mandibular centrals
(1) _____ crowns and roots of centrals and laterals
(1) _____ film placed vertically in holding blocks

	L	R

(1) _____ distal view of cuspids

(1) _____ PID positioned next to aiming ring, rod

(1) _____ proper time exposure set

(1) _____ patient positioned with chin up

Expose mandibular canine/cuspid

(1) _____ crown and root of canine, first premolar

(1) _____ film placed vertically in holding block

(1) _____ indicator rod and aiming ring in position

(1) _____ PID positioned next to aiming ring

(1) _____ proper time exposure set

(1) _____ patient positioned with chin up

Expose mandibular premolar

(1) _____ crown and root of first and second premolar

(1) _____ distal of canine

(1) _____ film placed horizontal in holding block

(1) _____ PID positioned next to aiming ring, rod

(1) _____ proper time exposure set

(1) _____ patient positioned with chin up

Expose mandibular molars

(1) _____ crown and root three-molar area

(1) _____ distal of second premolar/bicuspid

(1) _____ film placed horizontal in holding block

(1) _____ PID positioned next to aiming ring, rod

(1) _____ proper time exposure set

(1) _____ patient positioned with chin up

Total points for mandibular exposures

8 Dismiss the Patient (7 points)

(1) _____ remove collar and drape

(1) _____ reposition patient, dismiss patient

(1) _____ collect films for processing

(1) _____ remove gloves, wash hands

(1) _____ record treatment on patient's chart

(1) _____ don utility gloves, spray-wipe-spray lead drape

(1) _____ disinfect, sterilize and clean up in usual manner;
remove gloves, wash hands

(100)   Total points

COMPETENCY EVALUATION SHEET

P R O C E D U R E   5 9

Processing Dental Radiographs

Student Name _____ Date _____

GRADING PROTOCOL: Student is awarded the number of points indicated on the evaluation sheet for completing steps
successfully.

Total possible points = 100 points
80% needed for passing = 80 points

Total points this test _____ pass _____ fail _____

	PEER REVIEW	TEACHER REVIEW

POINTS

Manual

1 Prepare Films for Processing (10 points)

(2) _____ remove barrier shields at chairside, or don overgloves, use safelight,
set out paper towel
(2) _____ remove waterproof coverings in darkroom
(2) _____ isolate films in lightproof container
(2) _____ place wrappings and gloves into contaminated trash container
(2) _____ resume light, prepare to process   _____   _____

2 Assemble Equipment and Material (5 points)

(2) _____ obtain and mark developing rack
(3) _____ check area for spills or dirt   _____   _____

3 Prepare the Chemicals (10 points)

(1) _____ check freshness, level of solutions, replenish, if needed
(1) _____ replenish fixer before developer
(1) _____ stir solutions, separate rod for each solution
(2) _____ check temperature of developer, adjust if needed
(2) _____ check chart for developing time
(2) _____ set timer for development
(1) _____ clean up area for spills or dirt   _____   _____

4 Place Films on the Developing Rack (No White Light) (10 points)

(3) _____ hold films by edge
(2) _____ place on lowest clip of rack
(3) _____ alternate sides in filling rack
(2) _____ check for holding security   _____   _____

5 Place Films in the Developer (10 points)

(3) _____ place rack with films in solution
(2) _____ move or shake for a few seconds to remove air bubbles
(2) _____ check solution covering all film, films not touching sides
(3) _____ set timer in accordance with temperature   _____   _____

6 Rinse Films in Water (10 points)

(2) _____ lift rack from developer to water tank
(2) _____ let rack drip excess off
(2) _____ place rack with films into water bath
(2) _____ agitate or move rack around in water for a few seconds
(2) _____ raise rack, let solution drip into water bath   _____   _____

7 Place Films in the Fixer (10 points)

(3) _____ place rack with films into fixer, raise and lower five times
(3) _____ set timer for three minutes
(2) _____ agitate frequently
(2) _____ at timer signal, raise rack, drip into water   _____   _____

8 Place Films in the Water Bath (5 points)

(3) _____ place rack with film into water bath
(2) _____ let running water bathe films for 10 minutes   _____   _____

9 Dry Films (In Either Light) (5 points)

(1) _____ raise rack with films, drip into water bath
(2) _____ wash rack with films under running water stream
(1) _____ place rack with films on drying rack hook/rail
(1) _____ clean up area   _____   _____

Automatic Processing

10 Prepare Films (Without White Light) (10 points)

(1) _____ don overgloves, use safelight, set out paper towel
(2) _____ remove waterproof coverings
(1) _____ use hemostat to take film out of paper wrapper (optional)
(2) _____ place film into lightproof container
(2) _____ replace hemostat into dry forceps holder, or shake film into
            lightproof container
(2) _____ place waterproof coverings and gloves into contaminated trash container   _____   _____

11 Prepare Equipment (In White Light) (5 points)

(2) _____ check solution levels, replenish, if needed
(1) _____ replenish fixer before developer
(1) _____ check temperature of solutions
(1) _____ adjust machine controls (if not automatically regulated)   _____   _____

12 Process Films (5 points)

(1) _____ use no white light
(1) _____ place film onto roller
(2) _____ space films intermittently
(1) _____ permit machine to process film   _____   _____

13 Prepare Films for Display (5 points)

(1) _____ retrieve processed films
(2) _____ place films on marked developing rack, or place films into mount
(2) _____ clean up area   _____   _____

(100)   Total points   _____   _____

COMPETENCY EVALUATION SHEET

P R O C E D U R E   6 0

Mounting Dental Radiographs

Student Name _____ Date _____

GRADING PROTOCOL: Student is awarded the number of points indicated on the evaluation sheet for completing steps successfully.

Total possible points = 100 points
80% needed for passing = 80 points

Total points this test _____ pass _____ fail _____

	PEER REVIEW	TEACHER REVIEW

POINTS

1 Assemble Equipment and Materials (5 points)

(1) _____ choose a clean, dry area
(2) _____ wash and dry hands
(2) _____ arrange materials for use   _____   _____

2 Prepare Films for Mounting (10 points)

(4) _____ identify films
(4) _____ mark mount, record number if using film numbering system
(2) _____ don gloves (optional)   _____   _____

3 Locate Pimple (Bump) or Dimple (Concave) (5 points)

(5) _____ arrange films with dimple up or arrange films with pimple up   _____   _____

4 Arrange Films (5 points)

(2) _____ use film landmarks to select exposure
(2) _____ arrange films in sequential order on paper
(1) _____ prepare to mount   _____   _____

5 Mount Molar Bitewings (7 points)

	L	R

(1) _____ coronal view of both arches   _____   _____
(1) _____ three-molar area visible   _____   _____
(1) _____ occlusal plane center of film   _____   _____
(1) _____ distal of second premolar/bicuspid   _____   _____
(1) _____ ascending ramus to distal edge   _____   _____
(1) _____ bifurcation of mandibular molars on bottom of film   _____   _____
(1) _____ thicker, heavier teeth toward distal   _____   _____
Total points for molar bitewing mounting   _____   _____

6 Mount Premolar or Bicuspid Bitewings (7 points)

(1) _____ coronal view both arches   _____   _____
(1) _____ occlusal plane center of film   _____   _____

L R

(1) _____ both bicuspids, first molar area
(1) _____ distal of canine/cuspid
(1) _____ partial view second molar
(1) _____ bifurcation of mandibular molars on bottom of film
(1) _____ maxillary sinus on top of film
Total points for premolar/bicuspid bitewing

7 Mount Maxillary Incisors (7 points)

(1) _____ film in vertical position
(1) _____ two large central incisors
(1) _____ mesial portions of laterals
(1) _____ crowns and roots fully shown
(1) _____ nasal septum, fossae
(1) _____ incisive foramen
(1) _____ incisal edge toward center of mount
Total points for maxillary incisor

8 Mount Maxillary Canine or Cuspid (7 points)

(1) _____ film in vertical position
(1) _____ crown and root fully shown
(1) _____ distal part of lateral
(1) _____ mesial view of first premolar/bicuspid
(1) _____ large lingual cusp on premolar/bicuspid
(1) _____ possible view of maxillary sinus
(1) _____ incisal edge toward center of mount
Total points for maxillary canine/cuspid

9 Mount Maxillary Premolars or Bicuspids (7 points)

(1) _____ film in horizontal position
(1) _____ crowns and roots of both
(1) _____ maxillary sinus
(1) _____ distal part of lateral, mesial view of first molar
(1) _____ full lingual cusps
(1) _____ thicker heavier teeth toward distal
(1) _____ occlusal plane toward center of mount
Total points for maxillary premolars/bicuspids

10 Mount Maxillary Molars (7 points)

(1) _____ film in horizontal position
(1) _____ crowns and roots three-molar area
(1) _____ maxillary sinus, maxillary tuberosity
(1) _____ second premolar and distal first premolar
(1) _____ full lingual cusps on premolars
(1) _____ thicker, heavier teeth toward distal
(1) _____ occlusal plane toward center of mount
Total points for maxillary molars

11 Mount Mandibular Incisors (7 points)

(1) _____ film in vertical position
(1) _____ crowns and roots of centrals and laterals
(1) _____ laterals slightly wider than centrals

	L	R

(1) _____ distal view of cuspids   ____   ____
(1) _____ dense mandibular bone   ____   ____
(1) _____ lingual foramen   ____   ____
(1) _____ incisal edge toward center of mount   ____   ____
         Total points for mandibular incisors   ____   ____

12 Mount Mandibular Cuspid or Canine (7 points)

(1) _____ film in vertical position   ____   ____
(1) _____ crown and root of canine   ____   ____
(1) _____ first premolar and partial second   ____   ____
(1) _____ small lingual cusps   ____   ____
(1) _____ dense mandibular bone   ____   ____
(1) _____ distal view of lateral   ____   ____
(1) _____ incisal edge toward center of mount   ____   ____
         Total points for mandibular canine or cuspid   ____   ____

13 Mount Mandibular Premolars or Bicuspids (7 points)

(1) _____ film in horizontal position   ____   ____
(1) _____ crown and root of first and second premolar   ____   ____
(1) _____ small lingual cusps, dense mandibular bone   ____   ____
(1) _____ distal of canine   ____   ____
(1) _____ bifurcation of molars   ____   ____
(1) _____ occlusal plane toward center of mount   ____   ____
(1) _____ thicker, heavier teeth toward distal   ____   ____
         Total points for mandibular bicuspids/premolars   ____   ____

14 Mount Mandibular Molars (7 points)

(1) _____ film in horizontal position   ____   ____
(1) _____ crown and root three-molar area   ____   ____
(1) _____ ascending ramus to distal   ____   ____
(1) _____ distal of second premolar   ____   ____
(1) _____ bifurcation of molar roots   ____   ____
(1) _____ thicker, heavier teeth toward distal   ____   ____
(1) _____ occlusal plane toward center of mount   ____   ____
         Total points for mandibular molars   ____   ____

15 Clean up the Area (5 points)

(2) _____ review mounted series for errors
(2) _____ place films in patient's records
(1) _____ clean up area   ____   ____

(100)   Total points   ____   ____

COMPETENCY EVALUATION SHEET

PROCEDURE 61

Opening and Closing the Dental Business Office

Student Name _____ Date _____

GRADING PROTOCOL: Student is awarded the number of points indicated on the evaluation sheet for completing steps successfully.

Total possible points = 100 points
80% needed for passing = 80 points

Total points this test _____   pass _____   fail _____

	PEER REVIEW	TEACHER REVIEW

POINTS

1 Open the Office (10 points)

(4) _____ turn on lighting
(4) _____ activate air conditioning
(2) _____ check freshness and cleanliness of lab coat   _____   _____

2 Perform Desk Duties (15 points)

(3) _____ check answering service or phone machine
(3) _____ check incoming fax correspondence
(3) _____ check and post daily schedule
(3) _____ pull and complete patients' charts, records
(3) _____ activate computer, or prepare daily master log sheet   _____   _____

3 Prepare Reception Room (10 points)

(2) _____ dust reception room furniture
(2) _____ check magazine dates, conditions
(2) _____ fresh flowers, accessories
(2) _____ check supplies for patient comfort
(2) _____ clean child's corner   _____   _____

4 Sort Mail (10 points)

(2) _____ place unopened personal mail on doctor's desk
(1) _____ place relative correspondence on doctor's desk
(1) _____ place journals, ads of interest on doctor's desk
(2) _____ take laboratory cases to lab area, mark incoming chart
(1) _____ place payment for future processing
(2) _____ place statements with invoice file for processing
(1) _____ review and handle "junk" mail   _____   _____

5 Clean Reception Room and Desk Area (10 points)

(2) _____ set schedule for thorough cleaning
(3) _____ disinfect surfaces

(3) _____ move furniture, sweep, dust
(2) _____ disinfect children's toys   _____   _____

6 Complete Desk Work (15 points)

(3) _____ pull charts and records for next day
(3) _____ prepare schedule for following day
(3) _____ complete confirmation calls
(3) _____ complete financial postings
(3) _____ prepare deposit slip and bag   _____   _____

7 Freshen Reception Room (10 points)

(4) _____ pick up magazines, trash, toys
(3) _____ empty trash receptacles
(3) _____ empty and wash ashtrays (if applicable)   _____   _____

8 Complete Mail Transactions (10 points)

(4) _____ use weight and postage meter for correspondence
(3) _____ prepare lab cases
(3) _____ send out fax correspondence   _____   _____

9 Close Area (10 points)

(2) _____ make hard copy of transaction, turn off computer
(2) _____ set answering machine or service
(2) _____ remove trash bags to collection area
(1) _____ turn down air conditioner or heater
(1) _____ turn off lights and machines
(2) _____ secure area   _____   _____

(100)   Total points   _____   _____

COMPETENCY EVALUATION SHEET

PROCEDURE 62

Opening and Closing the Dental Operatory

Student Name _____ Date _____

GRADING PROTOCOL: Student is awarded the number of points indicated on the evaluation sheet for completing steps successfully.

Total possible points = 100 points
80% needed for passing = 80 points

Total points this test _____ pass _____ fail _____

	PEER REVIEW	TEACHER REVIEW

POINTS

Opening the Operatory

1 Prepare for Work (10 points)

(5) _____ arrive early
(5) _____ remove home clothes, don PPE clothing _____ _____

2 Prepare Operatory (10 points)

(2) _____ check posted daily schedule
(2) _____ dust operatory, check supplies
(2) _____ place barrier shields
(2) _____ flush lines, freshen water flow
(1) _____ prepare or check barrier placements
(1) _____ scan for acceptability, freshness _____ _____

3 Prepare Sterilizing Area (10 points)

(1) _____ turn on dry heat sterilizer
(2) _____ prepare trays for coming appointment
(2) _____ gather necessary records, lab cases, x-rays
(2) _____ check water supply in autoclave
(1) _____ check supplies, ultrasonic
(2) _____ make up solutions, spray bottles _____ _____

4 Prepare Darkroom (10 points)

(3) _____ Check cleanliness
(4) _____ check solutions, replenish
(3) _____ remove, mount, file any dry x-rays _____ _____

5 Prepare Laboratory Area (10 points)

(3) _____ activate machines, tanks, compressor
(2) _____ check supplies
(3) _____ review work order
(2) _____ clean up area, file completed cases _____ _____

Closing the Operatory

6 Clean Operatory Area (10 points)

(1) _____ don utility gloves and PPE
(2) _____ disinfect all surfaces, areas, hoses
(2) _____ flush lines with water, disinfectant
(1) _____ clean or replace traps
(2) _____ remove contaminated barrier shields
(1) _____ remove and reline trash containers
(1) _____ return all charts, records, and x-rays to desk   _____   _____

7 Clean Sterilizing Area (10 points)

(3) _____ clean, disinfect, and sterilize all equipment and items
(3) _____ clean ultrasonic cleaner and solutions, if needed
(2) _____ drain,clean, and change autoclave water reservoir, if needed
(2) _____ clean up area, gather trash, tie bundles, reline containers   _____   _____

8 Clean Laboratory Area (10 points)

(1) _____ clean up area
(2) _____ turn off machines
(1) _____ replace supplies
(2) _____ drain air compressor tank, oxygen, and nitrous tank hoses
(2) _____ check lab orders for next day
(2) _____ gather trash, tie bundle, reline containers   _____   _____

9 Clean Darkroom Area (10 points)

(2) _____ clean up spills
(4) _____ wash, dry, and replace racks; or turn off automatic developing machine
(2) _____ place lid on manual tank, remove cover on automatic machine
(2) _____ empty trash, tie bundle, replace liner   _____   _____

10 Change Clothing (10 points)

(2) _____ wash, disinfect gloves, remove
(2) _____ remove PPE, place in laundry bag
(2) _____ take laundry bag to pick up area
(2) _____ take trash to pick up area
(2) _____ wash hands   _____   _____

(100)   Total points   _____   _____

COMPETENCY EVALUATION SHEET

P R O C E D U R E 6 3

Telephone Techniques

Student Name _____ Date _____

GRADING PROTOCOL: Student is awarded the number of points indicated on the evaluation sheet for completing steps successfully.

Total possible points = 100 points
80% needed for passing = 80 points

Total points this test _____ pass _____ fail _____

	PEER REVIEW	TEACHER REVIEW

POINTS

1 Assemble Equipment and Materials (10 points)

(1) _____ gather pen or pencil, note pad
(1) _____ keep area neat and clutter free
(2) _____ answer phone right away
(1) _____ speak clearly and distinctly with empty mouth
(2) _____ identify office and speaker
(2) _____ identify caller
(1) _____ use caller's name frequently

2 Emergency Call Technique (10 points)

(3) _____ stay calm
(3) _____ identify caller
(2) _____ identify emergency and timeliness
(2) _____ offer assistance

3 Appointment Call Technique (10 points)

(2) _____ identify caller, need, and purpose
(1) _____ inquire to availability
(2) _____ offer selection of time
(2) _____ repeat time and date at end of call
(2) _____ let caller hang up
(1) _____ send appointment card if time permits

4 Incoming Inquiry Call Technique (10 points)

(2) _____ identify caller and problem
(2) _____ offer to provide information
(2) _____ suggest hold button, 30 seconds, or call back
(2) _____ identify caller on hold, give information
(2) _____ let caller hang up

5 Personal and Professional Call Technique (10 points)

(4) _____ identify caller
(3) _____ inform doctor of call
(3) _____ channel call or call back

6 Appointment Confirmation and Recall Technique (10 points)

(3) _____ identify office and speaker
(2) _____ confirm appointment, not remind
(3) _____ make recall appointments, offer selection
(2) _____ make on-call appointment   _____   _____

7 Ordering Supplies Call Technique (10 points)

(4) _____ have list ready
(3) _____ identify office and speaker
(3) _____ place order, date card   _____   _____

8 Outgoing Inquiries Call Technique (10 points)

(3) _____ identify office and speaker
(2) _____ check on invoices or bills
(3) _____ inquire into delivery or lab cases
(2) _____ make record of call, results   _____   _____

9 Collection Call Technique (10 points)

(2) _____ get doctor's permission
(2) _____ make at reasonable hour
(2) _____ be polite, identify office
(2) _____ state conditions, wait for reply
(2) _____ record results of call on patient's chart   _____   _____

10 Followup Call Technique (10 points)

(3) _____ identify office and speaker
(3) _____ inquire progress of patient
(2) _____ listen to conversation
(2) _____ let patient hang up   _____   _____

(100)   Total points   _____   _____

COMPETENCY EVALUATION SHEET

PROCEDURE 64

One Write Bookkeeping System

Student Name _____ Date _____

GRADING PROTOCOL: Student is awarded the number of points indicated on the evaluation sheet for completing steps successfully.

Total possible points = 100 points
80% needed for passing = 80 points

Total points this test _____ pass _____ fail _____

	PEER REVIEW	TEACHER REVIEW

POINTS

1 Assemble Equipment and Material (10 points)

(2) _____ place clean master day sheet on pegboard
(1) _____ date and number page, write hard with ballpoint pen
(1) _____ align shingled charge slip or receipt forms
(2) _____ have receipt number in sequence
(2) _____ gather ledger cards
(2) _____ place deposit slip on column   _____   _____

2 Register the Patient (10 points)

(2) _____ write account and patient name on form
(2) _____ write receipt number on master sheet
(2) _____ determine old balance from ledger card
(2) _____ note old balance on master sheet and charge slip form
(2) _____ remove charge slip, clip on patient file   _____   _____

3 Record Procedure and Charges (10 points)

(2) _____ accept charge slip from patient
(4) _____ insert ledger card under receipt slip
(4) _____ record procedure completed or charge   _____   _____

4 Record Payment (10 points)

(1) _____ request payment
(1) _____ accept payment from patient
(2) _____ record amount given on payment column and deposit column
(2) _____ signify if payment by cash or check
(2) _____ if no payment, mark zero or line in payment column
(2) _____ remove ledger card, tear off receipt card   _____   _____

5 Make Future Appointments (10 points)

(2) _____ notice when next appointment is required
(2) _____ set date and time with patient

(2) _____ write date and time on bottom of receipt slip
(2) _____ give receipt or appointment slips to patient
(2) _____ place charge slip in patient's file   _____   _____

6 Record Mail and Walk-in Payments (10 points)

(2) _____ pull patient ledger cards
(2) _____ place ledger card on next line
(2) _____ write MAIL on receipt number line
(2) _____ write ROA by whom on procedure line
(2) _____ remove ledger card, return to file   _____   _____

7 Assemble Insurance Superbill (10 points)

(2) _____ remove shingled slips, insert insurance superbill
(1) _____ record patient's old balance
(1) _____ remove entire superbill, clip to patient's chart
(1) _____ accept completed superbill from dentist in operatory
(2) _____ write in procedure, charges made, and the next appointment
(2) _____ give patient two copies, place one in patient's file
(1) _____ replace shingle receipt or charge slips   _____   _____

8 Fill Out Deposit Slip (10 points)

(3) _____ total cash and charge columns
(3) _____ total cash pile and stamped checks
(2) _____ reconcile amounts, place in deposit bag
(2) _____ place deposit slip into bag   _____   _____

9 Reconcile Receipts (10 points)

(3) _____ total each column
(3) _____ fill in proof of posting figures at bottom of page
(2) _____ check figures; when correct, remove sheet
(2) _____ place sheet in loose-leaf book   _____   _____

10 Clean Up Area (10 points)

(2) _____ check patient treatment records for data, return
(2) _____ review ledger cards, return to file
(2) _____ place ledger card file in safe, fireproof container
(2) _____ put away loose-leaf book of daily master pages
(2) _____ clean up area   _____   _____

(100)   Total points   _____   _____

COMPETENCY EVALUATION SHEET

PROCEDURE 65

Processing a Dental Insurance Claim

Student Name _____ Date _____

GRADING PROTOCOL: Student is awarded the number of points indicated on the evaluation sheet for completing steps successfully.

Total possible points = 100 points
80% needed for passing = 80 points

Total points this test _____ pass _____ fail _____

Using the patient information from the Assignment Sheet on Dental Records (Mary Ellen Young) and the dentist information from section B of Figure 11–2, make out a claim form for an initial examination (00110), complete intraoral radiographic examination (00210), and adult prophylaxis (01110). Fees may be estimated. Write in all appropriate signature lines.

	PEER REVIEW	TEACHER REVIEW

POINTS

1 Assemble Equipment and Materials (10 points)

(3) _____ collect needed items
(3) _____ specify if form for claim or pre-authorization
(4) _____ type or write in company name and address   _____ _____

2 Complete Patient Section (20 points)

(8) _____ list patient's statistical information
(6) _____ list employer's information
(6) _____ list spouse's information   _____ _____

3 Complete Attending Dentist Section (20 points)

(4) _____ list dentist's name and address
(8) _____ type in dentist's statistical information
(8) _____ answer treatment questions   _____ _____

4 Complete Examination and Treatment Section (20 points)

(4) _____ list tooth number and description of service
(4) _____ list date of service, procedure code, and fee
(4) _____ complete list of all services
(4) _____ total fees
(4) _____ fill in tooth diagram, if needed   _____ _____

5 Obtain Signatures (10 points)

(5) _____ get patient's signature, or type in signature on file
(4) _____ obtain dentist's signature and date
(1) _____ make copy of form   _____ _____

6 Prepare Envelope (10 points)

(3) _____ type name and address of insurance company
(2) _____ place claim form in envelope
(2) _____ include radiographs, if required
(3) _____ apply proper postage, mail   _____   _____

7 Clean Up Area (10 points)

(4) _____ mark patient's chart and insurance log
(2) _____ place copy of claim form in patient's file
(4) _____ put all materials away   _____   _____

(100)   Total points   _____   _____

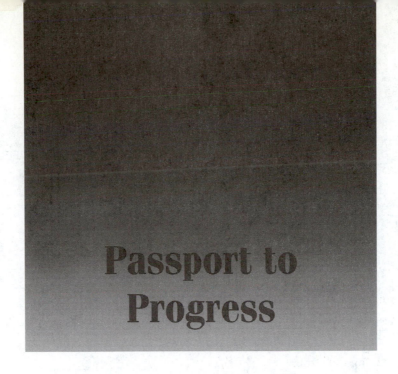

Passport to Progress

Name _____ Academic Year _____

Procedure Assignment Competency	Lesson Date	Testing Date	Pass/Fail/ Incomplete

Unit 1 The Dental Profession

A1.1	The Professional Dental Team (Careers)	_____	_____	_____
A1.2	The Role of the Dental Assistant	_____	_____	_____
A1.3	Qualities of the Dental Assistant	_____	_____	_____
A1.4	Ethics for the Dental Assistant	_____	_____	_____
A1.5	Dental Jurisprudence—Legal Considerations	_____	_____	_____
A1.6	Job Sources	_____	_____	_____
A1.7	Composing a Resume and Cover Letter	_____	_____	_____
A1.8	Completing a Job Application Form	_____	_____	_____
A1.9	Demonstrating Job Interview Skills	_____	_____	_____
	Unit 1 Post Test			

Unit 2 Emergency Care and First Aid

A2.1	Emergency Care Preparation	_____	_____	_____
P1	Measuring and Recording Vital Signs	_____	_____	_____
P2	Assisting the Choking Victim	_____	_____	_____
P3	Cardiopulmonary Resuscitation	_____	_____	_____
P4	Assisting with a Shock Emergency	_____	_____	_____
	Unit 2 Post Test	_____	_____	_____

Unit 3 Infection Control and Hazard Management

P5	Hand-washing Technique	_____	_____	_____
P6	Donning and Disposing Clinical Attire	_____	_____	_____
P7	Ultrasonic Cleaning	_____	_____	_____
P8	Operation of an Autoclave	_____	_____	_____
P9	Operating a Dry Heat Sterilizer	_____	_____	_____

P10	Using Chemicals as Disinfectants and Sterilizers	___	___	___
P11	Cleanup of Operatory Equipment Techniques	___	___	___
A3.1	Hazard and Fire Control	___	___	___
	Unit 3 Post Test	___	___	___

Unit 4 Basic Dental Fundamentals

A4.1	Tooth Anatomy	___	___	___
A4.2	Tooth Surfaces	___	___	___
A4.3	Tooth Numbering Systems	___	___	___
A4.4	Charting Teeth	___	___	___
A4.5	Operative Hand Instruments	___	___	___
P12	Transfer of Instruments	___	___	___
P13	Dental Rotary Instruments	___	___	___
	Unit 4 Post Test	___	___	___

Unit 5 Chairside Fundamentals

P14	Preparing and Dismissing the Patient	___	___	___
P15	Evacuate and Rinse	___	___	___
P16	Assisting with Local Anesthesia Administration	___	___	___
P17	Preparing Dental Liners and Cements	___	___	___
P18	Placement and Removal of the Tofflemire Retainer	___	___	___
	Unit 5 Post Test	___	___	___

Unit 6 Chairside Assisting

P19	Assisting with the Preliminary Examination	___	___	___
P20	Assisting with Alginate Impressions	___	___	___
P21	Assisting with Dental Prophylaxis	___	___	___
P22	Assisting with Topical Fluoride Application	___	___	___
P23	Assisting with Sealant Application	___	___	___
P24	Brushing and Flossing Techniques Instruction	___	___	___
P25	Diet and Nutrition Counseling	___	___	___
P26	Assisting with Dental Dam Application	___	___	___
P27	Assisting with Anterior Restoration	___	___	___
P28	Assisting with Amalgam Posterior Restoration	___	___	___
P29	Assisting with Composite Posterior Restoration	___	___	___
P30	Finishing and Polishing of Amalgam Restorations	___	___	___
P31	Assisting with Tooth Bleaching Appointments	___	___	___
	Unit 6 Post Test	___	___	___

Unit 7 Chairside Specialties

P32	Assisting with the Initial Exam and Preventive Techniques in Pediatric Dentistry	___	___	___
P33	Assisting with Pulp Treatment and Protective Covers	___	___	___
P34	Assisting with Space Maintainers (Visits 1 & 2)	___	___	___
P35	Assisting with the Endodontic Examination	___	___	___
P36	Assisting with Root Canal Therapy	___	___	___
P37	Assisting with Prosthodontic Impressions (Visit 2)	___	___	___
P38	Assisting with Try In and Delivery Appointments	___	___	___
P39	Assisting with Fixed Crowns (Visit 1)	___	___	___
P40	Assisting with Fixed Crowns (Final Visit)	___	___	___
	Unit 7 Post Test			

Unit 8 Dental Specialties

P41	Assisting with the Orthodontic Preliminary Examination	_____	_____	_____
P42	Assisting with the Placement of Orthodontic Bands	_____	_____	_____
P43	Assisting with Cementation of Brackets	_____	_____	_____
P44	Assisting with Arch Wire and Ligature Placement	_____	_____	_____
P45	Assisting with Arch Wire, Band, and Bracket Removal	_____	_____	_____
P46	Assisting with Multiple Extractions and Suture Removal	_____	_____	_____
P47	Assisting with Minor Tissue Surgery	_____	_____	_____
P48	Assisting with Periodontal Exam and Prophylaxis	_____	_____	_____
P49	Assisting with Gingivectomy and Removal of Periodontal Packing	_____	_____	_____
	Unit 8 Post Test	_____	_____	_____

Unit 9 Dental Laboratory Procedures

P50	Fabrication of Study Models	_____	_____	_____
P51	Separation of Models and Impression	_____	_____	_____
P52	Trimming Gypsum Models	_____	_____	_____
P53	Articulation of Study Models	_____	_____	_____
P54	Construction of Base Plates and Occlusal Rims	_____	_____	_____
P55	Construction of Custom Trays	_____	_____	_____
P56	Assisting with Fabrication of Temporary Crowns	_____	_____	_____
P57	Preparing Laboratory Cases for Shipping	_____	_____	_____
	Unit 9 Post Test	_____	_____	_____

Unit 10 Dental Radiation

A10.1	Radiation Safety Knowledge	_____	_____	_____
A10.2	Radiation Film Knowledge	_____	_____	_____
P58	Exposure of Intraoral Radiographs—Bisecting and Paralleling Techniques	_____	_____	_____
P59	Processing Dental Radiographs	_____	_____	_____
P60	Mounting Dental Radiographs	_____	_____	_____
A10.3	Analyzing Dental Radiographs	_____	_____	_____
	Unit 10 Post Test	_____	_____	_____

Unit 11 Business Procedures

P61	Opening and Closing the Dental Business Office (Receptionist)	_____	_____	_____
P62	Opening and Closing the Dental Operatory (Chairside)	_____	_____	_____
P63	Telephone Techniques	_____	_____	_____
A11.1	Appointment Scheduling	_____	_____	_____
A11.2	Patient Dental Records	_____	_____	_____
A11.3	Records Management	_____	_____	_____
P64	One Write Bookkeeping System	_____	_____	_____
P65	Processing a Dental Insurance Claim	_____	_____	_____
A11.4	Checking Accounts	_____	_____	_____
	Unit 11 Post Test	_____	_____	_____

Student Signature _____ Instructor Signature _____

Date _____ Date _____

Index